Blood Cells

Blood Cells

A Practical Guide

Barbara J. Bain MBBS, FRACP, FRCPath

Professor in Diagnostic Haematology
St Mary's Hospital Campus of Imperial College Faculty of Medicine, London
and Honorary Consultant Haematologist,
St Mary's Hospital, London

FIFTH EDITION

WILEY Blackwell

Contents

Preface

Blood Cells has been written with both the practising haematologist and the trainee in mind. My aim has been to provide a guide for use in the diagnostic haematology laboratory, covering methods of collection of blood specimens, blood film preparation and staining, the principles of manual and automated blood counts and the assessment of the morphological features of blood cells. My objective has been that the practising haematologist should find this book sufficiently comprehensive to be a reference source while, at the same time, the trainee haematologist and biomedical scientist should find it a straightforward and practical bench manual. I hope that the medically trained haematologist will gain a fuller understanding of the scientific basis of an important segment of laboratory haematology, while the laboratory scientist will understand more of the purpose and clinical relevance of laboratory tests. I trust it is not too ambitious to hope to be 'all things to all men'. This edition has been expanded to keep it as comprehensive and up-to-date as possible and includes more guidance on the further tests that should be performed for any given provisional diagnosis. However, microscopy and the automated full blood count remain the core of the book. My overriding purpose has been to show that microscopy not only provides the essential basis of our haematological practice, but can also lead to the excitement of discovery. The decline in the number of blood films made and the increasingly heavy clinical commitments of any haematologist who is not purely a laboratory haematologist make this book more than ever necessary. I thought that the fourth edition, published eight years ago, would be the last, but it seemed a pity to stop when there are still new things to be learnt about the circulating blood cells. If I succeed in sending the reader back to the microscope with renewed interest and enthusiasm I shall be well satisfied.

B.J.B. 2015

Acknowledgements

I should like to thank those who critically reviewed parts of this and previous editions of this book, including Carol Briggs who reviewed Chapter 2 of this edition. I should also like to thank the many colleagues who provided blood films for photography, or provided other images; they are individually acknowledged in the figure legends. I am grateful also to those others, numbering many hundreds, with whom I have discussed interesting and difficult diagnostic problems over the last 43 years. I should like to acknowledge Dr Helen Dodsworth without whose suggestion to an editor this book might not have happened. Finally, I should like to remember and acknowledge those who taught me to examine blood films, particularly but not only the late Professor Sir John Dacie, the late Professor David Galton, the late Professor Sunitha Wickramasinghe and the fortunately still surviving Professor Daniel Catovsky.

List of abbreviations

aCML	atypical chronic myeloid leukaemia	FITC	fluorescein isothiocyanate
ACTH	adrenocorticotropic hormone	FRC	red cell fragments
AD	autosomal dominant	G6PD	glucose-6-phosphate dehydrogenase
AE1	anion exchanger 1	G-CSF	granulocyte colony-stimulating factor
AIDS	acquired immune deficiency syndrome	GM-CSF	granulocyte-macrophage colony-
AIHA	autoimmune haemolytic anaemia		stimulating factor
ALL	acute lymphoblastic leukaemia	GPI	glycosylphosphatidylinositol
AML	acute myeloid leukaemia	Hb	haemoglobin concentration
ANAE	α-naphthyl acetate esterase	Hct	haematocrit
ANBE	α-naphthyl butyrate esterase	HDW	haemoglobin distribution width
AR	autosomal recessive	HELLP	haemolysis, elevated liver enzymes and
ATLL	adult T-cell leukaemia/lymphoma		low platelet count (syndrome)
ATP	adenosine triphosphate	HEMPAS	hereditary erythroid multinuclearity with
B-PLL	B-lineage prolymphocytic leukaemia		positive acidified serum test
CAE	chloroacetate esterase	HES	hypereosinophilic syndrome
CBC	complete blood count	HHV6	human herpesvirus 6
CD	cluster of differentiation	HIV	human immunodeficiency virus
CDA	congenital dyserythropoietic anaemia	HLA	histocompatibility locus antigen
CDC	Centers for Disease Control	HPC	haemopoietic progenitor cells
CEL	chronic eosinophilic leukaemia	HPFH	hereditary persistence of fetal
CGL	chronic granulocytic leukaemia		haemoglobin
CHCM	cellular haemoglobin concentration mean	HPLC	high performance liquid chromatography
	(Technicon H.1 series counters)	HTLV-1	human T-cell lymphotropic virus 1
CLL	chronic lymphocytic leukaemia	HTLV-2	human T-cell lymphotropic virus 2
CLL/PL	CLL, mixed cell type	ICSH	International Committee (now Council)
CLSI	Clinical and Laboratory Standards		for Standardization in Haematology
	Institute	Ig	immunoglobulin
CML	chronic myelogenous leukaemia	IG	immature granulocytes
CMML	chronic myelomonocytic leukaemia	IPF	immature platelet fraction
CMV	cytomegalovirus	IL	interleukin
CPD	cell population data	IMI	immature myeloid information
CTP	C-reactive protein	IRF	immature reticulocyte fraction
CV	coefficient of variation	ITP	idiopathic (autoimmune)
DDAVP	1-deamino-8-D-arginine vasopressin		thrombocytopenic purpura
DIC	disseminated intravascular coagulation	JMML	juvenile myelomonocytic leukaemia
DNA	deoxyribonucleic acid	LCAT	lecithin-cholesterol acyl transferase
EBV	Epstein–Barr virus	LDH	lactate dehydrogenase
EDTA	ethylenediaminetetra-acetic acid	LDW	lymphocyte distribution width
EMA	eosin-5-maleimide	LE	lupus erythematosus (cells)
ESR	erythrocyte sedimentation rate	LHD	low haemoglobin density
ET	essential thrombocythaemia	LI	lobularity index (Siemens instruments)
FAB	French–American–British (classifications	LUC	large unstained cells (Siemens
	of haematological neoplasms)		instruments)
FBC	full blood count	MALT	mucosa-associated lymphoid tissue
FDA	Food and Drug Administration	MCH	mean cell haemoglobin
FISH	fluorescence *in situ* hybridisation	MCHC	mean cell haemoglobin concentration

M-CSF	macrophage colony-stimulating factor
MCV	mean cell volume
MDS	myelodysplastic syndrome/s
MDS/MPN	myelodysplastic/myeloproliferative neoplasm
MDW	monocyte distribution width
MGG	May–Grünwald–Giemsa (stain)
MIRL	membrane inhibitor of reactive lysis
MLV	mean lymphocyte volume
MMV	mean monocyte volume
MNV	mean neutrophil volume
MPC	mean platelet component concentration
MPM	mean platelet mass
MPO	myeloperoxidase
MPV	mean platelet volume
MPXI	mean peroxidase index (Siemens instruments)
MRV	mean reticulocyte volume
MSCV	mean sphered cell volume
NAP	neutrophil alkaline phosphatase
NASA	naphthol AS acetate esterase
NASDA	naphthol AS-D acetate esterase
NCCLS	National Committee on Clinical Laboratory Standards (now renamed Clinical and Laboratory Standards Institute, CLSI)
NDW	neutrophil distribution width
NK	natural killer (cell)
NRBC	nucleated red blood cell
PAS	periodic acid–Schiff (reaction)
PCDW	platelet component distribution width
PCH	paroxysmal cold haemoglobinuria
PCR	polymerase chain reaction
Pct/PCT	plateletcrit
PCV	packed cell volume
PDW	platelet distribution width
Peg-rHuMGDF	polyethylene glycol recombination human megakaryocyte growth and development factor
PHA	phytohaemagglutinin
P-LCR	platelet large cell ratio
PLL	prolymphocytic leukaemia
PMDW	platelet mass distribution width

PNH	paroxysmal nocturnal haemoglobinuria
POEMS	polyneuropathy, organomegaly, endocrinopathy, M protein, skin changes (syndrome)
PRV	polycythaemia rubra vera
PV	polycythaemia vera
RAEB	refractory anaemia with excess of blasts
RARS	refractory anaemia with ring sideroblasts
RBC	red blood cell count
RCMD	refractory cytopenia with multilineage dysplasia
RCUD	refractory cytopenia with unilineage dysplasia
RDW	red cell distribution width
RNA	ribonucleic acid
RSf	Red cell Size factor
RT-PCR	reverse transcriptase polymerase chain reaction
SBB	Sudan black B
SD	standard deviation
SI	Système International
SIFD	sideroblastic anaemia, immune deficiency, fever, developmental delay (syndrome)
SLE	systemic lupus erythematosus
SLVL	splenic lymphoma with villous lymphocytes
TAM	transient abnormal myelopoiesis
TdT	terminal deoxynucleotidyltransferase
TNCC	total nucleated cell count
T-PLL	T-lineage prolymphocytic leukaemia
TRAP	tartrate-resistant acid phosphatase
TTP	thrombotic thrombocytopenic purpura
UWBC	uncorrected white blood cell count
WBC	white blood cell count
WHIM	warts, hypogammaglobulinaemia, infections, myelokathexis (syndrome)
WHO	World Health Organization
WIC	WBC in the impedance channel (Cell-Dyn instruments)
WNR	white cell nucleated channel
WOC	WBC in the optical channel (Cell-Dyn instruments)

Note to the reader

Unless otherwise stated, all photomicrographs have been stained with a May–Grünwald–Giemsa stain and have been photographed with a ×100 objective, giving a final magnification of approximately ×912.

About the companion website

This book is accompanied by a companion website:

www.wiley.com/go/bain/bloodcells

The website includes:

• Multiple Choice Questions

• Extended Matching Questions

CHAPTER 1

Blood sampling and blood film preparation and examination

Obtaining a blood specimen

Performing an accurate blood count and correctly interpreting a blood film require that an appropriate sample from the patient, mixed with the correct amount of a suitable anticoagulant, is delivered to the laboratory without undue delay. No artefacts should be introduced during these procedures.

The identity of the patient requiring blood sampling should be carefully checked before performing a venepuncture. This is usually done by requesting the patient to state surname, given name and date of birth and, for hospital inpatients, by checking a wristband to verify these details and, in addition, the hospital number. To reduce the chance of human error, bottles should not be labelled in advance. The person performing the phlebotomy must conform to local guidelines, including those for patient identification. Although traditionally more attention has been given to patient identification in relation to blood transfusion, it should be noted that wrong treatment has also followed the misidentification of patients from whom samples are taken for a blood count and identification must also be taken seriously in this field. More secure identification of inpatients can be achieved by the use of electronic devices in which the patient's identity is scanned in from a barcoded wristband by means of a hand-held device.

Patients should either sit or lie comfortably and should be reassured that the procedure causes only minimal discomfort; they should not be told that venepuncture is painless, since this is not so. It is preferable for apprehensive patients to lie down. Chairs used for venepuncture should preferably have adjustable armrests so that the arm can be carefully positioned. Armrests also help to ensure patient safety, since they make it harder for a fainting patient to fall from the chair. I have personally observed one patient who sustained a skull fracture when he fainted at the end of a venepuncture and fell forward onto a hard floor, and two other patients, neither previously known to be epileptic, who suffered epileptiform convulsions during venepuncture. Such seizures may not be true epilepsy, but consequent on hypoxia following brief vagal-induced cessation of heart beat [1]. If venepunctures are being performed on children or on patients unable to cooperate fully, then the arm for venepuncture should be gently but firmly immobilized by an assistant. Gloves should be worn during venepuncture, for the protection of the person carrying out the procedure. Non-latex gloves must be available if either the phlebotomist or the patient is allergic to latex. The needle to enter the patient must not be touched, so that it remains sterile.

In some circumstances, the patient should rest prior to venesection. In endurance athletes being tested for a 'biological passport', 10 minutes' rest in a seated position has been found to be sufficient for the haemoglobin concentration (Hb) and haematocrit (Hct) to fall to a stable level [2].

Peripheral venous blood

In an adult, peripheral venous blood is most easily obtained from a vein in the antecubital fossa (Fig. 1.1) using a needle and either a syringe or an evacuated tube. Of the veins in the antecubital region, the median cubital vein is preferred since it is usually large and well anchored in tissues, but the cephalic and basilic veins are also often satisfactory. Other forearm veins can be used, but they are frequently more mobile and therefore more difficult to penetrate. Veins on the dorsum of the wrist and hand often have a poorer flow and performing venepuncture at these sites is more likely to lead to bruising. This is also true of the anterior surface of the wrist where, in addition, venepuncture tends to be more painful and where there is more risk of damaging vital structures. Foot veins are not an ideal site for venepuncture and it is rarely necessary to use them. Injuries that have been associated with obtaining a blood sample from the antecubital fossa

Blood Cells A Practical Guide, Fifth Edition. By Barbara J. Bain © 2015 John Wiley & Sons, Ltd. Published 2015 by John Wiley & Sons, Ltd.
Companion Website: www.wiley.com/go/bain/bloodcells

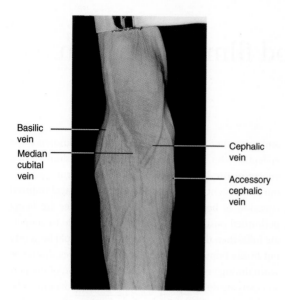

Basilic
vein

Median
cubital
vein

Cephalic
vein

Accessory
cephalic
vein

Fig. 1.1 Anterior surface of the left arm showing veins most suitable for venepuncture.

include damage to the lateral antebrachial cutaneous nerve [3] and inadvertent arterial puncture. Complications are more likely with the less accessible basilic vein than with the median antecubital or the cephalic vein. If anterior wrist veins have to be used, there is a risk of damage to the radial or ulnar nerve or artery. Use of foot veins is more likely to lead to complications, e.g. thrombosis, infection or poor healing.

When a vein is identified it is palpated to ensure it is patent. A patent vein is soft and can be compressed easily. A thrombosed vein feels cord-like and is not compressible. An artery has a thicker wall and is pulsatile. If a vein is not visible (in some dark-skinned or overweight people) it is identified by palpation after applying a tourniquet to achieve venous distension. If veins appear very small, warming of the arm to produce vasodilatation helps, as does tapping the vein and asking the patient to clench and unclench the fist several times.

It should be noted that pathogenic bacteria can be cultured from reusable tourniquets and it is prudent practice to use disposable tourniquets, at least for patients at particular risk of infection [4].

The arm should be positioned on the armrest so that the vein identified is under some tension and its mobility is reduced. The skin should be cleaned with 70% ethanol or 0.5% chlorhexidine and allowed to dry, to avoid stinging when the skin is penetrated. A tourniquet is applied

to the arm, sufficiently tightly to distend the vein, but not so tightly that discomfort is caused. Alternatively, a sphygmomanometer cuff can be applied and inflated to diastolic pressure, but the use of a tourniquet is usually quicker and simpler. If it is particularly important to obtain a specimen without causing haemoconcentration, e.g. in a patient with suspected polycythaemia, the tourniquet should be left on the arm only long enough to allow penetration of the vein. Otherwise it can be left applied while blood is being obtained, to ensure a continuing adequate flow of blood. It is preferable that the tourniquet is applied for no more than a minute, but the degree of haemoconcentration may not be great, even after 10 minutes' application. In one study the increase of the Hb and the red blood cell count (RBC) was about 2% at 2 and at 10 minutes [5]. However, in another study Hb rose by 9 g/l by 3 minutes and RBC and Hct by a corresponding amount [6].

Blood specimens can be obtained with a needle and an evacuated tube (see below) or with either a needle or a winged blood collection cannula (a 'butterfly') and a syringe. A winged cannula may reduce the chance of injury to nerves [7] and is certainly preferable for small veins and difficult sites. A 19 or 20 gauge needle is suitable for an adult and a 21 or 23 gauge for a child or an adult with small veins. When using a syringe, the plunger should first be moved within the barrel of the syringe to ensure that it will move freely. Next the needle is attached to the syringe, which, unless small, should have a side port rather than a central port. The guard is then removed. The needle is now inserted into the vein with the bevel facing upwards (Fig. 1.2). This may be done in a single movement or in two separate movements for the skin and the vein, depending on personal preference and on how superficial the vein is. With one hand steadying the barrel of the syringe so that the needle is not accidentally withdrawn from the vein, blood is withdrawn into the syringe using minimal negative pressure. Care should be taken not to aspirate more rapidly than blood is entering the vein, or the wall of the vein may be drawn against the bevel of the needle and cut off the flow of blood. If the tourniquet has not already been released, this must be done before withdrawing the needle. Following removal of the needle, direct pressure is applied to the puncture site with cotton wool or a sterile gauze square, the arm being kept straight and, if preferred, somewhat elevated. Adhesive plaster should not be applied until pressure has been sustained for long enough for bleeding from the puncture site to have stopped.

Evacuated tube systems include Vacutainer (Beckton-Dickinson) and Vacuette (Greiner Bio-One). When blood is taken into an evacuated tube the technique of venepuncture is basically similar. A double-ended needle is screwed into a holder, which allows it to be manipulated for venepuncture (Fig. 1.3). Alternatively, a winged cannula can be attached to an evacuated tube, using a plastic holder into which an adaptor is screwed. Once the vein has been entered, an evacuated tube is inserted into the holder and is pushed firmly so that its rubber cap is penetrated by the needle, breaking the vacuum and causing blood to be aspirated into the tube (Fig. 1.4). Evacuated tubes are very convenient if multiple specimens are to be taken, since several evacuated tubes can be applied in turn. Only sterile vacuum

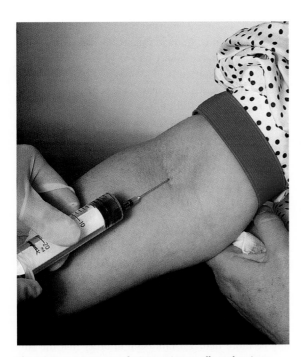

Fig. 1.2 Venepuncture technique using needle and syringe.

The needle should be removed from the syringe before expelling the blood into the specimen container, great care being taken to avoid self-injury with the needle. The needle should be put directly into a special receptacle for sharp objects without resheathing it, unless the needle incorporates a special device that can be flicked into place without risk to the fingers. The blood specimen is expelled gently into a bottle containing anticoagulant and is mixed gently by inverting the container four or five times. Forceful ejection of the blood can cause lysis. Shaking should also be avoided. The specimen container is then labelled with the patient's name and identifying details and, depending on the hospital's standard operating procedure, possibly also with a bar-code label, which is also applied to the request form and subsequently to the blood film. The time of venepuncture should also be recorded on the bottle. Bottles should not be labelled in advance away from the patient's bedside as this increases the chances of putting a blood sample into a mislabelled bottle. Recording the time of venepuncture is important both to allow the clinician to relate the laboratory result to the condition of the patient at the time and also to allow the laboratory to check that there has been no undue delay between venepuncture and performing the test.

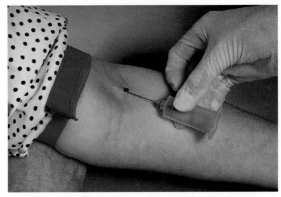

Fig. 1.3 Venepuncture technique using an evacuated container; the distal end of the needle has been screwed into the holder and the proximal needle has then been unsheathed and inserted into a suitable vein.

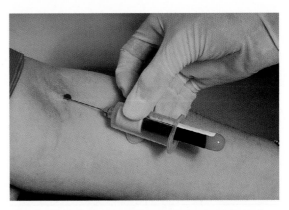

Fig. 1.4 Venepuncture technique using an evacuated container; the evacuated container has been inserted into the holder and forced onto the sharp end of the needle.

tubes should be used for obtaining blood specimens. In children and others with very small veins, an appropriately small vacuum tube should be used so that excessive pressure does not cause the vein to collapse. Once all necessary specimen tubes have been filled, the needle is withdrawn from the vein, still attached to the holder. To reduce the possibility of a needle-prick injury it is necessary to either: (i) use a specially designed device that permits the needle to be discarded with a single-hand technique; (ii) remove the needle from the holder with a specially designed safe device; or (iii) throw away the holder with the needle. The tubes of blood should be mixed promptly. When blood samples are obtained with an evacuated tube system the anticoagulant from one tube may contaminate another. Heparin may interfere with coagulation tests, ethylenediaminetetra-acetic acid (EDTA) with calcium measurements and fluoride with haematological investigations. It is therefore advised, by the NCCLS (National Committee on Clinical Laboratory Standards, now renamed the Clinical and Laboratory Standards Institute) that samples be taken in the order shown in Table 1.1.

If there is a need for a large specimen or a large number of specimens, either an evacuated tube system or a syringe and winged cannula should be used. In the latter case the tubing is pinched off to allow several syringes in turn to be attached. This technique is also useful in children and when small veins make venepuncture difficult. A blood specimen should not be taken from a vein above the site of an intravenous infusion, since dilution can occur. However, venepuncture below the site of an infusion is not associated with clinically significant inaccuracy.

'Capillary blood'

It is often necessary to obtain blood by skin puncture in babies and infants and in adults with poor veins.

Table 1.1 NCCLS* recommended order for taking blood samples [8].

Blood culture tubes
Plain glass tubes for serum samples
Sodium citrate tubes
Gel separator tubes/plain plastic tubes for serum
Heparin tubes/heparin gel separator tubes
EDTA tubes
Fluoride tubes for glucose

*National Committee of Clinical Laboratory Standards, now renamed the Clinical and Laboratory Standards Institute

EDTA, ethylenediaminetetra-acetic acid.

'Capillary' or, more probably, largely arteriolar blood may be obtained from a freely flowing stab wound made with a sterile lancet on the plantar surface of a warmed and cleansed heel (babies less than 3 months of age and infants), the plantar aspect of the big toe (infants) or a finger, thumb or ear lobe (older children and adults). The correct site for puncture of the heel is shown in Fig. 1.5. The lateral or posterior aspect of the heel should not be used in a baby, as the underlying bone is much closer to the skin surface than it is on the plantar aspect. In older patients a finger (excluding the fifth finger) or the thumb is preferred to an ear lobe, since bleeding from the ear lobe may be prolonged in a patient with a haemostatic defect, and pressure is difficult to apply. The palmar surface of the distal phalanx is the preferred site on a digit, since the underlying bone is closer to the skin surface on other aspects. The middle or ring finger of the non-dominant hand is preferred; puncture of these digits is less painful than puncture of the index finger. In adults, skin punctures should ideally be more than 1.5 mm deep in order that the lancet passes through the dermal–subcutaneous junction where the concentration of blood vessels is greatest,

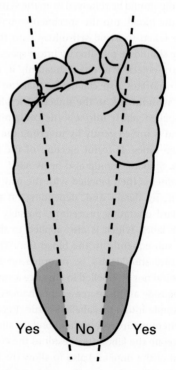

Fig. 1.5 The areas of the foot of a baby or infant that are suitable for obtaining capillary blood.

permitting a free flow of blood. Lancets used for heel puncture in full-term babies must not exceed 2.4 mm in length, since this is the depth below the skin of the calcaneal bone. Much shorter lancets are available and should be selected for use in premature babies. Osteomyelitis of the calcaneal bone has resulted from inadvertent puncture of the bone [9]. Previous puncture sites should be avoided, to reduce the risk of infection. Safety lancets, with a blade that retracts permanently after first use, have been developed in order to reduce the risk of accidental injury to phlebotomy staff. They are available in sizes appropriate for adults and children, infants and premature neonates.

Capillary samples should be obtained from warm tissues so that a free flow of blood is more readily obtained. If the area is cool then it should be warmed with a wet cloth, no hotter than 42°C. The skin should then be cleansed with 70% isopropanol and dried with a sterile gauze square (since traces of alcohol may lead to haemolysis of the specimen). The first drop of blood may be diluted with tissue fluid and should be wiped away with a sterile gauze square. Flow of blood may be promoted by gentle pressure, but a massaging or pumping action should not be employed, since this may lead to tissue fluid being mixed with blood.

Capillary blood can be collected into glass capillary tubes. These can be coated with EDTA, but tubes containing heparin are not suitable for full blood count (FBC) specimens since cellular morphology and staining characteristics are altered. Disposable pipettes complete with diluent, suitable for both automated and manual counts, are commercially available. Caution is necessary if glass capillary tubes are used, because of the risk of injury to the person obtaining the blood sample [10]. Caution should also be employed in the use of spring-loaded skin-prick devices, since transmission of hepatitis B from one patient to another has occurred when there has been a failure to change the platform as well as the lancet between patients [11]. However, automated lancets do ensure a standardised depth of penetration. Use of one proprietary automated incision device (Tenderfoot) has been reported to cause less bruising and to be associated with less haemolysis of capillary samples than when the device is not used [12, 13].

Platelet counts performed on capillary blood are often lower than are those on venous blood [14] and other parameters may also vary (see Chapter 5). The precision of measurement of Hb on a single drop of capillary blood

is poor and it is therefore recommended that several drops be put into an EDTA-containing tube [15].

Cord blood

Blood samples can be obtained from the umbilical cord immediately after birth. Cord blood is best obtained with a syringe and needle after removing any blood from the surface of the cord with a gauze square. Expressing blood from the cut end of the cord can introduce Wharton's jelly into the blood sample, with subsequent red cell agglutination. Haematological parameters on cord blood are not necessarily the same as those obtained from capillary or venous specimens from the neonate.

Fetal blood sampling

Blood samples can be obtained from a fetus by cordocentesis and can be diagnostically useful. A blood count and film can be useful not only when a haematological disorder is suspected, but when a fetus is being investigated because of dysmorphic features detected on ultrasound examination [16].

Obtaining a blood specimen from other sites

It may sometimes be necessary to obtain blood from the femoral vein or from indwelling cannulae in various sites. When blood is obtained from a cannula, the first blood obtained may be diluted by infusion fluid or contaminated with heparin and should be discarded. In infants, blood can be obtained from scalp veins or jugular veins.

Anticoagulant and specimen container

The anticoagulant of choice for blood count specimens is one of the salts of EDTA. K_2EDTA, K_3EDTA and Na_2EDTA have all been used. The preferred anticoagulant, recommended by the International Council (then Committee) for Standardization in Haematology (ICSH), is K_2EDTA in a final concentration of 1.5–2.2 mg/ml [17]. Both dry EDTA and EDTA in solution are in use. If screw-capped tubes are being used, a solution has the advantage that mixing of blood specimens is easier, so clotted specimens are less common. However, if a dry evacuated tube system is used, in which the inside of the tube is coated with the anticoagulant, poor mixing is not a problem. It should also be noted that some parameters are altered by dilution and, if too little blood is taken into a tube, dilution may be appreciable. Excess

EDTA also has deleterious effects on cell morphology in stained blood films. Na$_2$EDTA is less soluble than the potassium salts. K$_3$EDTA causes undesirable cell shrinkage, which is reflected in a lower microhaematocrit (see Chapter 2).

Many laboratories use automated blood counting instruments with a sampling device that is able to perforate the rubber cap of a blood specimen container, thus reducing unnecessary handling of blood. To take advantage of this it is necessary that not only evacuated tubes but also all blood containers have rubber caps that can be penetrated and resealed without permitting leakage.

Guidelines

Guidelines for the procedure of venepuncture [8] and for the protection of phlebotomists and laboratory workers from biological hazards [18] were published by the NCCLS and are still valid. It is recommended that 'standard precautions' proposed by the Centers for Disease Control (CDC), previously referred to as 'universal precautions', be applied to phlebotomy. This policy means that all blood specimens are regarded as potentially infectious. The following specific recommendations are made [18]:

1 Gloves should preferably be worn for all phlebotomy; their use is particularly important if the phlebotomist has any breaks in the skin, if the patient is likely to be uncooperative, if the phlebotomist is inexperienced or if blood is being obtained by skin puncture.
2 Gloves should be changed between patients.
3 An evacuated tube system should be used in preference to a needle and syringe.
4 If a needle and syringe have to be used and it is then necessary to transfer blood to an evacuated tube, the rubber stopper should not be removed. The stopper should be pierced by the needle and blood should be allowed to flow into the tube under the influence of the vacuum. To avoid the possibility of a self-inflicted wound the evacuated tube **must not be held in the hand** during this procedure, but instead should be placed in a rack.

Needle-prick injury

Precautions should be taken to avoid needle-prick (needle-stick) injuries. Hepatitis B can be readily transmitted by such injury, particularly when the patient is hepatitis B e antigen positive. Overall transmission rates of

7–30% have been reported following needle-prick injuries involving infected patients. If the patient is e antigen positive, the rate of transmission is of the order of 20% if hepatitis B immunoglobulin is given after the injury and about 30–40% if it is not given [19, 20]. Reported rates of transmission of hepatitis C have varied from 0 to 7%, with a mean of 1.8% [21]; however, when sensitive techniques are used, the rate of transmission has been found to be about 10% [22]. Transmission occurs only from patients who are positive for hepatitis C viral RNA [21]. Human immunodeficiency virus (HIV) is much less readily transmitted than hepatitis B or C, but a risk does exist. In 3430 needle-prick injuries reported up to 1993 the overall transmission rate was 0.46% [23]. Other infections that have been transmitted occasionally by needle-prick injury include malaria, cryptococcosis, tuberculosis, viral haemorrhagic fever and dengue fever [24–28].

A risk of injury and viral transmission also exists if glass capillary tubes are used for blood collection, and alternative blood collection devices have therefore been advised by the USA's Food and Drug Administration (FDA) [10].

Because it has proved impossible to eliminate needle-stick injuries totally, all hospitals should have agreed policies for meeting this eventuality. Both laboratory managers and occupational health services have a responsibility in this regard. Staff who are performing venepunctures should be offered vaccination against hepatitis B and the adequacy of their antibody response should be verified; if a needle-prick injury from a known hepatitis B–positive source occurs, the antibody titre should be checked and a booster vaccination should be given if necessary [18]. Phlebotomists with an inadequate antibody response to vaccination should, in the event of a needle-prick injury from an infected source, be offered hepatitis B immunoglobulin. Phlebotomists who have chosen not to be vaccinated should be offered hepatitis B immunoglobulin and vaccination should again be offered. Antiretroviral prophylaxis should be offered to those exposed to a risk of HIV exposure through needle-stick injury and ideally should be administered within a few hours of exposure; the risk of infection becoming established is reduced but not eliminated [29]. Prophylaxis offered was previously zidovudine alone, but at least triple agent antiretroviral therapy is now recommended. Current CDC recommendations can be found on the CDC's website (http://www.cdc.gov/hiv/risk/other/occupational.html). The use of nevirapine is not recommended because of the possibility of serious toxicity [30].

There appears to be no effective post-exposure prophylaxis for hepatitis C infection [21], but the consensus view is that interferon therapy is indicated in acute infection, including that acquired by needle-stick injury. Interferon alpha-2b in a dose of 5 million units daily for 4 weeks followed by the same dose three times a week for a further 20 weeks has been found to be efficacious [31]. Unless all new staff are routinely tested for HIV, occupational health services should consider at least offering storage of serum samples so that baseline HIV testing is possible in the event of a subsequent needle-prick injury. If this policy is not followed, serum storage should be offered in the event of a needle-prick injury from a seropositive source or from a source of unknown HIV status.

Specimen mixing

The blood specimen must be adequately mixed before making a blood film or performing a blood count. Mixing for one minute on a mechanical rotating mixer is sufficient [32]. Manual inversion (10 times) is also satisfactory as long as any refrigerated samples are first brought to room temperature [32].

Making a blood film

A blood film may be made from non-anticoagulated (native) blood, obtained either from a vein or a capillary, or from EDTA-anticoagulated blood. Chelation of calcium by EDTA hinders platelet aggregation so that platelets are evenly spread and their numbers can be assessed more easily (Fig. 1.6). Films prepared from capillary blood usually show prominent platelet aggregation (Fig. 1.7) and films from native venous blood often show small aggregates (Fig. 1.8). Films prepared from native venous or capillary blood are free of artefacts due to storage or the effects of the anticoagulant. A few laboratories still use such films as a matter of routine, but otherwise their use is obligatory for investigating abnormalities such as red cell crenation or white cell or platelet aggregation that may be induced by storage or EDTA. Conversely, making a blood film from EDTA-anticoagulated blood after arrival of the blood specimen in the laboratory has the advantage that some of the artefacts that may influence the validity of results obtained from automated instruments are more likely to be detected, e.g. the formation of fibrin strands, aggregation of platelets or agglutination of red cells induced by cold agglutinins. Good laboratory practice includes recording the date and time the specimen is received in the laboratory and making a film shortly after receipt of the specimen. In this way the length of any delay in transit is known and attribution of morphological changes to prolonged storage of EDTA-anticoagulated blood ('storage artefact', see Chapter 3) can be confirmed.

Blood films are prepared and examined on only a proportion of the specimens on which a blood count is performed. Consensus guidelines are available that suggest appropriate indications for the examination of a film [33].

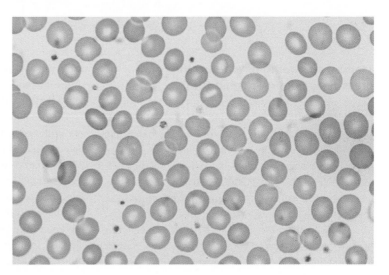

Fig. 1.6 A blood film from ethylenediaminetetra-acetic acid (EDTA)-anticoagulated blood showing an even distribution of platelets.

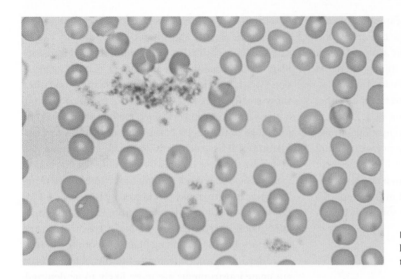

Fig. 1.7 A blood film from non-anticoagulated capillary blood showing the aggregation of platelets that usually occurs.

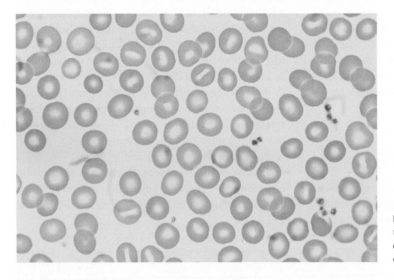

Fig. 1.8 A blood film from non-anticoagulated venous blood showing the minor degree of platelet aggregation that usually occurs.

Manual spreading of a blood film on a glass slide (wedge-spread film)

Glass slides must be clean and free of grease. They should not be too porous or background staining is increased [34]. A spreader is required and must be narrower than the slide. If a coverslip is to be applied, the spreader must also be narrower than the coverslip so that cells at the edge of the blood film are covered by the coverslip and can be easily examined microscopically. A spreader can be readily prepared by breaking the corner off a glass slide after incising it with a diamond pen; this provides a smooth-edged spreader that is large enough to be manipulated easily. Spreaders made by cutting transverse pieces from a slide are inferior since they are more difficult to handle and have at least one rough edge that may damage gloves or fingers.

The laboratory worker spreading blood films should wear gloves. A drop of blood (either native or anticoagulated) is placed near one end of the slide. Anticoagulated blood from screw-top containers can be applied to the slide using a capillary tube, which is then discarded. A drop of blood from specimen containers with penetrable lids can be applied to the slide by means of a special device that perforates the lid. The spreader is applied at an angle of 25–30°, in front of the drop of blood, and is drawn back into it (Fig. 1.9). Once the blood has run along its back edge,

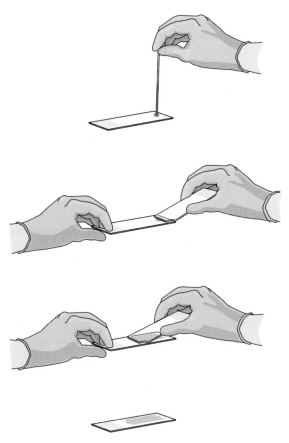

the spreader is advanced with a smooth, steady motion so that a thin film of blood is spread over the slide. If the angle of the spreader is too obtuse or the speed of spreading is too fast, the film will be too short. An experienced operator learns to recognise blood with a higher than normal Hct, which is more viscous and requires a more acute angle to make a satisfactory film and, conversely, blood with a lower than normal Hct, which requires a more obtuse angle. The spreading technique should produce a film of blood with a fairly straight tail. The film should be at least 2.5 cm long and should stop at least 1 cm from the end of the slide. A film of the shape of a thumbprint means that, when observing the film microscopically and moving across the film, the observer moves from an area that is optimal for identification of cells to an area that is too thick. It is important that the spreader is wiped clean with a dry tissue or gauze square after each use since it is otherwise possible to transfer abnormal cells from one blood film to another (Fig. 1.10).

As soon as slides are made they should be labelled with the patient's name and the date or with an identifying number. Small numbers of slides can be labelled with a diamond marker or by writing details on the thick part of the film. The fastest way to label large numbers of slides is with a methanol-resistant pen or by writing in pencil on the frosted end of a slide. Slides that are frosted at one end on **both** sides are useful because they avoid waste of staff time ensuring that the slide is the right way up. Blood films should be dried rapidly.

Fig. 1.9 The method of spreading a blood film.

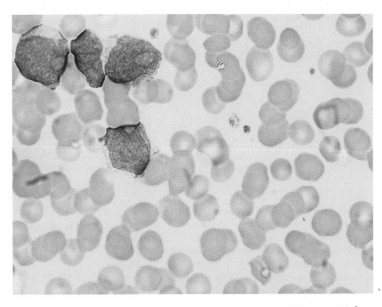

Fig. 1.10 Blast cells from a patient with acute leukaemia that have been inadvertently transferred to the blood film of another patient by the use of an inadequately cleaned spreader.

A hot-air blower or a fan to increase air circulation can be useful. If films are dried slowly, there is shrinkage of cells that can lead to the appearance of cytoplasmic blebs and villi, bipolar lymphocytes, hyperchromatic nuclei and inapparent nucleoli [28]; these changes can occur not only in normal cells but also in neoplastic cells so that their characteristic features are less apparent.

Fig. 1.11 shows a well-spread film in comparison with examples of poor films resulting from faulty technique.

Unless otherwise stated, this book deals with morphology as observed in wedge-spread films. Most of the photographs are of manually spread films, which were prepared from recently collected EDTA-anticoagulated blood.

Other methods of spreading thin films
Automated spreading of blood films
Wedge-spread films can be prepared by mechanical spreaders, which can be integrated into a staining machine or an automated full blood counter. A film of

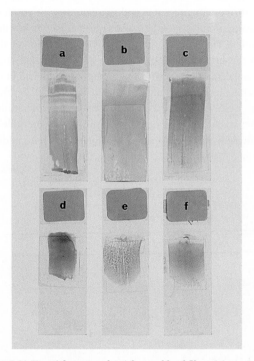

Fig. 1.11 Unsatisfactory and satisfactory blood films: (a) uneven pressure has produced ridges; (b) too broad and too long – the edges and the tail of the film cannot be examined adequately; (c) too long and streaked by an uneven spreader; (d) too thick and short due to the wrong angle or speed of spreading; (e) even distribution of blood cells has been interrupted because the slide was greasy; (f) satisfactory.

blood one cell thick can also be spread on a glass slide by centrifugation in a specially designed centrifuge, but this method is little used.

Films from blood with a very high Hct
If blood has a very high Hct, e.g. Hct > 0.60, Hb > 200 g/l, it can be impossible to make a good blood film, even if the angle and the speed of spreading are adjusted. Mixing a drop of blood and a drop of either saline or blood group AB plasma reduces viscosity so that a film can be made in which details of red cell morphology can be appreciated.

Buffy coat films
Buffy coat films are useful to concentrate nucleated cells, e.g. to look for low-frequency abnormal cells or bacteria. A tube of anticoagulated blood is centrifuged and a drop of the buffy coat is mixed with a drop of autologous EDTA-anticoagulated plasma and spread in the normal manner.

Thick films
Thick films are required for examination for malarial parasites and certain other parasites, the red cells being lysed before the film is examined. Parasites are much more concentrated in a thick film, so that searching for them requires less time. To make a thick film, several drops of native or EDTA-anticoagulated blood are placed in the centre of a slide and stirred with a capillary tube or an orange stick into a pool of blood of such a thickness that typescript or a watch face can be read through the blood (Fig. 1.12). The blood film is not fixed but, after drying, is placed directly into an aqueous Giemsa stain so that lysis of red cells occurs; this allows the organisms to be seen more clearly.

Unstained wet preparations
Unstained wet preparations are useful for searching for motile parasites such as microfilariae, which can be seen agitating the red cells. A drop of anticoagulated blood is placed on a slide and covered with a coverslip.

Fixation, staining and mounting

Fixation
Following air drying, thin films are fixed in absolute methanol for 10–20 minutes. It is important not to proceed to fixation until the blood film is dry. Premature fixation of a damp film leads to a characteristic artefact, when the

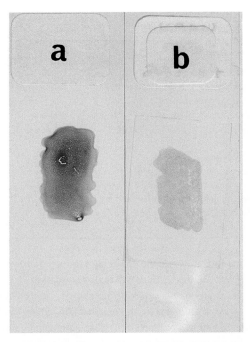

Fig. 1.12 Thick films for examination for malarial parasites: (a) unstained film showing the correct thickness of the film of blood; and (b) film stained without fixation, causing lysis of red cells.

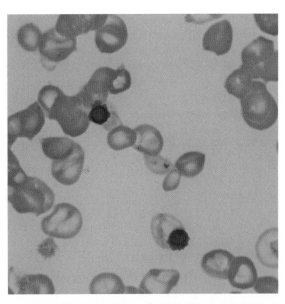

Fig. 1.13 A blood film that has been fixed before drying was complete. It is important not to confuse the apparent leaking of nuclear contents into the cytoplasm, which is an artefactual change, with dyserythropoiesis.

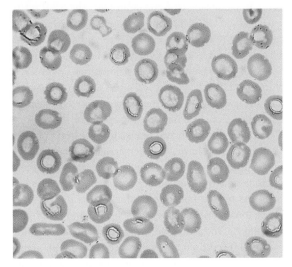

Fig. 1.14 Artefactual changes produced by 5% water in the methanol used for fixation.

contents of the nucleus appear to leak into the cytoplasm (Fig. 1.13). Poor fixation, also with characteristic artefactual changes, occurs if there is more than a few per cent of water in the methanol (Fig. 1.14); this renders interpretation of morphology, particularly red cell morphology, impossible and, if the film is not examined carefully, can give a mistaken impression of hypochromia. In warm, humid climates it may be necessary to change methanol solutions several times a day. Similar artefactual changes can be produced by condensation on slides. In humid climates, slides should be fixed as soon as they are thoroughly dry. A hot-air blower can be used to accelerate drying. In any circumstances, prolonged delay in fixation should be avoided as this can lead to alteration in the staining characteristics of the film, which can acquire a turquoise tint.

Staining

There is little consistency between laboratories in the precise stain used to prepare a blood film for microscopic examination, but the multiple stains in use are based on the Romanowsky stain, developed by the Russian protozoologist in the late nineteenth century [35]. Romanowsky used a mixture of old methylene blue and eosin to stain the nucleus of a malarial parasite purple and the cytoplasm blue. Subsequently, Giemsa modified the stain, combining methylene azure and eosin. The stain most commonly used in the UK is a combination of Giemsa's stain with May–Grünwald stain; it is therefore designated the May–Grünwald–Giemsa (MGG) stain. The stain most commonly used in North America is Wright's stain, which contains methylene blue and eosin; the methylene blue has been heated, or 'polychromed', to produce analogues of methylene blue. Sometimes this is combined with Giemsa's stain to give a Wright–Giemsa stain, which is generally held to give superior results. It has been demonstrated by chromatography that dyes prepared by traditional organic chemistry methods are not pure, dyes sold under the same designation containing a variable mixture of five to ten dyes [36]. Variation between different batches prepared by the same manufacturer also occurs.

The essential components of a Romanowsky-type stain are: (i) a basic or cationic dye, such as azure B, which conveys a blue-violet or blue colour to nucleic acids (binding to the phosphate groups of deoxyribonucleic acid (DNA) and ribonucleic acid (RNA)) and to nucleoprotein, to the granules of basophils and, weakly, to the granules of neutrophils; and (ii) an acidic or anionic dye, such as eosin, which conveys a red or orange colour to haemoglobin and the eosinophil granules and also binds to cationic nuclear protein, thus contributing to the colour of the stained nucleus. A stain containing azure B and eosin provides a satisfactory Romanowsky stain [35], as does a mixture of azure B, methylene blue and eosin [36]. The ICSH reference method for the Romanowsky stain [37], which uses pure azure B and eosin Y, gives very satisfactory results but such pure dyes are expensive for routine use. Satisfactory and reasonably consistent staining can be achieved using good-quality commercial stains and an automated staining machine. This method has been used for staining the majority of blood films photographed for this book.

Traditionally, cytoplasm that stains blue and granules that stain purple have both been designated 'basophilic', and granules that stain violet or pinkish-purple have been designated 'azurophilic'. In fact all these hues are achieved by the uptake of a single basic dye such as azure B or A. 'Acidophilic' and 'eosinophilic' both refer to uptake of the acidic dye, eosin, although 'acidophilic' has often been used to describe cell components staining pink, and 'eosinophilic' to describe cell components staining orange. The range of colours that a Romanowsky stain should produce is shown in Table 1.2.

Staining must be performed at the correct pH. If the pH is too low, basophilic components do not stain well. Leucocytes are generally pale, with eosinophil granules a brilliant vermilion. If the pH is too high, uptake of the basic dye may be excessive leading to general overstaining; it becomes difficult to distinguish between normal and polychromatic red cells, eosinophil granules are deep

Table 1.2 Characteristic staining of different cell components with a Romanowsky stain.

Cell component	Colour
Chromatin (including Howell-Jolly bodies)	Purple
Promyelocyte granules and Auer rods	Purplish-red
Cytoplasm of lymphocytes	Blue
Cytoplasm of monocytes	Blue-grey
Cytoplasm rich in RNA (i.e. 'basophilic cytoplasm')	Deep blue
Döhle bodies	Blue-grey
Specific granules of neutrophils. granules of lymphocytes, granules of platelets	Light purple or pink
Specific granules of basophils	Deep purple
Specific granules of eosinophils	Orange
Red cells	Pink

blue or dark grey, and the granules of normal neutrophils are heavily stained, simulating toxic granulation.

Stain solutions may need to be filtered shortly before use, to avoid stain deposit on the blood film, which can be confused with red cell inclusions. If an automated staining machine is used, superior results are usually achieved with a dipping technique, in which the entire slide is immersed in the stain, than with a flat-bed stainer, in which staining solution is applied to a horizontal slide. The latter type of staining machine is more prone to leave stain deposits on the slides and, if the blood film is too long or badly positioned, some parts of it may escape staining.

Destaining an MGG-stained blood film can be done by flooding the slide with methanol, washing in water and then repeating the sequence until all the stain has gone. This can be useful if only a single blood film is available and a further stain, e.g. an iron stain, is required.

Staining for malarial parasites

The detection and identification of malarial parasites are facilitated if blood films are stained with a Giemsa (or Leishman) stain at pH 7.2. At this pH, cells that have been parasitised by either *Plasmodium vivax* or *Plasmodium ovale* have different tinctorial qualities from non-parasitised cells and are easily identified. The inclusions in parasitised cells are also evident (see Chapter 3).

Mounting

If films are to be stored, mounting gives them protection against scratching and gathering of dust. As stated above, the coverslip should be sufficiently wide to cover the edges of the blood film. A neutral mountant that is miscible with xylene is required.

As an alternative to mounting, blood films can be sprayed with a polystyrene or acrylic resin.

If films are not to be stored, a thin film of oil can be smeared on the stained slide to permit microscopic examination at low power before adding a drop of oil to permit examination with the oil immersion lens.

Storage of slides

Ideal patient care and continuing education of haematology staff dictate that blood films should be stored as long as possible, preferably for some years. Unfortunately, the very large numbers of blood specimens now being processed daily by most haematology laboratories means that this is often difficult. The most economical way to store slides is in metal racks in stacking drawers. Labels showing the patient's name, the date and the laboratory number should be applied in such a way that they can be read when the slides are in storage. Slides that have been freshly mounted should be stored in cardboard trays or stacked in racks, separated from each other by wire loops, until the mountant has hardened and dried. When the mountant is no longer sticky, slides can be stacked closely together for maximum economy of space. Glass slides are heavy and if large numbers are to be stored the floor of the room may need to be strengthened.

When a patient has a bone marrow aspiration performed, a blood film should always be stored permanently with bone marrow films so that when it is necessary to throw out old peripheral blood films to make room for new ones, at least this film is available for review. A laboratory should also maintain a separate file of teaching slides. These should include examples of rare conditions and typical examples of common conditions.

Setting up and using a microscope

All laboratory workers should learn to set up a microscope correctly early in the course of their training. The following is the correct procedure for setting up a binocular microscope.

1 If you need to move or lift the microscope do so using only the arm (Fig. 1.15). Sit at the microscope and make sure that the height is correct for comfortable viewing. Adjust the chair or the height of the microscope above the bench, as necessary.

2 Plug in the electric lead and switch on the mains power supply.

3 Turn on the microscope.

4 Turn up the rheostat until there is a comfortable amount of light.

5 Lower the stage and rotate the × 10 objective into place; it will click when it engages.

6 Select a slide and place it on the stage, being careful to place it with the blood film and coverslip uppermost. Handle the slide only by its edges. Secure the slide with the levers provided for this purpose.

7 Raise the condenser as high as it will go.

8 Open the field diaphragm and the condenser aperture diaphragm fully.

9 Move the stage until the film of blood is beneath the objective, in the beam of light.

10 Raise the stage, looking at the slide from the side or the front rather than using the oculars (eyepieces), until the slide almost touches the objective.

11 Adjust the position of the oculars so that they match your interpupillary distance and look at the slide through the oculars, making sure that the light is at a comfortable level.

12 Lower the slide slowly using the coarse focus knob until the slide comes into focus.

13 Using the coarse and then the fine focus, focus on the slide with your right eye to the right ocular then, without moving the slide, rotate the ring on the left ocular so that the image recorded by your left eye is also sharp. (With some microscopes it is possible to adjust both oculars.)

14 Close the field iris diaphragm fully. The field iris diaphragm is near the lamp and controls the area of illumination.

15 Lower the condenser until the edge of the field iris diaphragm comes into focus. Check that the aperture in the field iris diaphragm is centred and, if it is not, centre it using the two centring screws on the condenser.

16 Adjust the focus by moving the condenser so that the edges of the diaphragm appear faintly blue rather than faintly red (Köhler illumination).

17 Open the field iris aperture so that the whole field of view is illuminated but no wider. If it is opened too wide, stray light will enter the field of view (particularly important for photography, for which purpose the diaphragm can be closed further till only the photographic frame is illuminated).

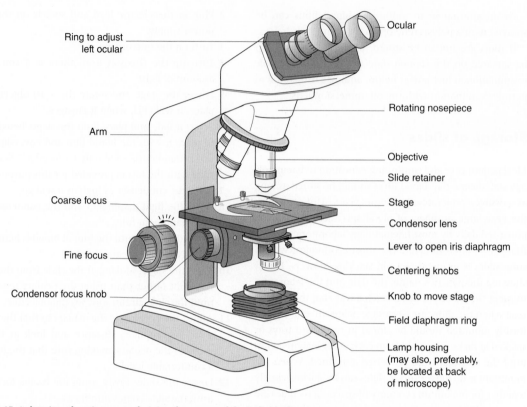

Ring to adjust left ocular

Ocular

Arm

Rotating nosepiece

Objective

Slide retainer

Coarse focus

Stage

Condensor lens

Lever to open iris diaphragm

Fine focus

Centering knobs

Condensor focus knob

Knob to move stage

Field diaphragm ring

Lamp housing (may also, preferably, be located at back of microscope)

Fig. 1.15 A drawing of a microscope showing the names of the individual parts.

18 Using the appropriate lever or ring, close the condenser aperture diaphragm to about 70–80% of the numerical aperture marked on the objective. A condenser scale near the lever or ring permits this to be done. This aperture controls the angular aperture of the cone of light that reaches the condenser lens. The more you close this aperture the less light there is and the lower the resolution, but the greater the contrast and depth of focus. For optimal optics, the condenser aperture iris should be reset for each objective.

19 Examine the slide with the × 10 objective,* then rotate in a × 40 objective. Readjust the focus and the condenser aperture iris and adjust the field iris diaphragm so that only the field of view is illuminated. Re-examine the slide.

20 Before using an oil immersion lens, rotate out the non-oil objective and put a drop of immersion oil in the centre of the slide. Rotate in an oil immersion objective, e.g. × 60 or × 100, and focus, using the coarse and then the fine focus and adjust the condenser aperture iris. Be careful not to rotate in any objective other than an oil immersion objective while there is a drop of oil on the slide. If you are not sure if an objective is for oil immersion or not, read its label. Do not use excess oil and do not mix two different types of oil. Do not overfill a bottle of oil or oil will get on your fingers.

21 After examining a slide with an oil immersion objective, gently wipe the oil from the objective and from the slide. If the slide has been freshly mounted, remove the oil gently so that the coverslip is not accidentally removed, removing enough of the oil that

*Note: microscopes used by haematology laboratories do not usually have a × 4 objective fitted, unless histological sections are also being examined. If a × 4 objective is to be used, e.g. for examining a trephine biopsy section, swing out the condenser before viewing the slide.

a non-oil lens will not be contaminated if the slide is again placed on a microscope stage. Removing oil from slides does not require lens tissues; ordinary tissues are satisfactory. Non-mounted blood films are not advised but, if they are used, be careful to minimise scratching of the blood film when removing oil.

22 When you have finished working, rotate back in the lowest power objective and lower the stage. Remove traces of oil from any oil immersion lens using methanol and lens tissues. Turn down the rheostat before turning off the microscope. Do not leave the microscope turned on when you are away from your workstation; in some poorly designed microscopes the lamp is very close to the field diaphragm and prolonged heat will damage the leaves of the diaphragm.

23 Keep the microscope clean. Dust can be removed with a small brush. Lenses should be cleaned only with lens tissues. These can be moistened with methanol (or a mixture of 3 parts methanol to 7 parts ether).

24 Cover the microscope with a dust cover when not in use.

Identifying the source of a problem and preventing problems

1 If there is no light, check that the light beam has not been deflected to a camera.

2 If you cannot focus on a blood film, check if the slide is upside down and make sure that there are not two coverslips instead of one. Some microscopes have a 'stop' on the coarse focus; if necessary, release it. Rarely, very thick slides may make it impossible to focus with a high power lens if a cover slip is mounted. Unsuitably thick coverslips can have the same effect.

3 If you cannot see the image clearly, clean the slide using tissues and methanol. Sealed methanolsoaked squares of tissue used to prepare the arm for venepuncture are convenient for cleaning slides and avoid the need to have a bottle of methanol in the microscopy laboratory. If cleaning the slide does not help, clean the objective gently using a lens tissue and methanol. Do not use xylene unless you are unable to get the lens clean with methanol.

4 If you wear spectacles you will find that it is impossible to use a microscope with bifocal or varifocal lenses. Modern plastic spectacle lenses are easily scratched and if there is an antiglare coating to the lenses this can also be scratched. Be sure that the oculars have a protective rubber guard if you are using spectacles with this type of lens or lens coating.

Examining a blood film

1 Check the label of the slide (patient identity and date).

2 Examine the film macroscopically for unusual characteristics.

3 Adjust the microscope as above and examine the film microscopically, examining the edges and the tail and then the whole film under low power, e.g. × 10 objective.

4 Next examine the whole film with a × 40 or × 50 objective. This is the most important part of the film examination as it is possible to scan the entire film to note any rare abnormal cells. Be systematic: look specifically at red cells, white cells and platelets.

5 Perform a differential count, if indicated.

6 Examine with an oil immersion lens only if there is some particular reason to do so.

TEST YOUR KNOWLEDGE

Visit the companion website for MCQs and EMQs on this topic:
www.wiley.com/go/bain/bloodcells

References

1 Roddy SM, Ashwal S and Schneider S (1983) Venipuncture fits: a form of reflex anoxic seizure. *Pediatrics*, **72**, 715–717.

2 Ahlgrim C, Pottgiesser T, Robinson N, Sottas PE, Ruecker G and Schumacher YO (2010) Are 10 min of seating enough to guarantee stable haemoglobin and haematocrit readings for the athlete's biological passport? *Int J Lab Haematol*, **32**, 506–511.

3 Sander HWE, Conigliari MF and Masdeu JC (1998) Antecubital phlebotomy complicated by lateral antebrachial cutaneous neuropathy. *N Engl J Med*, **339**, 2024.

4 Golder M, Chan CL, O'Shea S, Corbett K, Chrystie IL and French G (2000) Potential risk of cross-infection during peripheral-venous access by contamination of tourniquets. *Lancet*, **355**, 44.

5 Mull JD and Murphy WR (1993) Effects of tourniquet-induced stasis on blood determinations. *Am J Clin Pathol*, **39**, 134–136.

6 Lippi G, Salvagno GL, Montagnana M, Franchini M and Guidi GC (2006) Venous stasis and routine hematologic testing. *Clin Lab Haematol*, **28**, 332–337.

7 Ohnishi H, Watanabe M and Watanabe T (2012) Butterfly needles reduce the incidence of nerve injury during phlebotomy. *Arch Pathol Lab Med*, **136**, 352.

8 NCCLS. *H3-A4 – Procedure for the collection of diagnostic blood specimens by venipuncture: approved standard*, 4th edn. NCCLS, Wayne, PA, 1998.

9 Hammond KB (1980) Blood specimen collection from infants by skin puncture. *Lab Med*, **11**, 9–12.

10 Anonymous (1999) Glass capillary tubes: joint safety advisory about potential risks. *Lab Med*, **30**, 299.

11 Polish LB, Shapiro CN, Bauer F, Klotz P, Ginier P, Roberto RR *et al.* (1992) Nosocomial transmission of hepatitis B virus associated with the use of a spring-loaded finger-stick device. *N Engl J Med*, **326**, 721–725.

12 Vertanen H, Laipio ML, Fellman V, Brommels M and Viinikka L (2000) Hemolysis in skin puncture samples obtained by using two different sampling devices from preterm infants. Paper presented at 24th World Congress of Medical Technology, Vancouver, Canada.

13 Vertanen H, Fellman V, Brommels M and Viinikka L (2000) An automatic incision device causes less damages to the heels of preterm infants. Paper presented at 24th World Congress of Medical Technology, Vancouver, Canada.

14 Brecher G, Schneiderman M and Cronkite EP (1953) The reproducibility and constancy of the platelet count. *Am J Clin Pathol*, **23**, 15–26.

15 Conway AM, Hinchliffe RF and Anderson LM (1998) Measurement of haemoglobin using single drop of skin puncture blood: is precision acceptable? *J Clin Pathol*, **51**, 248–250.

16 Forestier F, Hohlfeld P, Vial Y, Olin V, Andreux J-P and Tissot J-D (1996) Blood smears and prenatal diagnosis. *Br J Haematol*, **95**, 278–280.

17 ICSH Expert Panel on Cytometry (1993) Recommendations of the International Council for Standardization in Haematology for ethylenediaminetetraacetic acid anticoagulation of blood for blood cell counting and sizing. *Am J Clin Pathol*, **100**, 371–372.

18 NCCLS. *M29-A – Protection of laboratory workers from instrument biohazards and infectious disease transmitted by blood, body fluids, and tissue: approved guideline*. NCCLS, Wayne, PA, 1997.

19 Masuko K, Mitsui T, Iwano K, Yamazaki C, Aikara S, Baba K *et al.* (1985) Factors influencing postexposure immunoprophylaxis of hepatitis B viral infection with hepatitis B immune globulin. High deoxyribonucleic acid polymerase activity in the inocula of unsuccessful cases. *Gastroenterology*, **88**, 151–155.

20 Seeff LB, Wright EC, Zimmerman HJ, Alter HJ, Dietz AA, Felsher BF *et al.* (1978) Type B hepatitis after needle-stick exposure: prevention with hepatitis B immune globulin. A final report of the Veterans Administration Cooperative study. *Ann Intern Med*, **88**, 285–293.

21 Ramsay ME (1999) Guidance on the investigation and management of occupational exposure to hepatitis C. *Commun Dis and Public Health*, **4**, 258–262.

22 Mitsui T, Iwano K, Masuko K, Yamazaki C, Okamoto H, Tsuda F *et al.* (1992) Hepatitis C virus infection in medical personnel after needlestick accident. *Hepatology*, **126**, 1109–1114.

23 Heptonstall J, Gill ON, Porter K, Black MB and Gilbart VL (1993) Health care workers and HIV: surveillance of occupationally acquired infection in the United Kingdom. *Commun Disease Rep*, **3**, 147–153.

24 Bending MR and Maurice PD (1980) Malaria: a laboratory risk. *Postgrad Med J*, **56**, 344–345.

25 Glaser JB and Garden A (1985) Inoculation of cryptococcosis without transmission of the acquired immunodeficiency syndrome. *N Engl J Med*, **312**, 266.

26 Kramer F, Sasse SA, Simms JC and Leedom JM (1993) Primary cutaneous tuberculosis after a needlestick injury from a patient with AIDS and undiagnosed tuberculosis. *Ann Intern Med*, **119**, 594–595.

27 Advisory Committee on Dangerous Pathogens. *Management and control of viral haemorrhagic fevers*. The Stationery Office, London, 1996.

28 De Wazières B, Gil H, Vuitton DA and Dupond JL (1998) Nosocomial transmission of dengue from a needlestick injury. *Lancet*, **351**, 498.

29 Katz MH and Gerberding JL (1997) Postexposure treatment of people exposed to the human immunodeficiency virus through sexual contact or injection drug use. *N Engl J Med*, **336**, 1097–1100.

30 Gottlieb S (2001) Nevirapine should not be prescribed for needlestick injuries. *BMJ*, **322**, 126.

31 Jaeckel E, Cornberg M, Wedemeyer H, Sanantonio T, Mayer J, Zankel M *et al.* (2001) Treatment of acute hepatitis C with interferon alfa-2b. *N Engl J Med*, **345**, 1452–1457.

32 Ashenden M, Clarke A, Sharpe K, d'Onofrio G, Allbon G and Gore CJ (2012) Preanalytical mixing of whole-blood specimens in the context of the Athlete Passport. *J Clin Pathol*, **65**, 8–13.

33 The International Consensus Group for Haematology Review (2005) Suggested criteria for action following automated CBC and WBC differential analysis. *Lab Haematol*, **11**, 83–90.

34 Nguyen D and Diamond L. *Diagnostic hematology: a pattern approach*. Butterworth-Heinemann, Oxford, 2000.

35 Wittekind D (1979) On the nature of the Romanowsky dyes and the Romanowsky–Giemsa effect. *Clin Lab Haematol*, **1**, 247–262.

36 Marshall PN, Bentley SA and Lewis SM (1975) A standardized Romanowsky stain prepared from purified dyes. *J Clin Pathol*, **28**, 920–923.

37 ICSH (1984) ICSH reference method for staining blood and bone marrow films by azure B and eosin Y (Romanowsky stain). *Br J Haematol*, **57**, 707–710.

CHAPTER 2

Performing a blood count

In the past, blood counts were performed by slow and labour-intensive manual techniques using counting chambers, microscopes, glass tubes, colorimeters, centrifuges and a few simple reagents. The only tests done with any frequency were estimations of haemoglobin concentration (Hb), packed cell volume (PCV) and white blood cell count (WBC). Hb was estimated by a method depending on optical density and was expressed as mass/volume, or even as a percentage in relation to a rather arbitrary 'normal' that represented 100%. PCV was a measurement of the proportion of a column of centrifuged blood that was occupied by red cells. Now expressed as a decimal fraction representing volume/volume, it was initially expressed as a percentage. White cells were counted microscopically in a diluted blood sample in a haemocytometer, a counting chamber of known volume. All cell counts were expressed as the number of cells in a unit volume. The red blood cell count (RBC) was performed occasionally, mainly when there was a need to make an estimate of red cell size. Platelets were counted, by light or phase-contrast microscopy, only when there was a clear clinical need. From the primary measurements relating to red cells other values were derived: the mean cell volume (MCV), mean cell haemoglobin (MCH) and mean cell haemoglobin concentration (MCHC). The formulae for these derived measurements are as follows:

$$MCV\,(fl) = \frac{PCV\,(l\,/\,l) \times 1000}{RBC\,(cells\,/\,l) \times 10^{-12}}$$

$$MCH\,(pg) = \frac{Hb\,(g\,/\,l)}{RBC\,(cells\,/\,l) \times 10^{-12}}\ OR$$

$$\frac{Hb\,(g\,/\,dl) \times 10}{RBC\,(cells\,/\,l) \times 10^{-12}}$$

$$MCHC\,(g\,/\,dl) = \frac{Hb\,(g\,/\,l)}{PCV\,(l\,/\,l) \times 10}\ \ OR\ \ \frac{Hb\,(g\,/\,dl)}{PCV\,(l\,/\,l)}$$

These and many other measurements are now made on automated and semi-automated instruments within minutes, using either modifications of the manual techniques or totally new technologies. Measurements are precise, i.e. repeated measurements on the same sample give very similar results. As long as the instruments are carefully calibrated and the blood has no unusual characteristics, measurements are also accurate, i.e. they give results that are very close to 'truth'. However, despite the widespread use of automated instruments, the manual techniques remain important both as reference methods and in the investigation of blood samples that appear to give anomalous test results on automated instruments. They also illustrate the principles that underlie various measurements.

Basic techniques

Haemoglobin concentration

To measure Hb, a known volume of carefully mixed whole blood is added to a diluent, which lyses red cells to produce a haemoglobin solution; lysis occurs because of the hypotonicity of the diluent, but may be accelerated by the inclusion in the diluent of a non-ionic detergent to act as a lytic agent. The Hb is then determined from the light absorbance (optical density) of the solution of haemoglobin or its derivative at a selected wavelength.

Cyanmethaemoglobin method

The International Committee (now Council) for Standardization in Haematology (ICSH) has recommended a reference method in which haemoglobin is converted to cyanmethaemoglobin (haemiglobincyanide) [1]. This method has three significant advantages:

1 Haemoglobin, methaemoglobin and carboxyhaemoglobin are all converted to cyanmethaemoglobin and are therefore included in the measurement. Of the forms of haemoglobin likely to be present in blood, only sulphaemoglobin – usually present in negligible amounts – is not converted to cyanmethaemoglobin, although carboxyhaemoglobin is more slowly converted than the other forms.

2 Stable secondary standards that have been compared with the World Health Organization (WHO) international standard are readily available for calibration [2].

Blood Cells A Practical Guide, Fifth Edition. By Barbara J. Bain © 2015 John Wiley & Sons, Ltd. Published 2015 by John Wiley & Sons, Ltd.
Companion Website: www.wiley.com/go/bain/bloodcells

3 Cyanmethaemoglobin has an absorbance band at 540 nm, which is broad and relatively flat (Fig. 2.1) and thus measurements can be made either on a narrow-band spectrophotometer or on a filter photometer or colorimeter that reads over a wide band of wavelengths. The reference method requires the addition of a diluent that contains: (i) potassium cyanide and potassium ferricyanide, to effect the conversion to methaemoglobin; (ii) dihydrogen potassium phosphate to lower the pH, accelerate the reaction, and allow the reading of light absorbance at 3 minutes rather than 10–15 minutes; and (iii) a non-ionic detergent, to accelerate cell lysis and reduce the turbidity due to precipitation of lipoproteins (and to a lesser extent red cell stroma), which is otherwise a consequence of the lower pH achieved by the dihydrogen potassium phosphate [2]. The absorbance of light by the solution is measured at 540 nm in a spectrophotometer. At this wavelength, the light absorbance of the diluent is zero; either water or, preferably, the diluent can be used as the blank. No standard is required, since the haemoglobin concentration can be calculated from the absorbance, given that the molecular weight and the millimolar extinction coefficient of haemoglobin are known. However, the wavelength of light produced by the instrument must be verified and the absorbance scale calibrated. A reference solution of cyanmethaemoglobin can be used for calibration.

Hb was once measured, in routine practice, by means of a photometer or colorimeter in which light of approximately 540 nm was produced by use of a yellow-green filter such as the Ilford 625. The light passing through the solution was detected by a photoelectric cell and the instrument scale showed either light absorbance or transmittance. Comparison of the instrument reading with that for a reference solution allowed calculation of the Hb; this was most conveniently done using a standard curve or a conversion table. Alternatively, the photometer could be calibrated to produce a direct readout of Hb. A reference cyanmethaemoglobin solution is suitable for verifying the accuracy of instruments of this type.

Certain characteristics of pathological blood samples may lead to inaccuracy in a cyanmethaemoglobin estimation of Hb. The presence of sulphaemoglobin will lead to slight underestimation of total haemoglobin concentration: 150 g/l will be measured as 148 g/l if 5% of haemoglobin is present as sulphaemoglobin [3]. The slow conversion of carboxyhaemoglobin to methaemoglobin leads to overestimation of the Hb if the test is read at 3 minutes, since carboxyhaemoglobin absorbs more light at 540 nm than does cyanmethaemoglobin. The maximum possible error that could be caused if 20% of the haemoglobin were in the form of carboxyhaemoglobin, a degree of abnormality that may be found in heavy smokers, would be 6% [3].

Spectrophotometers and photometers are both sensitive to the effect of turbidity, which may be caused by a high WBC, high concentrations of lipids or plasma proteins, or non-lysed red cells. Increased turbidity causes a factitiously elevated estimate of Hb. When the WBC is high, turbidity effects are circumvented by centrifugation or filtration of the solution prior to reading the absorbance. When turbidity is due to a high level of plasma protein (either when a paraprotein is present or when there is polyclonal hypergammaglobulinaemia resulting from severe chronic infection or inflammation), it can be cleared by the addition of either potassium carbonate or a drop of 25% ammonia solution. When turbidity is due to hyperlipidaemia, a blank can be prepared from the diluent and the patient's plasma or the lipid can be removed by diethyl ether extraction and centrifugation. The target cells of liver disease or red cells containing haemoglobin S or C may fail to lyse in the diluent and, again, increased turbidity produces a factitiously high reading of Hb. Occasionally, this phenomenon is observed without any identifiable abnormality in the red cells to account for it. Making a 1:1 dilution in distilled water ensures complete lysis of osmotically resistant cells.

The cyanmethaemoglobin method was modified for application in automated instruments by the use of various lytic agents and by reading absorbance after a shorter time or at a different wavelength.

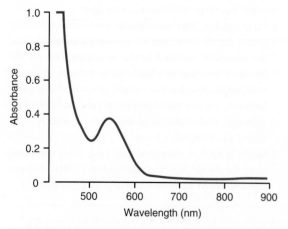

Fig. 2.1 Absorbance spectrum of cyanmethaemoglobin.

Other methods

Alternative methods of measuring Hb are not widely used except when they have been incorporated into haemoglobinometers. Such methods usually require standardisation by reference back to a cyanmethaemoglobin standard, but they otherwise avoid the use of cyanide, which is potentially toxic if released into the environment in large quantities.

Haemoglobin can be converted into a sulphated derivative with maximum absorbance at 534 nm by addition of sodium lauryl sulphate [4]. Conversion is almost instantaneous and methaemoglobin, but not sulphaemoglobin, is converted. This method correlates well with the reference method that is employed for calibration. This method is suitable for use with a spectrophotometer and has also been incorporated into several automated instruments.

Hb can also be measured following conversion to azidmethaemoglobin by the addition of sodium nitrate and sodium azide. This is the method employed by one portable haemoglobinometer (HemoCue, Clandon Scientific Ltd.), which employs measurements at two wavelengths, 570 and 880 nm, to permit compensation for turbidity. A modification of this instrument permits accurate measurements down to 0.1 g/l, so that it is also suitable for measurement of dilute solutions of haemoglobin, e.g. haemoglobin in fluid salvaged during surgery or haemoglobin in plasma or urine [5].

Hb can be measured as oxyhaemoglobin, in which case concentration of carboxyhaemoglobin, sulphaemoglobin and methaemoglobin will not be measured accurately. An artificial or secondary standard is needed. This method has been incorporated into directly reading haemoglobinometers, which are standardised to give the same result as a cyanmethaemoglobin method.

Hb can be measured as haematin produced under alkaline conditions. The alkaline–haematin method measures carboxyhaemoglobin, sulphaemoglobin and methaemoglobin, although it does not adequately measure haemoglobin F or haemoglobin Bart's, which are resistant to alkaline denaturation. An artificial standard is required. The acid–haematin method is less reliable and is not recommended.

Hb can be estimated without chemical conversion by measuring absorbance at 548.5 nm, at which wavelength deoxyhaemoglobin and oxyhaemoglobin both have the same optical density and that of carboxyhaemoglobin is not much less. Hb is calculated by comparison of absorbance with that of an artificial standard. Absorbance can also be integrated between 500 and 600 nm, the integral absorbance of oxyhaemoglobin, deoxyhaemoglobin and carboxyhaemoglobin being similar over this waveband.

New methods for the estimation of haemoglobin concentration have been introduced specifically for near-patient testing (see below).

Recommended units

The ICSH has recommended that Hb be expressed as g/l (mass concentration), or as mmol/l (molar concentration) in terms of concentration of the haemoglobin monomer. The conversion factor, if Hb is expressed in g/l, is 0.06206, i.e. an Hb of 120 g/l = 120 × 0.06206 mmol/l = 7.45 mmol/l. If Hb is expressed in molar concentration, then MCH and MCHC should also be expressed in this manner. An MCH of 27 pg is equivalent to 1.70 fmol. Similarly, an MCHC of 330 g/l (33 g/dl) is equivalent to 20 mmol/l. There are no clear practical advantages in expressing Hb as molar concentration and the potential for confusion and risk to patients if conversion to these units were to be attempted might be considerable. Laboratories in the great majority of countries express Hb as g/l or g/dl. This book will follow ICSH advice and use g/l.

Packed cell volume

The PCV is the proportion of a column of centrifuged blood that is occupied by red cells. Some of the measured column of red cells represents plasma that is trapped between red cells. The PCV is expressed as a decimal fraction representing l/l (litres/litre). The units may be stated or implied. The terms 'packed cell volume' and 'haematocrit' (Hct) were initially synonymous and were used interchangeably, but the ICSH has now recommended that PCV be reserved for estimates made by the traditional technique of centrifugation and Hct for estimates derived by other methods on automated instruments. The original method of measuring the PCV, as devised by Maxwell Wintrobe, required 1 ml of blood and prolonged (30 minutes to 1 hour) centrifugation in graduated glass tubes with a constant internal bore. This method, sometimes referred to as the macrohaematocrit, is the basis of the reference method [6], but for routine use it is cumbersome and slow. Since, for these reasons, it is no longer used in the diagnostic laboratory, it will not be discussed further. It has been replaced by the microhaematocrit, which has clinical usefulness by itself, can be combined with the Hb to derive an estimate of the MCHC, and can be used to calibrate automated counters.

Microhaematocrit

A small volume of blood is taken by capillarity into an ungraduated capillary tube (usually 75 mm long with an internal diameter of 1.2 mm), leaving about 15 mm unfilled. The end of the tube distant from the column of blood is sealed by heat, or by modelling clay or a similar product. It is then centrifuged for 5 or 10 minutes, at a high g value (for example 10 000–15 000 g) in a small, specially designed centrifuge, to separate the column of blood into red cells, buffy coat and plasma (Fig. 2.2). The PCV is read visually on a scale, the buffy coat of white cells and platelets being excluded from the measurement. The ICSH has published a selected method that employs 5 minutes' centrifugation [7]. A further 3 minutes' centrifugation is advisable if the sample is polycythaemic, in order to reduce the abnormal plasma trapping [8]. The microhaematocrit is usually measured on ethylenediaminetetra-acetic acid (EDTA)-anticoagulated venous blood, but it can also be performed on capillary blood if the sample is taken into a microhaematocrit tube, the interior of which is coated with heparin (2 iu). Plastic (polycarbonate) tubes are available and are safer than glass tubes.

A microhaematocrit can also be measured automatically by an instrument that is suitable for near-patient testing, which incorporates a centrifuge and an infrared analyser [9].

It should be noted that there are hazards associated with determining the microhaematocrit. Glass capillary tubes may break during insertion of modelling clay, leading to a penetrating injury and blood inoculation to the user. In one case human immunodeficiency virus (HIV) was transmitted and the house officer concerned subsequently developed the acquired immune deficiency syndrome (AIDS) [10,11]. Glass capillary tubes can also break during centrifugation, leading to a risk of injury and viral transmission [11].

The microhaematocrit has several sources of imprecision and inaccuracy. Because of the smallness of the tube, reading the level correctly can be difficult. Tubes may taper or be of an uneven bore. The seal is not flat, tending to be convex if modelling clay is used and concave if heat sealing is employed, although the error introduced by the type of seal is usually minor [12]. The amount of plasma trapping is usually around 1–3%, but is variable. It is less with longer periods of centrifugation and higher g values, but is also affected by other technical factors and by the characteristics of the blood sample (Table 2.1). It should be noted that in the USA blood is usually taken into K_3EDTA, and in the UK it is more usually taken into K_2EDTA; because of the cell shrinkage that occurs, the microhaematocrit with K_3EDTA is about 2% lower than with K_2EDTA [17]. The precision of the microhaematocrit can be improved by making at least three replicate measurements and taking the average; this is necessary when a manual PCV is used to calibrate an automated instrument. It has been recommended that, because of the increase in micro-haematocrit that occurs with deoxygenation, blood should be fully oxygenated when a microhaematocrit is used for calibration of an automated instrument [16].

Plasma trapping

Attempts have been made to make the microhaematocrit more accurate by 'correcting' the PCV for plasma trapping. A more accurate PCV means that an estimated MCV and MCHC are also more accurate. In experimental conditions this can be done by labelling plasma proteins with ^{131}I and determining the amount of radioactive isotope that is trapped in the red cell column. The correction may itself be inaccurate, since estimates of plasma trapping are lower when ^{131}I-labelled fibrinogen is used than when ^{131}I-labelled albumin is used [12]. Different studies have produced estimates varying from 1.3% to 3.2% for mean plasma trapping. Whether or not a plasma trapping correction is applied when calibrants for automated instruments are prepared will influence reference ranges for MCV, Hct and MCHC. The ICSH Committee on Cytometry reference method allows for the effect of plasma trapping

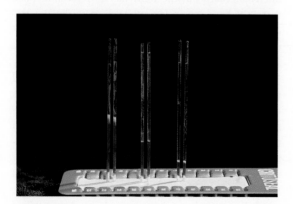

Fig. 2.2 Measurements of packed cell volume (PCV) by the microhaematocrit technique; paired tests from three patients are shown.

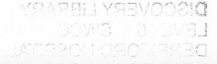

Table 2.1 Some factors affecting the microhaematocrit.

	Factors decreasing the microhaematocrit	Factors increasing the microhaematocrit
Consequent on dilution	Use of EDTA solution rather than dry EDTA (0.5% lower)	
Consequent on an alteration in the amount of trapped plasma	Longer period of centrifugation	Shorter period of centrifugation
	Increased centrifugal force (e.g. increased radius of centrifuge or increased speed of centrifugation)	Decreased centrifugal force
	Elevated ESR	Microcytosis (e.g. iron deficiency or thalassaemia trait)
		Sickle cell trait or sickle cell disease
		Spherocytosis
		Reduced flexibility of red cells on prolonged storage at room temperature
Consequent on red cell shrinkage	Excess EDTA [13,14]	
	K_3EDTA rather than K_2EDTA or Na_2EDTA [12] (about 2% lower)	K_2EDTA or Na_2EDTA
	Narrower tubes than recommended [15]	
	Soda lime tubes [15]	Borosilicate tubes
	Fully oxygenated blood [16]	Deoxygenated blood [16]

EDTA, ethylenediaminetetra-acetic acid; ESR, erythrocyte sedimentation rate

[18] (see below). One circumstance in which a plasma trapping correction is considered appropriate is when a microhaematocrit is being used for estimation of total red cell mass for the investigation of polycythaemia. Allowance should be made for the greater degree of plasma trapping of polycythaemic blood. It is suggested that if the PCV is less than 0.50 after centrifugation for 5 minutes, 2% correction should be applied; if it is greater than 0.50, a further 5 minutes' centrifugation should be carried out and the correction should be 3% [19].

Reference method
The ICSH reference method for the PCV [18] is based on determination of the Hb on whole blood and packed red cells, following centrifugation in a microhaematocrit centrifuge. The measurement on packed red cells is performed on cells obtained from the middle of the column of red cells where there is little trapping of plasma or white cell contamination. It therefore produces a measurement that does not include trapped plasma. The reference PCV is

$$\frac{\text{Standard whole blood haemoglobin concentration}}{\text{Packed red cell haemoglobin concentration}}$$

For blood with a normal haematocrit, a spun microhaematocrit is usually within 0.01 l/l of the reference PCV.

A 'surrogate reference method' using a microhaematocrit determined in borosilicate capillary tubes has also been proposed [20]. It also produces a measurement that is free of the effect of trapped plasma.

Other haematocrit methods
With automated instruments in current use, Hct is computed from the number and size of electrical impulses generated by red cells passing through a sensor (see below).

The red cell count
The red blood cell count (RBC), more usually referred to as the red cell count, was initially performed by counting red cells microscopically in a carefully diluted sample of blood contained in a counting chamber (haemocytometer) with chambers of known volume [21]. Although this method was capable of producing satisfactory results if great care was exercised, it proved very unreliable in routine use because of a high degree of imprecision, and it was also very time-consuming. For this reason the RBC and the variables derived from it were measured or calculated on only a minority of blood specimens.

More precise and therefore more clinically useful RBCs can be performed on single-channel semi-automated impedance counters, such as the Coulter Counter model ZM, which count cells in an accurately fixed and known volume of diluted blood as they pass through an aperture.

Although accurate setting of thresholds is needed, the instruments do not require calibration. The raw instrument cell counts produced are non-linear, with increasing cell concentration because of the greater likelihood of two cells passing through the aperture simultaneously (coincidence); depending on the instrument, coincidence correction may be an automatic function of the instrument or may be carried out by the user by reference to a table. White cells are also included in the RBC. Because red cells are normally at least 100-fold more numerous than white cells, the inaccuracy introduced by this is usually not great. RBCs determined on single-channel impedance counters are much more precise than those produced in counting chambers and they can also be produced with much less labour. They are therefore more clinically useful. They can be used with a manual Hb and PCV to calculate MCV and MCH, which are also much more precise than those derived from manual RBCs.

RBCs from single-channel semi-automated impedance counters can also be used to calibrate fully automated blood cell counters that count electrical impulses generated by red cells passing through a sensor. Automated instruments count of the order of 20 000–50 000 cells, so that the precision is again much greater than that of a haemocytometer count based on 500–1000 cells.

The reference method for the RBC employs a semi-automated single-channel aperture-impedance method, with accurate coincidence correction being achieved by extrapolation from counts on serial dilutions [22].

Derived red cell variables – red cell indices

Given the three measured variables (Hb, PCV/Hct and RBC), it is possible to derive the MCV, MCH and MCHC. When no plasma trapping correction is used, the MCV derived from a microhaematocrit will be an overestimate of the true value and the MCHC will be an underestimate. This is of no clinical consequence, since reference ranges will be derived in the same manner. The measured and derived variables that describe the characteristics of red cells are often referred to collectively as the red cell indices.

The white cell count

A manual white blood cell count (WBC), more usually referred to as a white cell count, is performed after diluting an aliquot of blood in a diluent that lyses red cells and stains the nuclei of the white cells [21]. White cells are counted microscopically in a haemocytometer with chambers of known volume. Nucleated red blood cells

(NRBC) cannot be readily distinguished from white cells in a counting chamber. If NRBC are present, their percentage can be counted on a stained blood film and the total nucleated cell count (TNCC) can be corrected. The manual WBC is imprecise, but this is of less practical importance than the imprecision of the RBC, since clinically important changes in WBC are usually of sufficient magnitude to be detected even with an imprecise method.

White cells can also be counted in diluted whole blood following red cell lysis, using a single-channel semi-automated impedance counter. In fully automated counters, white cells are counted by impedance technology or light scattering. Most automated counters are inadequate for counting very low numbers of white cells, e.g. for ensuring that units of blood products for transfusion have fewer than 5×10^6 white cells. In this circumstance, flow cytometry following staining of white cell nuclei with a deoxyribonucleic acid (DNA) stain is required [23].

The reference method for the WBC employs a semi-automated single-channel aperture-impedance method, with accurate coincidence correction being achieved by extrapolation from counts on serial dilutions [22]. The lower threshold is set between the noise produced by red cell stroma and the signals from leucocytes.

The platelet count

Platelets can be counted in a haemocytometer using either diluted whole blood (in which red cells can be either left intact or lysed) or platelet-rich plasma (prepared by sedimentation or centrifugation). If very large platelets are present, a whole-blood method is preferred to the use of platelet-rich plasma to avoid the risk of large heavy platelets being lost during preparative procedures. The use of platelet-rich plasma may be preferred if the platelet count is low. When the method leaves platelets intact, large platelets can be distinguished from small red cells by the platelet's shape, which may be oval rather than round, and by its irregular outline, with fine projections sometimes being visible. Use of ammonium oxalate, which lyses red cells, as a diluent produces a higher and more accurate count than use of formol-citrate, which leaves red cells intact [24]. Platelet counts are best performed on anticoagulated venous blood obtained by a clean venepuncture. Counts on blood obtained by finger-prick tend to be lower since some platelets adhere to endothelium of damaged vessels and aggregate, thus not being aspirated.

Platelets can be visualised in the counting chamber by light or phase-contrast microscopy. When using light microscopy, brilliant cresyl blue can be added to the diluent. This stains platelets light blue and facilitates their identification. On light microscopy, platelet identification is aided by their refractivity. It is easier to identify platelets by phase-contrast microscopy and such counts are therefore generally more precise.

Manual platelet counts are generally imprecise, particularly when the count is low. They are also very laborious, so that when this was the only technique available, counts were performed only when there was a clear clinical indication.

Platelets can be counted by semi-automated methods using impedance counters following the preparation of platelet-rich plasma. Coincidence correction and the use of two thresholds, to exclude both debris and contaminating red cells and white cells, are necessary. These techniques are also laborious and the several steps involved make them prone to error.

Laboratories with instrumentation suitable for an automated RBC but not an automated platelet count can estimate the platelet count indirectly by measuring the RBC and calculating the platelet count on the basis of the red cell:platelet ratio in a stained blood film.

However, the only satisfactory way to perform the number of platelet counts required by modern medical practice is with fully automated blood cell counters. Such instruments count platelets by either impedance, light-scattering or optical fluorescence technology. In a further refinement of the method, a fluorochrome-labelled monoclonal antibody to a platelet glycoprotein can be incorporated so that platelets are reliably distinguished from other small particles. Counts are generally precise, even at low levels, but unusual characteristics of the blood sample can cause inaccuracy (see Chapter 4). Manual haemocytometer counts or counting the red cell:platelet ratio in a blood film remain necessary in some patients with giant platelets, which, with many automated counters, cannot be distinguished from red cells.

Various proposals have been made for a reference method for the platelet count. The platelet count can be determined indirectly, using the reference method for the RBC and determining the red cell:platelet ratio on an automated instrument that is capable of distinguishing reliably between these two cell types. Alternatively, the platelet count can be determined by flow cytometry using a fluorochrome-labelled monoclonal antibody, such as CD41, CD42a or CD61, that binds specifically to platelets. Either a known amount of fluorescent beads can be used as a calibrant, or the ratio of red cells to fluorescent platelets can be determined and the platelet count can be calculated from a reference RBC [25–27]. The latter procedure is preferred, and is now the ICSH reference method [28], since dilution errors do not affect the count; a mixture of CD41 and CD61 directly-labelled antibodies is employed. It should be noted that, when there is an inherited platelet membrane defect with absence of one of the platelet glycoproteins, the relevant monoclonal antibody will not bind to platelets, hence the use of two antibodies. A similar flow cytometry technique has been recommended for routine platelet counts in severely thrombocytopenic patients, when an accurate platelet count is particularly important for determining whether or not a platelet transfusion is needed [29].

The differential white cell count

A differential white cell count is the assigning of leucocytes to their individual categories, this categorisation being expressed as a percentage or, when the WBC is available, as an absolute count. The ICSH recommends that the differential leucocyte count be expressed in absolute numbers [30] and this is strongly recommended. A differential count carried out by a human observer using a microscope is referred to as a manual differential count. It is usually performed on a wedge-spread film, the film being prepared either manually or with a mechanical film spreader. Automated differential counts are now generally performed by flow cytometry as part of a full blood count (FBC), differentiation between categories being based on the physical characteristics of the cells and sometimes on their biochemical characteristics. Depending on the specific automated analyser in use, a 'WBC' may be either a TNCC that also includes NRBC or, if the instrument is capable of recognising any NRBC present and excluding them from the total count, a true WBC. In the USA, the FBC is referred to as a complete blood count (CBC).

Cells that are normally present in the peripheral blood can be assigned to five or six categories, depending on whether non-segmented or band forms of neutrophils (see Chapter 3) are separated from segmented neutrophils or are counted with them. The differential count also includes any abnormal cells that may be present. NRBC can be included as a separate category in the differential count or, alternatively, their number can be expressed per 100 white cells. In the former case the uncorrected count is a TNCC rather than a WBC, and this is used for calculating absolute cell numbers. In the latter case, the TNCC is corrected to a WBC by subtracting the number of NRBC. Laboratories using automated instruments that produce a TNCC rather than a WBC should consistently follow one or other convention of expressing counts. It is probably better **not** to correct the TNCC to a WBC, but to calculate absolute counts from the TNCC and the percentage of each cell type, NRBC being included in the differential count. The advantage of this policy is that the TNCC is likely to be a precise measurement, whereas the ratio of NRBC to WBC, calculated by counting NRBC/100 WBC, is likely to be imprecise; it is better not to replace a precise measurement of the TNCC with an imprecise estimate of the WBC. However, the Clinical and Laboratory Standards Institute (CLSI) recommends that NRBC be expressed per 100 WBC [31]. Fortunately this problem is avoided by the most recent automated instruments, which can usually recognise and exclude NRBC from the WBC.

Differential white cell counts, like all laboratory tests, are subject to both inaccuracy and imprecision. Errors can be statistical in nature, distributional or interpretative. Manual differential counts are generally fairly accurate, but their precision is poor, whereas automated counts are generally fairly precise but are sometimes inaccurate.

Inaccuracy

With a manual differential count, inaccuracy or deviation from the true count results both from maldistribution and from misidentification of cells.

Maldistribution of cells

The different types of white cell are not distributed evenly over a slide. The tail of the film contains more neutrophils and fewer lymphocytes, whereas monocytes are fairly evenly distributed along the length of the film [32]. When large immature cells (blasts, promyelocytes and myelocytes) are present they are preferentially distributed at the edges of the film rather than in the centre and distally rather than proximally, in relation to lymphocytes, basophils, neutrophils and metamyelocytes [33]. The maldistribution of cells is aggravated if a film is too thin or if a spreader with a rough edge has been used. Various methods of tracking over a slide have been proposed to attempt to overcome errors due to maldistribution (Fig. 2.3). The method shown in Fig. 2.3a compensates for maldistribution between the body and the tail, but not for maldistribution between the centre and the edge, whereas the 'battlement' method shown in Fig. 2.3b tends to do the reverse, since the customary 100-cell differential count will not cover a very large proportion of the length of the blood film. A modified battlement track (Fig. 2.3c)

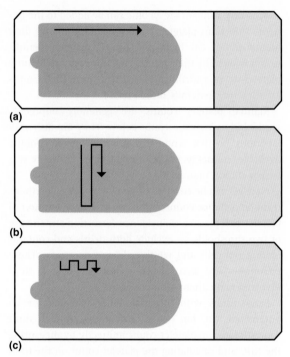

Fig. 2.3 Diagrams of blood films showing tracking patterns employed in a differential white blood cell count: (a) tracking along the length of the film; (b) battlement method; and (c) modified battlement method – two fields are counted close to the edge parallel to the edge of the film, then four fields at right angles, then two fields parallel to the edge and so on.

is a compromise between the two methods. In practice, the imprecision of a manual count is so great that a small degree of inaccuracy caused by maldistribution of cells is not of any great consequence. If there is white cell aggregation, the maldistribution of cells is so great that an accurate differential count is impossible.

Misidentification of cells and unidentifiable cells

Inaccuracy due to misidentification of cells is usually not great when differential counts are performed by experienced laboratory workers on high-quality blood films. An exception to this is the differentiation between band forms and segmented neutrophils. Criteria for making this distinction differ between laboratories, and there is also inconsistency in the application of the criteria within a laboratory because of an element of subjectivity. Occasionally it is also difficult to distinguish a monocyte from a large lymphocyte or a degranulated basophil from a neutrophil. Marked storage artefact renders a differential count very inaccurate; specifically, degenerating neutrophils may be misclassified as NRBC and preferential disintegration of neutrophils can cause a factitious elevation of the lymphocyte count. Inaccuracy can also be introduced into a count if many smear cells (see Chapter 3) are present and are not included in the count. If the smear cells are, for example, lymphocytes, then the percentage and absolute number of lymphocytes will be falsely low and the percentage and absolute number of all other cell types will be falsely high. Smear cells whose nature can be deduced can be counted with the category to which they belong. Otherwise smear cells and any other unidentifiable cells, if present in significant numbers, should be counted as a separate category or the percentage and absolute number of cells of all categories will be erroneous. In chronic lymphocytic leukaemia (CLL) it is possible to reduce the number of smear cells by adding one drop of albumin to four drops of blood before making the film.

Imprecision

The imprecision or lack of reproducibility of a count can be expressed as either the standard deviation (SD) or the coefficient of variation (CV) of replicate counts. The small number of cells conventionally counted in a manual differential count leads to poor precision [34]. When replicate counts are made of the percentage of cells of a given type among randomly distributed cells, the SD of the count is related to the square root of the number of cells counted. Specifically, the SD of the proportion of a given cell type, θ, is equal to [35]:

$$\sqrt{\frac{\Theta(1-\Theta)}{n}}$$

The 95% confidence limits of the proportion, i.e. the limits within which 95% of replicate counts would be expected to fall, are equal to θ ± 1.96 SD. The confidence limits of a given percentage of cells when 100 or more cells are counted are shown in Table 2.2. It will be seen that the confidence limits are wide. For example, the confidence limits of a 10% eosinophil count on a 100-cell differential count are 4–18%. The precision of the absolute count of any given cell count cannot be any better than the precision of the percentage but, if it is calculated from an automated WBC, which itself is quite a precise measurement, it is not a great deal worse. The imprecision of a manual differential count is greatest for those cells that are present in the smallest numbers, particularly the basophils. If it is diagnostically important to know whether or not there is basophilia, then it is necessary to improve precision by counting many more than the usual 100 cells (e.g. at least 200–500 cells). Similarly, if neutrophils constitute

Table 2.2 Ninety-five percent confidence limits of the observed percentage of cells when the total number of cells counted (n) varies from 100 to 10,000.*

Observed percentage of cells	Total number of cells counted (n)				
	100	200	500	1000	10 000
0	0–4	0–2	0–1	0–1	0–0.04
1	0–6	0–4	0–3	0–2	0.8–1.2
2	0–8	0–6	0–4	1–4	1.7–2.3
3	0–9	1–7	1–5	2–5	2.7–3.3
4	1–10	1–8	2–7	2–6	3.6–4.4
5	1–12	2–10	3–8	3–7	4.6–5.4
6	2–13	3–11	4–9	4–8	5.5–6.5
7	2–14	3–12	4–10	5–9	6.5–7.5
8	3–16	4–13	5–11	6–10	7.4–8.6
9	4–17	5–15	6–12	7–11	8.4–9.6
10	4–18	6–16	7–14	8–13	9.4–10.6
15	8–24	10–21	12–19	12–18	14.6–15.4
20	12–30	14–27	16–24	17–23	19.6–20.4
25	16–35	19–32	21–30	22–28	24.6–25.4
30	21–40	23–37	26–35	27–33	29.5–30.5
35	25–46	28–43	30–40	32–39	34.5–35.5
40	30–51	33–48	35–45	36–44	39.5–40.5
45	35–56	38–53	40–50	41–49	44.5–45.5
50	39–61	42–58	45–55	46–54	49.5–50.5

*Ranges for n = 100 to n = 1000 are derived from reference 34

only a small proportion of cells (e.g. in CLL), it is again necessary to count a larger number of cells to improve precision and determine whether there is neutropenia. Although the precision of a manual count could be improved by routinely counting more cells, it is not feasible in a diagnostic laboratory to routinely count more than 100 or, at the most, 200 cells. The poor precision of the count of cells present in the smallest numbers means that the reference limits for manual basophil and eosinophil counts include zero. It is therefore impossible, on the basis of a manual count, to say that a patient has basopenia or eosinopenia. It should also be noted that the precision of the band count is so poor that it is not generally very useful to count band cells separately from segmented neutrophils. A comment such as 'left shift' or 'increased band cells' can be made when such cells are clearly increased.

The CSLI has established a reference method for the differential count [31]. It uses a manually wedge-spread, Romanowsky-stained film. Two hundred cells are counted by each of two trained observers using a 'battlement' track (see Fig. 2.3b). The results are averaged to produce a 400-cell differential count, which is then divided by four.

The reticulocyte count

Reticulocytes are young red cells, newly released from the bone marrow, that still contain ribosomal ribonucleic acid (RNA). On exposure of unfixed cells to certain dyes, such as brilliant cresyl blue or 'new methylene blue', the ribosomes are precipitated and stained by the dye, to appear as a reticular network; as the cells are still living when exposed to the dye, this is referred to as supravital staining. With new methylene blue, red cells stain a pale greenish-blue while the reticulum stains bluish-purple.

The amount of reticulum in a reticulocyte varies from a large clump in the most immature cells (group I reticulocytes) to a few granules in the most mature forms (group IV reticulocytes) (Fig. 2.4). The difficulty in determining whether one or two dots of appropriately stained material represent RNA has led to various definitions of a reticulocyte being proposed. The minimum requirement varies from a single dot, through two or three dots to a minimum network. Since the majority of reticulocytes in the peripheral blood are group IV, the precise definition of a reticulocyte that is employed will have an appreciable effect on the reticulocyte count. The NCCLS (National Committee for Clinical Laboratory Standards, now the CLSI) classified as a reticulocyte 'any non-nucleated red cell containing two or more particles of blue-stained material corresponding to ribosomal RNA' [36]. This definition is also accepted by the ICSH [37].

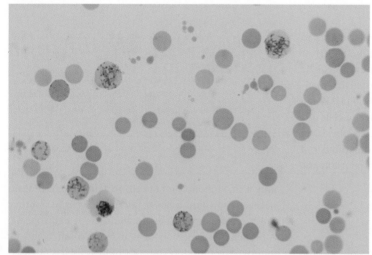

(a)

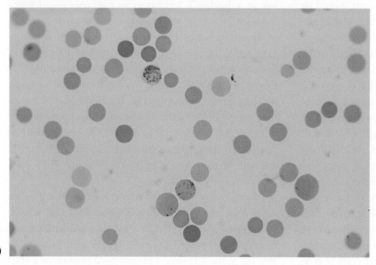

(b)

Fig. 2.4 Reticulocytes stained with new methylene blue. (a) A group I reticulocyte with a dense clump of reticulum, several group II reticulocytes with a wreath or network of reticulum and several group III reticulocytes with a disintegrated wreath of reticulum. (b) Group II, III and IV reticulocytes: the group IV reticulocyte has two granules of reticulum. There is also a cell with a single dot of reticulum. By some criteria this would also be classified as a reticulocyte. *Continued p. 27*

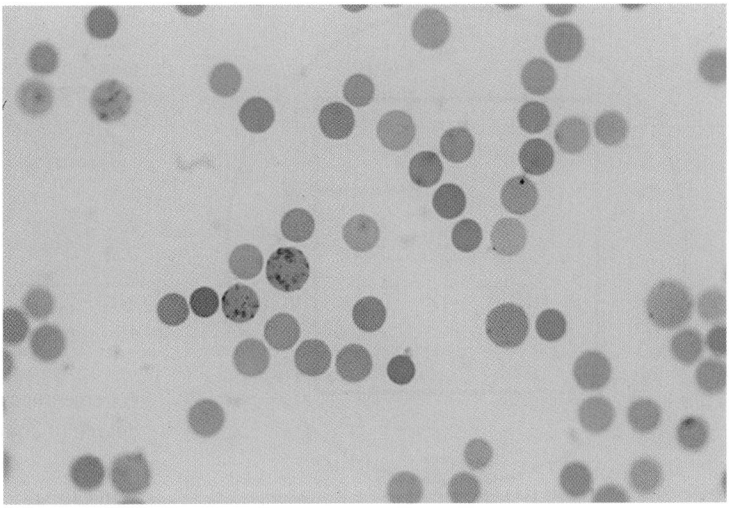

Fig. 2.4 *Continued* (c) Three reticulocytes and a Howell–Jolly body.

(c)

The RNA, which is responsible for forming the reticulum following supravital staining, gives rise, on Romanowsky-stained films, to diffuse cytoplasmic basophilia. The combination of cytoplasmic basophilia with the acidophilia of haemoglobin produces staining characteristics known as polychromasia. Not all reticulocytes contain enough RNA to cause polychromasia on a Romanowsky-stained film, but whether polychromatic cells correspond only to the least mature reticulocytes (equivalent to the group I reticulocytes) [38] or to all but the most mature reticulocytes (group I, II and III reticulocytes) [39] is not certain.

There are certain other inclusions that can be confused with the reticulum of reticulocytes. Methods of making the distinction are given in Table 2.3 and these other inclusions are discussed in more detail in Chapter 7. Cells containing Pappenheimer bodies, in particular, can sometimes be difficult to distinguish from late reticulocytes with only a few granules of reticulofilamentous material. If necessary, a reticulocyte preparation can be counterstained with a Perls stain to identify Pappenheimer bodies, or by a Romanowsky stain, to identify Howell–Jolly bodies. When a reticulocyte preparation is fixed in methanol and counterstained with a Romanowsky stain, the vital dye, e.g. the new methylene blue, is washed out during the methanol fixation. The reticulum is then stained by the basic component of the Romanowsky stain [40].

Reticulocytes are usually counted as a percentage of red blood cells. The use of an eyepiece containing a Miller ocular micrometer disc (Fig. 2.5) facilitates counting; reticulocytes are counted in the large squares and the total red cells in the small squares, which are

Table 2.3 The characteristic appearance of various red cell inclusions on a new methylene blue reticulocyte preparation.

Name	Nature	Appearance
Reticulum	Ribosomal RNA	Reticulofilamentous material or scanty small granules
Pappenheimer bodies	Iron-containing inclusions	One or more granules towards the periphery of the cell, may stain a deeper blue than reticulum, may be clustered
Heinz bodies	Denatured haemoglobin	Larger than Pappenheimer bodies, irregular in shape, usually attached to the cell membrane and may protrude through it, pale blue
Howell–Jolly bodies	DNA	Larger than Pappenheimer bodies, regular in shape, distant from the cell membrane, pale blue
Haemoglobin H inclusions	Denatured haemoglobin H	Usually do not form with the short incubation periods used for reticulocyte counts; if present they are multiple and spherical, giving a 'golf-ball' appearance; pale greenish-blue

DNA, deoxyribonucleic acid; RNA, ribonucleic acid

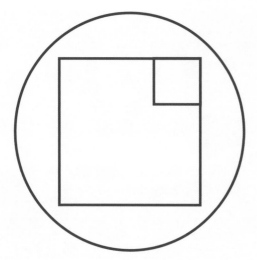

Fig. 2.5 The appearance of a Miller ocular micrometer for use in counting reticulocytes.

Table 2.4 The number of cells to be counted in the small square of a Miller graticule to achieve an acceptable degree of precision for the reticulocyte count.*

Reticulocyte count (%)	Approximate number of cells to be counted in small squares for CV of 10%	Equivalent to total count of
1–2	1000	9000
3–5	500	4500
6–10	200	1800
20–25	100	900

*From reference 37
CV, coefficient of variation

one ninth of the size of the large cells. If 20 fields are counted, the reticulocytes among about 2000 cells are counted and the reticulocyte percentage is equal to:

$$\frac{\text{Reticulocytes in 20 large squares} \times 100}{\text{Erythrocytes in 20 small squares} \times 9}$$

This method gives superior precision to counting the proportion of reticulocytes without an ocular insert [41]. Consecutive rather than random fields should be counted, since there is otherwise a tendency to subconsciously select fields with more reticulocytes [41]. It is also essential that the same principles of counting cells as are used in manual counting chamber counts are followed, i.e. the cells overlapping two of the four borders are not counted. Failure to follow this practice is thought to be the explanation of a bias towards lower counts that has been observed if a Miller disc is used [42]. The number of cells to be counted to achieve an acceptable degree of reproducibility increases as the percentage of reticulocytes falls. If a Miller graticule is used, the number of cells that should be counted to achieve a CV of about 10% is shown in Table 2.4 [37].

Reticulocyte counts have traditionally been expressed as a percentage. Since an RBC is generally available an absolute reticulocyte count, which gives a more accurate impression of bone marrow output, should be calculated. As an alternative, if an RBC is not available, a result that is more meaningful than

a percentage can be produced by correcting for the degree of anaemia as follows:

$$\text{Reticulocyte index} = \frac{\text{reticulocyte percentage} \times \text{observed Hct}}{\text{normal Hct}}$$

for example,

$$\text{Reticulocyte index} = \frac{1.2 \times 0.29}{0.45} = 0.77$$

This example shows that an apparently normal reticulocyte count can be demonstrated to be low if allowance is made for the presence of anaemia. This procedure and the use of an absolute reticulocyte count give similar information. A more complex correction [43] can be made that allows for the fact that in anaemic persons, under the influence of an increased concentration of erythropoietin, reticulocytes are released prematurely from the bone marrow and spend longer in the blood before becoming mature red cells. The reticulocyte index and the absolute reticulocyte count both give a somewhat false impression of bone marrow output in this circumstance. The reticulocyte production index [43] is calculated by dividing the reticulocyte index by the average maturation time of a reticulocyte in the peripheral blood at any degree of anaemia. Although the reticulocyte index and the reticulocyte production index have not found general acceptance, the concepts embodied in them should be borne in mind when reticulocyte counts are being interpreted.

Although the absolute reticulocyte count or one of the reticulocyte indices is to be preferred as an indicator of bone marrow output, the reticulocyte percentage has the advantage that it gives an indication of red cell lifespan. If a patient with a stable haemolytic anaemia has a reticulocyte count of 10%, it is apparent that 1 cell in 10 is no more than 1–3 days old.

Table 2.5 Units, abbreviations and symbols used for describing haematological variables.*

Variable	Abbreviation	Unit	Symbol
White blood cell count	WBC	number × 10^9/l	
Red blood cell count	RBC	number × 10^{12}/l	
Haemoglobin concentration	Hb	grams/litre **OR**	g/l, g/L†
		grams/decilitre **OR**	g/dl
		millimoles per litre	mmol/l
Haematocrit	Hct	litre/litre	l/l
Packed cell volume	PCV	litre/litre	l/l
Mean cell volume	MCV	femtolitre	fl
Mean cell haemoglobin	MCH	picograms **OR**	pg
		femtomoles	fm
Mean cell haemoglobin concentration	MCHC	grams/litre **OR**	g/l, g/L†
		grams/decilitre **OR**	g/dl
		millimoles per litre	mmol/l
Platelet count	Plt	number × 10^9/l	
Mean platelet volume	MPV	femtolitre	fl
Plateletcrit	Pct	litre/litre	l/l
Reticulocyte count	Retic	number × 10^9/l	
Erythrocyte sedimentation rate (Westergren, 1 hour)	ESR	millimitres, 1h	mm, 1h

*In addition, it should be noted that the approved abbreviation for 'international units' is iu (although IU is used for coagulation factors)
†g/L is preferred in the UK

The reticulocyte count is stable with storage of EDTA-anticoagulated blood at room temperature for up to 24 hours [44] and at 4°C for several days [37].

The CLSI reference method for the reticulocyte count is based on new methylene blue, with azure B being accepted as a suitable alternative [45].

Units and approved abbreviations

The ICSH has recommended standardised abbreviations for peripheral blood variables. These are shown together with the approved units of the Système International (SI) and their abbreviations in Table 2.5.

Automated image analysis

Pattern-recognition automated differential counters

CellaVision AB (Lund, Sweden) has produced pattern-recognition automated differential counters, the Diffmaster Octavia and its successor the CellaVision DM96, based on cell finding and microscopy of a May–Grünwald–Giemsa (MGG) or Wright–Giemsa stained blood film interpreted by a computer program employing neural networks [46,47]. Analysis of each slide takes about 5 minutes for the Octavia and about 3 minutes for the DM96. The identification of cells can be confirmed visually and, if necessary, altered. Images can be stored and used for review or teaching. The DM96 has been found to be faster than a trained laboratory scientist performing a routine differential count, with accuracy being similar [48]. The same company has also developed an image capture system that permits images to be captured in a small laboratory for transfer to a central laboratory on the same digital network; capture of images takes 17 minutes per 200 cells [49]. Information is available at www.cellavision.com.

Other pattern-recognition systems available include EasyCell assistant (Medica), HemaCam (Horn Imaging GmbH, Horiba medical) and HemoFAXS (TissueGnostics).

Automated blood cell counters

Principles of operation of automated haematology counters

The latest fully automated blood cell counters aspirate and dilute a blood sample and determine from 8 to more than 60 variables relating to red cells, white cells and platelets. Many counters are also capable of identifying a blood specimen (e.g. by bar-code reading), mixing it, transporting it to the sampling tube and checking it for adequacy of volume and absence of clots. Some are also linked to an automated film spreader. To avoid any unnecessary handling of blood specimens by instrument operators, sampling is usually by piercing a cap. Apart from the measurement of Hb, all variables depend on counting and sizing of particles, whether red cells, white cells or platelets, and some variables also require determining other characteristics of the particles. Particles can be counted and sized either by electrical impedance or by light scattering. Automated instruments have at least two channels. In one channel a diluent is added and red cells are counted and sized. In another channel a lytic agent is added, together with diluent, to reduce red cells to stroma, leaving the white cells intact for counting and also producing a solution in which Hb can be measured. Further channels are required for a differential WBC, which is often dependent on study of cells by a number of modalities, e.g. impedance technology with current of various frequencies, light scattering and light absorbance. A separate channel may be required for a reticulocyte count.

Automated instruments cannot recognise all the significant abnormalities that can be recognised by a human observer. They are therefore designed to produce accurate and precise blood counts on specimens that are either normal or show only numerical abnormalities or, with the most recent instruments, also contain NRBC; they are also designed to alert the instrument operator when the specimen has unusual characteristics that could either lead to an inaccurate measurement or require review of a blood film. This is often referred to as 'flagging'. Results should be flagged: (i) when the blood sample contains blast cells, granulocyte precursors (often referred to as immature granulocytes), NRBC or atypical lymphocytes; (ii) when there are giant or aggregated platelets or for any reason red cell and platelet populations cannot be separated; and (iii) when there is an abnormality likely to be associated with factitious results.

A new challenge to automated instruments is the production of accurate red cell indices, as well as total haemoglobin concentration, in patients who are infused with haemoglobin-based blood substitutes. This can be achieved with instruments, such as Siemens instruments, that measure size and haemoglobin concentration of individual red cells [50].

In the discussion of automated instruments, some instruments are included although they are no longer in general use because they demonstrate the principles of operation and illustrate the progressive improvement in technology that has occurred.

Beckman–Coulter instruments

Blood cells are extremely poor conductors of electricity. When a stream of cells in a conducting medium flows through a small aperture across which an electric current is applied (Fig. 2.6) there is a measurable increase in the electrical impedance across the aperture as each cell passes

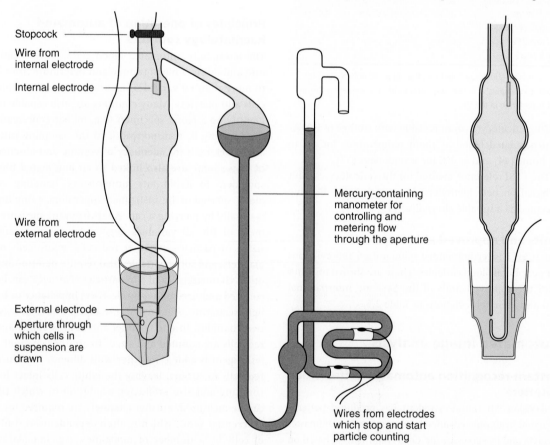

Stopcock
Wire from internal electrode
Internal electrode
Wire from external electrode
External electrode
Aperture through which cells in suspension are drawn
Mercury-containing manometer for controlling and metering flow through the aperture
Wires from electrodes which stop and start particle counting

Fig. 2.6 Semi-diagrammatic representation of part of Coulter Counter, model FN, showing the aperture tube and the manometer used for metering the volume of cell suspension counted. Right: diagrammatic representation of the cross-section of the aperture tube of an impedance counter.

through, this increase being proportional to the volume of conducting material displaced. The change in impedance is therefore proportional to the cell volume. Cells can thus be both counted and sized from the electrical impulses that they generate. This is the principle of impedance counting, which was devised and developed by Wallace Coulter in the late 1940s and 1950s and which ushered in the modern era of automated blood cell counting.

Aperture impedance is determined by capacitance and inductance as well as by resistance. Various factors apart from cell volume influence the amplitude, duration and form of the pulse, these being related to the disturbance of electrical lines of force as well as to the displacement of the conducting medium. Cell shape is relevant, as well as cell volume, so that cells of increased deformability, which can elongate in response to shear forces as they pass through the aperture, appear smaller than their actual size and rigid cells appear larger [51]. Furthermore, cells that pass through the aperture off centre produce aberrant impulses and appear larger than their actual size. Cells that recirculate through the edge of an electrical field produce an aberrant impulse, which is smaller than that produced by a similar cell passing through the aperture; a recirculating red cell can produce an impulse similar to that of a platelet passing through the aperture. Cells that pass through the aperture simultaneously, or almost so, are counted and sized as a single cell; the inaccuracy introduced requires correction, known as coincidence correction. Aberrant impulses can be edited out electronically. Sheathed flow or hydrodynamic focusing can direct cells to the centre of the aperture to reduce the problems caused both by coincidence and by aberrant impulses. Both sheathed flow and sweep flow behind an aperture can prevent recirculation of cells.

Impedance counters generally produce very precise measurements of cell volume and haemoglobin content and concentration. However, there are some inaccuracies inherent in the method, which are greater when cells are abnormal. The voltage pulse produced by a cell passing through the sensing zone can be regarded as the cell's electrical shadow, which suggests a particle of a certain size and shape. A normal red cell probably passes through the aperture in a fusiform or cigar shape [51], producing an electrical shadow similar to its actual volume, whereas a sphere produces an electrical shadow 1.5 times its actual volume [51]. A fixed rigid cell will appear larger than its actual volume. Furthermore, cell deformability is a function of haemoglobin

concentration within an individual cell. The effect of cell shape is not the same with all impedance counters. In one study the inaccuracy was greater with a Coulter STKR and a Cell-Dyn 3000 than with a Sysmex K-1000 and was not seen with a Sysmex NE-8000 [52].

Beckman–Coulter (previously Coulter) instruments initially measured Hb by a modified cyanmethaemoglobin method. For example, with the Coulter Counter S Plus IV, Hb was derived from the optical density at approximately 525 nm after a reaction time of 20–25 seconds. A cyanide-free reagent for Hb determination was subsequently introduced. Coulter instruments count and size red cells, white cells and platelets by impedance technology. Platelets and red cells are counted and sized in the same channel. The measurement of MCV and RBC allow the Hct to be derived, and the measurement of mean platelet volume (MPV) and the platelet count allow the derivation of an equivalent platelet variable, the plateletcrit (Pct). When the MPV is measured by impedance, it, and Pct, increase with storage of the blood. The MCH is derived from the Hb and the RBC. The MCHC is derived from the Hb, RBC and MCV. The variation in size of red cells is indicated by the red cell distribution width (RDW), which is the SD of individual measurements of red cell volume. The equivalent platelet variable is the platelet distribution width (PDW). There is often some overlap in size between small red cells and large platelets. Depending on the model of instrument, platelets and red cells may be separated from each other by a fixed threshold, e.g. at 20 fl, or by a moving threshold, or the data from counts between two thresholds, e.g. 2 and 20 fl, may be used to fit a curve, which is extrapolated so that platelets falling beyond these thresholds, e.g. between 0 and 70 fl, are also included in the count. White cells are counted in a separate channel, the Hb channel, following red cell lysis. With earlier instruments, NRBC present were mainly included in the 'WBC'. Histograms of volume distribution of white cells, red cells and platelets were provided (Fig. 2.7). A three-part differential count was based on impedance sizing following partial stripping of cytoplasm, the categories of white cell being granulocyte, lymphocyte and mononuclear cell.

Five-part differential Beckman–Coulter instruments including LH 750 and LH 780

The next generation of fully automated Coulter instruments – Coulter STKS, MAXM, HmX, Gen S, LH 750 and

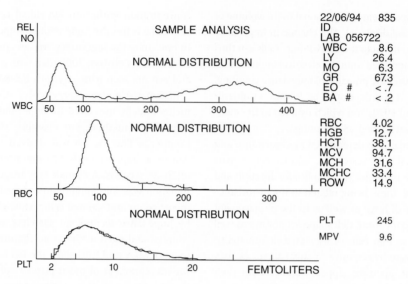

Fig. 2.7 Histograms produced by a Coulter S Plus IV automated counter showing volume distribution of white cells, red cells and platelets.

LH 780 – produce a five-part differential white cell count, which is based on various physical characteristics of white cells, following partial stripping of cytoplasm (Fig. 2.8 & Table 2.6). Three simultaneous measurements are made on each cell: (i) impedance measurements with low-frequency electromagnetic current, dependent mainly on cell volume; (ii) conductivity measurements with high-frequency (radiofrequency) electromagnetic current, which alters the bipolar lipid layer of the cell membrane allowing the current to penetrate the cells and is therefore dependent mainly on the internal structure of the cell, including nucleocytoplasmic ratio, nuclear density and granularity; (iii) forward light scattering at 10–70° when cells pass through a laser beam determined by the structure, shape and reflectivity of the cell. In later instruments (e.g. the Gen S, LH 750 and LH 780), the software permits further analysis of this data: conductivity measurements are corrected for the effect of cell volume so that they more accurately reflect internal cell structure and nucleocytoplasmic ratio – designated 'opacity'; light-scatter measurements are corrected for the effect of cell volume so that separation of different cell types is improved – designated 'rotated light scatter'. The abbreviation VCS (volume, conductivity, scatter) is used. Five cell populations are discriminated by three-dimensional cluster analysis based on cell volume, 'opacity' and rotated light scatter; clusters are separated by moving curvilinear thresholds. Clusters are represented graphically by plots of

cell volume against three discriminant functions derived from the data. Plots of size against discriminant function 1 (mainly derived from light scatter) separate cells into four clusters: neutrophils, eosinophils, monocytes and lymphocytes plus basophils (Fig. 2.8a). Basophils are located in the upper right-hand quadrant of the lymphocyte box. Plots of size against discriminant function 2 (mainly based on conductivity measurements with high-frequency electromagnetic current) separate cells into three clusters – lymphocytes, monocytes and granulocytes (Fig. 2.8b). A plot of size against discriminant function 3, obtained by gating out neutrophils and eosinophils, shows basophils as a cluster separate from lymphocytes and monocytes (Fig. 2.8c). In addition, there is a multicolour three-dimensional scatter plot.

In the case of the LH 750 and LH 780, precision is improved by counting white cells, red cells and platelets in triplicate and by extending the counting time if the WBC or platelet count is low. Particles greater than 35 fl after red cell lysis are counted as white cells. The instrument is able to count NRBC and corrects the WBC for NRBC interference [53]. Platelets are counted between 2 and 20 fl, but the curve is extrapolated to 70 fl to include large platelets. Reticulocytes can be counted in a separate mode (see below). A red cell variable, the mean sphered cell volume (MSCV), an artificial measurement in the reticulocyte channel, represents the average volume of sphered red cells in hypo-osmotic conditions [54]. Normally the MSCV is

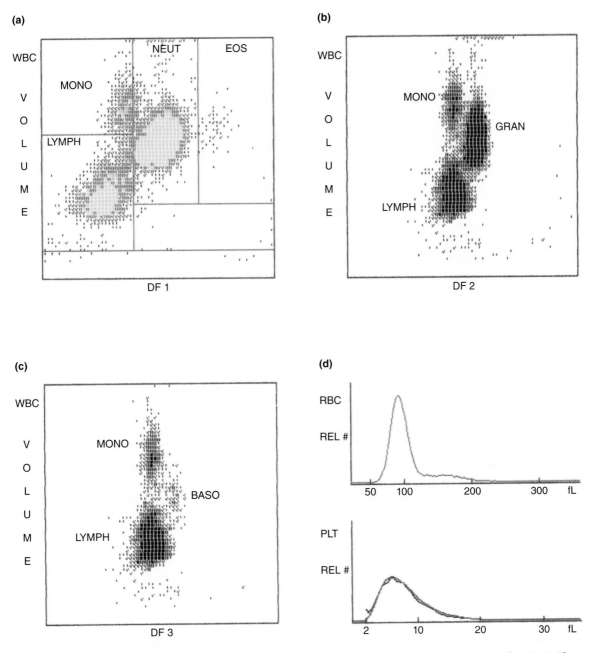

Fig. 2.8 Printouts of Coulter STKS automated counter. (a) Scatter plot of white cell volume against discriminant function 1. There are four white cell populations: NEUT, neutrophils; EOS, eosinophils; MONO, monocytes; and LYMPH, lymphocytes. (b) Scatter plots of white cell volume against discriminant function 2 showing three white cell populations: GRAN, neutrophils, eosinophils and basophils; MONO, monocytes; and LYMPH, lymphocytes. (c) Scatter plots of white cell volume against discriminant function 3 showing three white cell populations; BASO, basophils; MONO, monocytes; and LYMPH, lymphocytes. (d) Histogram showing size distribution of red cells and platelets.

Table 2.6 Technology employed in automated full blood counters performing 5–7-part differential counts.

Instrument	Technology
STKS, Gen S, LH 750, LH 780 and Unicel DxH800 (Beckman–Coulter)	(i) impedance with low frequency electromagnetic current (ii) conductivity with high frequency electromagnetic current (iii) laser light scattering
A^{c}T 5diff Analyzer (Beckman–Coulter)	(i) impedance measurements following differential lysis (ii) impedance technology and absorbance cytochemistry (after interaction with chlorazole black)
Sysmex SE-9000 (Sysmex Corporation)	(i) impedance with low frequency electromagnetic current (ii) impedance with high frequency electromagnetic current (iii) impedance with low frequency electromagnetic current at low and high pH
Sysmex XE-2100 (Sysmex Corporation)	(i) impedance with low frequency electromagnetic current (ii) impedance with radiofrequency electromagnetic current (iii) forward light scatter (iv) sideways light scatter (v) fluorescence intensity following interaction with a polymethine fluorescent dye
H.1 series, Advia 120 series (Bayer–Technicon, Siemens)	(i) light scattering following peroxidase reaction (ii) light absorbance following peroxidase reaction (iii) light scattering following stripping of cytoplasm from cells other than basophils by a lytic agent at low pH
Cell-Dyn 3500 (Abbott Diagnostics)	(i) forward light scatter (ii) narrow angle light scatter (iii) orthogonal light scatter (iv) polarised orthogonal light scatter
Cell-Dyn 4000 (Abbott Diagnostics)	As above plus (v) NRBC count following binding to fluorescent dye
ABX ABX Pentra 120Retic (Horiba ABX Diagnostics)	(i) impedance (ii) light absorbance following staining of granules with chlorazole black E (iii) impedance following preferential stripping of cytoplasm from basophils at low pH

greater than the MCV (of non-sphered cells) and an inversion of this relationship suggests the presence of spherocytosis or a similar abnormality of shape [54]. The MSCV has been noted to fall in athletes during training, correlating with evidence of haemolysis [55]. A red cell variable, designated low haemoglobin density (LHD), is produced by mathematical transformation of the MCHC; it has been found to correlate with the %Hypo on Siemens instruments (see below) and is a useful indicator of reduced iron availability, e.g. in patients with chronic kidney disease receiving erythropoietin [56]. A further calculated variable is the microcytic anaemia factor, Maf, (Hb × MCV)/100, which has been used for screening for iron depletion and iron-deficient erythropoiesis in athletes [57]. The LH750 has four flags for possible blast cells – NEBlast, LYBlast, MOBlast and VARIANT LY; these have been found to be collectively less sensitive (but more specific) than the four blast flags on Siemens ADVIA systems [58]. The Coulter Gen S, LH 750 and LH 780 VCS differential white cell data can be used as a flag for samples that are likely to contain malaria parasites [59,60]. An LH 750 statistical function

based on VCS lymphocyte data and platelet count can also be used as a flag for dengue fever [60].

In patients with acute leukaemia or suspected disseminated intravascular coagulation, the LH 750 platelet count shows a good correlation with the international reference method, but with the slope against the reference method indicating underestimation [61]. The MPV may be inaccurate (LH 750) in the presence of very large platelets as they are not recognised and are excluded from the measurement [62].

For the LH 750, the mean neutrophil volume (MNV), neutrophil distribution width (NDW), mean lymphocyte volume (MLV) and lymphocyte distribution width (LDW) can also be estimated from the VCS measurements. The MNV was found, in one study, to be superior to the WBC and the neutrophil percentage in the detection of sepsis in adults [63]. In a second study, MNV and NDW had better sensitivity and specificity than a manual band count, absolute neutrophil count and C-reactive protein (CRP) in the recognition of infection [64]. A further study found that MNV and mean monocyte volume (MMV) correlated with sepsis; these variables were less informative than interleukin 6 concentration, but showed similar sensitivity and specificity to CRP [65]. In a study in intensive care ward patients, NDW was found to discriminate patients with infection from those with acute inflammation and in this regard was superior to CRP and procalcitonin; all three variables could distinguish between localised and systemic infections [66]. In postoperative patients, an increased MNV and NDW were found in patients with infection in comparison with those without infection [67]. Children and adolescents with bacterial sepsis were found to have an increased NDW and LDW [68]. Similarly, using the LH 780, the MNV and NDW were found to be useful in the diagnosis of neonatal sepsis [69]. In a second study using the LH 750 and LH 755, MNV and CRP were found to be the most useful measurements in the diagnosis of neonatal sepsis [70].

Abnormalities in the measurements of mean neutrophil conductivity and mean neutrophil scatter on the LH 750, indicative of hypogranularity, can provide evidence of granulocytic dysplasia [71]. MNV may also be reduced [72].

The LH 750 and LH 780 incorporate a red cell size factor (RSf), which is based on the size of mature red cells and reticulocytes, using the formula $\sqrt{MCV^*MRV}$, i.e. the square root of the product of the MCV and the mean reticulocyte volume (MRV) [73]. Values correlate with the Ret-He of Sysmex instruments; they are low in iron deficiency and thalassaemia trait and are likely to fall when there is development of functional iron deficiency, e.g. in patients receiving erythropoietin therapy [73]. The LH 780 %LDH has been found to distinguish iron deficiency and anaemia of chronic disease with iron deficiency from iron-replete anaemia of chronic disease [74].

A curious blood film artefact has been reported with the LH 750 when avian red cells from a multiply punctured tube of reticulocyte control material were carried over to a subsequent patient sample, which was then used to make a film [75].

Beckman–Coulter Unicel DxH 800

The Beckman–Coulter Unicel DxH 800 provides an FBC, a 5-part differential count, a count of NRBC and a reticulocyte count. The differential count, including NRBC and 'immature granulocytes', is based on impedance (volume) and radiofrequency (conductivity) measurements plus five light-scatter measurements, this representing a further development of the VCS technology of earlier instruments (Fig. 2.9). Mean volume, variation in volume and other morphology-based information is produced for all

subpopulations, these measurements being collectively referred to as the 'cell population data' (CPD). The Hb is corrected when the uncorrected WBC (UWBC) is $11 \times 10^9/l$ or higher and the RBC is corrected when the UWBC is $140 \times 10^9/l$ or higher [76]. MCV, RDW and the RDW standard deviation (RDWSD) are corrected when the UWBC is $140 \times 10^9/l$ and there is evidence that white cells are interfering with the red cell histograms. The platelet count is based on measurements between 2 fl and 25 fl with a fitted curve to exclude red cell fragments. Platelet flags indicate the probability of giant platelets, platelet aggregates and interference at the lower or upper thresholds.

The flags on the DxH 800 have been assessed as more sensitive and more specific than those of the LH 750, with flagging of samples also being less common [77]. The DxH 800 shows superior sensitivity to blast cells to the LH 750 [78] and superior sensitivity and accuracy to the LH 780 in detecting and counting NRBC [76]. The DxH 800 has been found to be more accurate than the LH 780 in enumerating NRBC in adults [79] and more accurate than the Cell-Dyn Sapphire for enumerating NRBC in neonatal and paediatric samples [80]. It was found superior to the LH 750 and the Advia 2120 for the identification of NRBC in neonatal samples [81]. Findings in patients with sepsis are similar to those for the LH 750 and LH 780; MNV, NDW, MMV and monocyte distribution with (MDW) are increased, while most neutrophil light scatter measurements are reduced [82]. Cell population data for neutrophils and monocytes permit prediction of haemopoietic stem cell engraftment several days earlier than the absolute neutrophil count [83].

The DxH 800 has approximately 100% sensitivity and specificity in the detection of *P. vivax* malaria parasites, an abnormal signal being seen in the NRBC plot [84].

HematoFlow platform

The Beckman–Coulter Hematoflow platform virtually integrates a DxH 800 automated instrument and an FC500 flow cytometer using middleware to provide an FBC and a 16-part differential count [85,86]. The FC500 uses six directly labelled monoclonal antibodies (CD2, CD16, CD19, CD36, CD45 and CD294) in a five-colour single reagent, CytoDiff [85,86]. As an antibody-based platform, the Hematoflow system cannot count monocytes in patients with a congenital CD36 deficiency. Similarly, CD16-negative type III neutrophils in patients with paroxysmal nocturnal haemoglobinuria will not be recognised and will be categorised as immature granulocytes [87]. There is generally good agreement between

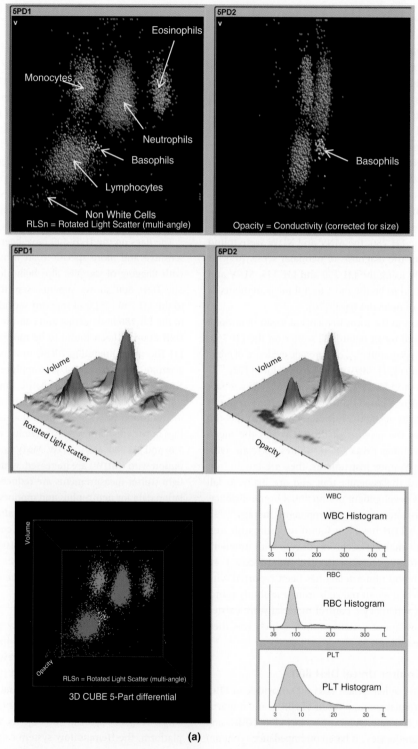

(a)

Fig. 2.9 Printouts from Beckman–Coulter DxH 800. (a) Scatter plots from the differential channel, five-part differential 1 (5PD1) and five-part differential 2 (5PD2), showing a plot of volume (v) against multi-angle rotated light scatter (RLSn) (left) and volume against opacity (right); in the corresponding three-dimensional representations (centre) the heights of the peaks reflect cell numbers; a composite three-dimensional plot (bottom left) can be rotated using a mouse to demonstrate different populations; histograms (bottom right)show the size of white blood cells (WBC), red blood cells (RBC) and platelets (PLT) in their respective channels; *Continued p. 37*

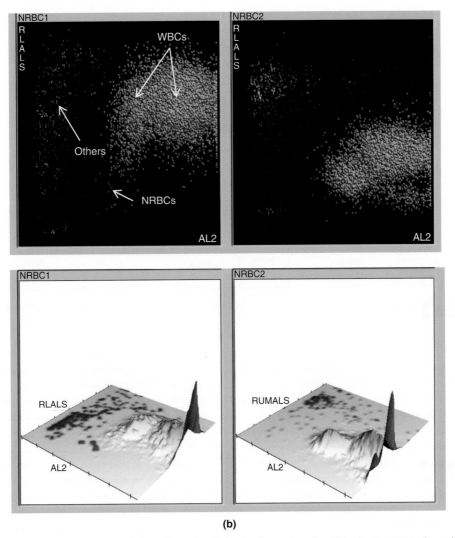

Fig. 2.9 *continued* (b) Two-dimensional and three-dimensional plots in the nucleated red blood cell (NRBC) channel showing the separation of NRBC from leucocytes; two light scatter measurements, RLAS (NRBC1, left) and RUMALS (NRBC2, right) are plotted against axial light loss (AL2), which measures the light absorbed as the cell passes through the flow cell (an indicator of cell size but also influenced by cellular transparency). By courtesy of Beckman–Coulter.

the differential counts of the XE-2100 and DxH 800, with the exception of basophil counts [86]. There are occasional instances of overestimation of monocytes and factitious basophilia has been observed in a patient in whom some lymphocytes were classified as basophils [86]. In one study, blast cells of acute myeloid leukaemia (AML) and B-lineage acute lymphoblastic leukaemia (ALL) were identified, but not blast cells of T-lineage ALL [85]. Others have found the system to be very sensitive for the detection of blast cells [87]. Much of

the published work required manual gating techniques and the recent introduction of a fully automated gating algorithm may have improved the quality of results.

A^{c}T 5diff counter

Another instrument marketed by Beckman–Coulter, the A^{c}T 5diff counter, performs a five-part differential count by means of measurements in two channels (Fig. 2.10 & Table 2.6). The WBC and the basophil count are determined by impedance measurements following differential

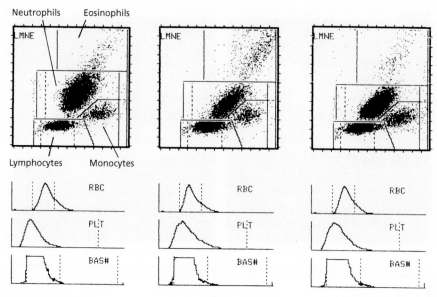

Fig. 2.10 Scatterplot and histograms produced by Beckman–Coulter A^{c}T 5diff counter: (a) normal; (b) sample with eosinophilia; (c) sample with monocytosis.

lysis, basophils being more resistant to stripping of cytoplasm in acid conditions. Other cell types are determined in a second channel using a combination of measurements of volume (by impedance technology) and absorbance cytochemistry (after interaction with chlorazole black). Chlorazole black binds to the granules of eosinophils (most strongly), neutrophils (intermediate) and monocytes (least strongly); lymphocytes are unstained. The principles underlying the differential count on this instrument have much in common with those employed in Siemens instruments (see below) and the technology employed is similar to that on certain Horiba instruments (see below). The instrument has a very small sample volume requirement, so is suitable for use with paediatric samples.

Information on Beckman–Coulter instruments is available on a company website, www.beckman.com.

Sysmex and other instruments incorporating impedance measurements

After the expiry of the initial patent of Coulter Electronics, impedance counters were introduced by a number of other manufacturers, among whom Sysmex Corporation is prominent. These instruments operate according to similar principles to those of Coulter instruments. Some instruments integrate the pulse heights from the red cell channel to produce Hct and derive the MCV from the RBC and Hct, while others do the reverse. Variables

measured are similar to those of Coulter analysers, often including a three-part or, with added technology, five- or six-part differential count. Platelets may be separated from red cells by fixed thresholds or moving thresholds and sometimes a platelet histogram is extrapolated beyond a threshold. The RDW on most instruments represents the SD of cell size measurements. Sysmex instruments give the option of CV as an index of RDW. Most impedance counters initially measured Hb by a modified cyanmethaemoglobin method, but this has now been largely replaced by cyanide-free methodology. For example, Sysmex instruments use a lauryl sulphate method.

Sysmex SE-9000

The Sysmex SE-9000 and later instruments have an Hb channel that is separate from the WBC channel. This permits the use of a strong lytic agent so that high WBCs are unlikely to interfere with Hb estimates. There are moving thresholds for both red cells and platelets, which are counted by impedance technology. As with earlier instruments, histograms of red cell, white cell and platelet volume distribution are provided (Fig. 2.11a). The MCV on this and certain other Sysmex instruments (K-1000 and NE-8000) has been noted to increase on deoxygenation and decrease on oxygenation [16]. The MCHC shows inverse changes. It is likely that the same effect would be observed with other automated counters, since the same phenomenon is observed with a microhaematocrit. The NE-8000 does not show the same inaccuracy in MCV and MCHC estimates with hypochromic cells as is seen with the Coulter STKR; for the K-1000, inaccuracy is intermediate [52].

The SE-9000 produces a five-part differential count by combining data from three channels (see Table 2.6). In the granulocyte–lymphocyte–monocyte channel leucocytes are separated from red cell ghosts and platelet clumps and are divided into three major clusters (Fig. 2.11b)

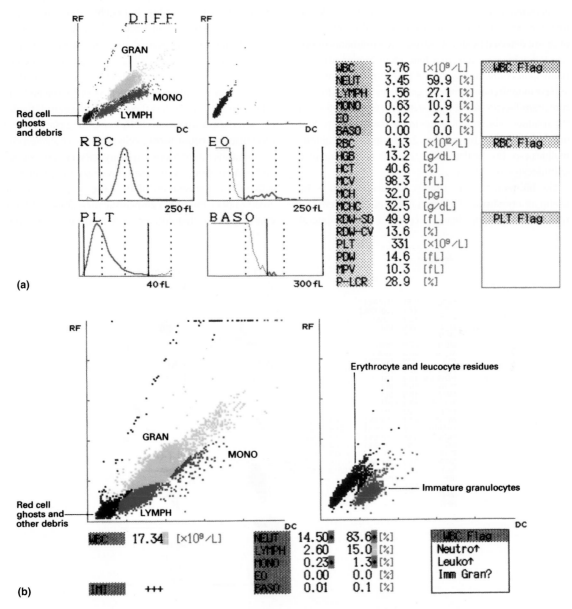

Fig. 2.11 Graphic output of Sysmex SE-9000 automated haematology analyser. (a) White cell scatter plots and red cell, platelet, eosinophil and basophil volume histograms on a normal sample. (b) White cell scatter plots – radiofrequency (RF) against direct current (DC) – of an abnormal sample with an increase of immature granulocytes. White cell populations shown are: GRAN, granulocytes; LYMPH, lymphocytes; MONO, monocytes (left); and immature granulocytes in a separate cluster from erythrocytes and residues of other leucocytes (right).

by a plot of radio-frequency capacitance measurements against direct current impedance measurements. Radio-frequency measurements depend on internal cellular structure – nucleocytoplasmic ratio, chromatin structure and cytoplasmic granularity – while direct current measurements depend on cell size. Eosinophils are detected by direct current measurements of cell size following exposure to a lytic agent at alkaline pH. Basophils are detected by direct current measurements of cell size following exposure to a lytic agent at acid pH. The neutrophil count is determined by subtracting basophil and eosinophil counts from the granulocyte count. Immature granulocytes can be separated from erythrocytes and the residues of other leucocytes in the immature myeloid information (IMI) channel (Fig. 2.11b, right). Any abnormalities can thus be flagged as: '? left shift', '? immature granulocytes' or '? Blasts'.

The immature myeloid index has been found to be useful as a predictor of a rise in CD34-positive stem cell numbers in patients being prepared for a peripheral blood stem cell harvest, and can serve as a trigger to start monitoring the number of CD34-positive cells [88].

Sysmex XE-2100

The Sysmex XE-2100 [89], introduced in 1999, incorporates fluorescence flow cytometry into a multichannel instrument that also utilises laser light, direct current (for impedance measurements) and radiofrequency current (for determining the internal structure of a cell) to perform a differential count (Fig. 2.12). A polymethine fluorescent dye combines with nucleic acids (nuclear DNA and RNA in cytoplasmic organelles) of 'permeabilised' cells. This instrument has the capacity to count reticulocytes, recognise and count RNA-containing platelets and recognise and count NRBC, cells with the characteristics of immature granulocytes (promyelocytes, myelocytes and metamyelocytes, IG) and haemopoietic progenitor cells (HPC). Recognition of the latter depends on the greater lipid content of cytoplasmic membranes of more mature cells, so that differential lysis can be used to lyse

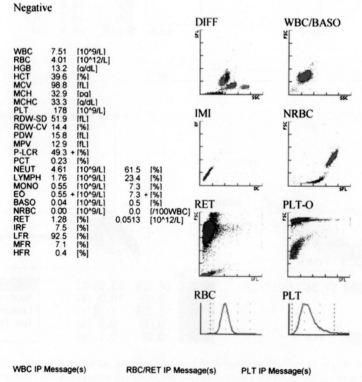

Fig. 2.12 Scatter plots and histograms of the Sysmex XE-2100 showing the leucocyte clusters (DIFF), the white cell count/basophil channel (WBC/BASO), immature granulocytes (IMI), nucleated red cell (NRBC), the reticulocyte channel (RET), the optical (fluorescent) platelet count (PLT-O) and red cell and platelet histograms (RBC and PLT).

mature cells and leave haemopoietic progenitor cells less damaged. Blast cells can be differentiated from less immature cells (Fig. 2.13). The XE-2100 can operate in CBC/DIFF mode, in which TNCC are counted and the presence of NRBC is flagged, or in NRBC mode, in which NRBC are counted and the WBC is computed by subtraction of NRBC from TNCC. This instrument also has the capacity to determine a platelet count by both impedance technology and an optical method, following interaction with a fluorescent dye – the latter in the reticulocyte channel. At low counts the optical-fluorescence platelet count is usually more accurate [90], whereas at high counts the linearity of the impedance count is better. Which count is more accurate when the count is low depends on the cause of the thrombocytopenia. Patients on chemotherapy may have WBC fragments,

leading to the optical count being an overestimate of the platelet count, whereas in patients with low platelet counts and large platelets, e.g. due to autoimmune thrombocytopenic purpura or thrombotic thrombocytopenic purpura, the optical count is generally more accurate. The instrument has a switching algorithm to select the most accurate platelet count and this should not be over-ridden [91]. In patients with acute leukaemia or suspected disseminated intravascular coagulation, platelet counts by the two methods show a good correlation with the international reference method, but the slope of the regression line indicates underestimation of the count [61]; erroneous counts are more likely when there is platelet activation. Inaccurate impedance counts can occur in the presence of red cell fragments or giant platelets. Inaccurate optical/fluorescence counts

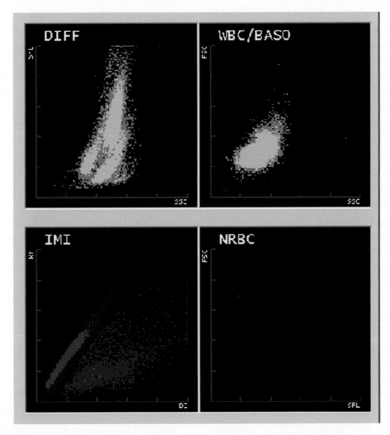

Fig. 2.13 Scatter plots of the Sysmex XE-2100 on a blood sample from a patient with acute myeloid leukaemia showing the leucocyte clusters (DIFF), the white cell count/basophil channel (WBC/BASO), immature myeloid information (IMI) and nucleated red cell (NRBC) scatter plots. The WBC was 38.2×10^9/l with flags for suspected blast cells and suspected immature granulocytes. The IMI scatter plot shows an abnormal population of blast cells and granulocyte precursors (red) and another population that represents mature granulocytes and the ghosts or erythrocytes (blue).

can occur when white cell fragments are present, e.g. in leukaemia. The immature platelet fraction (IPF) has been found to be increased in conditions of increased platelet turnover, e.g. autoimmune thrombocytopenic purpura, thrombotic thrombocytopenic purpura and pregnancy-associated hypertension [92]. The IPF is also predictive of recovery of bone marrow function following stem cell transplantation. In a specific geographical setting, pseudobasophilia plus thrombocytopenia was found to be highly predictive of dengue fever [93].

The XE-2100 is a multichannel instrument, the channels being as follows.

1 A haemoglobin channel using a strong lytic agent and a cyanide-free reagent (lauryl sulphate) for the measurement of Hb.
2 A red cell/platelet channel in which red cells and platelets are counted and sized by impedance technology, following hydrodynamic focusing; in addition to the usual red cell variables, mean platelet size, platelet distribution width (the width of the platelet size histogram at 20% of the peak height) and the percentage of large platelets (platelet large cell ratio, P-LCR, platelets larger than 12 fl expressed as a percentage) are provided. An increased percentage of large platelets has been observed in patients with hyperlipidaemia and this has been suggested as a possible risk factor for thrombosis [94]. An increase in MPV, PDW and P-LCR has been observed in autoimmune thrombocytopenic purpura in comparison with aplastic anaemia [95]. The MPV may be inaccurate, with impedance measurements, in the presence of very large platelets as they are excluded from the measurement [62]. Red cell variables include RBC-Y, which is the mean value of forward light scatter and is proportional to the haemoglobin content of red cells. Values tend to parallel the MCH.
3 A white cell differential channel in which neutrophils plus basophils, eosinophils, lymphocytes and monocytes are differentiated from each other, by cluster analysis, following interaction with a polymethine-based fluorescent dye; measurements made are of side light scatter (NEUT-X, indicative of the internal structure of cells), forward light scatter (indicative of cell size) and fluorescence intensity (NEUT-Y, indicative of DNA and RNA content and thus indicating the size of the nucleus). Immature granulocytes (promyelocytes, myelocytes and metamyelocytes) are counted in this channel. An increased percentage of immature

granulocytes has been found predictive of infection; however, although more predictive than the WBC, it was no better than the absolute neutrophil count [96]. NEUT-X is increased postpartum, in infection, following granulocyte colony-stimulating factor (G-CSF) therapy and in other circumstances when neutrophils appear hypergranular [97]. It is also increased in megaloblastic anaemia [98]. It may be decreased in myelodysplastic syndromes (MDS) and chronic myelomonocytic leukaemia (CMML), correlating with the microscopic observation of hypogranularity [97,98]. NEUT-Y is increased postpartum and may be decreased in MDS and CMML [97]. In one study scatter plots were sometimes abnormal in *P. vivax* malaria and, less often, in *P. falciparum* malaria, with cases showing pseudoeosinophilia [99]. In another study, abnormal scatter plots were found in *P. vivax, P. ovale* and *P. malariae* infection, but not in *P. falciparum* infection [100]. In patients with CLL, the automated lymphocyte count has been found to be reliable when compared with a manual count on albuminised blood films, and can thus replace the routine manual count [101]. The absolute neutrophil count has been found to be accurate and precise, even at low levels [102].

4 A white cell/basophil channel in which all cells except basophils are lysed so that basophils can be differentiated from other leucocytes by cluster analysis, using forward light scatter and side light scatter. In one study the basophil count showed poor correlation with flow cytometric counts with a correlation coefficient of 0.64, improving to 0.90 if samples with flags for abnormal white cells were excluded [103]. Pseudobasophilia was seen in 5/112 specimens [103].
5 An NRBC channel in which NRBC are differentiated from white cells and from red cell ghosts by cluster analysis based on fluorescence intensity and forward light scatter, following lysis of NRBC and interaction of cells with a fluorescent dye. NRBC are less fluorescent and scatter less light than leucocytes. Persisting NRBC in the peripheral blood following stem cell transplantation have been found to correlate with a significantly worse prognosis [104].
6 An IMI channel in which granulocyte precursors and putative HPC can be differentiated from mature leucocytes by cluster analysis based on impedance and radiofrequency current analysis following differential lysis. The absolute count of HPC has been found to be a clinically useful measurement for determining the

optimal timing for harvesting peripheral blood stem cells. Since the HPC count is quick and economical, it can be used to predict when it is worthwhile performing the more slow and expensive measurement of CD34-positive cells [105]. It should be noted that delay in performing the analysis leads to an appreciable decline in the count, e.g. 50% by three hours [106]. Flags for abnormal cells are produced by integrating information from the white cell differential channel and the IMI channel.

7 A reticulocyte channel (used only when the instrument is run in reticulocyte mode) in which platelets are also enumerated optically with an immature platelet count ('reticulated platelets') being determined by a fluorescence/optical method (see above); the fluorescent dye is a proprietary mixture of polymethine and oxazine. The reticulocyte channel can also be used to enumerate and monitor red cell fragments, by recognition of particles smaller than red cells with an RNA content less than that of a platelet, in patients with microangiopathic haemolytic anaemia [107,108]; there is a good correlation with microscopic counts [107]. Counts of red cell fragments should be done promptly as the count rises with storage [107]. The normal range for red cell fragments is less than 0.5%, with a value of less than 1% having a high negative predictive value [108]. This channel also measures reticulocyte haemoglobin content equivalent, Ret-He (estimated from forward light scatter, RET-Y), which is reduced with the onset of functional iron deficiency and responds rapidly to iron replacement. It also falls rapidly in patients hospitalised with pneumonia, representing an early sign of impaired haemoglobin synthesis resulting from inflammation [109]. The Ret-He, produced by transformation of the RET-Y and expressed in pg, gives similar information to Siemens instruments CHr in early iron deficiency and iron-restricted erythropoiesis, such as functional iron deficiency in a haemodialysis patient receiving erythropoietin [110,111]. It has been incorporated into an algorithm for the diagnosis of microcytic anaemias [112]. For further general information on the reticulocyte count, see above.

The 'reticulated platelet' count, the IPF, reflects thrombopoietic activity, correlating inversely with the platelet count in autoimmune thrombocytopenic purpura and being low in aplastic anaemia. An increase in the IPF% is predictive of bone marrow recovery following chemotherapy [113]. The IPF% is increased in liver disease; however, the IPF expressed as an absolute count is reduced in cirrhosis of the liver in comparison with values both in individuals without liver disease and in patients with fatty liver or chronic cirrhosis, indicating impairment of platelet production [114]. The IPF may be inappropriately increased in MDS [115].

Sysmex XE-2100D

The XE-2100D differs from the XE-2100 in not having channels for NRBC, reticulocytes and IMI. It thus provides an FBC and 5-part differential count only.

The MPV is method dependent; the XE-2100D gives significantly higher mean values for normal subjects than the Coulter LH 750, which in turn gives higher values than the Advia 2120; similar differences are seen with patient specimens [62].

Sysmex XE-5000

The Sysmex XE-5000, introduced in 2007, is the successor to the XE-2100. The additional functions, in comparison with the earlier instrument are: measurement of haemoglobin content and concentration of individual red cells permitting calculation of the percentage of hypochromic cells with a haemoglobin content less than 17 pg (%Hypo-He) and the percentage of hyperchromic red cells (%Hyper-He); estimation of the percentage of microcytes with a volume < 60 fl (%Micro-R) and the percentage of macrocytes with a volume > 120 fl (%Macro-R). The %Micro R is higher in thalassaemia heterozygosity than in mild or severe iron deficiency (while the immature reticulocyte fraction (IRF) is lower – but above normal) [116]. The %MicroR – the %Hypo He has been found useful in separating thalassaemia from iron deficiency in patients with no more than moderate anaemia; a value above 11.5 is strongly suggestive of thalassaemia [117]. In a further study, %MicroR – %Hypo He – RDW was found to be somewhat superior, with a cut-off of –7.6 being advised to maximise sensitivity [118]. The Ret-He and %Hypo-He were found to be useful in haemodialysis patients receiving erythropoietin for identifying those who would respond to iron therapy [119]; their usefulness was similar to that of related measurements on Siemens instruments. This instrument counts red cell fragments (FRC). There is a good correlation between microscopic and instrument counts, but with some overestimation on the part of the instrument, particularly when there is hypochromia

[120]. The XE-5000 has improved algorithms for flagging abnormal cells as 'blast cells', 'abnormal lymphocytes/lymphoblasts' or 'atypical lymphocytes' [121]; in one study it was found to give fewer false-positive flags than the XE-2100 for blast cells and abnormal/atypical lymphocytes, without an increase in false-negative flags, the need for film review thus being reduced [121]. In the same study the number of false-positive NRBC flags was increased, but was often negative on re-running [121]. In another study, however, in which three XE-5000 instruments were compared, reproducibility of the blast flag was found to be poor, as was sensitivity, with false negatives being seen in leucopenic samples [122]. Poor sensitivity to blast cells in leucopenia was confirmed in a further study of three instruments; lowering the thresholds for flagging and film review of specimens with a WBC less than 2×10^9/l was suggested [123].

Sysmex XN series

The Sysmex XN series are successors to the XE-5000. Changes include: the use of five fluorescence dyes in five different channels; introduction of a white cell nucleated channel (WNR) so that there is no longer a separate channel for NRBC; an improved white cell differential channel (WDF) so that a separate basophil channel is no longer needed; a white cell precursor channel (WPC), which is used for reflex testing when there is a positive blast/abnormal lymphocyte flag, and an additional fluorescent platelet channel (PLT-F), which incorporates a fluorescent RNA dye and permits the IPF to be estimated (it is used for reflex testing when there are abnormal red cell or platelet size histograms and permits an extended count when the platelet count is below a predetermined level). Immature granulocytes are quantified.

In an evaluation of the instrument, the following observations were made in comparison with the Sysmex XE-2100: NRBC are counted on all samples; positive flags for blast cells, 'abnormal lymphocytes' and 'atypical lymphocytes' are less frequent with no increase in false negatives; the need for blood film review is reduced by 49%; there is a low white cell count mode, use of which is suggested below a count of 0.5×10^9/l, in which an extended count gives improved precision for the differential count; turnaround time is improved by 10% [124]. In a comparison with a Beckman–Coulter DxH 800 and a Cell-Dyn Sapphire, the XN-2000 was found to be more sensitive in the detection of abnormal cells, including blast cells and NRBC [125].

Sysmex XT-2000i

The Sysmex XT-2000i is a compact, combined optical and impedance instrument suitable for small laboratories [126]. It has three detectors for forward light scatter, side light scatter and fluorescence, which are the basis of the five-part differential count, performed after staining with a polymethine dye. Red cell counts and platelet counts are performed by impedance measurements. Reticulocyte counts are performed in a supplementary mode after staining of RNA by polymethine; this mode also provides an optical platelet count.

Information about Sysmex instruments is available on a company website, www.sysmex.com.

Siemens instruments (previously Technicon then Bayer instruments)

A cell passing through a focused beam of light scatters the light, which may then be detected by photo-optical detectors placed lateral to the light beam. The degree of scatter is related to the cell size so that the cell can be both counted and sized. By placing a detector in the line of the light beam it is also possible to measure light absorbance. The light beam can be either white light or a high-intensity, coherent laser, which has superior optical qualities. The light detector can be either a photomultiplier or a photodiode, both of which convert light to electrical impulses that can be accumulated and counted.

H.1 series

The H.1 series of instruments – the H.1, H.2 and H.3 – are no longer current, but the later Advia series instruments are based on similar principles. Cells are counted and sized by light scattering, using white light for counting and sizing leucocytes and a laser for counting and sizing red cells and platelets. The red cells are isovolumetrically sphered, so that light scatter is not dependent on cell shape and can be predicted from the laws of physics. Cells move through a laser beam, and light scattered forward is measured at a narrow (2–3°) and a wider (5–15°) angle. A comparison of the two allows the computation of the size and haemoglobin concentration of individual red cells. Histograms showing the distribution of red cell volume and haemoglobin concentration are provided, together with a plot of volume against haemoglobin concentration (Fig. 2.14). The histogram of the cell volumes permits the derivation of the MCV, RDW and Hct.

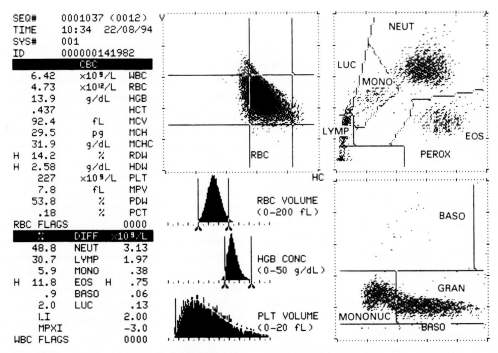

SEQ#   0001037 (0012)
TIME   10:34 22/08/94
SYS#   001
ID   000000141982

CBC		
6.42	×10⁹/L	WBC
4.73	×10¹²/L	RBC
13.9	g/dL	HGB
.437		HCT
92.4	fL	MCV
29.5	pg	MCH
31.9	g/dL	MCHC
H 14.2	%	RDW
H 2.58	g/dL	HDW
227	×10⁹/L	PLT
7.8	fL	MPV
53.8	%	PDW
.18	%	PCT
RBC FLAGS		0000

DIFF		×10⁹/L
48.8	NEUT	3.13
30.7	LYMP	1.97
5.9	MONO	.38
H 11.8	EOS H	.75
.9	BASO	.06
2.0	LUC	.13
	LI	2.00
	MPXI	–3.0
WBC FLAGS		0000

Fig. 2.14 Histograms and scatter plots of red cell volume and red cell haemoglobin concentration and white cell scatter plots produced by a Bayer-Technicon H.2 counter. In the peroxidase channel forward light scatter, largely determined by cell volume, is plotted against light absorbance, largely determined by the intensity of the peroxidase reaction. There are five white cell populations: NEUT, neutrophils; MONO, monocytes; LYMPH, lymphocytes; EOS, eosinophils; and LUC, large unstained cells, which are large, peroxidase-negative cells. In the basophil/lobularity channel forward light scatter, representing cell volume following differential cytoplasmic stripping, is plotted against high-angle light scatter, which is determined largely by cellular structure. There are three cell clusters, two of which overlap: BASO, basophils; MONONUC, mononuclear cells (lymphocytes and monocytes); and GRAN, granulocytes (neutrophils and eosinophils).

Similarly, the histogram of haemoglobin concentrations permits the derivation of the cellular haemoglobin concentration mean (CHCM) and the haemoglobin distribution width (HDW), the latter being indicative of the variation in haemoglobin concentration between individual cells. Hb is measured by a modification of conventional cyanmethaemoglobin methodology, and the MCH and MCHC are computed from the Hb, RBC and MCV. An optional lauryl sulphate method for Hb estimation is also available. The MCHC and CHCM are independently derived measurements, both representing the average haemoglobin concentration in a cell. They should give essentially the same result. This acts as an internal quality control mechanism, since errors in the estimation of Hb, e.g. resulting from a very high WBC, cause a discrepancy between these two measurements. It would be theoretically possible to omit the haemoglobin channel and compute Hb from the CHCM, RBC and MCV derived from light-scattering measurements.

The technology of the H.1 series of instruments appears to produce accurate estimations of MCV, Hct and MCHC, which agree well with reference methods [127,128]. It has been possible to avoid the inaccuracies of earlier light-scattering instruments (in which light scattering was influenced by cellular haemoglobin concentration as well as cell size) and the inaccuracies inherent in some impedance counters (in which the electrical shadow is influenced by cellular deformability as well as cell size). However, cells that cannot be isovolumetrically sphered, e.g. irreversibly sickled cells, will not be sized accurately. Similar measurements of two-angle light scatter permit platelets to be counted and sized. A Pct and PDW are also computed. Platelet counts using this technology appear to be superior, particularly when the count is low, to counts using impedance technology (Coulter or Sysmex) [27]. The MPV decreases on storage of the blood.

Hypochromic cells, as detected by these instruments, correlate with the observation of hypochromic cells on a blood film. The percentage is increased in iron deficiency and the anaemia of chronic disease. The percentage of hypochromic cells has been found to be very sensitive in the detection of functional iron deficiency in patients given erythropoietin, e.g. haemodialysis patients. Similar changes have been observed in iron-replete healthy volunteers and it has been suggested that this measurement might be useful in detecting illicit erythropoietin use by athletes [129]. However, in hospitalised patients, an increased percentage of hypochromic cells shows poor specificity for iron deficiency [130]. Hypochromic macrocytes have a different significance, being indicative of either dyserythropoiesis or an increased percentage of reticulocytes.

The red cell cytogram is diagnostically useful (see Chapter 8).

The differential count of the H.1 series is derived from two channels (see Table 2.6). The peroxidase channel uses white light and incorporates a cytochemical reaction in which the peroxidase of neutrophils, eosinophils and monocytes acts on a substrate, 4-chloro-1-naphthol, to produce a black reaction product, which absorbs light. Light scatter, which is proportional to cell size, is then plotted against light absorbance, which is proportional to the intensity of the peroxidase reaction (see Fig. 2.14). Neutrophils, eosinophils, monocytes and lymphocytes fall into four clusters, which are separated from each other and from cellular debris by a mixture of moving and fixed thresholds. A further cluster represents cells that are peroxidase-negative and larger than most lymphocytes, these being designated large unstained cells (LUC). In healthy subjects, LUC are mainly large lymphocytes, but abnormal cells such as peroxidase-negative blast cells, atypical lymphocytes, lymphoma cells, hairy cells, plasma cells and peroxidase-negative neutrophils can fall into this area. In the peroxidase channel, basophils fall in the lymphocyte area. They are separated from all other leucocytes in an independent basophil/lobularity channel, on the basis of their resistance to stripping of cytoplasm by a lytic agent in acid conditions. Basophils, sized by forward light scatter, are larger than the stripped residues of other cells (see Fig. 2.14). The basophil/lobularity channel is also used to detect the presence of blasts. Forward light scatter, which is proportional to cell size, is plotted against high-angle light scatter, which is a measure of increasing nuclear density and lobulation. Blasts are detected as a population with an abnormally low nuclear density. In addition, the 'lobularity index' (LI) is a measure of the ratio of the number of cells producing a lot of high-angle light scatter (lobulated neutrophils) to cells producing less high-angle light scatter (mononuclear cells, immature granulocytes and blasts).

Instruments of the H.1 series, in addition to flagging the presence of blasts, atypical lymphocytes, immature granulocytes and NRBC, produce two new white cell parameters – LI (described above) and the mean peroxidase index (MPXI). The latter is a measure of average peroxidase activity and is decreased in inherited peroxidase deficiency and also in acquired deficiency, as occurs in some MDS and myeloid leukaemias. A fall occurs during pregnancy, with a nadir at 20 weeks [131]. MPXI is increased in infection, in some myeloid leukaemias and MDS, in AIDS and in megaloblastic anaemia.

The later Siemens instrument, the Advia 120, operates on similar principles to the H.1 series instruments. The primary TNCC is provided by the basophil/lobularity channel rather than the peroxidase channel. There is improved cluster analysis in the basophil/lobularity channel, permitting more accurate flagging of the presence of NRBC (Figs 2.15 & 2.16). The platelet count is determined by two-dimensional analysis of size and refractive index, using laser light scatter at two angles; this has been found to produce a more accurate platelet count than that of the H.3 [132]. White cell flags are: ATYPS, NRBC, BLASTS, LS (left shift) and IG. Red cell flags are: MICRO, MACRO, ANISO, HYPER, HYPO, HCVAR, RBCF (red cell fragments) and RBCG (red cell ghosts). There is an expanded range of platelet parameters: mean platelet component concentration (MPC), platelet component distribution width (PCDW), mean platelet mass (MPM) and platelet mass distribution width (PMDW). Red cell ghosts and red cell fragments are separated from platelets and intact red cells on the basis of size and refractive index. Reference ranges have been published and it has been suggested that the MPC may be a useful indicator of platelet activation [133]. In a study comparing the Advia 120 basophil count with a flow cytometric count, poor correlation was observed with a correlation coefficient of 0.24, improving to 0.57 if samples with flags for abnormal white cells were excluded [103]. Pseudobasophilia was seen in 4/112 specimens [103]. This correlation

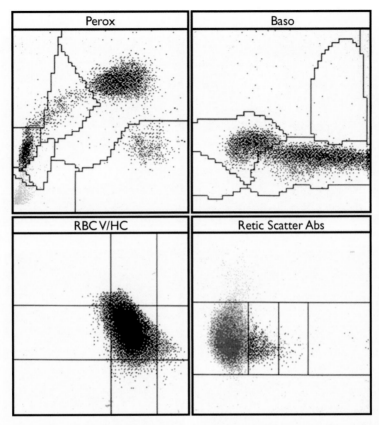

Fig. 2.15 Scatter plots produced by the Siemens Advia 120 on a normal blood sample, showing the peroxidase channel (top left, Perox), the basophil channel (top right, Baso), a plot of red cell size versus haemoglobin concentration (bottom left, RBC V/HC) and the reticulocyte channel scatter plot (bottom right, Retic Scatter Abs). In the Perox channel, the bottom left area is occupied by NRBC (on the left) and noise (on the right), platelet clumps appear in the area to the right of the lymphocyte box; in this channel basophils are located in the lymphocyte box. In comparison with H.1 series instruments, the Baso channel now has an area of noise (bottom) and a blast box (above and to the left of the noise box); the previous basophil box is divided into basophils (left) and 'Baso suspect' (right); on the extreme right, a narrow box is 'signals in saturation'.

was worse than was observed with a Cell-Dyn Sapphire instrument or a Sysmex XE-2100 [103]. In a comparison with three other instruments, the sensitivity of the Advia 120 blast flag (71%) was inferior to that of the XE-2100 and the DxH 800, and the specificity was the lowest of the four instruments [134]. LUC have not been found to be useful to predict numbers of haemopoietic progenitor cells [135].

The latest instrument in this series is the Advia 2120, which incorporates a cyanide-free haemoglobin method, enumeration of NRBC, correction of the TNCC to a WBC, and a reflex slide-spreader that adjusts for Hct and white cell count. The NRBC count is based on data from both the unstained area of the peroxidase chan-

nel and from a combination of data from the peroxidase channel and the basophil/lobularity channel. Sensitivity and specificity for the detection of NRBC were found to be 77.3% and 74.6%, respectively [136]. A platelet histogram measures particles between 0 and 60 fl, from which are calculated the MPV and the PDW. The calculated PCT, the product of the MPV and platelet count, is the volume of blood occupied by platelets. Other platelet variables are: the MPC, which is derived from the platelet component histogram (0–40 g/dl) and reflects platelet density; the MPM, calculated from the platelet dry mass histogram (0–5 pg); the LPLT, the count of platelets larger than 20 fl; and the percentage of large platelets (LPLT%). The MPV and MPC rise on storage, e.g. after

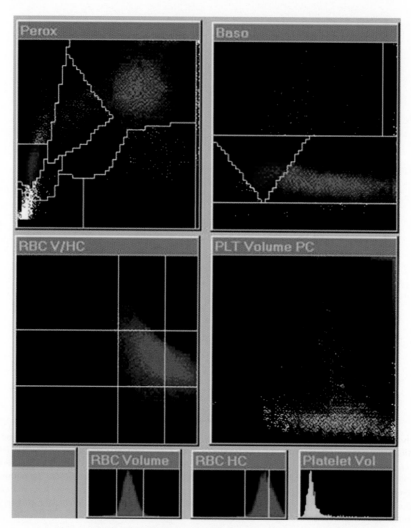

Fig. 2.16 Scatter plots and histograms produced by the Siemens Advia 120 on a blood sample from a patient with hereditary spherocytosis, showing the peroxidase channel (top left, Perox), the basophil channel (top right, Baso), a plot of red cell size versus haemoglobin concentration (centre left, RBC V/HC) and a plot of platelet size against platelet component (centre right, PLT volume PC). The y-axis in the PLT volume PC plot is the refraction index, proportional to the 'platelet component' (PC). At the bottom are histograms of red cell volume, red cell haemoglobin concentration (HC) and platelet volume. Note that there is a population of hyperdense cells representing spherocytes, apparent in the red cell cytogram and in the histogram of red cell haemoglobin concentration (RBC HC), crossing the right-hand haemoglobin concentration threshold in both plots. Red cell indices were RBC 3.55×10^{12}/l, Hb 109 g/l, Hct 0.32, MCV 89.2 fl, MCH 30.8 pg, MCHC 346 g/l and CHCM 396 g/l. By courtesy of Professor Gina Zini, Rome.

more than 3½ hours. In patients with acute leukaemia or suspected disseminated intravascular coagulation, the Advia 2120 platelet count shows a good correlation with the international reference method without any systematic error; erroneous counts are more likely when there is platelet activation [61]. Red cell fragments are detected and quantified in the platelet/red cell channel on the basis of a size of less than 30 fl and a refractive index of greater than 1.4; the normal range is less than 0.3% and a value of less than 1% has a high negative predictive value [108]. False elevation of the fragmented red cell count can result from the presence of very microcytic red cells [108]. There are four flags for the possible presence of blast cells – blast, 'basophil-no valley', ATYP and LUC; these have been found to be collectively more sensitive (and less specific) than the blast flags of the Beckman–Coulter LH750 analyser [58]. The CHret and HYPO% were found to be useful in haemodialysis patients receiving erythropoietin for identifying those who would respond to iron therapy [119]. The absolute neutrophil count of the Advia 2120i has been found to be accurate and precise, even at low levels [102]. LUC are increased in asymptomatic HIV-positive patients.

Information on Siemens instruments is available on a company website, www.healthcare.siemens.com.

Abbott (Cell-Dyn) instruments
Cell-Dyn 3500

The Cell-Dyn 3500 (Abbott Diagnostics) is a multichannel automated instrument incorporating both laser light-scattering and impedance technology. Hb is measured as cyanmethaemoglobin. Red cells, white cells and platelets are counted and sized by impedance technology following cytoplasmic stripping of white cells. Histograms of size distribution are provided (Fig. 2.17).

The WBC is also estimated in a light-scattering (laser) channel, which provides, in addition, an automated five-part differential count [137] (see Table 2.6). White cells mainly maintain their integrity and are hydrodynamically focused to pass in single file through the laser beam. In this channel, red cells are rendered transparent because their refractive index is the same as that of the sheath reagent. Four light-scattering parameters are measured:

1 Forward light scatter at 1–3° (referred to as 0° scatter), which is mainly dependent on cell size.
2 Narrow-angle light scatter at 7–11° (referred to as 10° scatter), which is dependent on cell structure and complexity.

3 Total polarised orthogonal light scatter at 70–100° (referred to as 90° scatter).
4 Depolarised orthogonal light scatter at 70–100° (referred to as 90°D scatter).

Scatter plots of white cell populations are provided (Fig. 2.18). Cells are first separated into granulocytes and mononuclear cells (Fig. 2.18a) on the basis of their lobularity and complexity. Next, granulocytes are separated into eosinophils and neutrophils on the basis of the unique ability of eosinophil granules to depolarise light (Fig. 2.18b). Next, the mononuclear cells are separated into monocytes, lymphocytes and degranulated basophils (basophil granules being soluble in the sheath reagent) on the basis of cell size and complexity (Fig. 2.18c). Finally, all five populations are indicated (colour coded) on a plot of lobularity against size (Fig. 2.18d). The identification of cell clusters with anomalous characteristics permits blasts, atypical lymphocytes, NRBC and immature granulocytes to be flagged.

The measurement of WBC by two technologies provides an internal quality control mechanism.

The WBC in the impedance channel (WIC) is falsely elevated if NRBC are present, whereas the WBC in the optical channel (WOC) excludes NRBC by means of a moving threshold. However, since the optical channel employs a less potent lytic agent, WOC may be falsely elevated when there are osmotically resistant red cells, as occurs with some neonatal blood samples. The likelihood of NRBC or osmotically resistant red cells is flagged and an algorithm selects the preferred result. If a suspicion of both NRBC and osmotically resistant cells is flagged, an extended period of lysis can be used to produce an accurate WOC.

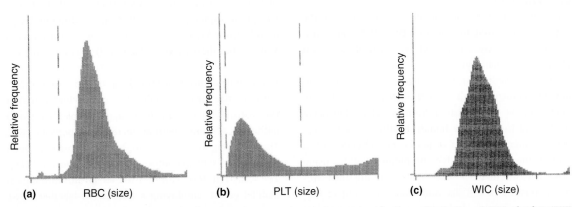

Fig. 2.17 Graphic output of Cell-Dyn 3500 automated counter, showing histograms of volume distribution of RBC, platelets (PLT) and white cells (WIC) derived from the impedance channel.

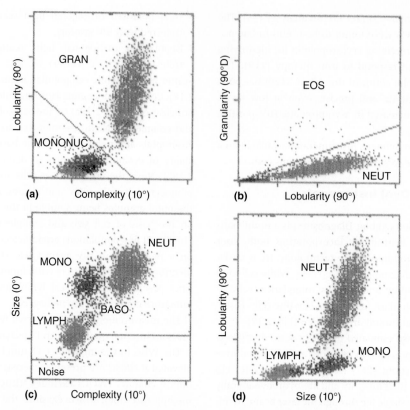

Fig. 2.18 Graphic output of a Cell-Dyn 3500 counter, showing white cell scatter plots derived from the white cell optical channel. (a) A plot of 90° scatter (indicating lobularity) against 10° scatter (indicating complexity) separates a granulocyte cluster from a mononuclear cluster. (b) 90°D (depolarised) scatter against 90° scatter separates the granulocyte cluster into eosinophils (which depolarise light) and neutrophils (which do not). (c) 0° scatter (related to size) against 10° scatter (related to complexity) separates the mononuclear cell cluster into lymphocytes, monocytes and degranulated basophils. (d) The five populations thus identified are shown on a plot of 90° scatter (related to lobularity) against 0° scatter (related to size). GRAN, granulocytes; MONONUC, mononuclear cells; NEUT, neutrophils; MONO, monocytes; LYMPH, lymphocytes; and EOS, eosinophils.

Cell-Dyn 4000

The Cell-Dyn 4000 incorporates, in addition to the variables measured by the Cell-Dyn 3500, an automated reticulocyte count and an erythroblast count [138,139]. Reticulocytes are recognised by analysis of both low-angle light scatter and green fluorescence following interaction with the DNA–RNA dye, CD4K530. They can be distinguished from platelets, leucocyte nuclei and Howell–Jolly bodies. Erythroblasts are recognised after interaction of permeabilised cells with a fluorescent DNA–RNA dye, propidium iodide, using three measurements – two light-scattering measurements relating to cell size and a measurement of red-fluorescence signals derived from erythroblast nuclei and damaged white cells. NRBC are distinguished from

platelets and from red cells with Howell–Jolly bodies or basophilic stippling. Since NRBC are enumerated separately from WBC, the Cell-Dyn is able to produce a WBC rather than a TNCC. The Cell-Dyn 4000 also gives a confidence estimate for the blast flag, which has been found to be clinically useful [140]. In addition, it incorporates a flag for non-viable white cells, which can alert the instrument operator to an aged sample [139] or a pathological sample with an increase in apoptotic cells. There is a flag for atypical lymphocytes, which has been found to be sensitive although not very specific [141]. The Cell-Dyn 4000 can be used for an immunological platelet count, employing a fluorescent-labelled CD61 monoclonal antibody [142]. This measurement correlates well with the reference (immunological) method.

It is a more expensive method, which is indicated for verifying low counts rather than being used on all specimens. It is indicated whenever the platelet count approaches a level that might trigger platelet transfusion (e.g. less than 20 or less than 10×10^9/l) and whenever there are giant platelets or significant numbers of red cell fragments or markedly microcytic cells [143]. This instrument has the possibility of an extended lyse period when red cells are incompletely lysed and an extended count mode for cytopenic samples. The Cell-Dyn 4000 can also be used to quantitate T cells, B cells and natural killer cells [144] and to quantitate fetal Rh D-positive cells in the circulation of an Rh D-negative mother, maternal blood being incubated with a monoclonal anti-D antibody conjugated to fluorescein isothiocyanate (FITC) [145]; however, these applications require downloading files for data analysis.

Cell-Dyn instruments have been observed to given abnormal patterns in some patients with *P. falciparum* or *P. vivax* malaria, as a result of the depolarisation of light by malaria pigment (haemozoin) [146]. This can serve to alert laboratory staff to this diagnosis, although not all haemozoin-positive samples are detected (1/10 missed in one study) [147].

Cell-Dyn Ruby

The Abbott Cell-Dyn Ruby is a fully optical instrument incorporating four detectors for polarised and depolarised light [126]. It performs a five-part differential count. An optional reticulocyte count can be performed after off-line staining with new methylene blue. There are two additional supplementary modes recommended for fragile white cells and lyse-resistant red cells respectively.

Cell-Dyn Sapphire

The Abbott Cell-Dyn Sapphire produces an FBC, a five-part differential leucocyte count and an NRBC count with an optional reticulocyte count. It incorporates four optical detectors for polarised and depolarised light and three fluorescence detectors. The type of laser and the reagents differ from those of earlier instruments, but the principles are the same. NRBC are enumerated following staining with the fluorochrome, propidium iodide; this also permits the provision of a viability index for white cells. The NRBC count has been found to be more accurate than that of the LH 780 or the DxH 800 [79]. Further optional tests are an immuno-platelet count

(using a CD61 monoclonal antibody) and a measurement of CD3-positive/CD4-positive and CD3-positive/CD8-positive T cells (using fluorochrome-labelled monoclonal antibodies). In patients with acute leukaemia or suspected disseminated intravascular coagulation, Cell-Dyn Sapphire platelet counts by all three methods show a good correlation with the international reference method, but with the slope of the regression line indicating underestimation of the count [61]; for the optical method, erroneous counts are more likely when there is platelet activation (which leads to loss of platelet granules). The RBC can be measured by an optical as well as an impedance method. Hb is measured by imidazole ligand chemistry. New red cell variables include %MIC (erythrocytes less than 60 fl), %MAC (erythrocytes greater than 120 fl), %HPO (erythrocytes with haemoglobin concentration less than 280 g/l), %HPR (erythrocytes with haemoglobin concentration greater than 410 g/l) and HDW. New reticulocyte variables include MCVr (mean volume of reticulocytes), MCHr (mean haemoglobin content of reticulocytes) and CHCr (mean haemoglobin concentration of reticulocytes). Red cell and reticulocyte variables show good correlation with equivalent variables on Siemens instruments, although there may be significant differences in mean values necessitating instrument-specific reference ranges [148]. Red cell and reticulocyte variables are not necessarily stable with time; MCH and MCHr are stable but within one day alterations in cell size mean that there is a rise in the MCV, MCVr and %HYO and a fall in the MCHC, CHCr and %HPR [148]. In a study comparing the basophil count of three instruments with a flow cytometric count, the Cell-Dyn Sapphire was found to be more accurate than the Sysmex XE-2100 or the Siemens Advia 120, although the correlation with the flow cytometric count was not ideal, the correlation coefficient being 0.81 or 0.87 if samples with flags for abnormal white cells were excluded [103]. This correlation was worse than was observed with a Cell-Dyn Sapphire instrument or a Sysmex XE-2100 [103]. Pseudobasophilia was seen in 4/112 specimens [103]. The blast flag on the Cell-Dyn Sapphire was found to be less sensitive than that of three other instruments, 65% in comparison with 71–94%, but the specificity was highest [134]. As with several earlier instruments, the Cell-Dyn Sapphire may show atypical polarisation events in patients with malaria, since the malaria pigment haemozoin shares with eosinophil granules the ability to depolarise light. The atypical signals appear on the neutrophil–eosinophil scatter plot in a different position from signals generated by eosinophil granules.

Cell-Dyn Emerald

This is a bench-top analyser providing 18 variables including RDW, MPV and a three-part differential count, which can be used as a point-of-care instrument [149]. Measurements are based on impedance and a non-cyanide method for Hb estimation. A very small blood sample is sufficient.

Information on Abbott instruments is available on a company website, www.abbottdiagnostics.com.

Horiba ABX instruments

Horiba instruments such as the ABX Pentra DX 120 and Pentra DX Nexus (Horiba ABX Diagnostics) are haematology analysers that have evolved from Helios Argos instruments. Red cells, white cells and platelets are counted and sized by impedance technology and histograms of size distribution are provided. The Hct is determined by summing the amplitudes of electrical signals generated by red cells, with a coincidence correction. Platelets are separated from red cells by a floating threshold between 18 fl and 25 fl. Hb is measured by one of two methods, either by a cyanmethaemoglobin method or by oxidation of haem iron followed by stabilisation to produce chromogenic substances that can be quantified. A five-part differential count is based on two channels in the Pentra DX120 (see Table 2.6). In one channel, light absorbance and impedance measurements are made, after interaction of cells with chlorazole black E, the active principle of Sudan black B (Fig. 2.19). This dye stains eosinophil granules most strongly, neutrophil granules somewhat less and monocyte granules more weakly; light absorbance of stained cells is determined both by the strength of staining of granules and the degree of complexity of the nucleus. In a second channel, basophils are differentiated from other white cells by impedance measurements following differential cytoplasmic stripping. Different white cell populations are displayed on a plot of light absorbance against impedance and are enumerated by cluster analysis (with moving thresholds). Three further abnormal white cell populations are enumerated, when present. 'Atypical lymphocytes' are both counted separately and included in the total lymphocyte count (in contrast to the Siemens instruments, where 'large unstained cells' are counted separately but excluded from the lymphocyte count). 'Large immature cells' (LIC) are counted separately but are also assigned to either the neutrophil category or the monocyte category, depending on their light absorbance. The 'atypical lymphocyte' (ATL) category may include not only atypical lymphocytes in conditions such as infectious mononucleosis, but also lymphoma cells, CLL cells, small blast cells and plasma cells. The LIC category may include myeloblasts, monoblasts, promyelocytes (including those present in acute promyelocytic leukaemia), myelocytes, metamyelocytes, lymphoblasts and lymphoma cells. The Pentra DX 120 counts NRBC following nuclear staining by thiazole orange, a fluorescent nucleic acid stain. This instrument also provides a reticulocyte count, RET H, RET M and RET L (high, medium and low fluorescence reticulocytes), MRV (mean reticulocyte volume) and RHC_C (reticulocyte haemoglobin content calculated). Immature reticulocytes are flagged. Immature granulocytes (IMG), immature monocytes (IMM) and immature lymphocytes (IML) are flagged.

The Pentra DX Nexus provides an extended differential count that includes IMG, IML and IMM, LIC and ATL. NRBC are quantified by fluorescence after binding to thiazole orange and the WBC is corrected. In addition to the reticulocyte count, IRF, MRV and RHC_C are provided. The RHCc correlates with the CHr of the Advia 2120 and could be useful in the detection of functional iron deficiency.

Information on Horiba instruments can be found on a company website, www.horiba-abx.com.

Nihon Kohden instruments

The Nihon Kohden instruments, Celltac *E* and Celltac *F*, have a red cell/platelet channel and a white cell/haemoglobin channel. A five-part differential count is based on laser light scatter at three angles: low forward angle (cell size), high forward angle (cell structure) and side angle (internal granularity). Hb can be measured by a cyanmethaemoglobin or a cyanide-free method.

Information is available on a company website, www.nihonkohden.com.

Mindray instruments

The Mindray BC-6800 Auto Hematology Analyzer uses laser light scatter at two angles plus fluorescence signals.

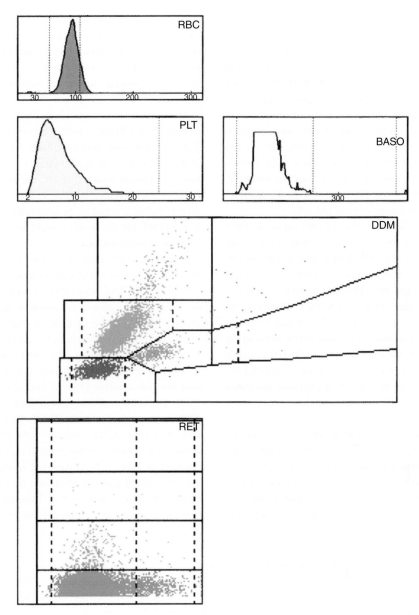

Fig. 2.19 Histograms of red cell (RBC) and platelet (PLT) size distribution and scatter plots of the differential white cell channel (DDM) and the reticulocyte channel (RET) of the Horiba ABX Pentra 120 analyser.

It produces an FBC, a five-part differential count, reticulocyte count, IRF, NRBC count, immature granulocyte count, high fluorescent cell (HFC) count (atypical lymphocytes and blast cells) and two flags, 'infected RBC?' and 'InR#' count, that may indicate the presence of malaria parasites.

Automated reticulocyte counts and reticulated platelet counts
Automated reticulocyte count

Most automated reticulocyte counts depend on the ability of various fluorochromes to combine with the RNA of reticulocytes. Fluorescent cells can then be counted in a flow cytometer. The fluorochromes also combine with DNA so that nucleated cells fluoresce. An alternative technology is based on staining of RNA by a non-fluorescent nucleic acid stain such as new methylene blue or oxazine 750. Reticulocytes are then detected by light scattering or light absorbance or by analysis of three different cell properties (Coulter instruments). White cells, NRBC and platelets can usually be separated from reticulocytes on the basis of gating for size and either their light scattering/absorbance or the intensity of their fluorescence. Reticulocyte counts can be expressed as an absolute count or as a percentage of total red cells.

Because of the large number of cells counted, automated reticulocyte counts are much more precise than manual counts. It was hoped that they might also be more accurate, since the subjective element in recognising late reticulocytes with only one or two granules of positively staining material is eliminated. However, the automated count is altered by: (i) the choice of fluorochrome; (ii) the duration of exposure of the blood to the fluorochrome; (iii) the temperature at which the sample is kept after mixing; and (iv) the setting of thresholds – the upper threshold to exclude fluorescing nucleated cells and the lower threshold to exclude background autofluorescence.

Similar considerations apply to automated reticulocyte counts using non-fluorescent nucleic acid stains. A reference range for an automated reticulocyte count is therefore specific to an instrument and method. Reference ranges that have been established show considerable variation. It is still necessary to consider the

manual count to decide whether a range represents 'truth'. Ideally, automated and manual counts should show a close correlation; mean counts should be similar, and the intercept on the y-axis of the regression line of automated counts on manual counts should be small.

Automated reticulocyte counts fall as the blood ages *in vitro*. This is likely to reflect reticulocyte maturation. It also occurs with manual counts but, because of the imprecision of the manual count, it is less likely to be noticed. If blood is stored at 4°C the reticulocyte count is stable for 72 hours, but if it is left at room temperature a 5% fall is noted by 24 hours and a 10% fall by 48 hours [150]. Ideally counts should be performed within 6 hours of venepuncture.

Automated reticulocyte counts can be performed on general purpose flow cytometers, such as the Becton Dickinson FACScan or the Coulter EPICS XL, or on a dedicated reticulocyte counter, such as the Sysmex R-1000, R-2000 or R-3000 (Fig. 2.20). Increasingly an automated reticulocyte counting capacity is incorporated into automated full blood counters, as in the Sysmex XE-2100 (see Fig. 2.12), the Bayer H.3 and the Advia series (Figs. 2.21–2.23), the Cell-Dyn 3500 and 4000, the later versions of the Coulter STKS, the Coulter MAXM, HmX, Gen S, LH750 and DxH 800 (Fig. 2.24), and the ABX Pentra 120 and Pentra DX Nexus. Technologies employed are summarised in Table 2.7. Automated reticulocyte counts vary in their degree of precision. In a comparison of five instruments, Doretto *et al.* found the imprecision was greatest for the Coulter LH750, followed in order

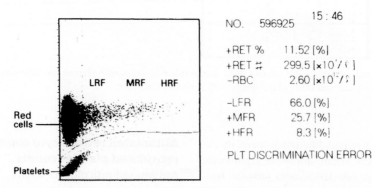

Fig. 2.20 Scatter plot of the reticulocyte count of the Sysmex R.3000. Cell volume is plotted against fluorescence intensity. A threshold separates red cells from platelets. Reticulocytes are divided into high fluorescence (HFR) representing the most immature reticulocytes, intermediate fluorescence (MFR) and low fluorescence (LFR) representing late reticulocytes.

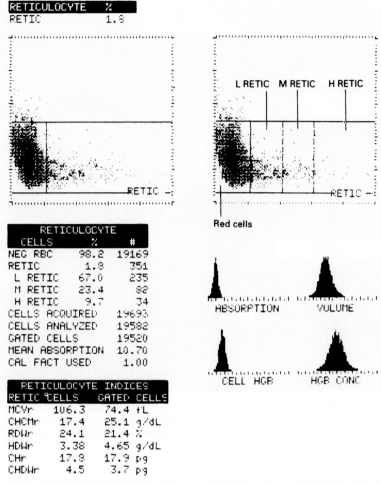

Fig. 2.21 Printout of a Bayer H.3 counter showing the scatter plot of the reticulocyte counting channel. The volume and haemoglobin content of reticulocytes and other red cells are determined by high- and low-angle light scattering and light absorbance is measured following uptake of a nucleic acid dye, oxazine 750. Six variables of potential clinical usefulness are measured for reticulocytes as well as for total red cells: MCV, CHCM (= MCHC), RDW, HDW (in g/dl), CH (= MCH) and CHDW (HDW in pg). Cell volume is plotted against light absorbance. Reticulocytes are divided into high absorbance (H RETIC) representing early reticulocytes, intermediate absorbance (M RETIC) and low absorbance (L RETIC) representing late reticulocytes.

by the ABX Pentra, Advia120, Sysmex XE-2100 and Cell-Dyn 4000 [151]. Reference intervals are instrument specific (*see* Table 5.20).

Automated reticulocyte counts can also be performed by image analysis of a blood film stained with new methylene blue [152].

The automated reticulocyte count, like the manual count, is useful in determining whether anaemia is caused by failure of bone marrow output or increased red cell destruction. Because of its greater precision, the automated reticulocyte count is also useful in monitoring the response to erythropoietin therapy in chronic renal failure, and in detecting bone marrow recovery following therapy for aplastic anaemia or following chemotherapy for malignant disease.

Reticulocyte immaturity

Automated reticulocyte counters can also provide various indices of reticulocyte immaturity, since intensity

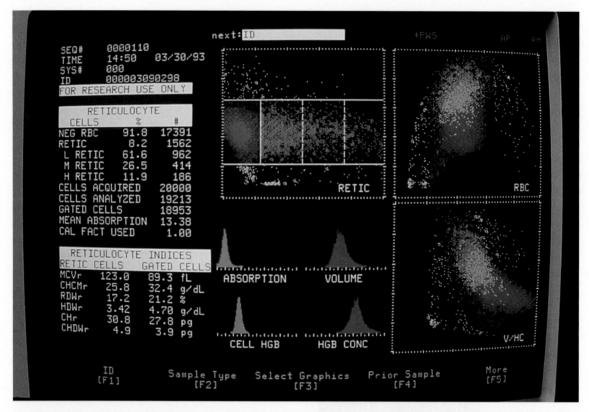

Fig. 2.22 Photograph of the colour monitor of a Bayer H.3 automated counter. The scattergram shows volume and haemoglobin content of reticulocytes (blue) in relation to size and haemoglobin content of other red cells (red) on both a Mie map and a red cell cytogram. This sample had a greatly increased reticulocyte count as a consequence of a haemolytic transfusion reaction.

of fluorescence or uptake of another nucleic acid stain is proportional to the amount of RNA in the cell. Instruments may divide reticulocytes into low, intermediate and high (or low and high) fluorescence/absorbance/light scatter, higher values indicating an increasing degree of immaturity. They may also give a mean measurement. The count of immature reticulocytes varies greatly between instruments and reference ranges are therefore instrument specific. For example, the Pentra 120 Retic immature reticulocyte fraction is higher than that of either the Sysmex XE-2100 or the Sysmex R-2000 [153] (see also Table 5.20). The reference range is also instrument specific for the mean reticulocyte volume. Such measurements are of clinical significance when considered in relation to the reference range for the instrument in question. In anaemia resulting from haemolysis or blood loss, the percentage of immature reticulocytes rises as the total reticulocyte count rises [154]. However, when there is dyserythropoiesis the percentage of immature reticulocytes may be elevated despite a normal or reduced total reticulocyte count. This has been observed, for example, in AML, MDS, megaloblastic anaemia and aplastic anaemia [154–156]. A disproportionate increase in immature reticulocytes indicates abnormal maturation of reticulocytes [155]. In other anaemias with little dyserythropoiesis but with a poor reticulocyte response, e.g. iron deficiency anaemia or the anaemia of chronic renal failure, the absolute reticulocyte count is reduced, but the percentage of immature reticulocytes is normal. The percentage of immature reticulocytes is increased, without anaemia or any increase in the reticulocyte percentage, in a significant proportion of patients with cardiac and pulmonary disease [157]. It has been suggested that this results from erythropoietin release as a response to hypoxia.

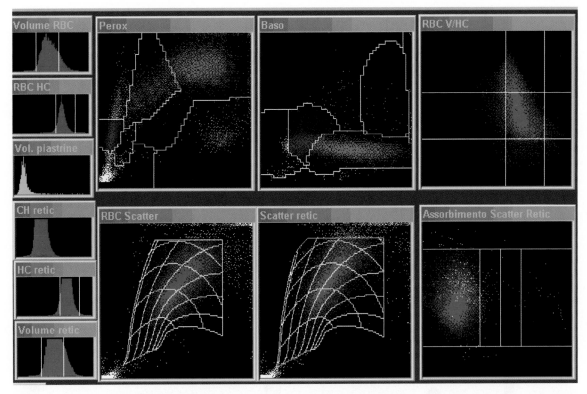

Fig. 2.23 Scatter plots and histograms produced by the Siemens Advia 120 on a blood sample from a patient with pure red cell aplasia showing reticulocytopenia. The red cell cytogram (RBC V/HC) shows that there is macrocytosis (increased signals above the upper volume threshold). Note that, in comparison with the increased reticulocytes seen in Fig. 2.22, there are virtually no reticulocytes (blue dots) in the bottom right plot of light absorption in the reticulocyte channel. The absolute reticulocyte count was very low, 9.2×10^9/l, with a reticulocyte percentage of 0.43. Red cells indices were RBC 2.14×10^{12}/l, Hb 68 g/l, Hct 0.21, MCV 99 fl, MCH 31.8 pg, MCHC 321 g/l, CHCM 325 g/l, RDW 21%. Note that because of heterogeneity of red cell size, the MCV at the upper limit of normal does not reflect the presence of the significant number of macrocytes that are seen in the red cell histogram and cytogram; instrument flags included macrocytosis +++ and anisocytosis ++. By courtesy of Professor Gina Zini.

When effective erythropoiesis is restored after a period of reduced output of red cells, e.g. following bone marrow transplantation or during recovery from chemotherapy, there is a rise in the percentage and absolute count of immature reticulocytes in advance of any rise in the total reticulocyte percentage, neutrophil count or platelet count [158]. Similarly, an increase in the percentage of immature reticulocytes predicts haemopoietic recovery when severe aplastic anaemia is treated with immunosuppressive therapy, occurring in advance of a rise in the neutrophil count or the total reticulocyte count [159]. The IRF has also been found to be useful in predicting the optimal time

for a peripheral blood stem cells harvest in some, but not all, studies [52].

Reticulated platelets

Young platelets, newly released from the bone marrow, contain significant amounts of RNA; they can be identified on a blood film after exposure of the blood to methylene blue. By analogy with reticulocytes, they have been called 'reticulated platelets'. Automated reticulocyte counters can be modified to measure reticulated platelets. The Sysmex R-3000 has been modified to measure both reticulated platelets and large platelets. Reticulated platelets can also

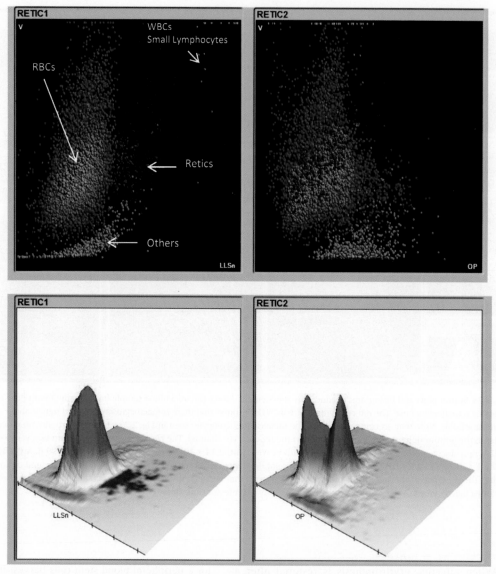

Fig. 2.24 Reticulocyte scatter plots and three-dimensional representations from Beckman–Coulter DxH 800 instrument on a sample of normal blood. In the plot of volume (v) against log of light scatter (LLSn) the reticulocyte and immature reticulocytes form clusters distinct from mature red cells and white cells (RETIC1, left). In the plot of volume against opacity (OP) the reticulocytes do not appear to separate (RETIC2, right), but in fact the software identifies them in three-dimensional analysis. By courtesy of Beckman–Coulter.

be enumerated on a flow cytometer after exposure to a fluorescent dye, such as thiazole orange, capable of binding to nucleic acids. The concentration of the fluorescent dye must be carefully judged to avoid binding to platelet components other than RNA [160]. It is also possible to use two-colour fluorescence, combining a nucleic acid stain with a fluorochrome-labelled platelet monoclonal antibody such as CD61 [161]. Reticulated platelets can now also be quantified on automated analysers.

In most studies, an increased percentage of reticulated platelets has been found to indicate that

Table 2.7 Technologies employed for automated reticulocyte counting in automated instruments [42,150].

Instrument	Fluorochrome or stain
Fluorescence-based methods	
R-1000, R-2000, R-3000, R-3500, SE-9000 and SE-9500 (Sysmex)	Auramine O
XE-5000 and XN (Sysmex)	A proprietary polymethine dye
Cell-Dyn 4000 (Abbott)	CD4K530 (light scatter and fluorescence intensity measurements)
XL (Beckman–Coulter)	Coriphosphine O
FACScan (Becton Dickinson)	Thiazole orange
Pentra 120 Retic and Pentra DX Nexus (Horiba ABX Diagnostics) [150]	Thiazole orange
Non-fluorescent RNA-binding agents	
H.3, Advia series (Siemens)	Oxazine 750 (absorbance measurement)
Cell-Dyn 3500 (Abbott)	New methylene blue (light scattering measurement)
STKS/MAXM/Gen S/DxH 800 (Beckman–Coulter)	New methylene blue (VCS: volume, conductivity and scatter measurements on ghosts of sphered cells)

thrombocytopenia results from increased platelet destruction rather than bone marrow failure, but there is some overlapping of results and conflicting data have also been published [160,162,163]. Following bone marrow transplantation [164], during recovery from chemotherapy and during treatment of thrombotic thrombocytopenic purpura [161] and autoimmune thrombocytopenic purpura, an increase in reticulated platelets heralds a rise in the platelet count.

Counts of reticulated platelets require instrument-specific reference ranges.

Near-patient testing

Blood gas analysers either measure Hb directly by spectrophotometry or calculate it from the Hct determined by conductivity measurements; such instruments often also measure many biochemical variables. In addition to blood gas analysers, there are various small instruments that are simple enough in their operation that they can be used for near-patient or point-of-care testing by individuals who are not fully trained biomedical

scientists, but have been specifically trained for this more limited role. Some instruments measure a number of variables whereas others measure only Hb. The HemoCue® (HemoCue AG, Wetzikon, Switzerland) measures Hb by an azide methaemoglobin reaction and photometry. HemoCue® WBC DIFF determines, in addition, the WBC and a five-part differential count. The iSTAT haematocrit cartridge (Abbott Point of Care) estimates Hct by conductivity measurement and calculates an Hb from the Hct. Extreme leucocytosis can give a falsely elevated measurement [165]. An estimate of Hb can also be made by comparing the intensity of colour of a drop of blood on filter paper with a colour scale [166]. This method is suitable for screening in peripheral clinics with no ready access to laboratories. It is available from Teaching Aids at Low Cost (www.talcuk.org). It is likely to be used particularly in developing countries, but also has potential as a test for screening blood donors prior to blood donation. The colour of a drop of blood can similarly be compared with coloured discs, as in the Lovibond Tintometer (www.tintometer.com).

Non-invasive methods

A novel instrument, the Hemoscan, is a portable instrument with a hand-held probe, which is placed beneath the tongue [167]. The probe emits light that reflects from the target tissue to a tiny camera. The instrument is said to produce an estimate of Hb, PCV and WBC. A similar principle underlies the Hemo-Monitor and the Astrim, which measure Hb non-invasively on the basis of light absorbance in the near-infrared range when a finger is inserted into the instrument [168,169]; estimates have been found to be comparable to laboratory measurements in most patients, but not in those with a paraprotein [169]. However, the correlation with standard methods and the accuracy do not appear to be sufficient at present for this to be a very useful advance [170]. The Pronto-7 (Masimo Corporation) also estimates Hb based on light absorption by a finger, giving results comparable to laboratory measurements [171]; SpO_2, pulse rate and perfusion index are also measured. Hb can also be measured non-invasively by inserting a finger within a ring-shaped sensor attached to a monitor in the NBM 200 and NBM 200MP (OrSense); the NBM 200 measures Hb and pulse rate, while the NBM 200MP also measures oxygen saturation. The Hb estimate is by means of light absorbance.

HemoGlobe is a novel adaption of a mobile phone, designed for use in underdeveloped countries, which estimates haemoglobin by pulse oximetry and converts the results into colour graphics: green for mild anaemia, yellow for moderate and red for severe.

http://releases.jhu.edu/2012/07/24/undergraduates-cellphone-screening-device-for-anemia-wins-250000-prize/

Storage of blood specimens prior to testing

If there is to be any delay in performing a blood count, the specimen should be stored at 4°C. Storage at room temperature increases the number of 'flags' and introduces inaccuracies. For example, with the Siemens H.1 and Advia series of instruments a left shift flag becomes very frequent, the MCV rises and the MCHC falls. Similarly, room temperature storage of samples for counts on a Cell-Dyn 3500 instrument was observed to cause an increased number of flags, a fall of the WBC as measured by the optical system (but not by the impedance system), a fall in the neutrophil percentage, a rise in the lymphocyte percentage, a rise in the MCV and a fall in the MCHC [172]. Platelet characteristics vary on storage. For example, with the Siemens Advia 120 there is a rise in the MPV and a fall in the MPC [133]. It is important for laboratory scientists to be familiar with the effects of storage on blood counts determined on the specific instrument in use.

TEST YOUR KNOWLEDGE

Visit the companion website for MCQs and EMQs
    on this topic:
www.wiley.com/go/bain/bloodcells

References

1 International Committee for Standardization in Haematology (1978) Recommendations for reference method for haemoglobinometry in human blood (ICSH Standard EP 6/2: 1977) and specifications for international haemiglobincyanide reference preparation (ICSH Standard EP 6/3: 1977). *J Clin Pathol*, **31**, 139–143.

2 Davis B and Jungerius B, on behalf of International Council for the Standardization of Haematology (ICSH) (2009) International Council for Standardization in Haematology technical report 1-2009: new reference material for haemiglobincyanide for use in standardization of blood haemoglobin measurements. *Int J Lab Hematol*, **32**, 139–141.

3 van Kampen EJ and Zijlstra WG (1983) Spectrophotometry of hemoglobin and hemoglobin derivatives. *Adv Clin Chem*, **23**, 199–257.

4 Lewis SM, Garvey B, Manning R, Sharp SA and Wardle J (1991) Lauryl sulphate haemoglobin: a non-hazardous substitute for HiCN in haemoglobinometry. *Clin Lab Haematol*, **13**, 279–290.

5 Morris LD, Pont A and Lewis SM (2001) Use of a new HemoCue system for measuring haemoglobin at low concentrations. *Clin Lab Haematol*, **23**, 91–96.

6 International Committee for Standardization in Haematology Expert Panel on Blood Cell Sizing (1980) Recommendation for reference method for determination by centrifugation of packed cell volume of blood. *J Clin Pathol*, **33**, 1–2.

7 ICSH (1982) Selected methods for the determination of the packed cell volume. In: van Assendelft OW & England JM (eds) *Advances in Hematological Methods: the blood count*. CRC Press, Boca Raton.

8 Guthrie DL and Pearson TC (1982) PCV measurement in the management of polycythaemic patients. *Clin Lab Haematol*, **4**, 257–265.

9 Weatherall MS and Sherry KM (1997) An evaluation of the Spuncrit™ infra-red analyser for measurement of haematocrit. *Clin Lab Haematol*, **19**, 183–186.

10 Aoun H (1989) When a house officer gets AIDS. *N Engl J Med*, **321**, 693–696.

11 Anonymous (1999) Glass capillary tubes: joint safety advisory about potential risks. *Lab Med*, **30**, 299.

12 Crosland-Taylor PJ (1982) The micro PCV. In: van Assendelft OW & England JM (eds) *Advances in Hematological Methods: the blood count*. CRC Press, Boca Raton.

13 Lampasso JA (1965) Error in hematocrit value produced by excessive ethylenediaminetetraacetate. *Am J Clin Pathol*, **44**, 109–110.

14 Pennock CA and Jones KW (1966) Effects of ethylenediaminetetra-acetic acid (dipotassium salt) and heparin on the estimation of packed cell volume. *J Clin Pathol*, **19**, 196–199.

15 Karlow MA, Westengard JC and Bull BS (1989) Does tube diameter influence the packed cell volume? *Clin Lab Haematol*, **11**, 375–383.

16 Bryner MA, Houwen B, Westengard J and Klein O (1997) The spun micro-haematocrit and mean cell volume are affected by changes in the oxygenation state of red blood cells. *Clin Lab Haematol*, **19**, 99–103.

17 Lines RW and Grace E (1984) Choice of anticoagulants for packed cell volume and mean cell volume determination. *Clin Lab Haematol*, **6**, 305–306.

18 Expert Panel on Cytometry of the International Council for Standardization in Haematology (2000) ICSH recommendation for the measurement of a reference packed cell volume. *Lab Haematol*, **7**, 148–170.

19 International Committee for Standardization in Haematology (1980) Recommended methods for measurement of red cell and plasma volume. *J Nucl Med*, **21**, 793–800.

20 Bull BS, Fujimoto K, Houwen B, Klee G, van Hove L and van Assendelt OW on behalf of the ICSH Expert Panel on Cytometry (2003) International Council for Standardization in Haematology (ICSH) Recommendations for "Surrogate Reference" Method for the Packed Cell Volume. *Lab Hematol*, **9**, 1–9.

21 Briggs C and Bain BJ (2012) Basic haematological techniques. In: Bain BJ, Bates I, Laffan MA and Lewis SM (eds) *Dacie and Lewis Practical Haematology*, 11th edn. Churchill Livingstone, Edinburgh.

22 International Council for Standardization in Haematology: Expert Panel on Cytometry (1994) Reference method for the enumeration of erythrocytes and leucocytes. *Clin Lab Haematol*, **16**, 131–138.

23 Barnett D, Goodfellow K, Ginnever J, Granger V, Whitby L and Reilly JT (2001) Low level leucocyte counting: a critical variable in the validation of leucodepleted blood transfusion components as highlighted by an external quality assessment study. *Clin Lab Haematol*, **23**, 43–51.

24 Lewis SM (1982) Visual haemocytometry. In: van Assendelt OW & England JM (eds) *Advances in Hematological Methods: the blood count*. CRC Press, Boca Raton.

25 Dickerhoff R and van Ruecker A (1995) Enumeration of platelets by multiparameter flow cytometry using platelet specific antibodies and fluorescent reference particles. *Clin Lab Haematol*, **17**, 163–172.

26 Tanaka C, Ishii T and Fujimoto K (1996) Flow cytometric platelet enumeration utilizing monoclonal antibody CD42a. *Clin Lab Haematol*, **18**, 265–269.

27 Harrison P, Horton A, Grant D, Briggs C and Machin S (2000) Immunoplatelet counting: a proposed new reference procedure. *Br J Haematol*, **108**, 228–235.

28 International Council for Standardization in Haematology: Expert Panel on Cytometry and International Society of Laboratory Haematology Task Force on Platelet Counting (2001) Platelet counting by the RBC/platelet method: a reference method. *Am J Clin Pathol*, **115**, 460–464.

29 Norris S, Pantelidou D, Smith D and Murphy MF (2003) Immunoplatelet counting: potential for reducing the use of platelet transfusions through more accurate platelet counting. *Br J Haematol*, **121**, 605–613.

30 International Council for Standardization in Haematology: Expert Panel on Cytometry (1995) Recommendation of the International Council for Standardization in Haematology on reporting differential leucocyte counts. *Clin Lab Haematol*, **17**, 113.

31 Clinical and Laboratory Standards Institute (2007) *Reference Leukocyte (WBC) Differential Count (Proportional) and Evaluation of Instrumental Methods; Approved Standard—Second Edition*. CLSI document H20-A, Clinical and Laboratory Standards Institute, Wayne, Pennsylvania.

32 Talstad I (1981) Problems in microscopic and automatic cell differentiation of blood and cell suspensions. *Scand J Haematol*, **26**, 398–406.

33 Davidson E (1958) The distribution of cells in peripheral blood smears. *J Clin Pathol*, **11**, 410–411.

34 Rümke CL (1960) Variability of results in differential cell counts on blood smears. *Triangle*, **4**, 154–157.

35 England JM and Bain BJ (1976) Total and differential leucocyte count. *Br J Haematol*, **33**, 1–7.

36 Koepke IF and Koepke JA (1986) *Reticulocytes. Clin Lab Haematol*, **8**, 169–179.

37 The Expert Panel on Cytometry of the International Council for Standardization in Haematology (1992) *ICSH Guidelines for Reticulocyte Counting by Microscopy of Supravitally Stained Preparations*. World Health Organization, Geneva.

38 Perrotta AL and Finch CA (1972) The polychromatophilic erythrocyte. *Am J Clin Pathol*, **57**, 471–477.

39 Crouch JY and Kaplow LS (1985) Relationship of reticulocyte age to polychromasia, shift cells, and shift reticulocytes. *Arch Pathol Lab Med*, **109**, 325–329.

40 Lowenstein ML (1959) The mammalian reticulocyte. *Int Rev Cytol*, **9**, 135–174.

41 Brecher G and Schneiderman MR (1950) A time-saving device for counting of reticulocytes. *Am J Clin Pathol*, **20**, 1079–1083.

42 Koepke JA (1999) Update on reticulocyte counting. *Lab Med*, **30**, 339–343.

43 Hillman RS and Finch CA (1969) The misused reticulocyte. *Br J Haematol*, **17**, 313–315.

44 Fannon M, Thomas R and Sawyer L (1982) Effect of staining and storage times on reticulocyte counts. *Lab Med*, **13**, 431–433.

45 NCCLS (2004) *Methods for Reticulocyte Counting (Automated Blood Cell counters, Flow Cytometry, and Supravital Dyes); Approved guideline—Second Edition*. NCCLS document H44-A2, Clinical and Laboratory Standards Institute, Wayne, Pennsylvania.

46 Kratz A, Bengtsson HI, Casey JE, Keefe JM, Beatrice GH, Grzybek DY et al. (2005) Performance evaluation of the CellaVision DM96 system: WBC differentials by automated digital image analysis supported by an artificial neural network. *Am J Clin Pathol*, **124**, 770–781.

47 Ceelie H, Dinkelaar RB and van Gelder W (2007) Examination of peripheral blood films using automated microscopy: evaluation of Diffmaster Octavia and Cellavision DM96. *J Clin Pathol*, **60**, 72–79.

48 Briggs C and Machin S (2012) Can automated blood film analysis replace the manual differential? *Int J Lab Hematol*, **34**, Suppl. 1, 6–7.

49 Smits SM and Leyte A (2014) Clinical performance evaluation of the CellaVision Image Capture System in the white blood cell differential on peripheral blood smears. *J Clin Pathol*, **67**, 168–172.

50 Kunicka J, Malin M, Zelmanovic D, Katzenberg M, Canfield W, Shapiro P and Mohandas N (2001) Automated quantification of hemoglobin-based blood substitutes in whole blood samples. *Am J Clin Pathol*, **116**, 913–919.

51 Rowan RM (1983) *Blood Cell Volume Analysis*. Albert Clark, London.

52 Paterakis GS, Laoutaris NP, Alexia SV, Siourounis PV, Stamulakatou AK, Premitis EE *et al.* (1993) The effect of red cell shape on the measurement of red cell volume. A proposed method for the comparative assessment of this effect among various haematology analysers. *Clin Lab Haematol*, **16**, 235–245.

53 Igout J, Fretigny M, Vasse M, Callat MP, Silva M, Willemont L *et al.* (2004) Evaluation of the Coulter LH750 haematology analyser compared with flow cytometry as the reference method for WBC, platelet and nucleated RBC count. *Clin Lab Haematol*, **26**, 1–7.

54 Zini G, d'Onofrio G, Garzia M and di Mario A (2005) *Citologia Ematologica in Automazione*. Verduci Editore, Rome.

55 Banfi G, Di Gaetano N, Lopez RS and Melegati G (2007) Decreased mean sphered cell volume values in top-level rugby players are related to the intravascular hemolysis induced by exercise. *Lab Hematol*, **13**, 103–107.

56 Urrechaga E (2010) The new mature red cell parameter, low haemoglobin density of the Beckman-Coulter LH750: clinical utility in the diagnosis of iron deficiency. *Int J Lab Hematol*, **32**, e144–150.

57 Dopsaj V, Martinovic J and Dopsaj M (2014) Early detection of iron deficiency in elite athletes: could microcytic anemia factor (Maf) be useful? *Int J Lab Hematol*, **36**, 37–44.

58 Shelat SG, Canfield W and Shibutani S (2010) Differences in detecting blasts between ADVIA 2120 and Beckman-Coulter LH750 hematology analyzers. *Int J Lab Hematol*, **32**, 113–116.

59 Fourcade C, Casbas MJ, Belaouni H, Gonzalez JJ, Garcia PJ and Pepio MA (2004) Automated detection of malaria by means of the haematology analyser Coulter GEN.S. *Clin Lab Haematol*, **26**, 367–372.

60 Sharma P, Bhargava M, Sukhachev D, Datta S and Wattal C (2014) LH750 hematology analyzers to identify malaria and dengue and distinguish them from other febrile illnesses. *Int J Lab Hematol*, **36**, 45–55.

61 Kim SY, Kim JE, Kim HK, Han KS and Toh CH (2010) Accuracy of platelet counting by automated hematologic analyzers in acute leukemia and disseminated intravascular coagulation: potential effects of platelet activation. *Am J Clin Pathol*, **134**, 634–647.

62 Latger-Cannard V, Hoarau M, Salignac S, Baumgart D, Nurden P and Lecompte T (2012) Mean platelet volume: comparison of three analysers towards standardization of platelet morphological phenotype. *Int J Lab Hematol*, **34**, 300–310.

63 Chaves F, Tierno B and Xu D (2005) Quantitative determination of neutrophil VCS parameters by the Coulter automated hematology analyzer. *Am J Clin Pathol*, **124**, 440–444.

64 Bagdasaryan R, Zhou Z, Tierno B, Rosenman D and Xu D (2007) Neutrophil VCS parameters are superior indicators for acute infection. *Lab Hematol*, **13**, 12–16.

65 Mardi D, Fwity B, Lobmann R and Ambrosch A (2010) Mean cell volume of neutrophils and monocytes compared with C-reactive protein, interleukin-6 and white blood cell count for prediction of sepsis and nonsystemic bacterial infections. *Int J Lab Hematol*, **32**, 410–418.

66 Charafeddine KM, Youssef AM, Mahfouz RA, Sarieddine DS and Daher RT (2011) Comparison of neutrophil volume distribution width to C-reactive protein and procalcitonin as a proposed new marker of acute infection. *Scand J Infect Dis*, **43**, 777–784.

67 Zhu Y, Cao X, Chen Y, Zhang K, Wang Y, Yuan K and Xu D (2012) Neutrophil cell population data: useful indicators for postsurgical bacterial infection. *Int J Lab Hematol*, **34**, 295–299.

68 Koenig S and Quillen K (2010) Using neutrophil and lymphocyte VCS indices in ambulatory pediatric patients presenting with fever. *Int J Lab Hematol*, **32**, 459–451.

69 Celik IH, Demirel G, Sukhachev D, Erdeve O and Dilman U (2013) Neutrophil volume, conductivity and scatter parameters with effective modeling of molecular activity statistical program gives better results in neonatal sepsis. *Int J Lab Hematol*, **35**, 82–87.

70 Bhargava M, Saluja S, Sindhuri U, Saraf A and Sharma P (2014) Elevated mean neutrophil volume+CRP is a highly sensitive and specific predictor of neonatal sepsis. *Int J Lab Hematol*, **36**, e11–e14.

71 Wiesent T, von Weikersthal L, Pujol N (2005) Automated detection of neutrophil dysplasia for the screening of myelodysplasia and myelodysplastic syndromes. *Blood*, **106**, 303b.

72 Miguel A, Orero M, Simon R, Collado R, Perez PL, Pacios A *et al.* (2007) Automated neutrophil morphology and its utility in the assessment of neutrophil dysplasia. *Lab Hematol*, **13**, 98–102.

73 Urrechaga E, Borque L and Escanero JF (2011) Analysis of reticulocyte parameters on the Sysmex XE 5000 and LH 750 analyzers in the diagnosis of inefficient erythropoiesis. *Int J Lab Hematol*, **33**, 37–44.

74 Urrechaga E, Unceta M, Borque L and Escanero JF (2012) Low hemoglobin density potential marker of iron availability. *Int J Lab Hematol*, **34**, 47–51.

75 Senzel L, Kube B, Lou M, Gibbs A, Ahmed T and Brent Hall (2013) Contamination of patient blood samples by avian RBCs from control material during automated hematology analysis. *Am J Clin Pathol*, **140**, 127–131.

76 Hedley BD, Keeney M, Chin-Yee I and Brown W (2010) Initial performance evaluation of the UniCel® DxH 800 Coulter® cellular analysis system. *Int J Lab Hematol*, **33**, 45–56.

77 Jean A, Boutet C, Lenormand B, Callat M-P, Buchonnet G, Barbay V *et al.* (2011) The new haematology analyzer DxH 800: an evaluation of the analytical performances and leucocyte flags, comparison with the LH 755. *Int J Lab Hematol*, **33**, 138–145.

78 Barnes PW, Eby CS and Shimer G (2010) Blast flagging with the UniCel DxH 800 Coulter Cellular Analysis System. *Lab Hematol*, **16**, 23–25.

79 Tan BT, Nava AJ and George TI (2011) Evaluation of the Beckman Coulter UniCel DxH 800, Beckman Coulter LH 780, and Abbott Diagnostics Cell-Dyn Sapphire Hematology

Analyzers on adult specimens in a tertiary care hospital. *Am J Clin Pathol*, **135**, 939–951.

80 Tan BT, Nava AJ and George TI (2011) Evaluation of the Beckman Coulter UniCel DxH 800 and Abbott Diagnostics Cell-Dyn Sapphire Hematology Analyzers on pediatric and neonatal specimens in a tertiary care hospital. *Am J Clin Pathol*, **135**, 929–938.

81 Kwon M-J, Nam M-H, Kim SH, Lim CS, Lee CK, Cho Y *et al.* (2011) Evaluation of the nucleated red blood cell count in neonates using the Beckman Coulter UniCel DxH 800 analyzer. *Int J Lab Hematol*, **33**, 620–628.

82 Park D-H, Park K, Park J, Park H-H, Chae H, Lim J *et al.* (2011) Screening of sepsis using leukocyte cell population data from the Coulter automatic blood cell analyzer DxH800. *Int J Lab Hematol*, **33**, 391–399.

83 Kahng J, Yahng SA, Lee JW, Kim Y, Kim M, Oh E-J *et al.* (2014) Novel markers of early neutrophilic and monocytic engraftment after hematopoietic stem cell transplantation. *Ann Lab Med*, **34**, 92–97.

84 Lee HK, Kim SI, Chae H, Kim M, Lim J, Oh EJ *et al.* (2012) Sensitive detection and accurate monitoring of *Plasmodium vivax* parasites on routine complete blood count using automatic blood cell analyzer (DxH800™). *Int J Lab Hematol*, **34**, 201–207.

85 Kim J-E, Kim B-R, Woo K-S and Han J-Y (2012) Evaluation of the leukocyte differential on a new automated flow cytometry hematology analyzer. *Int J Lab Hematol*, **34**, 547–550.

86 Park BG, Park C-J, Kim S, Yoon C-H, Kim D-H, Jang S and Chi H-S (2012) Comparison of the Cytodiff flow cytometric leucocyte differential count system with the Sysmex XE-2100 and Beckman Coulter UniCel DxH 800. *Int J Lab Hematol*, **34**, 584–593.

87 Jo Y, Kim SH, Koh K, Park J, Shim YB, Lim J *et al.* (2011) Reliable, accurate determination of the leukocyte differential of leukopenic samples by using hematoflow method. *Korean J Lab Med*, **31**, 131–137.

88 Gowans ID, Hepburn MD, Clark DM, Patterson G, Rawlinson PSM and Bowen DT (1999) The role of the Sysmex SE9000 immature myeloid index and Sysmex R2000 reticulocyte parameters in optimizing the timing of peripheral blood stem cell harvesting in patients with lymphoma and myeloma. *Clin Lab Haematol*, **21**, 331–336.

89 Ruzicka K, Veitl M, Thalhammer-Scherrer R and Schwarzinger I (2001) The new hematology analyzer Sysmex XE-2100; performance evaluation of a novel white blood cell differential technology. *Arch Pathol Lab Med*, **125**, 391–396.

90 Briggs C, Harrison P, Grant D, Staves J, and Machin SJ (2000) New quantitative parameters on a recently introduced automated blood cell counter—the XE 2100. *Clin Lab Haematol*, **22**, 345–350.

91 Briggs C, Kunka A and Machin SJ (2004) The most accurate platelet count on the Sysmex XE-2100. Optical or impedance? *Clin Lab Haematol*, **26**, 157–158.

92 Briggs C, Kunka S, Hart D, Oguni S and Machin SJ (2005) Assessment of an immature platelet fraction (IPF) in peripheral thrombocytopenia. *Br J Haematol*, **126**, 93–99.

93 Pai S (2012) Pseudobasophilia on the Sysmex-XE 2100: a useful screening tool for primary dengue infection in endemic areas. *Int J Lab Hematol*, **34**, Suppl. 1, 25.

94 Grotto HZW and Noronha JFA (2004) Platelet larger cell ratio (P-LCR) in patients with dyslipidemia. *Clin Lab Haematol*, **26**, 347–349.

95 Kaito K, Otsubo H, Usui N, Yoshida M, Tanno J, Kurihara E *et al.* (2005) Platelet size deviation width, platelet large cell ratio, and mean platelet volume have sufficient sensitivity and specificity in the diagnosis of immune thrombocytopenia, *Br J Haematol*, **128**, 698–702.

96 Ansari-Lari MA, Kickler TS and Borowitz MJ (2003) Immature granulocyte measurement using the Sysmex XE-2100. *Am J Clin Pathol*, **120**, 795–799.

97 Furundarena JR, Araiz M, Uranga M, Sainz MR, Agirre A, Trassorras M *et al.* (2010) The utility of the Sysmex XE-2100 analyzer's NEUT-X and NEUT-Y parameters for detecting neutrophil dysplasia in myelodysplastic syndromes. *Int J Lab Hematol*, **32**, 360–366.

98 Agorasti A, Nikolakopoulou E, Mitroglou V and Konstantinidou D (2012) The structural parameter NEUT-X in vitamin B12 deficiency. *Int J Lab Hematol*, **34**, Suppl. 1, 74.

99 Jain M, Gupta S, Jain J and Grover RK (2012) Usefulness of automated cell counter in detection of malaria in a cancer set up – our experience. *Indian J Pathol Microbiol*, **55**, 467–473.

100 Dubreuil P, Pihet M, Cau S, Croquefer S, Deguigne PA, Godon A *et al.* (2014) Use of Sysmex XE-2100 and XE-5000 hematology analyzers for the diagnosis of malaria in a non-endemic country (France). *Int J Lab Hematol*, **36**, 124–134.

101 Gulati GL, Bourne S, El Jamal SM, Florea AD and Gong J (2011) Automated lymphocyte counts vs manual lymphocyte counts in chronic lymphocytic leukemia patients. *Lab Med*, **42**, 545–548.

102 Amundsen EK, Urdal P, Hagve TA, Holthe MR and Henriksson CE (2012) Absolute neutrophil counts from automated hematology instruments are accurate and precise even at very low levels. *Am J Clin Pathol*, **137**, 862–869.

103 Amundsen EK, Henriksson CE, Holthe MR and Urdal P (2012) Is the blood basophil count sufficiently precise, accurate, and specific?: three automated hematology instruments and flow cytometry compared. *Am J Clin Pathol*, **137**, 86–92.

104 Otsubo H, Kaito K, Asai O, Usui N, Kobayashi M and Hoshi Y (2005) Persistent nucleated red blood cells in peripheral blood is a poor prognostic factor in patients undergoing stem cell transplantation. *Clin Lab Haematol*, **27**, 242–246.

105 Pollard Y, Watts MJ, Grant D, Chavda N, Linch DC and Machin SJ (1999) Use of the haemopoietic progenitor cell count of the Sysmex SE-9500 to refine apheresis timing of peripheral blood stem cells. *Br J Haematol*, **106**, 538–544.

106 Buttarello M and Plebani M (2008) Automated blood cell counts: state of the art. *Am J Clin Pathol*, **130**, 104–116.

107 Banno S, Ito Y, Tanaka C, Hori T, Fujimoto K, Suzuki T *et al.* (2005) Quantification of red blood cell fragmentation by the automated hematology analyzer XE-2100 in patients with living donor liver transplantation. *Clin Lab Haematol*, **27**, 292–296.

108 Lesesve J-F, Asnafi V, Braun F and Zini G (2012) Fragmented red blood cells automated measurement is a useful parameter to exclude schistocytes on the blood film. *Int J Lab Hematol*, **34**, 566–576.

109 Schoorl M, Snijders D, Schoorl M, Boersma WG and Bartels PC (2012) Temporary impairment of reticulocyte haemoglobin content in subjects with community-acquired pneumonia. *Int J Lab Hematol*, **34**, 390–395.

110 Franck S, Linssen J, Messinger M and Thomas L (2004) Potential utility of Ret-Y in the diagnosis of iron-restricted erythropoiesis. *Clin Chem*, **50**, 1240–1242.

111 Miwa N, Akiba T, Kimata N, Hamaguchi Y, Arakawa Y, Tamura T *et al.* (2010) Usefulness of measuring reticulocyte hemoglobin equivalent in the management of haemodialysis patients with iron deficiency. *Int J Lab Hematol*, **32**, 248–255.

112 Sudmann ÅA, Piehler A and Urdal P (2012) Reticulocyte hemoglobin equivalent to detect thalassemia and thalassemic hemoglobin variants. *Int J Lab Hematol*, **24**, 605–613.

113 Yamaoka G, Kubota Y, Nomura T, Inage T, Arai T, Kitanaka A *et al.* (2010) The immature platelet fraction is a useful marker for predicting the timing of platelet recovery in patients with cancer after chemotherapy and hematopoietic stem cell transplantation. *Int J Lab Hematol*, **32**, e208–e216.

114 Nomura T, Kubota Y, Kitanaka A, Kurokouchi K, Inage T, Saigo K *et al.* (2010) Immature platelet fraction measurement in patients with chronic liver disease: a convenient marker for evaluating cirrhotic change. *Int J Lab Hematol*, **32**, 299–306.

115 Sugimori N, Kondo Y, Shibayama M, Omote M, Takami A, Sugimori C *et al.* (2009) Aberrant increase in the immature platelet fraction in patients with myelodysplastic syndrome: a marker of karyotypic abnormalities associated with poor prognosis. *Eur J Haematol*, **81**, 54–60.

116 Urrechaga E, Borque L and Escanero JF (2011) Erythrocyte and reticulocyte parameters in iron deficiency and thalassaemia. *J Clin Lab Anal*, **25**, 223–228.

117 Urrechaga E, Borque L and Escanero JF (2011) The role of automated measurement of red cell subpopulations on the Sysmex XE 5000 analyzer in the differential diagnosis of microcytic anemia. *Int J Lab Hematol*, **33**, 30–36.

118 Urrechaga E, Borque L and Escanero JF (2011) The role of automated measurement of RBC subpopulations in differential diagnosis of microcytic anemia and β-thalassemia screening. *Am J Clin Pathol*, **135**, 374–379.

119 Buttarello M, Pajola R, Novello E, Rebeschini M, Cantaro S, Oliosi F *et al.* (2010) Diagnosis of iron deficiency in patients undergoing hemodialysis. *Am J Clin Pathol*, **133**, 949–954.

120 Chalvatzi K, Spiroglou S, Nikolaidou A and Diza E (2013) Evaluation of fragmented red cell (FRC) counting using Sysmex XE-5000 – Does hypochromia play a role? *Int J Lab Hematol*, **35**, 193–199.

121 Briggs CJ, Linssen J, Longair I and Machin SJ (2011) Improved flagging rates on the Sysmex XE-5000 compared with the XE-2100 reduce the number of manual film reviews and increase laboratory productivity. *Am J Clin Pathol*, **136**, 309–316.

122 Eilertsen H, Vøllestad NK and Hagve T-A (2013) The usefulness of blast flags on the Sysmex XE-5000 is questionable. *Am J Clin Pathol*, **139**, 633–640.

123 Pozdnyakova O and Dorfman DM (2013) Sysmex XE-5000 Blast Q Flag Analysis. *Am J Clin Pathol*, **140**, 918–919.

124 Briggs C, Longair I, Kumar P, Singh D and Machin S (2012) Performance evaluation of the Sysmex XN modular system. *J Clin Pathol*, **65**, 1024–1030.

125 Hotton J, Broothaers J, Swaelens C and Cantinieaux B (2013) Performance and abnormal cell flagging comparisons of three automated blood cell counters: Cell-Dyn Sapphire, DxH-800, and XN-2000. *Am J Clin Pathol*, **140**, 845–852.

126 Leers MPG, Goertz H, Feller A and Hoffmann JJML (2011) Performance evaluation of the Abbott CELL-DYN Ruby and the Sysmex XT-2000i haematology analysers. *Int J Lab Hematol*, **33**, 19–29.

127 Mohandas N, Kim YR, Tycko DH, Orlik J, Wyatt J and Groner W (1986) Accurate and independent measurement of volume and hemoglobin concentration of individual red cells by laser light scattering. *Blood*, **68**, 506–513.

128 von Feltan U, Furlan M, Frey R and Bucher U (1978) Test of a new method for hemoglobin determinations in automatic analysers. *Med Lab*, **31**, 223–231.

129 Breymann C, Rohling R, Krafft A, Huch A and Huch R (2000) 'Blood doping' with recombinant erythropoietin (rhEPO) and assessment of functional iron deficiency in healthy volunteers. *Br J Haematol*, **108**, 883–888.

130 Thomas C and Thomas L (2002) Biochemical markers and hematologic indices in the diagnosis of functional iron deficiency. *Clin Chem*, **8**, 1066–1076.

131 Tsakonas DP, Tsakona CP, Worman CP, Goldstone AH and Nicolaides KH (1994) Myeloperoxidase activity and nuclear segmentation of maternal neutrophils during normal pregnancy. *Clin Lab Haematol*, **16**, 337–342.

132 Chapman DH, Hardin J-A, Miers M, Moyle S and Kinney MC (2001) Reduction of the platelet review rate using two-dimensional platelet method. *Am J Clin Pathol*, **115**, 894–898.

133 Brummitt DR and Barker HF (2000) The determination of a reference range for new platelet parameters produced by the Bayer ADVIA™120 full blood count analyser. *Clin Lab Haematol*, **22**, 103–107.

134 Meintker L, Ringwald J, Rauh M and Krause SW (2013) Comparison of automated differential blood cell counts from Abbott Sapphire, Siemens Advia 120, Beckman

Coulter DxH 800, and Sysmex XE-2100 in normal and pathologic samples. *Am J Clin Pathol*, **139**, 641–650.

135 Greenfield HM, Sweeney DA, Newton RK, Leather A, Murray J, Angelica R *et al.* (2005) Estimation of haematopoietic progenitor cells in peripheral blood by the Advia 120 and BD vantage flow cytometer: a direct comparison for the prediction of adequate collections. *Clin Lab Haematol*, **27**, 287–291.

136 Kratz A, Maloum K, O'Malley C, Zini G, Rocco V, Zelmanovic D and Kling G (2006) Enumeration of nucleated red blood cells with the ADVIA 2120 Hematology System: an International Multicenter Clinical Trial. *Lab Hematol*, **12**, 63–70.

137 Cornbleet PJ, Myrick D, Judkins S and Levy R (1992) Evaluation of the CELL-DYN 3000 differential. *Am J Clin Pathol*, **98**, 603–614.

138 Kim YR, Yee M, Metha S, Chupp V, Kendall R and Scott CS (1998) Simultaneous differentiation and quantification of erythroblasts and white blood cells on a high throughput clinical haematology analyser. *Clin Lab Haematol*, **20**, 21–29.

139 Grimaldi E and Scopacasa F (2000) Evaluation of the Abbott CELL-DYN 4000 hematology analyzer. *Am J Clin Pathol*, **113**, 497–505.

140 Hoedemakers RMJ, Pennings JMA and Hoffmann JJML (1999) Performance characteristics of blast flaging on the Cell-Dyn 4000 haematology analyser. *Clin Lab Haematol*, **21**, 347–351.

141 Hoffmann JJML and Hoedemakers RMJ (2004) Diagnostic performance of the variant lymphocyte flag of the Abbott Cell-Dyn 4000 haematology analyser. *Clin Lab Haematol*, **26**, 9–13.

142 Gill JE, Davis KA, Cowart WJ, Nepacena FU and Kim Y-T (2000) A rapid and accurate closed-tube immunoassay for platelets on an automated hematology analyzer. *Am J Clin Pathol*, **114**, 47–56.

143 Kunz D, Kunz WS, Scott CS and Gressner AM (2001) Automated CD61 immunoplatelet analysis of thrombocytopenic samples. *Br J Haematol*, **112**, 584–592.

144 Molera T, Roemer B, del Mar Perera Alvarez M, Lemes A, de la Iglesia Iñigo S, Palacios G and Scott CS (2005) Analysis and enumeration of T cells, B cells and NK cells using the monoclonal antibody fluorescence capability of a routine haematology analyser (Cell-Dyn CD4000). *Clin Lab Haematol*, **27**, 224–234.

145 Little BH, Robson R, Roemer B and Scott CS (2005) Immunocytometric quantitation of foeto-maternal haemorrhage with the Abbott Cell-Dyn CD4000 haematology analyser. *Clin Lab Haematol*, **27**, 21–31.

146 Scott CS, Zyl D, Ho E, Meyersfeld D, Ruivo L, Mendelow BV and Coetzer TL (2003) Automated detection of malaria-associated intraleucocytic haemozoin by Cell-Dyn CD4000 depolarization analysis. *Clin Lab Haematol*, **25**, 77–86.

147 Hänscheid T, Romão R, Grobusch MP, Amaral T and Melo-Cristino J (2011) Limitation of malaria diagnosis with the Cell-Dyn® analyser: not all haemozoin-containing monocytes are detected or shown. *Int J Lab Hematol*, **33**, e14–e16.

148 Ermens AA, Hoffmann JJ, Krokenberger M and Van Wijk EM (2012) New erythrocyte and reticulocyte parameters on CELL-DYN Sapphire: analytical and preanalytical aspects. *Int J Lab Hematol*, **34**, 274–282.

149 Khoo T-L, Xiros N, Guan F, Orellana D, Holst J *et al.* (2013) Performance evaluation of the Abbott CELL-DYN Emerald for use as a bench-top analyzer in a research setting. *Int J Lab Hematol*, **35**, 447–456.

150 Lacombe F, Lacoste L, Vial J-P, Briais A, Reiffers J, Boisseau MR and Bernard P (1999) Automated reticulocyte counting and immature reticulocyte fraction measurements. *Am J Clin Pathol*, **112**, 677–685.

151 Doretto P, Biasioli B, Casolari B, Pasini L, Bulian P, Buttarello M *et al.* (2011) Conteggio reticulocitario automizzato: valutazione NCCLS H-44 ed ICSH su 5 strumenti. In: Cenci A and Cappelletti P (eds) *Appunti di Ematologia di Laboratorio*. MAF Servizi Editore, Turin.

152 Riley RS, Ben-Ezra JM and Tidwell A (2001) Reticulocyte enumeration: past & present. *Lab Med*, **10**, 599–608.

153 Briggs C, Grant D and Machin SJ (2001) Comparison of the automated reticulocyte counts and immature reticulocyte fraction measurements obtained with the ABX Pentra 120 Retic blood cell analyzer and the Sysmex XE-2100 automated haematology analyzer. *Lab Haematol*, **7**, 1–6.

154 Watanabe K, Kawai Y, Takeuchi K, Shimizu N, Iri H, Ikeda Y and Houwen B (1994) Reticulocyte maturity as an indicator for estimating qualitative abnormality of erythropoiesis. *J Clin Pathol*, **47**, 736–739.

155 Daliphard S, Bizet M, Callat MP, Beufe S, Latouche JB, Soufiani H and Monconduit M (1993) Evaluation of reticulocyte subtype distribution in myelodysplastic syndromes. *Am J Hematol*, **44**, 210–220.

156 Torres Gomez A, Casano J, Sanchez J, Madrigal E, Blanco F and Alvarez MA (2003) Utility of reticulocyte maturation parameters in the differential diagnosis of macrocytic anemias. *Clin Lab Haematol*, **25**, 283–288.

157 Kendall RG, Mellors I, Hardy J and McArdle B (2001) Patients with pulmonary and cardiac disease show an elevated proportion of immature reticulocytes. *Clin Lab Haematol*, **23**, 27–31.

158 Grotto HZW, Vigoritto AC, Noronha JFA and Lima GALM (1999) Immature reticulocyte fraction as a criterion for marrow engraftment. Evaluation of a semi-automated reticulocyte counting method. *Clin Lab Haematol*, **23**, 285–287.

159 Sica S, Sora F, Laurenti L, Piccirillo N, Salutari P, Chiusolo P *et al.* (1999) Highly fluorescent reticulocyte count predicts haemopoietic recovery after immunosuppression for severe aplastic anaemia. *Clin Lab Haematol*, **21**, 387–389.

160 Robinson M, Machin S, Mackie I and Harrison P (2000) *In vivo* biotinylation studies: specificity of labelling of reticulated platelets by thiazole orange and mepacrine. *Br J Haematol*, **108**, 859–864.

161 Robinson M, Mackie I, Machin S and Harrison P (2000) Technological methods: two colour analysis of reticulated platelets. *Clin Lab Haematol*, **22**, 211–213.

162 Romp KG, Peters WP and Hoffman M (1994) Reticulated platelet counts in patients undergoing autologous bone marrow transplantation: an aid in assessing marrow recovery. *Am J Hematol*, **46**, 319–324.

163 Kurata Y, Hayashi S, Kiyoi T, Kosugi S, Kashiwagi H, Honda S and Tomiyama Y (2001) Diagnostic value of tests for reticulated platelets, plasma glycocalicin, and thrombopoietin levels for discriminating between hyperdestructive and hypoplastic thrombocytopenia. *Am J Clin Pathol*, **115**, 656–664.

164 Koh K-R, Yamane T, Ohta K, Hino M, Takubo T and Tatsumi N (1999) Pathophysiological significance of simultaneous measurement of reticulated platelets, large platelets and serum thrombopoietin in non-neoplastic thrombocytopenic disorders. *Eur J Haematol*, **63**, 295–301.

165 Huisman A and de Vooght K (2012) Differences in point-of-care versus central laboratory hemoglobin level due to extreme leucocytosis. *Int J Lab Hematol*, **34**, Suppl. 1, 119.

166 Lewis SM, Scott GJ and Wynn KJ (1998) An inexpensive and reliable new haemoglobin colour scale for assessing anaemia. *J Clin Pathol*, **51**, 21–24.

167 Anonymous (2000) Hemoglobin, hematocrit, and WBCs in the microcirculation. *Lab Med*, **31**, 440–441.

168 Berrebi A and Fine I (1999) Non-invasive measurement of hemoglobin/hematocrit over a wide clinical range using a new optical signal processing method. *Blood*, **94**, Suppl. 1, Part 2, 10b.

169 Kinoshita Y, Yamane T, Takubo T, Kanashima H, Kamitani T, Tatsumi N and Hino M (2002) Measurement of hemoglobin concentrations using the Astrim™ non-invasive blood vessel monitoring apparatus. *Acta Haematol*, **108**, 109–110.

170 Saigo K, Imoto S, Hashimoto M, Mito H, Moriya J, Chinzei T *et al.* (2004) Noninvasive monitoring of hemoglobin: the effects of WBC counts on measurement. *Am J Clin Pathol*, **121**, 51–55.

171 Shah N, Osea EA and Martinez GJ (2014) Accuracy of noninvasive hemoglobin and invasive point-of-care hemoglobin testing compared with a laboratory analyzer. *Int J Lab Hematol*, **36**, 56–61.

172 Wood BL, Andrews J, Miller S and Sabath DE (1999) Refrigerated storage improves the stability of the complete blood count and automated differential. *Am J Clin Pathol*, **112**, 687–695.

CHAPTER 3
Morphology of blood cells

Examining the blood film

Blood films should be examined in a systematic manner, as follows.

1 Patient identification should be checked and confirmed and the microscope slide matched with the corresponding full blood count (FBC) report. The sex and age of the patient should be noted, since the blood film cannot be interpreted without this information. In a multiracial community it is also helpful to know the ethnic origin of the patient.

2 The film should be examined macroscopically to confirm adequate spreading and to look for any unusual spreading or staining characteristics. The commonest macroscopic abnormality is an increased blue coloration caused by hypergammaglobulinaemia (Fig. 3.1) due either to a paraprotein, e.g. in multiple myeloma and related conditions, or to a reactive increase in immunoglobulins, e.g. in cirrhosis or rheumatoid arthritis. Abnormal staining characteristics are also caused by the presence of foreign substances such as heparin, which conveys a pink tinge, or the vehicles of certain intravenous drugs. Occasionally, macroscopic abnormalities are caused by precipitation of cryoglobulin, gross red cell agglutination, platelet clumping or the presence of clumps of tumour cells (Figs 3.2–3.4).

3 The film should be examined microscopically, using a microscope correctly set up to give optimal illumination. Examination should take place first under a low power (e.g. with the × 10 or × 25 objective) and then with a higher power (× 40 or × 50 objective) with an eyepiece magnification of × 10 or × 12. It is only necessary to use oil immersion and a × 100 objective when observation of fine detail is required or when searching for malaria

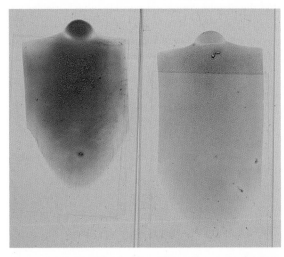

Fig. 3.1 Blood film of a patient with multiple myeloma (left) compared with another blood film stained in the same batch (right). The deeper blue staining occurs because the high concentration of immunoglobulin leads to increased uptake of the basic component of the stain.

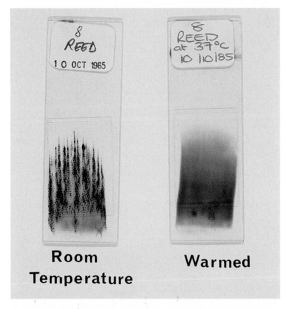

Fig. 3.2 Blood films from a patient with a potent cold agglutinin. The left-hand film, which shows marked agglutination, was prepared from ethylenediaminetetra-acetic acid (EDTA)-anticoagulated blood that had been standing at room temperature. The right-hand film, which shows no macroscopic agglutination, was prepared from blood warmed to 37°C.

Blood Cells A Practical Guide, Fifth Edition. By Barbara J. Bain © 2015 John Wiley & Sons, Ltd. Published 2015 by John Wiley & Sons, Ltd.
Companion Website: www.wiley.com/go/bain/bloodcells

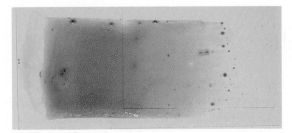

Fig. 3.3 Blood film from a patient with multiple myeloma showing cryoglobulin precipitates. Courtesy of Dr Sue Fairhead, London.

parasites. Laboratories using unmounted films may find it useful to have a × 50 oil immersion objective in addition to a × 100. It should be noted that some immersion oils can cause contact dermatitis and care should therefore be exercised in their use [1]. The use of a relatively low power is important since it allows rapid scanning of a large part of the film and facilitates the detection of abnormal cells when they are present at a low frequency. It is also useful in the appreciation of rouleaux

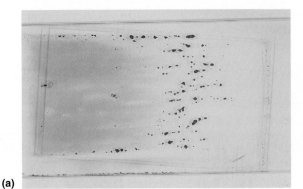

(a)

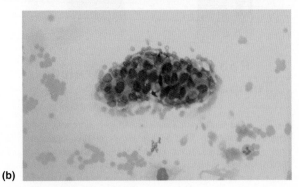

(b)

Fig. 3.4 Blood film showing visible aggregates of tumour cells: (a) macroscopic photograph of slide; (b) photomicrograph, low power, showing that the visible masses are clumps of tumour cells. Courtesy of Dr Sue Fairhead.

and red cell and white cell agglutination. Examination of the blood film must also include examination of the edges and the tail, since large abnormal cells and clumps of cells are often distributed preferentially in these areas. Platelet aggregates and fibrin strands, if present, are often found in the tail of the film.

On placing a film under the microscope, the first decision to be made is whether or not it is suitable for further examination. Spreading, fixation and staining must be satisfactory and there should be no artefactual changes produced by excess ethylenediaminetetra-acetic acid (EDTA) or prolonged storage. It is unwise to give an opinion on an inadequate blood film. A well-spread film should have an appreciable area where cells are a monolayer, i.e. where they are touching but not overlapping. White cells should be distributed regularly without undue concentration along the edges or in the tail, such as occurs when the film is spread too thinly. Granulocytes are found preferentially along the edges and in the tail of a wedge-spread film and lymphocytes are preferentially in the centre, but in a carefully spread film the difference is not great.

Blood films should be examined for platelet aggregates (Fig. 3.5), which may cause the platelet count to be falsely low, or fibrin strands (Fig. 3.6), which indicate partial clotting of the sample with the likelihood that the platelet count and possibly other variables are invalid. Platelets that have discharged their granules following aggregation may appear as pale blue masses not immediately identifiable as platelets.

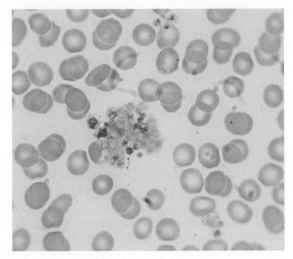

Fig. 3.5 Platelet aggregate in a blood film. Following aggregation, some of the platelets have discharged their granule contents and thus appear grey.

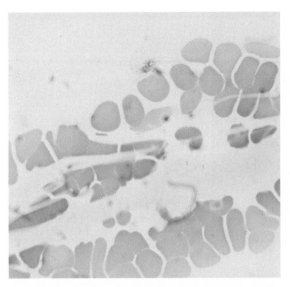

Fig. 3.6 Fibrin strands in a blood film from a patient with a hypercoagulable state. The fibrin strands are very weakly basophilic and cause deformation of the red cells between which they pass. Fibrin strands can also form when there has been partial clotting of a blood specimen because of difficulty in venepuncture.

Storage-induced and other artefacts

Blood films should be made without delay, but laboratories that receive specimens by post or transported from a distance should be aware of the changes induced by storage. Prolonged storage of EDTA-anticoagulated blood causes loss of central pallor simulating spherocytosis [2], crenation or echinocytic changes in red cells (Fig. 3.7), degeneration of neutrophils (see Fig. 3.7) and lobulation of some lymphocyte nuclei (Fig. 3.8). Excess EDTA may itself cause crenation of red cells and also accelerates the development of storage changes. Degenerating neutrophils may have a similar appearance to apoptotic neutrophils formed *in vivo* (see Fig. 3.103) or may be completely amorphous. If there has been prolonged delay in the blood specimen reaching the laboratory, e.g. 3 days or more, most of the neutrophils will have degenerated and the white blood cell count (WBC) will have fallen as a consequence. If an inexperienced laboratory worker does not recognise the storage artefact and attempts to perform a differential count, a factitious neutropenia and lymphocytosis will be recorded. Inexperienced observers may also misclassify neutrophils with a single rounded nuclear mass as nucleated red blood cells (NRBCs). Storage also leads to

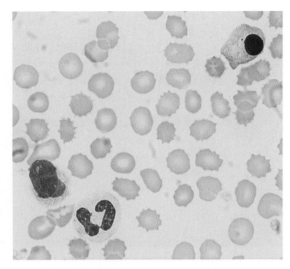

Fig. 3.7 Blood film showing storage artefact – crenation (echinocytosis), a disintegrated cell and a neutrophil with a rounded pyknotic nucleus.

artefactual changes in other components of the automated blood count.

Another unusual artefactual change is produced by accidentally heating samples, e.g. by transporting a blood specimen in a hot car [3]. This causes dramatic fragmentation of red cells (Fig. 3.9), which can be confused with hereditary pyropoikilocytosis.

Artefacts may also be attributable to drugs administered to patients. For example, polyoxyethylated castor

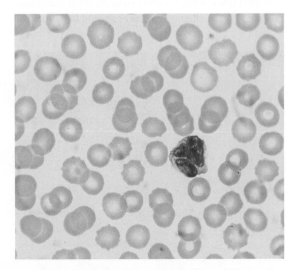

Fig. 3.8 Blood film showing storage artefact – mild crenation and lobulation of a lymphocyte nucleus.

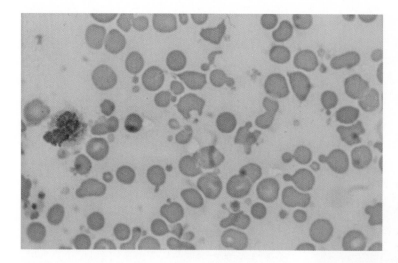

Fig. 3.9 Blood film from a blood specimen that has been transported in a hot motor vehicle, showing red cell budding and fragmentation.

oil, used to solubilise paclitaxel, causes large clear areas between cells, rouleaux formation and red cell aggregates [4].

If a blood film is regarded as suitable for further examination, then all cell types and also the background staining should be evaluated systematically. Increased background staining is usually due to an increase in immunoglobulins, either polyclonal or monoclonal. Abnormalities that may be noted between cells include crystals of monoclonal cryoglobulin [5,6] (Figs 3.10 & 3.11), amorphous cryoglobulin deposits (Fig. 3.12) and amorphous or fibrillar deposits that represent abnormal mucopolysaccharide that circulates in the blood of patients with malignant disease [7]. The film appearances should be compared

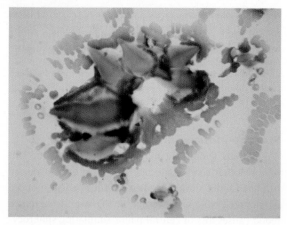

Fig. 3.10 Low power view of a blood film showing large cryoglobulin crystals.

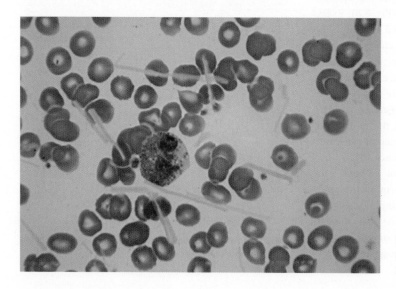

Fig. 3.11 Blood film showing crystals of cryoglobulin. By courtesy of Dr Poormina Kumar, London.

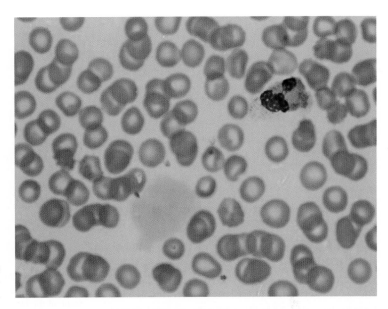

Fig. 3.12 Blood film showing an amorphous deposit of cryoglobulin; there is also phagocytosed cryoglobulin within the neutrophil.

with the FBC and a judgement made as to whether the WBC, haemoglobin concentration (Hb), mean cell volume (MCV) and platelet count are consistent with the film, or whether there is some unusual feature that could invalidate them. If the FBC and the film are inconsistent with each other, then the blood specimen should be inspected and the FBC – and if necessary the film – should be repeated. Such discrepancies may be due to: (i) a poorly mixed or partly clotted specimen; (ii) a specimen that is too small so that the instrument has aspirated an inadequate volume; or (iii) the blood film and FBC being derived from different blood specimens. If such technical errors are eliminated, discrepancy may be due to an abnormality in the specimen such as hyperlipidaemia or the presence of a cold agglutinin. Hyperlipidaemia may be suspected when there are blurred red cell outlines (Fig. 3.13) and red cell agglutinates are often present in the film when there is a cold agglutinin (Fig. 3.14). The validation of the blood count by comparison with the blood film and by other means is dealt with in Chapter 4.

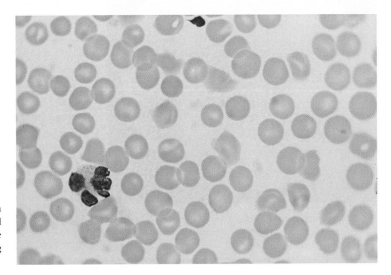

Fig. 3.13 Blood film from a patient with hyperlipidaemia showing misshapen red cells with fuzzy outlines and blurring of the outline of the lobes of a neutrophil resulting from the high concentration of lipids.

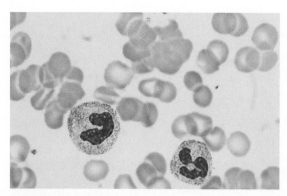

Fig. 3.14 Red cell agglutinates in the peripheral blood film of a patient with a high titre cold agglutinin.

Erythrocytes

The majority of normal red cells or erythrocytes are disciform in shape (Fig. 3.15) [8]; a minority are bowl-shaped. On a stained peripheral blood film they are approximately circular in outline and show only minor variations in shape and moderate variations in size (Fig. 3.16). The average diameter is about 7.5 μm. In the area of a film where cells form a monolayer, a paler central area occupies approximately the middle third of the cell.

The normal shape and flexibility of a red cell are dependent on the integrity of the cytoskeleton to which the lipid membrane is bound. An abnormal shape can be caused

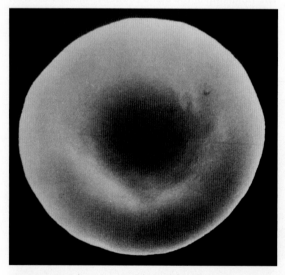

Fig. 3.15 Scanning electron micrograph of a normal red cell (discocyte). Courtesy of Professor Aaron Polliack, Jerusalem, from Hoffbrand and Pettit [8].

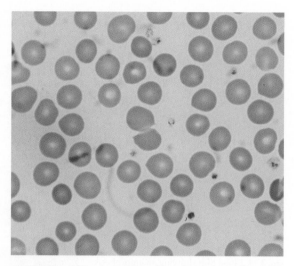

Fig. 3.16 Blood film of a healthy subject showing normal red cells and platelets. The red cells show little variation in size and shape. Some of the platelets show granules dispersed through the cytoplasm, while others have a granulomere and a hyalomere.

by a primary defect of the cytoskeleton or membrane or be secondary to red cell fragmentation or to polymerisation, crystallisation or precipitation of haemoglobin. The red cell membrane is a lipid bilayer crossed by several transmembrane proteins, most importantly protein 3 and the glycophorins. The principal protein of the cytoskeleton is spectrin; heterodimers composed of α and β spectrin chains assemble into spectrin tetramers, which are bound to other spectrin tetramers to form a complex network. The cytoskeletal network is bound to the lipid bilayer by interactions of spectrin β chain with ankyrin and the transmembrane protein, band 3, and interactions of spectrin α and β chains with actin, protein 4.1 and the transmembrane protein, glycophorin C; the interaction of ankyrin with band 3 is modulated by protein 4.2 while the interaction of spectrin and actin is stabilised by interaction with protein 4.1 and adducin (see Fig. 3.36) [9].

Certain terms used to describe red cell morphology require definition. Two terms are used to describe cells of normal morphology: (i) normocytic, which means that the cells are of normal size; and (ii) normochromic, which means that the cells have the normal concentration of haemoglobin and therefore stain normally. Other descriptive terms imply that the morphology is abnormal and they should therefore not be used, when reporting blood films, to describe normal physiological variation. For example, the cells of a neonate should not be reported as 'macrocytic' since it is normal for the cells of a neonate to be larger than those of an adult. Similarly, the red cells of a healthy pregnant woman should not be reported as showing 'anisocytosis' or 'poikilocytosis', since no abnormality is present. Policy differs between laboratories as to whether every normal film is reported as being normocytic and normochromic or whether a comment on the red cell morphology is made only when it is abnormal or when it is particularly significant that it is normal. Either policy is acceptable as long as it is consistently applied and clinical staff are aware of it. If a patient is anaemic but the red cells are normocytic and normochromic, it is useful to say so since this narrows the diagnostic possibilities.

Anisocytosis

Anisocytosis is an increase in the variability of erythrocyte size beyond that which is observed in a normal healthy subject. Anisocytosis is a common, non-specific abnormality in haematological disorders. In automated instrument counts, an increase in the red cell distribution width (RDW) (see Chapter 2) is indicative of anisocytosis.

Microcytosis

Microcytosis is a decrease in the size of the erythrocytes. Microcytes are detected on a blood film by a reduction of red cell diameter to less than 7–7.2 μm (Fig. 3.17). The nucleus of a small lymphocyte, which has a diameter of approximately 8.5 μm, is a useful guide to the size

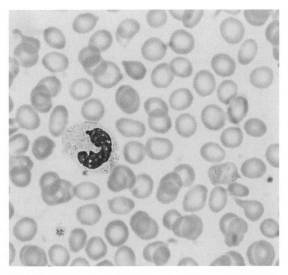

Fig. 3.17 Microcytosis in a patient with β thalassaemia trait; the MCV was 62 f1. The blood film also shows mild hypochromia, anisocytosis and poikilocytosis.

of a red cell. Microcytosis may be general or there may be a population of small red cells. If all or most of the red cells are small there is a reduction in the MCV, but a small population of microcytes can be present without the MCV falling below the reference range. Some of the causes of microcytosis are listed in Table 3.1.

Table 3.1 Some causes of microcytosis.

Inherited
β thalassaemia heterozygosity (β thalassaemia trait, β thalassaemia minor)
β thalassaemia homozygosity or compound heterozygosity (β thalassaemia major or intermedia)
δβ and γδβ thalassaemia heterozygosity or δβ thalassaemia homozygosity
Haemoglobin Lepore heterozygosity or homozygosity
Hereditary persistence of fetal haemoglobin homozygosity and some instances of heterozygosity (e.g. due to KLF1 inactivating mutation)
α^0 thalassaemia heterozygosity
α^+ thalassaemia homozygosity or, to a lesser extent, heterozygosity
Haemoglobin Constant Spring, haemoglobin Paksé and haemoglobin Quong Sze heterozygosity
Haemoglobin H disease
Sickle cell heterozygosity [10, 11] (disputed, see Chapter 8)
Haemoglobin C heterozygosity [10, 11] and homozygosity
Sickle cell/haemoglobin C disease [12]
Haemoglobin E heterozygosity [13] and homozygosity [14]
Haemoglobin D-Punjab (D-Los Angeles) heterozygosity
Heterozygosity for other rare abnormal haemoglobins producing thalassaemia-like conditions (e.g. haemoglobin Tak, haemoglobin Indianapolis)
Congenital sideroblastic anaemia
Atransferrinaemia
Ferrochelatase deficiency (erythropoietic protoporphyria) [15]
Hepatoerythropoietic porphyria [16]

(continued)

Table 3.1 (*Continued*)

Associated with iron overload but with absent bone marrow iron [17]
Associated with elliptocytosis [18]
Hereditary pyropoikilocytosis (as a result of red cell fragmentation)
Inherited iron malabsorption plus defect in incorporation of iron [19]
Acaeruloplasminaemia [20]
Copper deficiency [21]
Haem oxygenase deficiency [22]
Homozygosity [23] or compound heterozygosity [24] for *SLC11A2* gene encoding divalent metal transporter 1
Homozygosity for mutation in *GLRX5* gene encoding glutaredoxin [25] (one patient)
Bi-allelic mutation in the *TMPRSS6* gene (leading to iron-refractory iron deficiency anaemia) [26]
Majeed syndrome (congenital dyserythropoietic anaemia with osteomyelitis and dermatosis due to *LPIN2* mutation) [27]
Acquired
Iron deficiency (including bone marrow iron deficiency in pulmonary haemosiderosis)
Anaemia of chronic disease
Myelodysplastic syndromes, particularly but not only associated with acquired haemoglobin H disease [28]
Secondary acquired sideroblastic anaemia (e.g. caused by various drugs; some cases of lead poisoning and some cases of copper deficiency [29]
  or zinc excess with functional copper deficiency, e.g. ingestion of zinc-containing coins as a feature of mental illness) [30–32];?
  hyperzincaemia with hypercalprotectinaemia (nature of anaemia not specified) [33]
Hyperthyroidism [34]
Ascorbic acid deficiency (rarely) [35]
Cadmium poisoning [36]
Aluminium poisoning
Antibody to erythroblast transferrin receptor [37]

The red cells of healthy children are smaller than those of adults, whereas those of neonates are much larger, so that cell size must be interpreted in the light of the age of the subject. Microcytosis is uncommon in neonates but can occur in α thalassaemia disorders and when iron deficiency results from intrauterine blood loss; it is also likely that microcytosis is present at birth in congenital sideroblastic anaemia and atransferrinaemia. As a group, Black people have smaller red cells than Caucasians; this is likely to be largely the result of a high prevalence of α thalassaemia trait, together with a lower prevalence of β thalassaemia trait, haemoglobin C trait and other haemoglobinopathies that are associated with microcytosis, rather than to any intrinsic ethnic difference in red cell size.

Macrocytosis

Macrocytosis is an increase in the size of erythrocytes. The erythrocytes of neonates show a considerable degree of macrocytosis if they are assessed in relation to those of adults. Fetal red cells are also much larger than those of adults. A slight degree of macrocytosis is also seen as a physiological feature of pregnancy [38] and in older adults [39].

Macrocytosis is recognised on a blood film by an increase in cell diameter (Fig. 3.18). It may be a generalised change, in which case the MCV will be raised, or it may affect only a proportion of the red cells. Macrocytes may be round or oval in outline, the diagnostic significance being somewhat different. Some of the causes of macrocytosis are listed in Table 3.2.

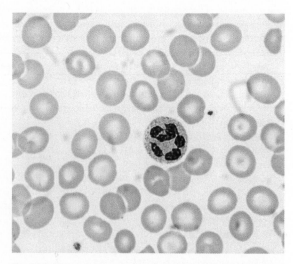

Fig. 3.18 Macrocytosis associated with liver disease; the MCV was 105 fl. Several target cells are also present.

Table 3.2 Some causes of macrocytosis.

Associated with reticulocytosis Haemolytic anaemia Haemorrhage	Ethanol intake Liver disease Phenytoin therapy Some cases of copper deficiency [45] Arsenic poisoning [46] ? Familial macrocytosis [47]

Associated with megaloblastic erythropoiesis
Vitamin B_{12} deficiency and inactivation of vitamin B_{12} by chronic
    exposure to nitric oxide
Folic acid deficiency, antifolate drugs (including methotrexate,
    pentamidine, pyrimethamine and trimethoprim and including
    methotrexate administered intrathecally [40]), cough mixture abuse [41]
Scurvy
Drugs interfering with DNA synthesis – used as anticancer
    drugs, immunosuppressive agents and in the treatment of the
    acquired immune deficiency syndrome (including doxorubicin,
    daunorubicin, azathioprine, mercaptopurine, cyclophosphamide,
    cytarabine, fluorouracil, hydroxycarbamide, procarbazine,
    tioguanine, zidovudine and stavudine)
Imatinib or sunitinib therapy (not only due to vitamin B_{12}
    deficiency) [42,43]
Rare inherited defects of DNA synthesis (including hereditary orotic
    aciduria, thiamine-responsive anaemia, Wolfram syndrome (also
    known as DIDMOAD – **D**iabetes **I**nsipidus, **D**iabetes **M**ellitus
    Optic **A**trophy and **D**eafness – syndrome), and the Lesch–Nyhan
    syndrome)
	Associated with macronormoblastic erythropoiesis
	Some congenital dyserythropoietic anaemias, particularly type I
	Pure red cell aplasia of infancy (Blackfan–Diamond syndrome),
	    including a *forme fruste* with macrocytosis only [48]
	Aplastic anaemia
	Maternally inherited sideroblastic anaemia [49]
	Pearson syndrome
	Anorexia nervosa [50]
	Genetic haemochromatosis [51]
	Erythroblastic synartesis [52]

**Associated with megaloblastic or macronormoblastic
erythropoiesis**
Myelodysplastic syndromes including refractory anaemia with ring
    sideroblasts
Some acute myeloid leukaemias
Multiple myeloma and monoclonal gammopathy of undetermined
    significance [44]
	Uncertain mechanism
	Cigarette smoking [39]
	Chronic obstructive pulmonary disease
	Trisomy 18 [53]
	Trisomy 21 (Down syndrome) [53,54]
	Triploidy [53,55]
	Familial autoimmune/lymphoproliferative disorder [56]
	Development of antibodies to thrombopoietin [57]
	
	Factitious
	Cold agglutinins
	Delay in measuring MCV in some types of hereditary stomatocytosis,
	    particularly hereditary cryohydrocytosis [58]
	Marked delay in measuring MCV with certain automated counters
	    (see Chapter 4)

MCV, mean cell volume

Hypochromia

Hypochromia is a reduction of the staining of the red cell (Fig. 3.19); there is an increase in central pallor, which occupies more than the normal approximate one-third of the red cell diameter. Hypochromia may be general or there may be a population of hypochromic cells. Severe hypochromia may be reflected in a reduction in the mean cell haemoglobin concentration (MCHC), but the sensitivity of this measurement to hypochromia depends on the method by which it is measured. Any of the conditions leading to microcytosis may also cause hypochromia, although in some subjects with α or β thalassaemia trait the blood film shows microcytosis without appreciable hypochromia and, in rare patients with copper deficiency, hypochromia is associated with macrocytosis [45]. Red cells of healthy children are often hypochromic if assessed in relation to the appearance of the red cells

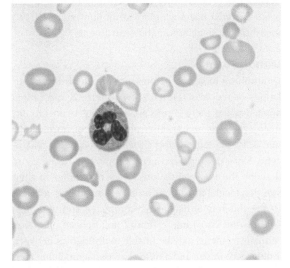

Fig. 3.19 Hypochromic red cells in a patient with iron deficiency anaemia. The film also shows anisochromasia.

of adults. Since the intensity of staining of the red cell is determined by the thickness of the cell as well as by the concentration of haemoglobin, hypochromia can also be noted in cells that are thinner than normal, whether or not they have a normal volume and haemoglobin concentration; such cells are designated 'leptocytes'.

Hyperchromia

The term 'hyperchromia' is rarely used in describing blood films. It can be applied when cells are more intensely stained than normal, but it is more useful to indicate why a cell is hyperchromic. Spherocytes and irregularly contracted cells stain more intensely than normal; the MCHC may be increased, indicating that the hyperchromia is related not only to a change in the shape of the cell but also to a true increase in the intracellular haemoglobin concentration. Some macrocytes are thicker than normal and this causes them to be hyperchromic without any increase in haemoglobin concentration; central pallor may be totally lacking.

Anisochromasia

Anisochromasia describes an increased variability in the degree of staining or haemoglobinisation of the red cell (see Fig. 3.19). In practice, it usually means that there is a spectrum of staining from hypochromic to normochromic. Anisochromasia commonly indicates a changing situation, such as iron deficiency developing or responding to treatment or anaemia of chronic disease developing or regressing. Anisochromasia is reflected in an elevated haemoglobin distribution width (HDW) measured by some automated instruments.

Dimorphism

Dimorphism indicates the presence of two distinct populations of red cells (Fig. 3.20). The term is most often applied when there is one population of hypochromic, microcytic cells and another population of normochromic cells, the latter being either normocytic or macrocytic. Since the term is a general one, it is necessary to describe the two populations. They may differ in their size, haemoglobin content or shape and this is relevant to the differential diagnosis. Automated counters may confirm the visual impression of dimorphism, although some instruments may be unable to distinguish between a difference in size and a difference in haemoglobin concentration. Causes of a dimorphic film included iron deficiency anaemia (following administration of iron or

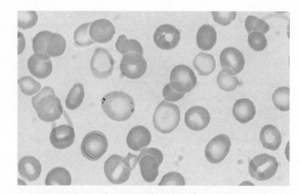

Fig. 3.20 A dimorphic peripheral blood film from a patient with sideroblastic anaemia as a feature of a myelodysplastic syndrome (MDS). One population of cells is normocytic and normochromic while the other is microcytic and hypochromic. One of the poorly haemoglobinised red cells contains some Pappenheimer bodies.

blood transfusion), sideroblastic anaemia, the heterozygous state for hereditary sideroblastic anaemia, macrocytic anaemia post-transfusion, double deficiency of iron and either vitamin B_{12} or folic acid, unmasking of iron deficiency following treatment of megaloblastic anaemia and delayed transfusion reactions. Rare causes include mosaicism for β thalassaemia trait associated with a constitutional chromosomal abnormality [59] and chimaerism post-stem cell transplantation when either the donor or the host has microcytosis with a genetic basis.

Polychromasia

Polychromasia or polychromatophilia describes red cells that are pinkish-blue as a consequence of uptake both of eosin, by haemoglobin, and of basic dyes, by residual ribosomal ribonucleic acid (RNA). Since reticulocytes are cells in which ribosomal RNA takes up a vital dye to form a visible reticulum, it will be seen that there is likely to be a relationship between reticulocytes and polychromatic cells. Both are immature red cells newly released from the bone marrow. However, the number of polychromatic cells in a normal blood film is usually less than 0.1% [60], considerably less than the normal reticulocyte count of around 1–2%. On average, in patient samples, the reticulocyte count is about double the visual estimate of polychromatic cells [61]. This is because only the most immature (grade I) reticulocytes are polychromatic. In conditions of transient or persistent haemopoietic stress, when erythropoietin levels are high, immature reticulocytes are released from the bone marrow. They are

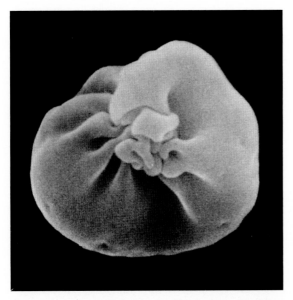

Fig. 3.21 Scanning electron microscopy of a reticulocyte. Courtesy of Professor Aaron Polliack, from Hoffbrand and Pettit [8].

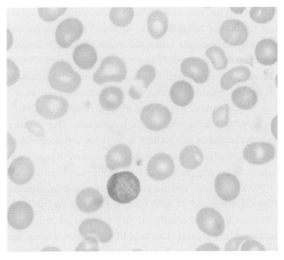

Fig. 3.22 A polychromatic cell that is also larger than a normal cell; it may be designated a polychromatic macrocyte. The film also shows anisocytosis and poikilocytosis.

considerably larger than mature erythrocytes and, as a consequence of a reduced haemoglobin concentration, are less dense. On average their diameter is about 28% greater than that of a mature erythrocyte [60]. On scanning electron microscopy they have an irregular, multilobated surface (Fig. 3.21). They are readily recognised, in May–Grünwald–Giemsa (MGG)-stained films, by their greater diameter, their lack of central pallor and their polychromatic qualities (Fig. 3.22). They are often referred to as 'polychromatic macrocytes'. Sometimes the irregular shape apparent on electron microscopy can also be discerned by light microscopy (Fig. 3.23). Late reticulocytes, which are the only forms present in the blood of haematologically normal subjects, are cup-shaped and only slightly larger than mature erythrocytes. They are therefore difficult to recognise on an MGG-stained film.

The total number of reticulocytes, the proportion of early reticulocytes and the number of polychromatic

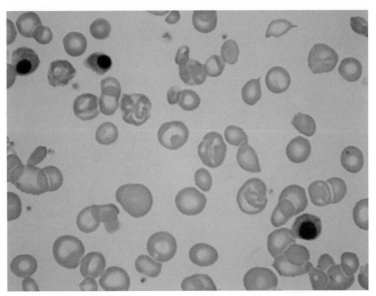

Fig. 3.23 Blood film showing polychromatic macrocytes in a patient with sickle cell anaemia, illustrating the highly irregular shape of reticulocytes.

macrocytes increase as a physiological response to increasing altitude or other hypoxic stimulus and as a normal response to anaemia when there are no factors limiting erythropoiesis. In severely anaemic patients, a lack of polychromasia is significant. It is absent in pure red cell aplasia and in aplastic anaemia, and is inconspicuous in the anaemia of chronic disease and often in renal failure when the erythropoietin response is inadequate. The absence of polychromasia in a patient with sickle cell anaemia or other haemolytic anaemia is important since it may indicate complicating parvovirus B19-induced red cell aplasia.

Polychromatic erythrocytes are increased in primary myelofibrosis and in metastatic carcinoma of the bone marrow. In these conditions the number of polychromatic cells is greater than would be expected from the degree of anaemia and the polychromatic cells may be abnormal – more deeply basophilic than normal and not always increased in size [36].

When the reticulocyte count is increased, automated counters show an increased MCV and RDW. Bayer H.1 series instruments show, in addition, an increased HDW and reticulocytes are seen as hypochromic macrocytes on the red cell cytogram (see Fig. 3.64).

Poikilocytosis

A cell of abnormal shape is a poikilocyte. Poikilocytosis is therefore a state in which there is an increased proportion of cells of abnormal shape. High altitude produces some degree of poikilocytosis in haematologically normal subjects [62]. Poikilocytosis is also a common, often non-specific abnormality in many haematological disorders. It may result from the production of abnormal cells by the bone marrow or from damage to normal cells after release into the blood-stream. If poikilocytosis is very marked, diagnostic possibilities include primary or secondary myelofibrosis, congenital and acquired dyserythropoietic anaemias, hereditary pyropoikilocytosis (Fig. 3.24) and haemoglobin H disease (Fig. 3.25). Extreme poikilocytosis with microcytosis was noted in a child with compound heterozygosity for a *DMT1* mutation [24]. Patients with Gaucher disease have been found to have an increased proportion of poikilocytes, 2.9%, compared to 1% in controls, the forms seen being dacrocytes, elliptocytes, echinocytes and schistocytes [63]. The presence of poikilocytes of certain specific shapes, e.g. spherocytes or elliptocytes, may have a particular significance (see below).

It is important not to confuse deformation of red cells due to a plasma abnormality with true poikilocytosis. The presence of cryoglobulin can lead to remarkable deformation of red cells (Fig. 3.26). Because the cryoglobulin may be only weakly basophilic it may not be readily apparent. The appearance of something extraneous indenting red cells provides a clue.

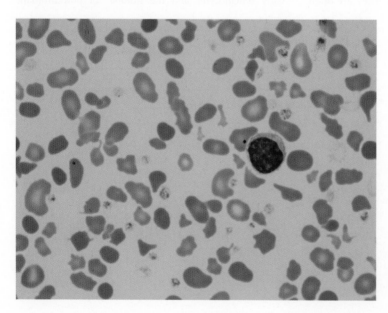

Fig. 3.24 Blood film showing striking poikilocytosis in a patient with hereditary pyropoikilocytosis. With thanks to Dr Mike Leach, Glasgow.

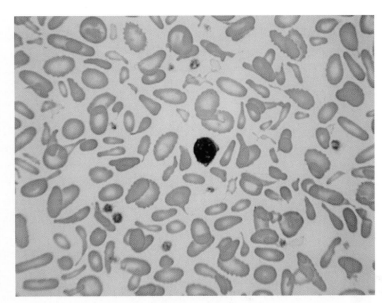

Fig. 3.25 Blood film showing striking poikilocytosis in a patient who has co-inherited hereditary elliptocytosis and the genotype of haemoglobin H disease ($\alpha^{TSaudi}\alpha/\alpha^{TSaudi}\alpha$). Elliptocytes are prominent among the numerous poikilocytes.

Spherocytosis

Spherocytes are cells that, rather than being disciform, are spherical or near-spherical in shape (Fig. 3.27) [64]. They are cells that have lost membrane without equivalent loss of cytosol, as a consequence of an inherited or acquired abnormality of the red cell cytoskeleton and membrane. In a stained blood film, spherocytes lack the normal central pallor. The diameter of a sphere is less than that of a disc-shaped

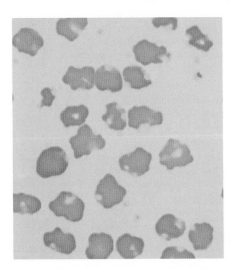

Fig. 3.26 Blood film showing deformation of red cells by a precipitated cryoglobulin.

object of the same volume, and thus a spherocyte may appear smaller than a discocyte. It is preferable, however, to restrict the term 'microspherocyte' to cells of reduced volume rather than merely reduced diameter. Macrospherocytes may be a feature of hereditary stomatocytosis (over-hydrated variant); they result from osmotic swelling. In examining a blood film for the presence of spherocytes it is important to examine that part of the film where the cells are just touching, since normal cells may lack central pallor near the tail of the film. Overlapping cells can also give a false impression of spherocytosis. Spherocytes do not stack well into rouleaux.

The distinction between spherocytes and irregularly contracted cells (see below) is important since the diagnostic significance is different.

Some of the causes of spherocytosis are shown in Table 3.3. There are a variety of underlying mechanisms. In hereditary spherocytosis there is an abnormality of the cytoskeleton with a secondary destabilisation and loss of membrane. In acquired conditions, spherocytosis can result from direct damage to the red cell membrane, e.g. by heat (Fig. 3.28), clostridial toxins (Fig. 3.29) or snake venoms. Loss of membrane can follow antibody coating of the cell by alloantibodies (Fig. 3.30), autoantibodies or drug-induced antibodies; the macrophages of the reticuloendothelial system recognise immunoglobulin or complement on the surface of the cell and remove pieces

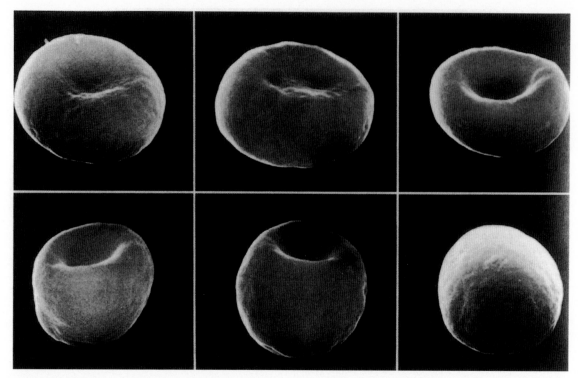

Fig. 3.27 Scanning electron micrography of spherocytes and forms intermediate between discocytes and spherocytes. From Bessis [64].

Table 3.3 Some causes of spherocytosis.

Conditions that may be associated with numerous spherocytes	Conditions that may be associated with smaller numbers of spherocytes
Hereditary spherocytosis	*As an isolated feature*
Warm autoimmune haemolytic anaemia	Immediate transfusion reaction
Delayed haemolytic transfusion reaction	Acute cold autoimmune haemolytic anaemia
ABO haemolytic disease of the newborn and, to a lesser extent, Rh haemolytic disease of the fetus and newborn	Chronic cold haemagglutinin disease
	Penicillin-induced haemolytic anaemia
Administration of anti-D to Rh D-positive patients, e.g. in the treatment of autoimmune thrombocytopenic purpura	Acute attacks of paroxysmal cold haemoglobinuria
	Infusion of large amounts of intravenous lipid [68]
Passenger lymphocyte syndrome following solid organ transplantation (e.g. anti-A, anti-B, anti-E antibodies)	Pyrimidine 5'-nucleotidase deficiency[†] [69]
Drug-induced immune haemolytic anaemia (innocent bystander mechanism)	*In association with other poikilocytes*
	Normal neonate
Clostridium perfringens sepsis	Hyposplenism
Zieve syndrome[*]	Sickle cell anaemia
Low erythrocyte ATP caused by phosphate deficiency [65, 66]	Microangiopathic haemolytic anaemia (microspherocytes)
Snake-bite-induced haemolysis	Mechanical haemolytic anaemia (microspherocytes)
Bartonellosis (Oroya fever)	Hereditary elliptocytosis with transient severe manifestations in infancy [70]
Fresh-water drowning or intravenous infusion of water	Hereditary pyropoikilocytosis (including homozygosity for mutations causing hereditary elliptocytosis)
Burns (microspherocytes)	
Sulphuric acid exposure (microspherocytes) [67]	Rh null phenotype

ATP, adenosine triphosphate
[*]irregularly contracted cells may be more characteristic
[†]spherocytes may be spiculated

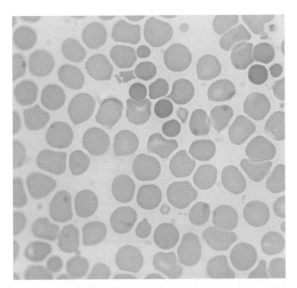

Fig. 3.28 Blood film of a patient with severe burns showing spherocytes, microspherocytes and red cells that appear to be budding off very small spherocytic fragments.

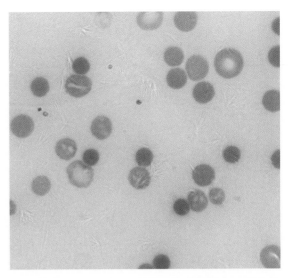

Fig. 3.29 Blood film of a patient with clostridial septicaemia showing many spherocytes. Courtesy of the late Professor Harry Smith.

of membrane. When red cells fragment, those fragments with a relative lack of membrane form microspherocytes; this is the mechanism of formation of spherocytes in microangiopathic haemolytic anaemia, mechanical haemolytic anaemia and hereditary pyropoikilocytosis. Erythrocytes stored for transfusion become spheroechinocytes as the blood ages (see below). Rarely, marked spherocytosis has been described in hypophosphataemia, e.g. in liver disease [65], in acute diabetic ketoacidosis [66] and during over-vigorous correction of hyperphos-

phataemia [71]; the mechanism is likely to be adenosine triphosphate (ATP) depletion. In Heinz body haemolytic anaemias, although most abnormal cells are irregularly contracted cells (see below), there are usually also some spherocytes.

Irregularly contracted cells

Irregularly contracted cells lack central pallor and appear smaller and denser than normal erythrocytes without being as regular in shape as spherocytes (Fig. 3.31).

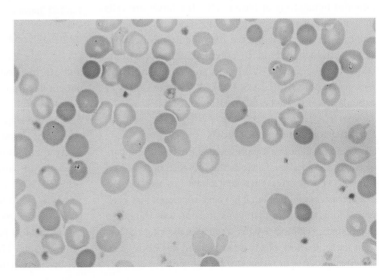

Fig. 3.30 Spherocytes in the peripheral blood film of an iron deficient patient who suffered a delayed transfusion reaction due to an anti-Rh D antibody; the film is dimorphic, showing a mixture of the recipient's hypochromic microcytic cells and the donor cells, which have become spherocytic.

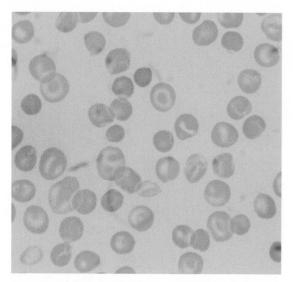

Fig. 3.31 Blood film of a patient with haemoglobin C disease showing irregularly contracted cells and several target cells.

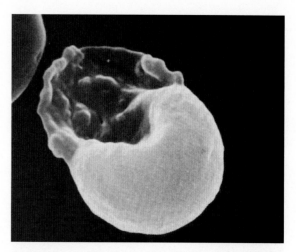

Fig. 3.32 Scanning electron micrograph showing a hemi-ghost cell containing Heinz bodies. Courtesy of Dr T.K. Chan and colleagues, Hong Kong, and the *British Journal of Haematology* [72].

Irregularly contracted cells are formed when there is oxidant damage to erythrocytes, or damage to red cell membranes by precipitation of unstable haemoglobin or free α or β chains. Blood films showing irregularly contracted cells often also show some spherocytes; these are formed when a red cell inclusion, such as a Heinz body, has been removed by the pitting action of splenic macrophages with associated loss of red cell membrane. Keratocytes (see below) may likewise be present as a result of the removal of a Heinz body. Blood films showing irregularly contracted cells may also show ghost cells and also hemighosts or blister cells. The latter are cells in which most of the haemoglobin has precipitated in half of the cell leaving the red cell membranes in apposition with each other in the other half of the cell; Heinz bodies may be present in the clear area as well as in the rest of the cell (Figs 3.32 & 3.33) [72]. Some causes of irregularly contracted cells are shown in Table 3.4.

Elliptocytosis and ovalocytosis

Elliptocytosis indicates the presence of increased numbers of elliptocytes and ovalocytosis the presence of increased numbers of ovalocytes. These terms have not been used in any consistent manner, but it has been suggested that a cell with a long axis more than twice its short axis should be designated an elliptocyte while a cell with the long axis less than twice its short axis is designated an ovalocyte [75]. When elliptocytes or ovalocytes are numerous (Fig. 3.34)

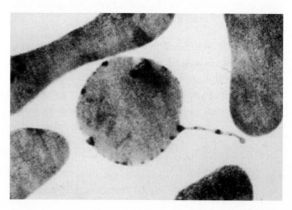

Fig. 3.33 Transmission electron micrograph showing a hemi-ghost cell containing Heinz bodies. Courtesy of Dr T.K. Chan and colleagues, Hong Kong, and the *British Journal of Haematology* [72].

and are the dominant abnormality it is likely that the patient has an inherited abnormality affecting the red cell cytoskeleton, such as hereditary elliptocytosis. Smaller numbers of elliptocytes or ovalocytes may be seen in iron deficiency, in some patients with β thalassaemia heterozygosity and homozygosity, megaloblastic anaemia, primary myelofibrosis and myelodysplastic syndromes (MDS) and occasionally in inherited red cell enzyme abnormalities, e.g. pyruvate kinase deficiency; in these conditions it is likely that elliptocytes reflect dyserythropoiesis. Elliptocytosis in MDS has been linked to an acquired deficiency of protein 4.1 [76]. In Papua New Guinea, ovalocytosis has been associated with Gerbich negativity and a specific

Table 3.4 Some conditions that are associated with irregularly contracted cells.

Conditions that may be associated with numerous irregularly contracted cells
Haemoglobin C disease
Haemoglobin C/β thalassaemia
Sickle cell/haemoglobin C disease
Unstable haemoglobins
Acute haemolysis in G6PD deficiency or other abnormalities of the pentose shunt
Severe oxidant stress (drugs or chemicals), e.g. dapsone therapy or copper sulphate poisoning, in patients without abnormalities of the pentose shunt
Zieve syndrome
Wilson disease [73]
Conditions that may be associated with smaller numbers of irregularly contracted cells
Minor haemolytic episodes in G6PD deficiency
Moderate oxidant stress in patients without abnormalities of the pentose shunt
Defects in glutathione biosynthesis
Neonatal glutathione peroxidase deficiency (which is probably secondary to transient deficiency of selenium, an essential co-factor)
Haemoglobin C trait
Unstable haemoglobins
β thalassaemia trait
Haemoglobin H disease
Haemoglobin E disease or trait
Hereditary xerocytosis (dehydrated variant of hereditary stomatocytosis)
Congenital dyserythropoietic anaemia type II [74]

G6PD, glucose-6-phosphate dehydrogenase

mutation in the gene encoding glycophorin C [77]. Macrocytic ovalocytes or oval macrocytes are characteristic of megaloblastic anaemia and South-East Asian ovalocytosis and are also seen in dyserythropoiesis, e.g. in primary myelofibrosis. Elliptocytes are biconcave and thus are capable of forming rouleaux.

In a group of Thai patients, ovalocytosis was found to be a feature of homozygosity for mutations in the *SLC4A1* gene that lead to distal renal tubular acidosis [78]. The gene encodes the erythrocyte membrane protein, anion exchanger 1 (AE1) and the shorter AE1 protein found in renal tubules. Homozygotes for the G701D mutation and compound heterozygotes for G701D/A858D have ovalocytes comprising about a quarter of their red cells; they have compensated haemolysis but can develop anaemia and reticulocytosis during periods of metabolic acidosis. The compound heterozygotes also have small numbers of pincered cells and schistocytes. Homozygotes and compound heterozygotes who are also heterozygous for haemoglobin E have ovalocytes comprising about two-thirds of red cells. Heterozygotes for G701D are haematologically normal unless they also carry haemoglobin E or α+ thalassaemia, in which case they also have ovalocytes. However, a heterozygote for A858D had 20% ovalocytes and also had acanthocytes, echinocytes and schistocytes [78]. A compound heterozygote for G701D and the in-frame deletion of the same gene that leads to South-East Asian ovalocytosis, who also had α+ thalassaemia, had haemolytic anaemia aggravated by acidosis, whereas simple heterozygotes for South-East Asian ovalocytosis do not have haemolysis [78].

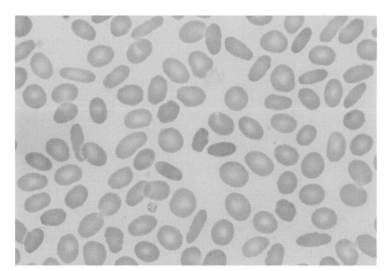

Fig. 3.34 Blood film of a patient with hereditary elliptocytosis showing elliptocytes and ovalocytes.

Teardrop cells (dacrocytes)

Teardrop or pear-shaped cells (dacrocytes) (Fig. 3.35) occur when there is bone marrow fibrosis or severe dyserythropoiesis and also in some haemolytic anaemias. They are particularly characteristic of megaloblastic anaemia, thalassaemia major and myelofibrosis – either primary myelofibrosis or myelofibrosis secondary to metastatic carcinoma or other bone marrow infiltration. In both thalassaemia major and primary myelofibrosis, the proportion of teardrop cells decreases following splenectomy, suggesting either that they are the product of extramedullary haemopoiesis or that they are formed when the spleen causes further damage to abnormal red cells. Teardrop cells that are present in occasional cases of autoimmune haemolytic anaemia [79], Heinz body haemolytic anaemia and β thalassaemia major are likely to be the result of the action of splenic macrophages on abnormal erythrocytes, resulting from the removal of part of the red cell, Heinz bodies or α chain precipitates. Teardrop poikilocytes are common in patients with erythroleukaemia [80].

Spiculated cells

The terminology applied to spiculated cells is confused. In particular, the term 'burr cell' has been used by different authors to describe different cells and therefore is better abandoned. The terminology of Bessis [64] is recommended since it is based on careful study of abnormal cells by scanning electron microscopy and is clear and relatively easy to apply. Bessis divided spiculated cells into echinocytes, acanthocytes, keratocytes and schistocytes.

Echinocytes

Echinocytes are erythrocytes that have lost their disc shape and are covered with 10–30 short blunt spicules of fairly regular form (Figs 3.36 & 3.37). The main causes of echinocytosis are shown in Table 3.5. Echinocytes may be produced *in vitro* by exposure to fatty acids and certain drugs or simply by incubation. The end stage of a discocyte–echinocyte transformation is a spheroechinocyte. A spheroechinocyte is also formed when a spherocyte undergoes an echinocytic change and, similarly, other abnormally shaped cells, e.g. acanthocytes, can undergo an echinocytic change.

When donor blood is stored for transfusion, cells become spheroechinocytes (Fig. 3.38) as lysolecithin is formed and as ATP concentration decreases; membrane lipid, both cholesterol and phospholipid, is then lost when microvesicles containing small amounts of haemoglobin are shed from the tips of the spicules. When blood is transfused and there is resynthesis of ATP, many of the cells revert to cup-shaped stomatocytes rather than to discocytes; those that have lost a lot of membrane remain spherocytic.

In vivo, echinocyte formation may be related to increased plasma fatty acids (such as occurs during heparin therapy), ATP depletion and lysolecithin formation. During echinocyte formation there is entry of calcium into cells with polymerisation of spectrin. Echinocytosis is reversible *in vitro* and *in vivo*, e.g. by suspending cells in fresh plasma or by allowing ATP resynthesis.

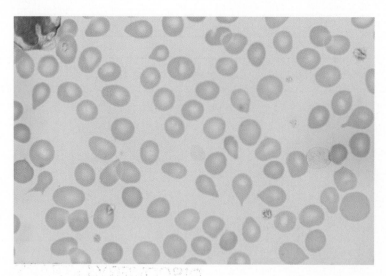

Fig. 3.35 Blood film of a patient with primary myelofibrosis showing teardrop poikilocytes (dacrocytes).

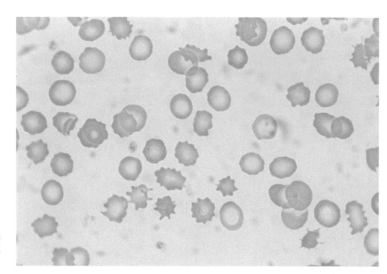

Fig. 3.36 Echinocytes in the peripheral blood film of a patient with chronic renal failure.

In laboratories that make films from EDTA-anticoagulated blood rather than fresh blood, by far the most common cause of echinocytosis is delay in making the blood film (see Fig. 3.7). This storage artefact, often referred to as 'crenation', is likely to be caused by a fall in ATP or by lysolecithin formation. Echinocytosis, other than as an artefactual change, is quite uncommon. The prevalence is greater in neonates [84]. Echinocytes are normal in a pre-term neonate [85]. Echinocytosis can occur in liver disease [84], but acanthocytosis (see below) is more common. It can occur in the early stages of the haemolytic–uraemic syndrome, but subsequently echinocytosis resolves leaving only the features of microangiopathic haemolytic anaemia. A very rare haemolytic anaemia resulting from a mutation in *SLC2A1* is characterised by echinocytosis [86]. Echinocytosis, other than as a storage artefact, is probably most common in critically ill patients with multiorgan failure including both hepatic and renal failure. On multivariate analysis, echinocytosis (mainly reflecting hepatic and renal impairment) is predictive of mortality in hospitalised patients [87].

Echinocytosis observed following the development of hypophosphataemia in patients on parenteral feeding is attributable to a fall in ATP concentration and this may also be the mechanism operating when echinocytes develop in hereditary pyruvate kinase deficiency and

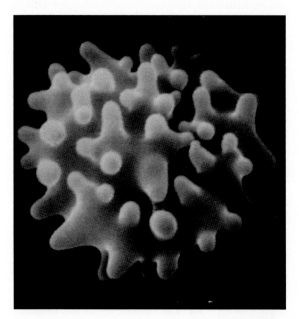

Fig. 3.37 Scanning electron micrograph of an echinocyte. Courtesy of Professor Aaron Polliack, from Hoffbrand and Pettit [8].

Table 3.5 Some causes of echinocytosis.

Storage artefact
Liver disease, particularly with co-existing renal failure
Nutritional or other phosphate deficiency [71]
Pyruvate kinase deficiency
Phosphoglycerate kinase deficiency
Aldolase deficiency [81]
Decompression phase of diving [82]
Haemolytic–uraemic syndrome
Following burns
Following cardiopulmonary bypass
Splenic haemangioma [83]
Post-transfusion (spheroechinocytes)

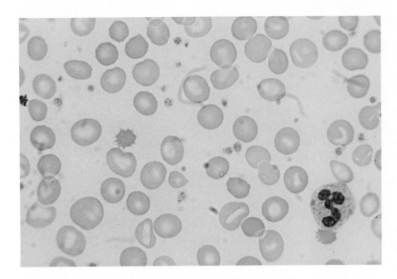

Fig. 3.38 Spheroechinocyte in a peripheral blood film made from blood taken shortly after a blood transfusion. The spheroechinocyte is a transfused cell.

in phosphoglycerate kinase deficiency. Echinocytosis occurring in hypothermic, heparinised patients on cardiopulmonary bypass has been attributed to a rise of free fatty acid concentration. The echinocytosis that has been noted as a delayed response in severely burned patients may be the result of lipid abnormalities.

Acanthocytes

Acanthocytes are cells of approximately spherical shape bearing between 2 and 20 spicules that are of unequal length and distributed irregularly over the red cell surface (Figs 3.39–3.46). Some of the spicules have club-shaped rather than pointed ends. Causes of acanthocytosis are shown in Table 3.6. Acanthocyte formation probably results from a preferential expansion of the outer leaflet of the lipid bilayer that comprises the red cell membrane [99]. Acanthocytes cannot form rouleaux.

Unlike echinocytosis, acanthocytosis is not reversible on suspending cells in fresh plasma. In acanthocytosis associated with abetalipoproteinaemia or liver disease, the cholesterol:phospholipid ratio in the red cells is increased. This is in contrast to the target cells associated with liver disease in which the cholesterol and phospholipid concentrations rise in parallel.

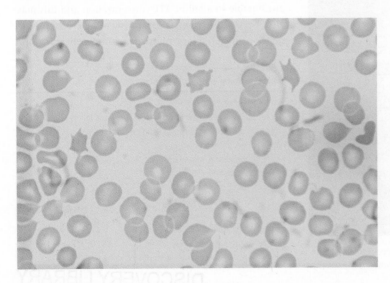

Fig. 3.39 Acanthocytes in the peripheral blood film of a patient with anorexia nervosa.

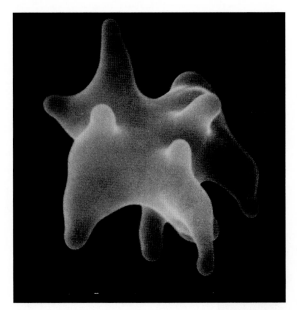

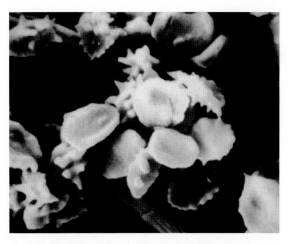

Fig. 3.42 Scanning electron micrograph showing acanthocytes in a patient with the McLeod phenotype. By courtesy of Dr Guy Lucas, Manchester.

Fig. 3.40 Scanning electron micrograph of an acanthocyte. Courtesy of Professor Aaron Polliack, from Hoffbrand and Pettit [8].

Acanthocytosis as an inherited phenomenon is associated with a number of different syndromes and its presence may help in their diagnosis. It was first described in association with retinitis pigmentosa, degenerative neurological disease, fat malabsorption and abetalipoproteinaemia [100]. Acanthocytosis

can similarly be observed in inherited hypobetalipoproteinaemia. A low percentage of acanthocytes is observed in Anderson disease, an inherited lipid malabsorption syndrome [98].

Subsequent to its description in abetalipoproteinaemia, acanthocytosis was recognised in association with several rare degenerative neurological diseases with normal β lipoproteins [101,102]. These conditions have been collectively designated neuroacanthocytosis [88]

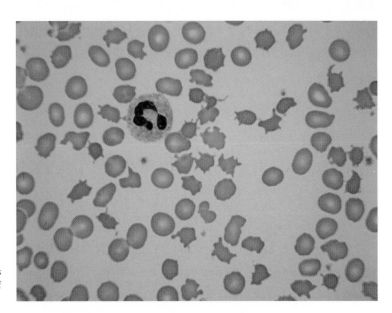

Fig. 3.41 Blood film showing acanthocytes in choreo-acanthocytosis. By courtesy of Dr Peter Bain, London.

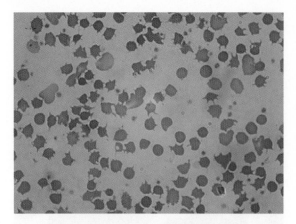

Fig. 3.43 Medium power view of a blood film showing acanthocytes resulting from homozygosity for the A858D mutation in the *SLC4A1* gene. Courtesy of Dr Lesley Bruce, Bristol.

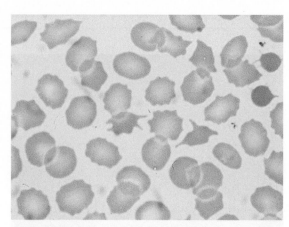

Fig. 3.44 Unusually numerous acanthocytes in the peripheral blood film of a haematologically normal subject who has had a splenectomy. The film also shows a target cell.

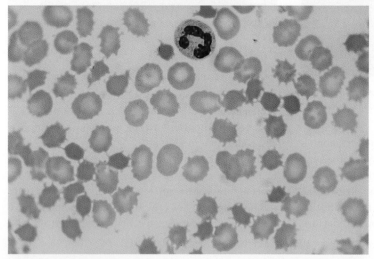

Fig. 3.45 Numerous acanthocytes in the blood film of a patient with abetalipoproteinaemia.

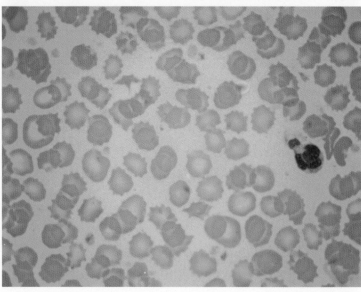

Fig. 3.46 Numerous acanthocytes in the blood film of a baby with infantile pyknocytosis.

Table 3.6 Some causes of acanthocytosis.

Conditions associated with large numbers of acanthocytes

Inherited

Hereditary abetalipoproteinaemia (*MTP* mutation, AR)

Hereditary hypobetalipoproteinaemia (some cases; *APOB* mutation, AR)

Associated with degenerative neurological disease (neuroacanthocytosis) with normal lipoproteins

   Choreoacanthocytosis (*VPS13A* mutation, AR) [88]

   McLeod red cell phenotype (*KX* mutation, sex-linked recessive)

   Huntingdon-like disease 2* (*JPH3* mutation, AD)

   Pantothenate-kinase associated neurodegeneration, HARP syndrome (hypoprebetalipoproteinaemia, acanthocytosis, retinitis pigmentosa and pallidal degeneration)* (*PANK2* mutation, AR) [89]

In(Lu) red cell phenotype (Lu(a-b-), *KLF1* haploinsufficiency) [90]

Associated with abnormal band 3 of red cell membrane (*SLC4A1* mutation, AR) [91–93]

Medium chain acyl-CoA dehydrogenase deficiency (*ACADM* mutation, AR) [94]

Hereditary high red cell membrane phosphatidylcholine haemolytic anaemia [95] (which probably represents hereditary xerocytosis)

Acquired

Hypobetalipoproteinaemia caused by malnutrition or lipid deprivation

'Spur cell' haemolytic anaemia associated with liver disease (usually associated with alcoholic cirrhosis but also occasionally with severe viral hepatitis, neonatal hepatitis, cardiac cirrhosis, haemochromatosis or advanced Wilson disease)

Infantile pyknocytosis

Vitamin E deficiency in premature neonates

Myelodysplastic syndromes [96]

Conditions associated with small numbers of acanthocytes

Inherited

Heterozygotes for the McLeod phenotype

Pyruvate kinase deficiency

Woronet trait

Dyserythropoiesis associated with a *GATA1* mutation [97]

Anderson disease (*SARIB* mutation, AR) [98]

Acquired

Post-splenectomy and hyposplenism

Anorexia nervosa and starvation

Myxoedema and panhypopituitarism

*Some cases have acanthocytes. AD, autosomal dominant; AR, autosomal recessive

(Fig. 3.41). The acanthocytes may be more apparent on a wet preparation [103]. Most cases of neuroacanthocytosis result from mutation in the *VPS13A* gene [104] and others from mutation in *JP3* (junctophilin 3), *KX* (McLeod phenotype) or *PANK2* [88,89,105]. Some cases

of the McLeod phenotype (Fig. 3.42) not only lack Kell antigens, but also have chronic granulomatous disease as the result of a contiguous gene syndrome; female carriers of this mutation have two populations of red cells, one acanthocytic and one not. The In(Lu) red cell phenotype, in which there is absent or reduced expression of Lu and several other blood group antigen systems [106], results from haploinsufficiency of a transcription factor gene. Acanthocytosis has also been associated with a deficiency of *SLC4A1*-encoded band 3 protein resulting from homozygosity for a P868L [91] or an A858D mutation [92,93] (Fig. 3.43); Omani Arab homozygotes for the A858D mutation have striking acanthocytosis and echinocytosis with occasional ovalo/elliptocytes; heterozygotes have smaller numbers (15–20%) of acanthocytes with a minimal tendency to ovalocytosis [92]; Indian homozygotes for the A858D mutation were described as having hereditary spherocytosis, but published photographs indicate that acanthocytosis is the dominant feature [93].

Keratocytes

Keratocytes (or horned cells) (Fig. 3.47) are cells with pairs of spicules – usually two but sometimes four or six – which have been formed by the fusion of opposing membranes to form a pseudovacuole with subsequent rupture of the membrane at the cell surface. They are formed when there is mechanical damage to red cells, e.g. by fibrin strands or a malfunctioning cardiac prosthesis. They have been observed in schistocytic haemolytic anaemias including microangiopathic haemolytic anaemia, in disseminated intravascular coagulation and in renal disease, e.g. glomerulonephritis, uraemia and following renal transplantation. They can also result from removal of a Heinz body (Fig. 3.48) [107].

Prekeratocytes are erythrocytes that retain central pallor and have a sharply defined submembranous vacuole. They are believed to give rise to a keratocyte through rupture of the vacuole. They are most characteristic of iron deficiency, but are also present in β thalassaemia trait, anaemia of chronic disease and microangiopathic haemolytic anaemia [108].

Schistocytes

Schistocytes are fragments of red cells. In healthy adult subjects they do not exceed 0.2% of red cells, but in neonates they may be up to 1.9% and in premature neonates up to 5.5% [109].

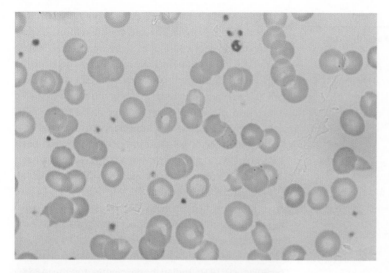

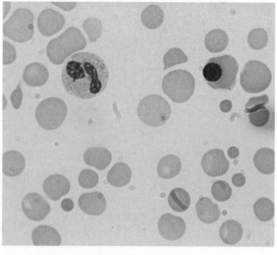

Fig. 3.47 Keratocytes in the peripheral blood film of a patient with microangiopathic haemolytic anaemia.

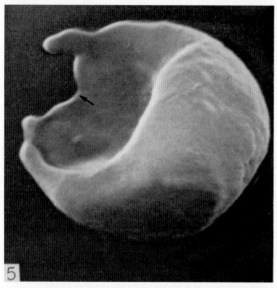

Fig. 3.48 Scanning electron micrograph of a keratocyte, formed by removal of a Heinz body. Courtesy of Dr M. Amare and colleagues and the *British Journal of Haematology* [107].

Fig. 3.49 Fragments including microspherocytes in the peripheral blood film of a patient with the haemolytic–uraemic syndrome. The film also shows polychromasia and a nucleated red blood cell (NRBC).

Schistocytes are formed either by fragmentation of abnormal cells, e.g. in hereditary pyropoikilocytosis, or following mechanical, toxin- or heat-induced damage of previously normal cells (Fig. 3.49). When resultant on mechanical damage, schistocytes often coexist with keratocytes. Many schistocytes are spiculated. Others have been left with too little membrane for their cytoplasmic volume and therefore have formed microspherocytes (spheroschistocytes). In burned patients,

schistocytes may be microdiscocytes as well as microspherocytes (see Fig. 3.92). An uncommon form of red cell fragment, a linear or filamentous structure, is observed in sickle cell anaemia [110] (Fig. 3.50). The commonest causes of schistocyte formation are microangiopathic and mechanical haemolytic anaemias, collectively known as schistocytic haemolytic anaemia. Schistocytes may be a feature of MDS [111] and are common in patients with erythroleukaemia [80].

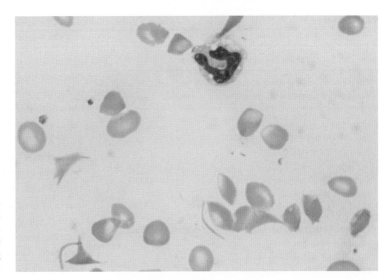

Fig. 3.50 The blood film of a patient with sickle cell anaemia showing linear red cell fragments and increased numbers of irregularly contracted cells; the latter feature resulted from a severe pulmonary sickling crisis at the time the film was made.

An International Council for Standardization in Haematology (ICSH) guideline provides criteria for the recognition and enumeration of schistocytes in schistocytic haemolytic anaemias [109]. For this purpose they advise the inclusion of fragments with sharp angles and straight borders, small crescents, helmet cells, keratocytes and microspherocytes, the latter only in the presence of other characteristic cells [109]. Quantification is per 1000 erythrocytes, with more than 1% schistocytes being regarded as significant. Quantification is only relevant when schistocytosis is the dominant morphological abnormality.

Red cell fragments can also be quantified by several automated haematology analysers, for example the Sysex XE-2100 and the Bayer Advia 120. This can be used for screening for schistocytic haemolytic anaemias, although false negative results may be obtained when there is macrocytosis [109].

Target cells

Target cells have an area of increased staining, which appears in the middle of the area of central pallor (Fig. 3.51). Target cells are formed as a consequence of there being redundant membrane in relation to the volume of the cytoplasm. They may also be thinner than normal cells. *In vivo* they are bell-shaped and this can be demonstrated on scanning electron microscopy (Fig. 3.52). They flatten on spreading to form the characteristic cell seen on light microscopy. Target cells may be microcytic, normocytic or macrocytic, depending on the underlying abnormality and the mechanism of their formation. Some of the causes of target cell formation are shown in Table 3.7. Target

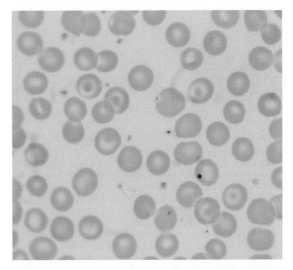

Fig. 3.51 Blood film of a haematologically normal patient who has had a splenectomy, showing target cells and a Howell–Jolly body.

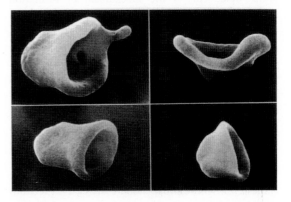

Fig. 3.52 Scanning electron micrographs of target cells. From Bessis [64].

Table 3.7 Some causes of target cell formation.

Conditions that are often associated with large numbers of target cells
Obstructive jaundice
Hereditary LCAT deficiency
Familial hypobetalipoproteinaemia [112]
Haemoglobin C disease
Sickle cell anaemia
Compound heterozygosity for haemoglobin S and haemoglobin C
Haemoglobin D disease
Haemoglobin O-Arab disease
Conditions that may be associated with moderate or small numbers of target cells
Parenchymal liver disease
Splenectomy and other hyposplenic states
Haemoglobin C trait
Haemoglobin S trait
Haemoglobin E trait and disease
Haemoglobin Lepore trait
β thalassaemia minor, intermedia and major
Haemoglobin H disease
Iron deficiency
Sideroblastic anaemia
Hereditary xerocytosis (dehydrated variant of hereditary stomatocytosis) [113]
Analphalipoproteinaemia [114] and hypoalphalipoproteinaemia [115]
Hereditary phytosterolaemia [116]
Acquired phytosterolaemia as a result of parenteral nutrition [116]

LCAT, lecithin-cholesterol acyl transferase

cells may also be an artefact, as a result of using dirty slides [117].

Target cells may be formed because of an excess of red cell membrane, as when there is excess membrane lipid. This is the mechanism of formation in obstructive jaundice, severe parenchymal liver disease and hereditary deficiency of lecithin-cholesterol acyl transferase (LCAT). The ratio of membrane cholesterol to cholesterol ester is increased. Red cells lack enzymes for the synthesis of cholesterol and phospholipid and for the esterification of cholesterol so that changes in the membrane lipids are passive, reflecting changes in plasma lipids. When LCAT activity is reduced, the ratio of cholesterol to cholesterol ester in the red cell membrane increases. There may also be an increase in total membrane cholesterol, with a proportionate increase in lecithin and with a decrease in ethanolamine. LCAT is synthesised in hepatocytes and so it may be reduced in liver disease. In obstructive jaundice very high levels of bile salts inhibit LCAT. This does not, however, appear to be the sole mechanism of target cell formation in obstructive jaundice, since patients may have target cells without their plasma being able to inhibit the LCAT activity of normal plasma. When target cells are formed as a result of plasma lipid abnormalities, they revert to a normal shape on being transfused into a subject with normal plasma lipids. If changes in membrane lipids that would normally cause target cell formation occur in patients with spherocytosis, the cells become more disciform; this phenomenon may be observed when a patient with hereditary spherocytosis develops obstructive jaundice.

An alternative mechanism of target cell formation is a reduction of cytoplasmic content without a proportionate reduction in the quantity of membrane. This is the mechanism of target cell formation in a group of conditions such as iron deficiency, thalassaemias and haemoglobinopathies in which target cells are associated with hypochromia or microcytosis. Target cells are much less numerous in iron deficiency than in thalassaemias. The reason for this is not clear.

Knizocyte
Knizocytes are triconcave erythrocytes, which may be seen in patients with liver disease [118].

Stomatocytosis
Stomatocytes are cells that, on a stained blood film, have a central linear slit or stoma (Fig. 3.53). Occasionally such cells are seen in the blood films of healthy subjects. On scanning electron microscopy or in wet preparations with the cells suspended in plasma they are cup- or bowl-shaped (Fig. 3.54). Stomatocytes can be formed *in vitro*, e.g. in response to low pH or exposure to cationic lipid-soluble drugs such as chlorpromazine; the change in shape is reversible. The end stage of a discocyte–stomatocyte transformation is a spherostomatocyte. Stomatocytosis results from a variety of membrane abnormalities but probably essentially from expansion of the inner leaflet of the lipid bilayer that comprises the red cell membrane [99]. In liver disease, stomatocyte formation has been attributed to an increase of lysolecithin in the inner layer of the red cell membrane. In hereditary spherocytosis and autoimmune

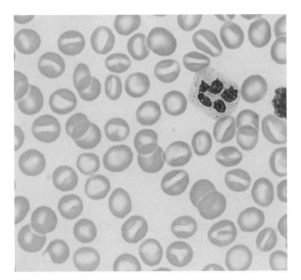

Fig. 3.53 Blood film in hereditary stomatocytosis showing stomatocytes.

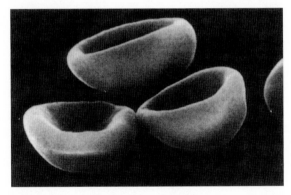

Fig. 3.54 Scanning electron micrograph of stomatocytes. From Bessis [64].

haemolytic anaemia, progressive loss of membrane leads to formation of stomatocytes, spherostomatocytes and spherocytes.

Stomatocytes have been associated with a great variety of clinical conditions [119,120] but an aetiological connection has not always been established. The commonest cause of stomatocytosis is alcohol excess and alcoholic liver disease; in these cases there is often associated macrocytosis and in those with very advanced liver disease there may also be triconcave cells [121]. The combination of stomatocytosis and macrocytosis is also seen in patients receiving hydroxycarbamide and occasionally in MDS. It is possible that

chlorpromazine exposure can cause stomatocytosis *in vivo* as well as *in vitro* since an association has been observed [120]. Certain inherited erythrocyte membrane abnormalities are characterised by stomatocytes, either alone in hereditary stomatocytosis and hereditary xerocytosis or in association with other abnormalities in Rh_{null} or Rh_{MOD} syndromes [122] and South-East Asian ovalocytosis. Ovalocytes and stomatocytes occur in homozygotes for mutations in the *SLC4A1* gene that cause distal renal tubular acidosis (see above). Stomatocytosis in hereditary high red cell membrane phosphatidylcholine haemolytic anaemia is associated with numerous target cells [95]; this condition is now thought to be identical to hereditary xerocytosis [123]. Stomatocytosis has been associated with some cases of hereditary haemolytic anaemia associated with adenosine deaminase overproduction [123]. Analphalipoproteinaemia (Tangier disease) [114] and hypoalphalipoproteinaemia [115] are associated with stomatocytosis. Increased stomatocytes have been reported in association with target cells in a single patient with familial hypobetalipoproteinaemia [112], but in the published photograph the target cells are much more convincing than the stomatocytes. LCAT deficiency shows both target cells and stomatocytes. An increased incidence of stomatocytosis has been reported in healthy Mediterranean (Greek and Italian) subjects in Australia [124]. This condition, designated Mediterranean stomatocytosis/macrothrombocytopenia, is now known to be a manifestation of hereditary phytosterolaemia [125]. Similar morphological features, also associated with haemolytic anaemia and thrombocytopenia, occur in association with parenteral nutrition with soy-based lipid emulsions [116].

Sickle cells

A sickle cell is a very specific type of cell that is confined to sickle cell anaemia and other forms of sickle cell disease. Sickle cells are crescent- or sickle-shaped with pointed ends (Fig. 3.55). The characteristic shape is very apparent on scanning electron micrography (Fig 3.56). The blood film in sickle cell anaemia may also show boat- or oat-shaped cells (Fig. 3.55) that are not pathognomonic for the presence of haemoglobin S but are highly suggestive. Other highly characteristic poikilocytes formed in the presence of haemoglobin S are SC poikilocytes, formed when

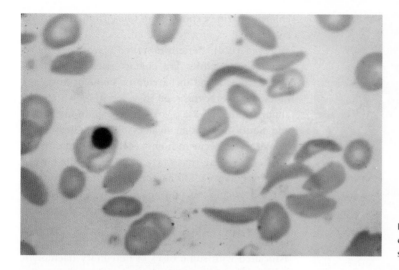

Fig. 3.55 Blood film of a patient with sickle cell anaemia showing sickle cells and boat-shaped cells.

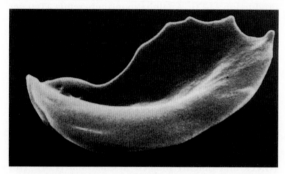

Fig. 3.56 Scanning electron micrograph of a sickle cell. From Bessis [64].

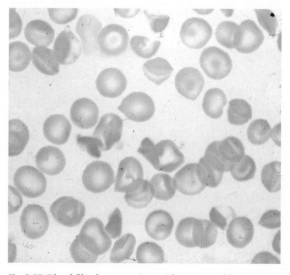

Fig. 3.57 Blood film from a patient with compound heterozygosity for haemoglobin S and haemoglobin C showing a characteristic SC poikilocyte.

both haemoglobin S and haemoglobin C are present (Fig. 3.57) and 'Napoleon hat cells' that are characteristic of haemoglobin S-Oman (Fig. 3.58). Very rarely a blood film from a patient with sickle cell trait shows sickle cells; this was observed as an *in vitro* artefact in a child with acute lymphoblastic leukaemia with a high white cell count, being attributed to oxygen consumption by the leukaemic cells [126].

Pincer cells

Pincer or mushroom-shaped cells are a feature of hereditary spherocytes resulting from deficiency of band 3 (Fig. 3.59). They are also common in erythroleukaemia [80]. Similar cells can be seen in oxidant-induced haemolysis, when they result from removal of two adjacent Heinz bodies.

Inclusions in erythrocytes
Howell–Jolly bodies

Howell–Jolly bodies (see Fig. 3.51) are medium-sized, round, cytoplasmic red cell inclusions that have the same staining characteristics as a nucleus and can be demonstrated to be composed of deoxyribonucleic acid (DNA). A Howell–Jolly body is a fragment of nuclear material. It can arise by karyorrhexis (the breaking up of a nucleus) or by incomplete nuclear expulsion, or can represent a chromosome that has separated from the mitotic spindle during

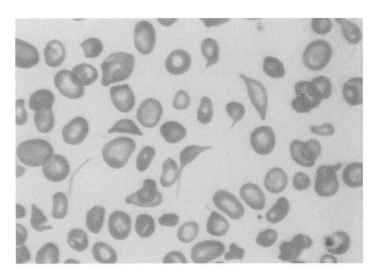

Fig. 3.58 Blood film of a patient with compound heterozygosity for haemoglobin S and haemoglobin S-Oman showing the 'Napoleon hat' red cells that are characteristic of haemoglobin S-Oman. Courtesy of Dr R.A. Al Jahdamy and colleagues, Oman.

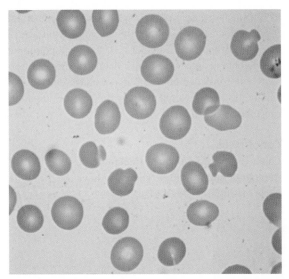

Fig. 3.59 Blood film of a patient with hereditary spherocytosis as a result of a band 3 mutation, showing pincer or mushroom cells.

abnormal mitosis. Some Howell–Jolly bodies are found in erythrocytes within the bone marrow in haematologically normal subjects but, since they are removed by the spleen, they are not seen in the peripheral blood. They appear in the blood following splenectomy and are also present in other hyposplenic states, including transient hyposplenic states resulting from reticulo-endothelial overload. They can be a normal finding in neonates (in whom the spleen is functionally immature). The rate of formation of Howell–Jolly bodies is increased in megaloblastic anaemias and, if the patient is also hyposplenic, large numbers of Howell–Jolly bodies will be seen in the peripheral blood.

Searching for Howell–Jolly bodies is a reliable technique for screening for significant hyposplenism, although a phase-microscopy pitted cell count is more sensitive and will also detect milder impairment of splenic function [127].

Basophilic stippling

Basophilic stippling (Fig. 3.60) or punctate basophilia describes the presence in erythrocytes of considerable numbers of small basophilic inclusions that are dispersed through the erythrocyte cytoplasm and can be demonstrated to be RNA. They are composed of aggregates of ribosomes; degenerating mitochondria and siderosomes may be included in the aggregates, but most such inclusions are negative with Perls acid ferrocyanide stain for iron. Very occasional cells with basophilic stippling can be seen in normal subjects. Increased numbers are seen in the presence of thalassaemia minor (particularly β thalassaemia trait and α thalassaemia trait due to haemoglobin Constant Spring), thalassaemia major, megaloblastic anaemia, unstable haemoglobins, haemolytic anaemia, dyserythropoietic states in general (including congenital dyserythropoietic anaemia, sideroblastic anaemia, erythroleukaemia and primary myelofibrosis), liver disease and poisoning by heavy metals such as lead, arsenic, bismuth, zinc, silver and mercury. Basophilic stippling is a prominent feature of hereditary deficiency of pyrimidine 5′-nucleotidase [128], an enzyme that is required for RNA degradation. Inhibition of this enzyme may also be responsible for the prominent basophilic stippling in some patients with lead poisoning. Similar findings have been reported in a putative deficiency of CPD-choline phosphotransferase, resulting in accumulation of the pyrimidine phosphodiester, CPD-choline [129].

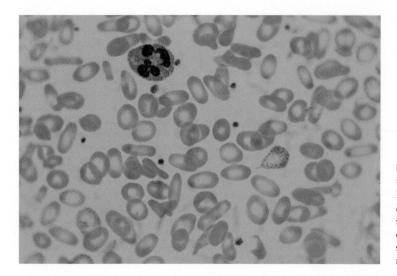

Fig. 3.60 Prominent basophilic stippling in the peripheral blood film of a patient who has inherited both β thalassaemia trait and hereditary elliptocytosis. The film also shows microcytosis and numerous elliptocytes and ovalocytes. One of the heavily stippled cells is a teardrop poikilocyte. Courtesy of Dr F. Toolis, Dumfries.

Pappenheimer bodies

Pappenheimer bodies (Fig. 3.61; see also Fig. 3.20) are basophilic inclusions that may be present in small numbers in erythrocytes; they often occur in small clusters towards the periphery of the cell and can be demonstrated to contain iron. They are composed of ferritin aggregates, or mitochondria or phagosomes containing aggregated ferritin. They stain on a Romanowsky stain because clumps of ribosomes are co-precipitated with the iron-containing organelles. A cell containing Pappenheimer bodies is a siderocyte. Reticulocytes often contain Pappenheimer bodies. Following splenectomy in a haematologically normal subject, small numbers of Pappenheimer bodies appear, these being ferritin aggregates. In pathological conditions, such as lead poisoning or sideroblastic anaemia, Pappenheimer bodies can also represent iron-laden mitochondria or phagosomes. If the patient has also had a splenectomy they will be present in much larger numbers.

Cabot rings

Cabot rings are remnants of microtubutes that formed the mitotic spindle [130]. They may have the form of a circle or a figure of eight (Fig. 3.62).

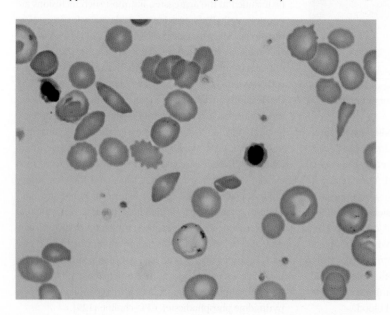

Fig. 3.61 Blood film from a patient with sickle cell anaemia showing an erythrocyte containing multiple Pappenheimer bodies. Their peripheral position and tendency to cluster are apparent.

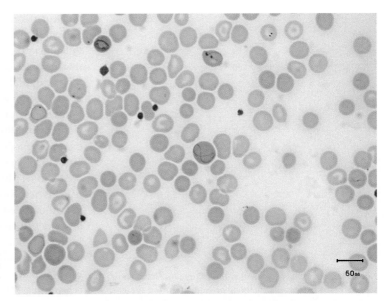

Fig. 3.62 Cabot rings in the blood film of a patient who had received the microtubule inhibitor paclitaxel, medium power. By courtesy of Dr Greg Hapgood, Melbourne.

Micro-organisms in erythrocytes

Both protozoan parasites and other micro-organisms can be seen within red cells (see below).

Crystals

Slender purple-violet crystals, often radially arranged, have been observed in red cells in congenital erythropoietic porphyria (Fig. 3.63) [131].

Circulating nucleated red blood cells

Except in the neonatal period and occasionally in pregnancy, the presence of NRBC (see Fig. 3.49) in the peripheral blood is abnormal, generally indicating hyperplastic erythropoiesis or bone marrow infiltration. In the

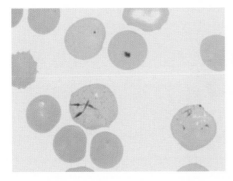

Fig. 3.63 Blood film of a patient with congenital erythropoietic porphyria showing radially arranged crystals in red cells. Courtesy of Dr Anna Merino and colleagues, Barcelona, and the *British Journal of Haematology* [131].

neonatal period, an increased number of NRBC are seen in premature neonates and when there is growth retardation or the neonate has experienced hypoxia. An increased NRBC count at birth with a rise rather than a fall in the neonatal period has been found to be predictive of intraventricular haemorrhage in premature babies [132]. Increased numbers of NRBC can also be seen in babies with Down syndrome. On multivariate analysis, NRBC are predictive of mortality in hospitalised patients (except in obstetric patients and patients with sickle cell disease) [87]. NRBC are also predictive of mortality in medical intensive care ward patients [133].

If both NRBC and granulocyte precursors are present the film is described as leucoerythroblastic. NRBC in the peripheral blood may be morphologically abnormal; e.g. they may be megaloblastic or show the features of iron deficient or sideroblastic erythropoiesis. An increased frequency of karyorrhexis in circulating NRBC may be seen in arsenic and lead poisoning [134] and in certain dyserythropoietic states such as erythroleukaemia and severe iron deficiency anaemia. Examination of a buffy coat film is helpful if assessment of morphological abnormalities in NRBC is required.

Red cell agglutination, rouleaux formation and red cell rosetting

Red cell agglutinates (see Fig. 3.14) are irregular clumps of cells whereas rouleaux (Fig. 3.64) are stacks of erythrocytes resembling a pile of coins.

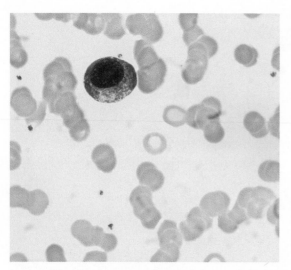

Fig. 3.64 Blood film of a patient with multiple myeloma showing increased rouleaux formation consequent on the presence of a paraprotein; the film also shows increased background staining and a circulating myeloma cell.

Reticulocytes may form agglutinates when their numbers are increased; this is a normal phenomenon. Mature red cells agglutinate when they are antibody-coated. Small agglutinates may be seen in warm auto-immune haemolytic anaemia. Agglutinates are more common in paroxysmal cold haemoglobinuria and in chronic cold haemagglutinin disease there may be massive agglutination (see Fig. 3.2).

Rouleaux formation is increased when there is an increased plasma concentration of proteins of high molecular weight. The most common causes are pregnancy (in which fibrinogen concentration is increased), inflammatory conditions (in which polyclonal immunoglobulins, α_2 macroglobulin and fibrinogen are increased) and plasma cell neoplasms such as multiple myeloma (in which increased immunoglobulin concentration is caused by the presence of a monoclonal paraprotein). Rouleaux formation may be artefactually increased if a drop of blood is left standing for too long on a microscope slide before the blood film is spread.

Abnormal clumping of red cells can also occur in patients receiving certain intravenous drugs that use polyethoxylated castor oils as a carrier (e.g. miconazole, phytomenadione and ciclosporin).

Rosetting of red cells around neutrophils (Fig. 3.65) is a rare phenomenon that is likely to be antibody mediated. It is sometimes an *in vitro* phenomenon and may be EDTA dependent [135]. It has been observed, together with erythrophagocytosis, in paroxysmal cold haemoglobinuria [136].

Leucocytes

Normal peripheral blood leucocytes are classified either as polymorphonuclear leucocytes or as mononuclear cells, the latter term indicating lymphocytes and monocytes. Polymorphonuclear leucocytes are also referred to as polymorphonuclear granulocytes, polymorphs or granulocytes. The term 'granulocyte' has also been used to refer more generally to both the mature polymorphonuclear leucocytes usually seen in the peripheral

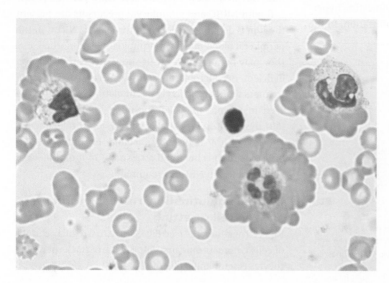

Fig. 3.65 Red cell rosetting.

blood and their granulated precursors. Polymorphs have lobulated nuclei, which are very variable in shape, hence 'polymorphic', and prominent cytoplasmic granules, which differ in staining characteristics between the three classes – neutrophil, eosinophil and basophil. Mononuclear cells may also have granules; in the case of the monocyte they are inconspicuous, whereas in the lymphocyte they are sometimes prominent but are not numerous. In pathological conditions and in certain physiological conditions, such as pregnancy and during the neonatal period, precursors of polymorphs may appear in the peripheral blood. A variety of abnormal leucocytes may also be seen in certain disease states. The terms 'polymorph' and 'granulocyte' should not be used to refer specifically to neutrophils, since these designations also includes eosinophils and basophils.

Granulocytes

The neutrophil

The mature neutrophil measures 12–15 μm in diameter. The cytoplasm is acidophilic with many fine granules. The visible granules are not the secondary granules of the neutrophil, which are below the level of resolution of the light microscope. Rather, they are primary granules that have altered their staining characteristics. Although they are not individually visible, it is the specific neutrophil granules that are responsible for the pink tinge of neutrophil cytoplasm. The nucleus has clumped chromatin and is divided into two to five distinct lobes by filaments, which are narrow strands of dense heterochromatin bordered by nuclear membrane (Fig. 3.66). The nucleus tends to follow an approximately circular form since in the living cell the nuclear lobes are arranged in a circle around the centrosome. In normal females a 'drumstick' may be seen protruding from the nucleus of a proportion of cells (Fig. 3.67). A normal neutrophil has granules spread evenly through the cytoplasm, but there may be some agranular cytoplasm protruding at one margin of the cell. This may represent the advancing edge of a cell in active locomotion.

Characteristics of the nucleus

The neutrophil band form and left shift

A cell that otherwise resembles a mature neutrophil but that lacks nuclear lobes (Fig. 3.68) is referred to as a neutrophil band form or a 'stab' form (from the German *Stabzelle* referring to a shepherd's staff or crook). The Committee for the Clarification of Nomenclature of Cells and Diseases of the Blood Forming Organs has defined a band cell as 'any cell of the granulocyte series which has a nucleus which could be described as a curved or coiled band, no matter how marked the indentation, if it does not completely segment the nucleus into lobes separated by a filament'. A filament is a thread-like connection with 'no significant nuclear material' [137]. A band is differentiated from a metamyelocyte (see below) by having an appreciable amount of nucleus with parallel sides. Small numbers of band cells are seen in healthy subjects. An increase in the number of band

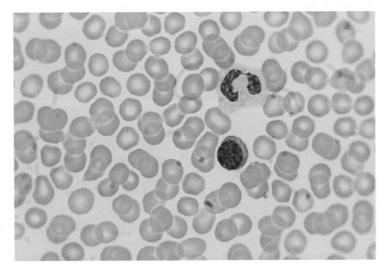

Fig. 3.66 Blood film of a healthy subject showing a normal polymorphonuclear neutrophil and normal small lymphocyte. The disposition of the nuclear lobes around the circumference of a circle is apparent.

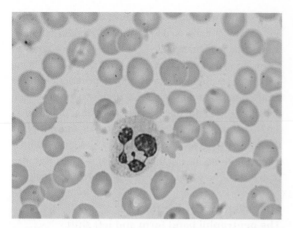

Fig. 3.67 Blood film of a healthy female showing a normal neutrophil with a drumstick.

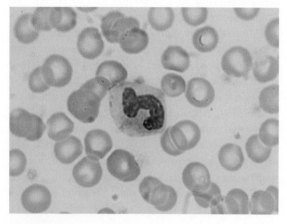

Fig. 3.68 A neutrophil band form. The nucleus is non-segmented and also has chromatin that is less condensed than that of the majority of segmented neutrophils.

cells in relation to normal neutrophils is known as a left shift. When a left shift occurs, neutrophil precursors more immature than band forms (metamyelocytes, myelocytes, promyelocytes and blast cells) may also be released into the blood. A left shift is a physiological occurrence in pregnancy. In the non-pregnant patient it often indicates a response to infection or inflammation, or some other stimulus to the bone marrow. A left shift, including even a few blast cells, is produced by the administration of cytokines such as granulocyte colony-stimulating factor (G-CSF) and granulocyte-macrophage colony-stimulating factor (GM-CSF).

The actual percentage or absolute number of band forms or the ratio of band forms to neutrophils that is regarded as normal is dependent on the precise definition of band form used and how the definition is applied in practice. Inconsistency between laboratories with regard to definition is common, as is variation between and within laboratories as to how definitions are applied. Band cell counts have been employed in the detection of infection in neonates, but again various definitions have been applied [138,139]. For example, Akenzua *et al.* [138] defined a (segmented) neutrophil as a cell with lobes separated by a thin filament whose width is less than one-third the maximum diameter of the lobes, whereas Christensen *et al.* [140] required the lobes to be separated by a definite nuclear filament. An increase in band forms in a neonate can be the result of bacterial infection (e.g. group B streptococcus or listeria) or congenital virus infection (e.g. cytomegalovirus or coxsackie virus) [85].

A left shift contributes to the Alvarado score for the presumptive diagnosis of acute appendicitis [141].

The neutrophil lobe count and right shift

In normal blood, most neutrophils have one to five lobes. Six-lobed neutrophils are rare. A right shift is said to be present if the average lobe count is increased or if there is an increased percentage of neutrophils with five or six lobes. The average lobe count of normal neutrophils varies between observers, with values of 2.5–3.3 obtained in different studies [142]. In practice, a formal lobe count is time-consuming and the presence of more than 3% of neutrophils with five lobes or more (Fig. 3.69) is a more practical indicator of right shift. This is also a more sensitive index of neutrophil hypersegmentation than the average lobe count and allows hypersegmentation to be detected in patients in whom a simultaneous increase in band forms means that the average lobe count is normal. A further index of right shift, which has been found to be more sensitive than either of the above, is the segmentation index:

$$\frac{\text{number of neutrophils with 5 lobes or more} \times 100}{\text{number of neutrophils with four lobes}}$$

Values of greater than 16.9 are abnormal [143]. A right shift or neutrophil hypersegmentation is seen in megaloblastic anaemia and in occasional patients with infection, uraemia or MDS. There is also a significant incidence in iron deficiency anaemia when other haematinic

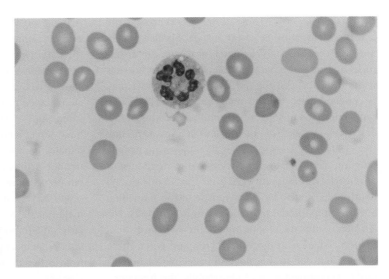

Fig. 3.69 A hypersegmented neutrophil showing seven nuclear lobes. The film also shows anisocytosis with both microcytes and macrocytes.

deficiencies are excluded [144]. Some hypersegmented neutrophils are seen following the administration of G-CSF [145]. Hypersegmented neutrophils are diploid cells; in patients with megaloblastic anaemia they are **not** derived from giant metamyelocytes [146]. Neutrophil hypersegmentation occurs as a rare hereditary characteristic with an autosomal dominant inheritance [147]. In the inherited condition known as myelokathexis there is neutropenia in association with a defect of neutrophil lobulation [148,149]. Neutrophils are hypersegmented with long chromatin filaments separating the lobes and with coarse, almost pyknotic chromatin; Döhle bodies, toxic granulation and neutrophil vacuolation have also been noted [149]. Rarely, a similar

anomaly is seen in MDS, but at least some of these cases differ from the inherited condition in that the hypersegmented neutrophils are tetraploid (Fig. 3.70).

The presence of macropolycytes with more than five lobes is not an indication of right shift since the increased number of lobes is the result of an increased DNA content rather than any abnormality of nuclear segmentation.

The neutrophil drumstick, sessile nodules and other nuclear projections

Some neutrophils in normal females have a drumstick-shaped nuclear appendage about 1.5 μm in diameter, which is linked to the rest of the nucleus by a filament

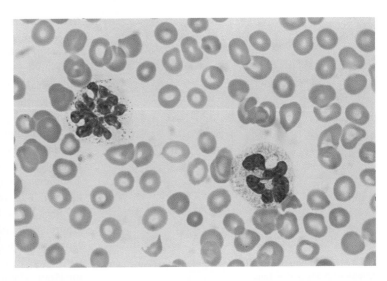

Fig. 3.70 Blood film of a patient with MDS showing two neutrophils. Both are macropolycytes and one shows a defect of nuclear segmentation resembling myelokathexis. The size of the cells and the amount of nuclear material suggest that they are tetraploid cells.

[150] (see Fig. 3.67). These drumsticks represent the inactive X chromosome of the female. Similar projections with central pallor (racquet forms) are not drumsticks and do not have the same significance. In cells without drumsticks, the inactive X chromosome may be condensed beneath the nuclear membrane, where it can be detected in some neutrophil band forms [151], or it may protrude from the nucleus as a sessile nodule (Fig. 3.71). Like drumsticks, sessile nodules are usually only found in females. In one study the frequency of drumsticks was found to vary from 1 in 38 to 1 in 200 neutrophils, and to be characteristic of the individual but also proportional to the lobe count [150,152]. If a left shift occurs, the proportion of cells with drumsticks reduces, whereas in macropolycytes, and when there is right shift due to megaloblastic anaemia or hereditary hypersegmentation of neutrophils, the frequency of drumsticks is increased.

The presence and frequency of drumsticks are related to the number of X chromosomes. They do not occur in normal males, in individuals with the testicular feminisation syndrome who are phenotypically female but genetically (XY) male, or in Turner's syndrome (XO) females. In XXY males with Klinefelter syndrome, drumsticks are found but in lower numbers than in females. Paradoxically, XXX females rarely have cells with double drumsticks and on average their lobe count and frequency of drumsticks are lower than those of normal females; they have an increased incidence of sessile nodules and it has been suggested that the presence of an extra X chromosome inhibits nuclear segmentation [153]. However, triploidy, with the karyotype 69,XXY, is associated with the presence of drumsticks and in addition the nuclei are large and show increased sessile nodules and thorn-like and club-shaped projections [154]. Females with an isochromosome of the long arms of the X chromosome have larger and more frequent drumsticks, whereas females with deletions from the X chromosome have smaller drumsticks [147]. Natural human chimaeras whose cells are a mixture of cells of male and female origin have a drumstick frequency consistent with a male/female mixture of neutrophils [152] and, similarly, an alteration of the drumstick count may be seen after bone marrow transplantation when bone marrow from a female has been transplanted into a male or vice versa.

The proportion of neutrophils with drumsticks and sessile nodules is reduced in women with chronic myelogenous leukaemia (CML), but returns to normal when the WBC falls on treatment [155].

The drumstick count (and the average lobe count) are reduced in Down syndrome [156].

In addition to drumsticks and sessile nodules, neutrophil nuclei may have other projections that can have the shape of clubs, hooks or tags. These projections can also be seen in the neutrophils of males. Increased nuclear projections can be a feature of MDS [157] (Fig. 3.72). The presence of several thread-like projections from the nuclei of most neutrophils is a characteristic feature of congenital trisomy 13 syndrome [158,159].

Other abnormalities of neutrophil nuclei

Other abnormalities of neutrophil nuclei are shown in Table 3.8. Reduced neutrophil segmentation that is not consequent on temporary bone marrow stimulation with release of immature cells is seen as an inherited anomaly (the Pelger–Huët anomaly) or as an acquired anomaly (the pseudo-Pelger–Huët or acquired Pelger–Huët anomaly). The Pelger–Huët anomaly was first described by Pelger in 1928 and its familial nature was recognised by Huët in 1931 [178]. It is inherited as an autosomal dominant characteristic with a prevalence between 1 in 100 and 1 in 10 000 in different communities [179]. It has been recognised in many ethnic groups including Caucasians, Black people, Chinese, Japanese and Indonesians. It results from a mutation in the *LBR* gene, at 1q42.1, encoding the lamin B receptor [180]. The abnormality is distinctive. The majority

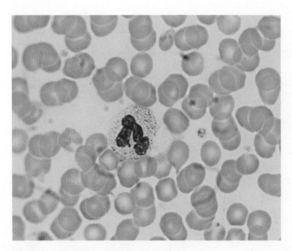

Fig. 3.71 Blood film of a healthy female showing a band neutrophil with a sessile nodule.

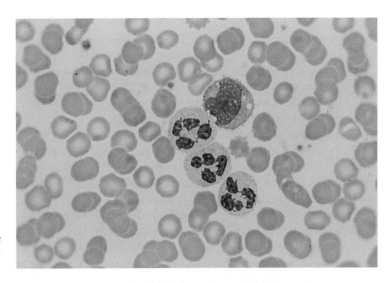

Fig. 3.72 Blood film of a patient with chronic myelomonocytic leukaemia showing neutrophils with abnormal nuclear projections.

Table 3.8 Some alterations and abnormalities that may be present in neutrophil nuclei.

Abnormality	Presence noted in
Left shift	Pregnancy, infection, hypoxia, shock
Hypersegmentation	Megaloblastic erythropoiesis
	Iron deficiency
	Uraemia
	Infection
	Hereditary neutrophil hypersegmentation
	Myelokathexis [148]
	Myelodysplastic syndrome [160]
Hyposegmentation	Pelger–Huët anomaly
	Specific granule deficiency [161]
	Severe congenital neutropenia due to *VPS45* mutation [162]
	Non-lobed neutrophils with other congenital anomalies (one case) [163]
	Acquired or pseudo-Pelger–Huët anomaly (myelodysplastic syndromes and acute myeloid leukaemia)
	Reversible drug-induced Pelger–Huët anomaly (mycophenolate mofetil, tacrolimus) [164]
Increased nuclear projections	Trisomy 13 syndrome [158]
	Associated with large platelets (single family) [165]
	Associated with a large Y chromosome (drumstick like) [166]
	Turner syndrome [167]
	As an isolated defect [168]
	Myelodysplastic syndromes [157]
Ring nuclei	Chronic myelogenous leukaemia [169]
	Acute myeloid leukaemia [170]
	Chronic neutrophilic leukaemia [171]
	Megaloblastic anaemia [172]
Botryoid nucleus	Heat stroke [173]
	Hyperthermia [174]
	Burns
Dense chromatin clumping	Myelodysplastic syndromes [175]
	Reversible effect of certain drugs (including mycophenolate mofetil)
	Myelokathexis [149]
Detached nuclear fragments	Dysplastic granulopoiesis due to HIV infection [176] or administration of drugs interfering with DNA synthesis [177], including chlorambucil, mycophenolate mofetil and tacrolimus

HIV, human immunodeficiency virus

of neutrophils have bilobed nuclei (Fig. 3.73a), the lobes being rounder than normal and the chromatin more condensed than would be expected for the degree of nuclear lobulation; a characteristic spectacle or *pince-nez* shape is common. Other nuclei are shaped like dumbells or peanuts (Fig. 3.73b). A small proportion of neutrophils, usually not more than 4%, have non-lobulated nuclei (Fig. 3.73c); they are distinguished from myelocytes by a lower nucleocytoplasmic ratio, the condensation of nuclear chromatin and the maturity of the cytoplasm. Subjects with the Pelger–Huët anomaly also show reduced lobulation of eosinophils and basophils [181]. In rare homozygotes with the Pelger–Huët anomaly all the neutrophils have round or oval nuclei. Neutrophils, eosinophils, basophils and monocytes are non-lobulated and there may also be mild neutropenia, giant platelets and mild thrombocytopenia [182]. Homozygotes may also show developmental delay, epilepsy and skeletal abnormalities [180], but most do not. The distinction between the Pelger–Huët anomaly and a left shift is important since heterozygosity for the inherited condition is of no clinical significance. If a left shift occurs in a patient with the Pelger–Huët anomaly the proportion of non-lobed neutrophils is further increased. If a subject with the Pelger–Huët anomaly develops megaloblastic erythropoiesis, a right shift occurs and neutrophils with three, four or even five lobes are seen [183]; megaloblastosis also causes loss of the characteristic dense clumping of the nuclear chromatin and drumsticks may become identifiable.

In another congenital anomaly, specific granule deficiency (previously designated lactoferrin deficiency), neutrophils with a marked reduction in the numbers of specific granules also have poorly lobulated or bilobed nuclei [161,184] (Fig. 3.74).

A single patient has been described in whom non-lobed neutrophils were associated with skeletal malformations, microthalmia and mental retardation [163].

The acquired Pelger–Huët anomaly (Fig. 3.75) is common in MDS and in acute myeloid leukaemias. It occurs occasionally in other haematological neoplasms, particularly primary myelofibrosis and during the evolution of CML. Features that help in making the distinction from the inherited Pelger–Huët anomaly are that the percentage of affected neutrophils is usually less and there is commonly an association with neutropenia, hypogranularity of neutrophils, Döhle bodies or dysplastic features in other lineages.

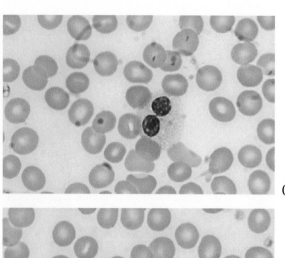 (a)

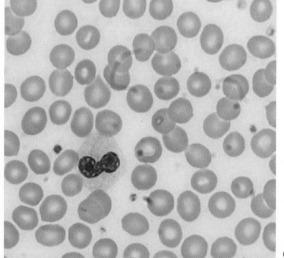 (b)

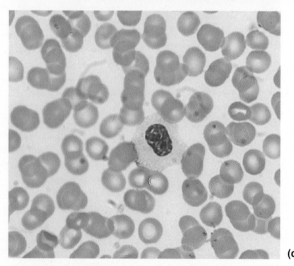 (c)

Fig. 3.73 Blood film of a patient with the inherited Pelger–Huët anomaly showing three neutrophils with: (a) bilobed nucleus; (b) peanut-shaped nucleus; and (c) non-lobed nucleus.

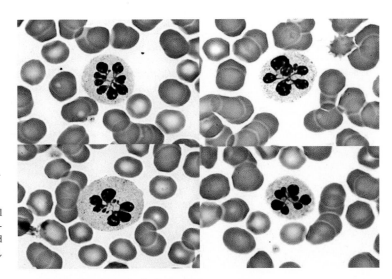

Fig. 3.79 Composite image of peripheral blood film from a patient with cocaine-induced hyperthermia showing botryoid nuclei. With thanks to Dr Patrick Ward, Duluth, Minnesota.

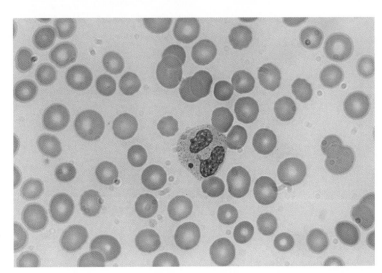

Fig. 3.80 Blood film of a patient on combination chemotherapy for lymphoma showing a neutrophil with a detached nuclear fragment (Howell–Jolly body-like inclusion).

inflammatory and autoimmune conditions or during cytotoxic chemotherapy [191]. Apoptosis should be distinguished from the morphologically similar degenerative changes that occur as an *in vitro* artefact on prolonged storage of blood.

Abnormalities of neutrophil cytoplasm

Abnormalities of neutrophil cytoplasm are summarized in Table 3.9.

Reduced granulation

Reduced granulation of neutrophils can occur as a congenital anomaly, e.g. in specific granule deficiency (see Fig. 3.74), but this is rare. It is usually an acquired abnormality, most often as a feature of MDS (Fig. 3.81). It has been found that a visual assessment that granules are reduced by two-thirds is a reproducible criterion applicable in making a diagnosis of MDS [157]. In HIV infection some neutrophils may show reduced granulation, but this is not as marked as in MDS. Reduced granulation may be apparent in severe infections, as a result of discharge of granules; residual granules may be prominent. Neutrophils produced in response to administration of G-CSF may be hypogranular [145]. Infusion of intravenous lipid can cause neutrophil swelling, degranulation and vacuolation persisting for 6–8 hours [217].

Table 3.9 Some alterations and abnormalities of neutrophil cytoplasm.

Abnormality		Presence noted in
Reduced granulation		Myelodysplastic syndromes and acute myeloid leukaemia
		Specific granule (lactoferrin) deficiency [161]
		Grey platelet syndrome (some families) [192]
		Severe congenital neutropenia due to *VPS45* mutation [162]
Increased granulation		'Toxic' granulation – pregnancy, infection, inflammation, G-CSF and GM-CSF therapy [193,194]
		Aplastic anaemia
		Hypereosinophilic syndromes
		Alder–Reilly anomaly
		Chronic neutrophilic leukaemia [171]
		Myelodysplastic syndromes (uncommonly) [195]
		Myelokathexis [149]
Abnormal granulation		Chédiak–Higashi syndrome and related anomalies [196,197]
		Pseudo-Chédiak–Higashi granules in haematological neoplasms
		Alder–Reilly anomaly
		Acute myeloid leukaemia [198] and myelodysplastic syndromes [195]
Auer rods		Acute myeloid leukaemia and myelodysplastic syndromes
Other crystalline inclusions		Acute myeloid leukaemia [199]
Vacuolation		Infection, G-CSF therapy, GM-CSF therapy
		Acute alcohol poisoning [200,201]
		Jordans anomaly [202]
		Carnitine deficiency
		Kwashiorkor [203]
		Myelokathexis (some families) [149,204]
Döhle bodies or similar inclusions		Infection, inflammation, burns, pregnancy, G-CSF therapy
		Myelodysplastic syndromes and acute myeloid leukaemia
		MYH9-related disorders (May–Hegglin anomaly, Fechtner [205] and Sebastian syndromes)
		Kwashiorkor [203]
		Myelokathexis [149]
Actin inclusions		Congenital abnormality associated with anaemia and grey skin [206]
Phagocytosed material	Bacteria and fungi	Bacterial and fungal infections
	Parasites	Leishmaniasis, malaria (rare)
	Cryoglobulin	Multiple myeloma and other cryoglobulinaemias
	Mucopolysaccharide	Various carcinomas [7]
		Wilms tumour
		Hirschsprung disease [207]
	Nucleoprotein	Systemic lupus erythematosus [208] ('LE cell')
	Melanin	Melanoma [209]
	Bilirubin crystals or amorphous deposits	Severe hyperbilirubinaemia [210,211]
	Cystine crystals	Cystinosis [212]
	Haemosiderin	Iron overload [213]
	Erythrocytes	Autoimmune haemolytic anaemia, paroxysmal cold haemoglobinuria [214], incompatible blood transfusion, potassium chlorate poisoning
	Platelets	*Citrobacter freundii* septicaemia [215], associated with EDTA-dependent platelet satellitism [216]

EDTA, ethylene diamine tetra-acetic acid; G-CSF, granulocyte colony-stimulating factor; GM-CSF, granulocyte macrophage colony-stimulating factor

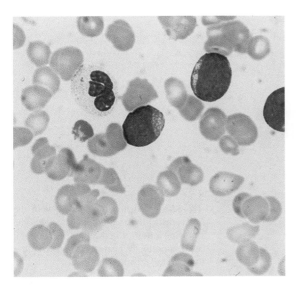

Fig. 3.81 Blood film of a patient with acute myeloid leukaemia (AML) showing three blasts and a hypogranular neutrophil.

Increased granulation

Increased granulation of neutrophils, with granules appearing both larger and more basophilic than normal, is designated toxic granulation (Fig. 3.82). When neutrophil maturation is normal, the azurophilic or primary granules become less strongly azurophilic as the cell matures so that, rather than staining reddish-purple, they stain violet or fail to stain at all. In a neutrophil showing toxic granulation the primary granules remain strongly azurophilic; this may be related to a higher concentration of acid mucosubstances than in normal neutrophils [218]. Degranulation may lead to neutrophils that show toxic granulation also having reduced numbers of granules. Although 'toxic' granulation is characteristic of infection it is non-specific, being seen also in the presence of tissue damage of various types. It is also a feature of normal pregnancy and occurs with cytokine therapy (G-CSF and GM-CSF) even in the absence of infection. In neonates, toxic granulation may signify bacterial infection, but it can also result from severe birth asphyxia, meconium aspiration or maternal chorioamnionitis (when the baby is not infected but cytokines cross the placenta) [85]. Other causes of heavy neutrophil granulation are shown in Figs 3.83 and 3.84 and in Table 3.9.

Abnormal granulation and Auer rods

Abnormal neutrophil granulation is seen in a number of inherited conditions including the Chédiak–Higashi syndrome and the heterogeneous group of conditions giving rise to the Alder–Reilly anomaly (Table 3.10). The Alder–Reilly anomaly occurs as an isolated abnormality, in association with an abnormal peroxidase [220] and as a feature of Tay–Sachs disease, Batten–Spielmeyer–Vogt disease and the mucopolysaccharidoses. The abnormal neutrophils may have heavy granulation resembling toxic granulation or there may be large, clearly abnormal granules (see Fig. 3.84). In the Chédiak–Higashi syndrome (Fig. 3.85) the abnormal granules are quite variable in their staining characteristics and some

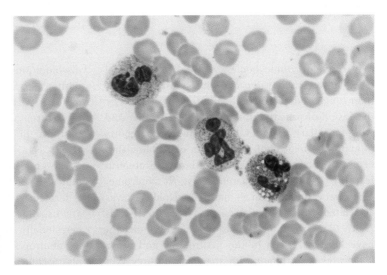

Fig. 3.82 Three neutrophils in the peripheral blood film of a patient with bacterial infection showing toxic granulation and vacuolation.

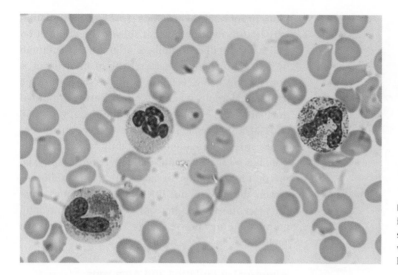

Fig. 3.83 Blood film of a patient with the idiopathic hypereosinophilic syndrome showing a normal neutrophil, a neutrophil with abnormally heavy granulation and a hypogranular band eosinophil.

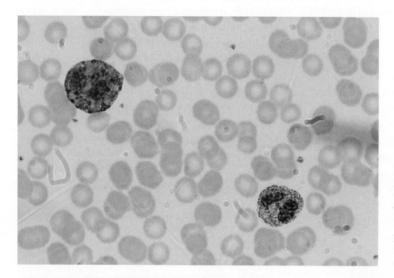

Fig. 3.84 Blood film of a patient with the Maroteaux–Lamy syndrome showing the Alder–Reilly anomaly of neutrophils. The neutrophil has granules that resemble 'toxic' granules. The other granulocyte is probably an eosinophil with granules having very abnormal staining characteristics. Courtesy of Mr Alan Dean, Nottingham.

may resemble Döhle bodies; at the ultrastructural level, however, they are abnormal granules rather than rough endoplasmic reticulum, being formed by the fusion of primary granules with each other and with secondary granules. There have been reports of abnormal neutrophil granulation resembling that of the Chédiak–Higashi syndrome but with atypical features [196]. In an apparently distinct syndrome, abnormal granulation of all mature myeloid cells was associated with bile duct atresia and livedo reticularis [211]. Giant bright blue inclusions composed of actin have been described in the neutrophils and other leucocytes of an infant with anaemia and grey skin

discoloration [206] (Fig. 3.86) and in a second infant without associated abnormalities [221]. Occasional patients with MDS or AML have giant granules in neutrophils, which are morphologically similar to those of the Chédiak–Higashi syndrome [198] (Fig. 3.87).

The Auer rod that is seen in haematological malignancies, specifically AML and some subtypes of MDS, is formed by fusion of primary granules. Auer rods are usually confined to blast cells (Fig. 3.88) but occasionally they are seen in maturing cells, including neutrophils (Fig. 3.89), which are part of the neoplastic clone.

Table 3.10 Inherited conditions in which leucocytes have abnormal granules or cytoplasmic inclusions.

Abnormality	Associated features	Morphology of granules or inclusions	Nature of granules or inclusions	Nature of cells affected
Chédiak–Higashi anomaly*	Anaemia, neutropenia, thrombocytopenia, jaundice, neurological abnormalities, recurrent infections	Giant granules with colour ranging from grey to red	Giant secondary (specific) granules	Neutrophil, eosinophil, basophil, monocyte, lymphocyte, melanocyte, renal tubular cell, many other body cells
Alder–Reilly anomaly*†	Tay-Sachs disease, mucopolysaccharidoses (Hunter syndrome,** Sanfilippo syndrome, Morquio syndrome, Scheie syndrome, Maroteaux-Lamy syndrome, β glucuronidase deficiency), multiple sulphatase deficiency [219], associated with abnormal myeloperoxidase [220]	Dark red or purple inclusions that may resemble toxic granules, inclusions or vacuoles in lymphocytes	Mucopoly-saccharide or other abnormal carbohydrate	Neutrophil, eosinophil, basophil, monocyte (rarely), lymphocyte; in Maroteaux–Lamy syndrome platelets also have abnormal granules
MYH9-related disorders including May–Hegglin anomaly‡	Thrombocytopenia, giant platelets	Resemble Döhle bodies but larger and more angular	Amorphous areas of cytoplasm containing structures related to ribosomes	Neutrophil, eosinophil, basophil, monocyte

*autosomal recessive
†Hunter syndrome is sex-linked recessive
‡autosomal dominant

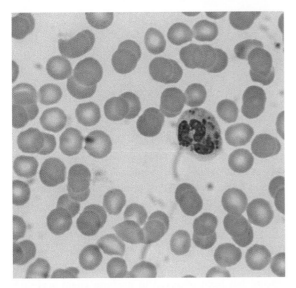

Fig. 3.85 Blood film of a patient with the Chédiak–Higashi syndrome showing a neutrophil with giant and abnormally staining granules. Courtesy of Dr J. McCallum, Kirkaldy.

Vacuolation

Neutrophil vacuolation is most often an acquired abnormality. It can occur as the result of the fusion of granules with a phagocytic vacuole with subsequent exocytosis of the contents of the secondary lysosome. This is usually a feature of infection (see Fig. 3.82) and partial degranulation of the neutrophil may also be apparent. In neonates, vacuolation can occur as a result of necrotising enterocolitis or candidiasis as well as bacterial infection [85]. Vacuolation of neutrophils can also occur as a toxic effect following ethanol ingestion [200] (Fig. 3.90), but this is much less often observed than ethanol-induced vacuolation of myeloid precursors; the vacuolation is attributed both to invagination of the membrane with inclusion of plasma and to mitochondrial swelling and disruption [201]. Intravenous lipid infusion can cause neutrophil vacuolation [217]. Neutrophil vacuoles are particularly large and distinct in paroxysmal cold haemoglobinuria, when they result from lysis of a phagocytosed erythrocyte. Colchicine toxicity causes vacuolation [190]. Neutrophil vacuolation

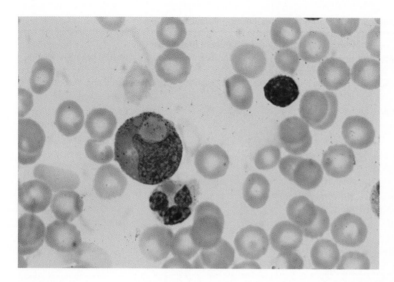

Fig. 3.86 Bone marrow film of a patient with giant actin inclusions (Brandalise syndrome) showing blue inclusions in a neutrophil and a promyelocyte. Similar inclusions were present in peripheral blood neutrophils and also in eosinophils, basophils, monocytes and lymphocytes. Courtesy of Dr R.C. Ribeiro, Memphis.

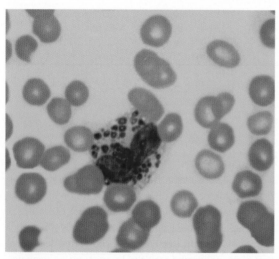

Fig. 3.87 Blood film of a patient with MDS showing pseudo-Chédiak–Higashi granules in a neutrophil.

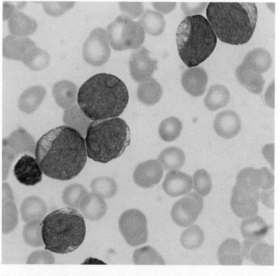

Fig. 3.88 Peripheral blood film of a patient with AML showing blasts, one of which contains an Auer rod.

can occur in hepatic failure. Neutrophil vacuolation is a feature of acquired neutrophil dysplasia associated with a 17p–chromosome anomaly.

Neutrophil vacuolation as the result of an inherited abnormality is rare. It occurs, together with vacuolation of neutrophil precursors, monocytes and some eosinophils, basophils and lymphocytes, in a familial defect designated Jordans anomaly [202,222]; cells contain neutral lipid that is stainable with oil red O and the vacuoles are due to dissolution of lipid [222]. Jordans' original patients may have had carnitine deficiency, which is

known to cause lipid storage myopathy with lipid vacuoles in neutrophils [223]. Similar lipid vacuoles in neutrophils occur in neutral lipid storage disease (also known as triglyceride storage disease with impaired long-chain fatty acid oxidation and as Dorfman–Chanarin syndrome [224,225]). Two genetic defects can cause neutral lipid storage disease, mutation of *ABHD5* and mutation of *PNPLA2*. Neutrophil vacuolation, together with acanthocytosis, has been observed in medium chain acyl-CoA dehydrogenase deficiency [94]. Neutrophil vacuolation is also observed in some families with myelokathexis

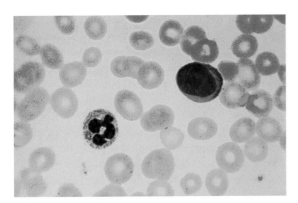

Fig. 3.89 Blood film of a patient with AML showing a blast cell and a mature neutrophil that contains an Auer rod. By courtesy of Professor Daniel Catovsky, London.

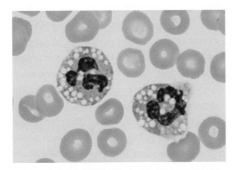

Fig. 3.90 Blood film of a patient with a heavy alcohol intake showing prominent vacuolation of neutrophils. Courtesy of Dr Wendy Erber, Perth, Australia.

[204] and in the WHIM (warts, hypogammaglobulinae-mia infections and myelokathexis) syndrome. Neutrophil vacuolation occurs in specific granule deficiency.

Döhle bodies and similar inclusions

Döhle bodies are small, pale blue or blue-grey cytoplas-mic inclusions, single or multiple, often found towards the periphery of the cell (Fig. 3.91). They usually measure only 1–2 μm in diameter but may be up to 5 μm. At the ultrastructural level, they are composed of strands of rough endoplasmic reticulum, frequently arranged in parallel manner, together with glycogen granules [226]. Their ribosomal component is indicated by pink staining with a methyl green–pyronin stain and by destruction by ribonuclease; they are better seen in films made from non-anticoagulated blood [227]. Döhle bodies are associated with pregnancy, infective

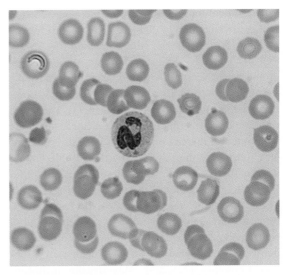

Fig. 3.91 Blood film of a patient with septicaemia showing a Döhle body in a neutrophil.

and inflammatory states, burns (Fig. 3.92) and adminis-tration of cytokines such as G-CSF and GM-CSF. They may be seen in MDS and AML, and have been described in pernicious anaemia, polycythaemia vera, CML, haemolytic anaemia, granulomatosis with polyangiitis (previously Wegener's granulomatosis), and following use of anti-cancer chemotherapeutic agents [228].

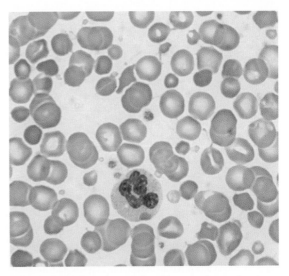

Fig. 3.92 Blood film of a patient with severe burns showing a prominent Döhle body. The red cells also show abnormalities attributable to burns.

Large inclusions resembling Döhle bodies, often numerous and sharply defined, are a feature of the *MYH9*-related disorders; these include the May–Hegglin anomaly, Alport syndrome, Epstein syndrome, Fechtner syndrome and Sebastian syndrome, see Table 8.13) and are also characterised by thrombocytopenia and giant platelets (Fig. 3.93). The inclusions are often spindle- or crescent-shaped, randomly distributed in the cell rather than near the cell margin, and more intensely staining than Döhle bodies. At the ultrastructural level these inclusions differ from the Döhle bodies of reactive states; they appear as an amorphous area largely devoid of organelles, often incompletely surrounded by a single strand of rough endoplasmic reticulum and containing a few dense rods and spherical particles, which are probably ribosomes [226,229]. May–Hegglin inclusions are composed largely of a mutant form of the non-muscle myosin heavy chain IIa protein [230]. They are devoid of glycogen granules [226].

In normal subjects, Döhle bodies are rare. In one study they were seen in 3 of 20 healthy subjects with an average frequency of 0.1 per 100 cells [228]. In pregnancy, the number of Döhle bodies per 100 cells increases in parallel with the WBC [227]; the increased frequency persists into the postpartum period.

Exogenous neutrophil inclusions

Since neutrophils are phagocytes they may contain inclusions that represent phagocytosed material such as microorganisms or cryoglobulin. Malaria pigment is occasionally observed in neutrophils (Fig. 3.94) but is more commonly present in monocytes. Less often malaria parasites are present (Fig. 3.95). Cryoglobulin (Fig. 3.96) may be seen as single or multiple round, weakly basophilic inclusions or as a single large inclusion that displaces the nucleus. Phagocytosis of cryoglobulin occurs *in vitro*, when the blood is left standing, rather than *in vivo* [231]. A greyish-purple deposit that was not a cryoglobulin but probably represented immune complexes has been reported in a patient with splenic lymphoma with villous lymphocytes [232]. Abnormal mucopolysaccharide that circulates in the blood of patients with malignant disease may be ingested by neutrophils [7]. The formation of lupus erythematosus (LE) cells is usually an *in vitro* phenomenon, but they may be seen in the peripheral blood (Fig 3.97), e.g. in patients with severe lupus erythematosus (SLE) [208]. Square or rectangular crystals of cystine can be seen in peripheral blood leucocytes in cystinosis but are more readily detected with phase-contrast microscopy [212]. Large cytoplasmic inclusions were observed in a case of colchicine poisoning [233]. Refractile golden yellow haemosiderin inclusions were observed in a patient with thalassaemia major who had iron overload and sepsis [213].

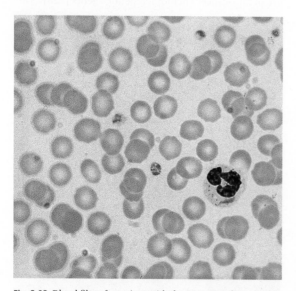

Fig. 3.93 Blood film of a patient with the May–Hegglin anomaly showing a May–Hegglin inclusion, which resembles a Döhle body. Large platelets are also apparent. Courtesy of Dr Norman Parker, London.

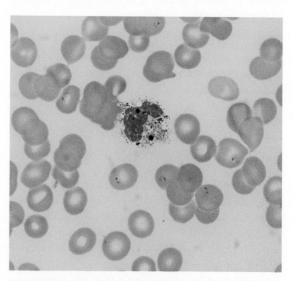

Fig. 3.94 Blood film of a patient with *Plasmodium falciparum* malaria showing malaria pigment in a neutrophil and ring forms of the parasite within red cells.

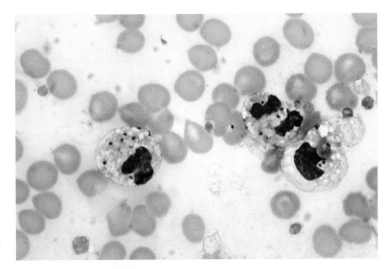

Fig. 3.95 Blood film of a patient with malaria showing microgametes of *Plasmodium vivax* that have been phagocytosed by neutrophils.

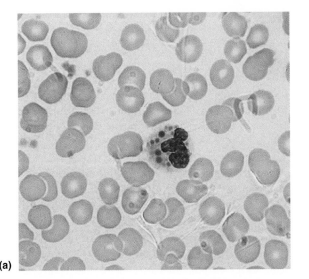

(a)

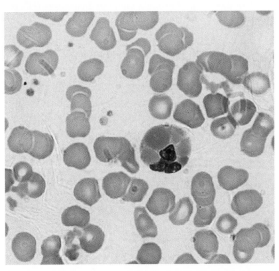

(b)

Fig. 3.96 Blood film of a patient with cryoglobulinaemia showing cryoglobulin that has been ingested by neutrophils and appears as: (a) small round inclusions; and (b) large masses filling the cytoplasm and displacing the nucleus. Some extracellular cryoglobulin is also present. Courtesy of Mr Alan Dean.

Neutrophils may also ingest red cells, a phenomenon referred to as erythrophagocytosis. This has been observed in autoimmune haemolytic anaemia, paroxysmal cold haemoglobinuria, during acute exacerbations of chronic cold haemagglutinin disease, in other patients with a positive direct antiglobulin test and in haemolysis induced by snake-bite, both with and without a positive direct antiglobulin test [234]. It is also seen in patients with defective red cells, as in sickle cell anaemia and sickle cell/haemoglobin C disease, and in any severe haemolytic anaemia due to an intrinsic red cell defect. One patient has been reported with severe haemolytic anaemia and extreme erythrophagocytosis by neutrophils (a third of neutrophils phagocytic) in the absence of a detectable autoantibody but responsive to corticosteroids and splenectomy [235]. Erythrophagocytosis has been reported in a patient given G-CSF and GM-CSF; the latter agent appeared to be the principal cause [236]. Abnormal neutrophils showing marked erythrophagocytosis were reported

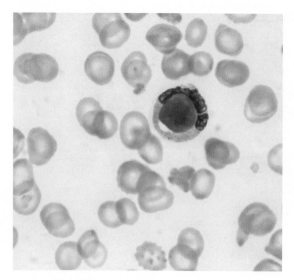

Fig. 3.97 Blood film showing a lupus erythematosus (LE) cell that has formed spontaneously.

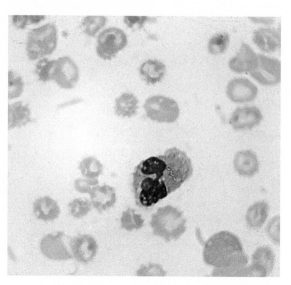

Fig. 3.99 The blood film of a young baby showing a neutrophil containing refractile bilirubin crystals. By courtesy of Dr Sudharma Vidyatilake, Colombo.

in a patient with chronic myelomonocytic leukaemia (CMML) [237].

Ingestion of melanin has been seen in patients with metastatic melanoma (Fig. 3.98). Rarely bilirubin crystals are seen within neutrophils of infants and children with a markedly elevated plasma bilirubin; they are refractile and faintly yellow (Fig. 3.99);

they have been found to form *in vitro* when EDTA-anticoagulated blood is allowed to stand for at least 30 minutes [238]. Coarse bright green cytoplasmic inclusions were reported in two patients with liver failure [239].

Other abnormalities of neutrophil morphology
Macropolycytes

A macropolycyte is about twice the size of a normal neutrophil (Fig. 3.100); its diameter is 15–25 μm rather than 12–15 μm and analysis of its DNA content shows that it is tetraploid rather than diploid, the number of lobes present being increased proportionately. Some macropolycytes are binucleated (Fig. 3.101). Occasional macropolycytes are seen in the blood of healthy subjects. Increased numbers are seen in an inherited (autosomal dominant) condition in which 1–2% of neutrophils are giant with 6- to 10-lobed nuclei, or with twin mirror-image nuclei [240]. Increased numbers, together with rather non-specific dysplastic features, have been described in DiGeorge syndrome [241]. Macropolycytes, including binucleated cells, have been observed following the administration of G-CSF [193] and are present in increased numbers in megaloblastic anaemia. In megaloblastic anaemia they have a DNA content varying between diploid and tetraploid [146]; in contrast to hypersegmented neutrophils, they are derived from giant metamyelocytes. They have

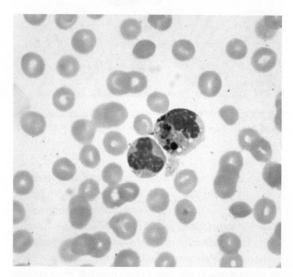

Fig. 3.98 Blood film showing a neutrophil containing melanin in a patient with widely disseminated malignant melanoma. By courtesy of Dr John Luckit, London, and the late Dr David Swirsky.

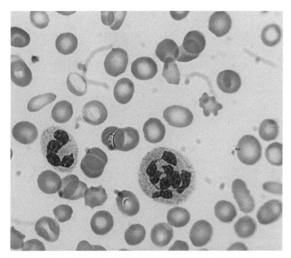

Fig. 3.100 Blood film of a patient with MDS showing a macropolycyte, which is twice the size of the adjacent normal neutrophil. The nucleus is also twice normal size and shows increased nuclear segmentation; it is likely that this is a tetraploid cell. In addition the film shows anisochromasia.

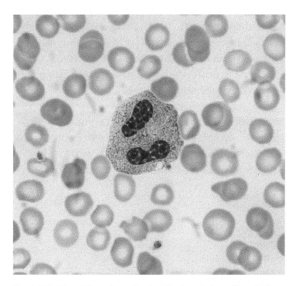

Fig. 3.101 Blood film of a patient with chronic lymphocytic leukaemia (CLL) and reversible chlorambucil-induced myelodysplasia showing a binucleated tetraploid neutrophil. Courtesy of the late Dr P.C. Srivastava.

also been reported in chronic infection, CML and other myeloproliferative neoplasms, and following the administration of cytotoxic drugs and antimetabolites. Most macropolycytes have nuclear and cytoplasmic staining characteristics that are the same as those of other neutrophils, but in megaloblastic anaemia macropolycytes

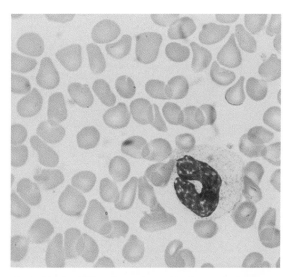

Fig. 3.102 Blood film of a patient with the acquired immune deficiency syndrome (AIDS) showing a hypogranular (probably tetraploid) giant metamyelocyte.

may be seen that have a more open chromatin pattern and do not have an increased number of lobes [242]. Patients with HIV infection may have not only binucleate macropolycytes and macropolycytes with an open chromatin pattern but also circulating giant metamyelocytes (Fig. 3.102), cells that are characteristic of megaloblastic anaemia and are usually seen only in the bone marrow.

Necrobiotic (apoptotic) neutrophils and other myeloid cells

Necrobiotic neutrophils are cells that have died in the peripheral blood by a process known as apoptosis or 'programmed cell death'. Occasionally such cells are seen in the blood of healthy subjects and are recognised by their dense, homogeneous (pyknotic) nuclei, which eventually become completely round or fragment into multiple dense masses; the cytoplasm shows prominent acidophilia (Fig. 3.103). Infection is the most common cause of increased numbers of apoptotic neutrophils [243]. In invasive meningococcal disease, the number of apoptotic neutrophils correlates with the severity of infection [244]. Some patients with AML have numerous necrobiotic myeloid cells (Fig. 3.104). If blood is left at room temperature for a long time, a similar change can occur as an *in vitro* artefact. Leucocytes that have degenerated to the extent that nuclear material is no longer apparent have been designated necrotic; this is generally an artefact consequent on prolonged storage.

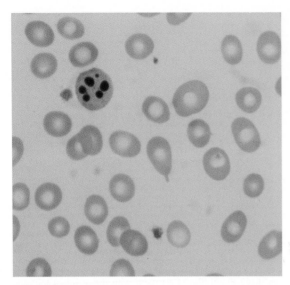

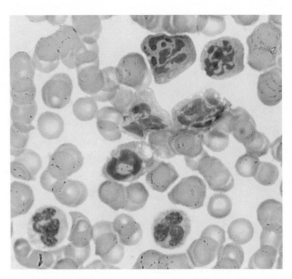

Fig. 3.103 Blood film of a patient with megaloblastic anaemia showing an apoptotic neutrophil. The chromatin has condensed and the nucleus has fragmented into rounded pyknotic masses. The film also shows anisocytosis, macrocytosis and a teardrop poikilocyte.

Fig. 3.104 Blood film of a patient with AML showing five apoptotic leukaemic cells.

Neutrophil aggregation

Aggregation of neutrophils with or without aggregation of platelets develops *in vitro* in some patients when EDTA-anticoagulated blood is allowed to stand. In some patients this may be the end stage of platelet satellitism. This is an antibody-mediated time-dependent phenomenon, which is not of any clinical significance although it may lead to erroneous automated WBCs. Neutrophil aggregation has also been observed as a transient phenomenon in associ-

ation with infectious mononucleosis [245] and in acute bacterial infection (Fig. 3.105). Occasionally, it is observed in a patient over many months or years and may then be associated with autoimmune disease (Fig. 3.106).

In some patients when the cause is a cold-acting antibody, red cell agglutinates coexist.

Neutrophil or other leucocyte fragments

Occasionally circulating fragments of neutrophil cytoplasm are present in patients with sepsis [246] or in patients to whom G-CSF has been administered [145].

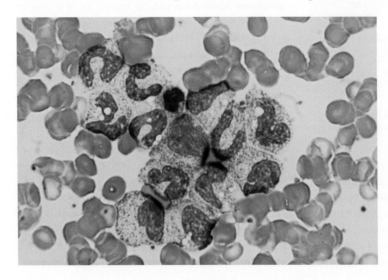

Fig. 3.105 Blood film of a patient with overwhelming sepsis showing neutrophil aggregation, left shift, toxic granulation and neutrophil vacuolation.

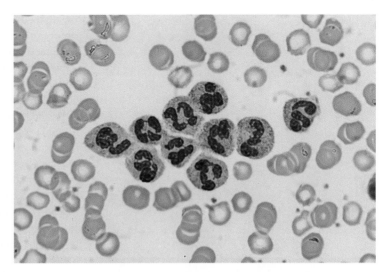

Fig. 3.106 Blood film of a patient with rheumatoid arthritis showing neutrophil aggregation caused by a cold antibody. In this patient, *in vitro* neutrophil aggregation was observed for more than a decade and often led to inaccurate automated white cell counts (WBCs).

Fragmentation of neutrophils has been observed, in association with microangiopathic haemolytic anaemia, in a patient with clot formation at the tip of a dialysis catheter [247]. The mechanism is likely to have been mechanical damage to neutrophils. Neoplastic cells, such as leukaemic blast cells, are more prone to fragmentation than are normal cells and leucocyte fragmentation is not infrequently observed in AML (see Fig. 4.2).

The eosinophil

The eosinophil (Fig. 3.107) is slightly larger than the neutrophil, with a diameter of 12–17 μm. The nucleus

is usually bilobed but occasional nuclei are trilobed, the average lobe count being about 2.3. In females, eosinophils may have drumsticks (Fig. 3.108), but as the frequency of drumsticks is related to the degree of lobulation of the nucleus they are quite infrequent. Eosinophil granules are spherical and considerably larger than those of neutrophils; they pack the cytoplasm and stain reddish-orange. The cytoplasm of eosinophils is weakly basophilic, ribosomes and rough endoplasmic reticulum being more abundant than

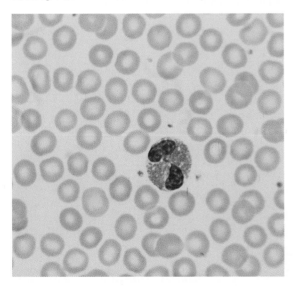

Fig. 3.107 An eosinophil in the peripheral blood film of a healthy subject.

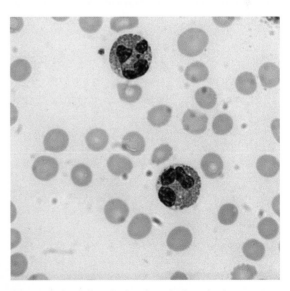

Fig. 3.108 Blood film of a female with idiopathic hypereosinophilic syndrome (HES) showing two eosinophils, one of which has a drumstick.

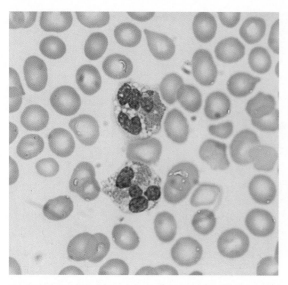

Fig. 3.109 Blood film of a patient with idiopathic HES showing eosinophil hypersegmentation. Both eosinophils have nuclei with four lobes.

in mature neutrophils; when degranulation occurs the pale blue cytoplasm is visible. Very occasional eosinophils in healthy subjects contain some granules with basophilic staining characteristics.

Abnormalities of eosinophil nuclei

Eosinophils may show nuclear hypersegmentation (Fig. 3.109), hyposegmentation (Fig. 3.110) or ring-shaped nuclei (Fig. 3.111). Hypersegmentation can occur in megaloblastic anaemia. It can also be a hereditary phenomenon [248]; in one family hypersegmented eosinophils were also poorly granulated [249] without any apparent clinical defect. Increased lobulation has also been reported, together with decreased numbers of eosinophils, in Down syndrome [156,250]. Increased lobulation is a feature of myelokathexis including the WHIM syndrome [149]. Reduced eosinophil lobulation occurs in the Pelger–Huët anomaly (see Fig. 3.110) and has also been observed in specific granule deficiency [161].

Hypersegmentation, hyposegmentation and ring-shaped nuclei can all occur as acquired abnormalities. Hyposegmentation of eosinophil nuclei occurs as an acquired phenomenon in myeloproliferative neoplasms, including primary myelofibrosis, and in MDS (Fig. 3.112). In the latter group of disorders the chromatin may be clumped and the nuclei entirely or largely non-lobed [251]; this may be regarded as an acquired Pelger–Huët anomaly confined to eosinophils. Patients with eosinophilic leukaemia may have both hypersegmented and hyposegmented eosinophils. Hyposegmented eosinophils can be seen in reactive eosinophilia [252]. Ring eosinophils are seen in a variety of conditions [253]; they appear to have no specific diagnostic significance. Howell–Jolly body-like inclusions, likely to be drug induced, have been observed in one patient [254].

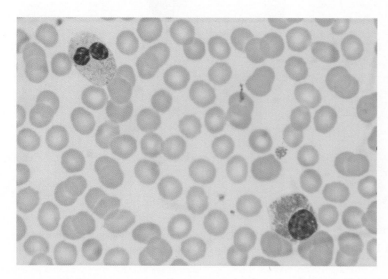

Fig. 3.110 Blood film of a patient with the inherited Pelger–Huët anomaly showing a bilobed neutrophil and a nonlobed eosinophil.

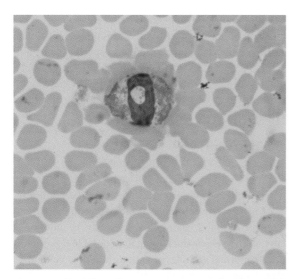

Fig. 3.111 Blood film of a patient with cyclical oedema with eosinophilia showing an eosinophil with a ring-shaped nucleus.

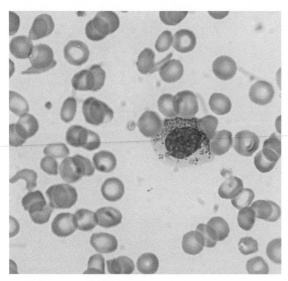

Fig. 3.112 Blood film of a patient with MDS showing a non-lobulated and hypogranular eosinophil.

Abnormalities of eosinophil granules and cytoplasm

Abnormal eosinophil granules may be seen, together with abnormal neutrophil granules, in a variety of inherited conditions including the Chédiak–Higashi syndrome (Fig. 3.113) and the Alder–Reilly anomaly (see Fig. 3.84 and Table 3.10). In the Alder–Reilly

anomaly, eosinophil granules may be grey-green or purple on Romanowsky staining [178]. In the Chédiak–Higashi syndrome, some granules are blue-grey. Eosinophils in GM1 gangliosidosis type 1 (β galactosidase 1 deficiency) can have both abnormally staining granules and vacuolation [255] (Fig. 3.114). A further abnormality, confined to eosinophils and

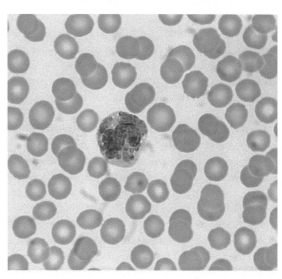

Fig. 3.113 Blood film of a patient with the Chédiak–Higashi syndrome showing an abnormally granulated eosinophil. Courtesy of Dr J. McCallum.

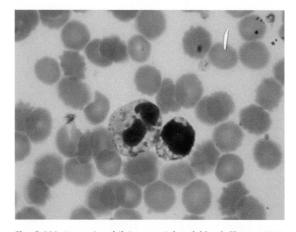

Fig. 3.114 An eosinophil in a peripheral blood film in GM1 ganglosidosis (β galactosidase deficiency) showing vacuolation and abnormal granules; the lymphocyte is also vacuolated. Courtesy of Dr Jiří Pavlů, London.

basophils, has been noted in one family, the inheritance being autosomal dominant [248]; inclusions were grey or grey-blue. Cytoplasmic inclusions are present in eosinophils in the May–Hegglin anomaly [226] and in the actin inclusion (Brandalise) syndrome [206].

In acquired disorders of granulopoiesis it is not uncommon to see eosinophils in which some granules have basophilic staining characteristics. These are immature granules, sometimes designated 'pro-eosinophilic granules'. Such cells are increased in frequency in CML (Fig. 3.115), chronic eosinophilic leukaemia and certain categories of AML in which eosinophils are part of the leukaemic clone, particularly cases of acute myelomonocytic leukaemia with eosinophilia associated with inversion of chromosome 16. In all the above cases the abnormal granules are shown on ultrastructural examination to be eosinophil granules with unusual staining characteristics, but in some patients with CML there are also hybrid cells with a mixture of granules of eosinophil type and basophil type [256].

In acquired disorders, eosinophils may be vacuolated or wholly or partly agranular. Hypogranularity could result from defective formation of eosinophil granules in dysmyelopoietic states, but since it is usually accompanied by vacuolation it appears likely that in most instances it results from degranulation.

Vacuolation and hypogranularity are seen in some but not all cases of chronic eosinophilic leukaemia. However, the changes are quite non-specific, being also sometimes seen in reactive eosinophilia. For example, among seven patients with eosinophilia associated with B and T lymphoblastic leukaemia or lymphoma five had cytologically abnormal eosinophils [252].

The basophil

The basophil (Fig. 3.116) is of similar size to the neutrophil (10–14 μm in diameter). The nucleus is usually obscured by purple-black granules, which are intermediate in size between those of the neutrophil and those of the eosinophil. Basophil nuclei may be non-lobulated in the Pelger–Huët anomaly (Fig 3.117). Basophils have abnormal granules in various inherited conditions (Fig. 3.118; also see Table 3.10).

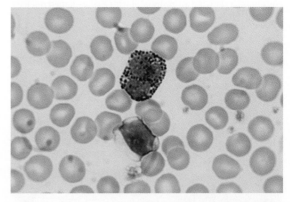

Fig. 3.116 A basophil and a small lymphocyte in the peripheral blood film of a healthy subject.

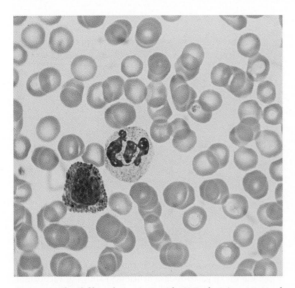

Fig. 3.115 Blood film of a patient with CML showing a normal neutrophil and an eosinophil with some basophilic granules.

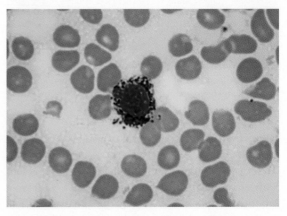

Fig. 3.117 Blood film of a patient with the inherited Pelger–Huët anomaly showing a hypolobated basophil.

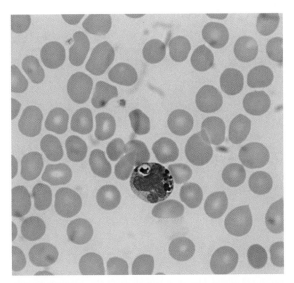

Fig. 3.118 Blood film of a patient with the Chédiak–Higashi syndrome showing an abnormal basophil. Courtesy of Dr J. McCallum.

Granules can be reduced in number in myeloproliferative neoplasms and MDS (Fig. 3.119), and degranulation can occur in acute allergic conditions (such as urticaria and anaphylactic shock) and during post-prandial hyperlipidaemia. A reduction in the number of granules can also be artefactual since basophil granules are highly water soluble.

Cytoplasmic inclusions are present in the May–Hegglin anomaly [226].

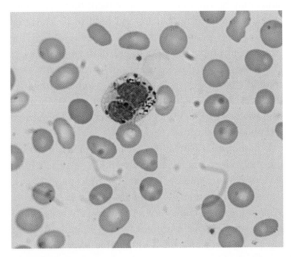

Fig. 3.119 Blood film of a patient with MDS showing a hypogranular basophil.

Lymphocytes and plasma cells

The lymphocyte

Peripheral blood lymphocytes vary in diameter from 10 to 16 μm. The smaller lymphocytes (10–12 μm), which predominate, usually have scanty cytoplasm and a round or slightly indented nucleus with condensed chromatin (Fig. 3.120). The larger lymphocytes (12–16 μm), which usually constitute about 10% of circulating lymphocytes, have more abundant cytoplasm and the nuclear chromatin is somewhat less condensed (Fig. 3.121). The smaller lymphocytes are usually circular in outline, whereas larger ones may be somewhat irregular. The cytoplasm, being weakly basophilic, stains pale blue. Lymphocytes may have small numbers of azurophilic granules, which

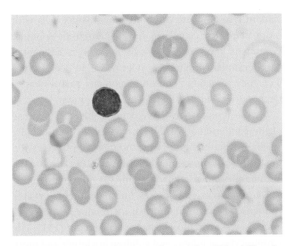

Fig. 3.120 A small lymphocyte in the peripheral blood film of a healthy subject.

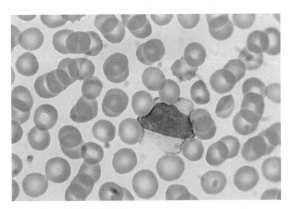

Fig. 3.121 A large lymphocyte in the peripheral blood film of a healthy subject.

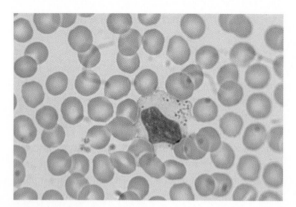

Fig. 3.122 A large granular lymphocyte in the peripheral blood film of a healthy subject.

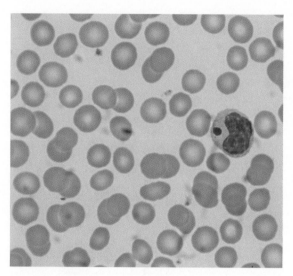

Fig. 3.123 Blood film of a patient with the Chédiak–Higashi syndrome showing a lymphocyte with a large cytoplasmic inclusion. Courtesy of Dr J. McCallum.

contain lysosomal enzymes; occasional larger cells with more abundant cytoplasm have a dozen or so quite prominent granules. Such cells have been designated 'large granular lymphocytes' (Fig. 3.122). In healthy subjects they sometimes constitute as many as 10–15% of lymphocytes, but usually they are less frequent.

Mature lymphocytes have a nucleolus but, because of the condensation of the chromatin, it is not usually visible in small lymphocytes. In large lymphocytes the nucleolus can sometimes be discerned. Because of the chromatin condensation, it is similarly difficult to detect sex chromatin in lymphocytes, but sometimes it is visible condensed beneath the nuclear membrane in the larger lymphocytes with more dispersed chromatin [151]. The lymphocytes of infants and children are larger and more pleomorphic than those of adults. In general, the functional subsets of lymphocytes cannot be distinguished morphologically, but lymphokine-activated cytotoxic T cells and natural killer cells are found within the population of large granular lymphocytes.

Morphological abnormalities of lymphocytes in inherited conditions

Inclusions may be found in lymphocytes in the Chédiak–Higashi syndrome and Alder–Reilly anomaly (see Table 3.10). In the Chédiak–Higashi syndrome the lymphocyte inclusions can be very large (Fig. 3.123), but in the Alder–Reilly anomaly (Fig. 3.124) they are only a little larger than the granules of normal large granular lymphocytes. Heterozygous carriers of the Chédiak–Higashi syndrome may also have lymphocyte inclusions, but only in a small proportion of cells [257].

Occasionally, in the Alder–Reilly anomaly, inclusions are found in lymphocytes in the absence of neutrophil abnormalities. Lymphocyte inclusions are usually found when the Alder–Reilly anomaly is consequent on Tay–Sachs disease or on the mucopolysaccharidoses, although they are rare in Morquio syndrome. Heterozygous carriers for Tay–Sachs disease may have lymphocyte inclusions [178], but in a much lower proportion of lymphocytes than in homozygotes. Alder–Reilly inclusions may be round or comma-shaped; they are sometimes surrounded by a halo, and tend to be clustered at one pole of the cell (see Fig. 3.124a). When the Alder–Reilly anomaly is due to one of the mucopolysaccharidoses the inclusions stain polychromatically with toluidine blue (see Fig. 3.124b), but when the underlying cause is Tay–Sachs disease they do not. GM gangl, osidosis (galactosidase deficiency) may have abnormal lymphocyte inclusions (Fig. 3.125).

Lymphocyte vacuolation occurs in many inherited metabolic disorders including I-cell disease (Fig. 3.126), sialidosis (mucolipidosis type I), the mucopolysaccharidoses, Jordans anomaly, Niemann–Pick disease type A, Wolman disease, cholesteryl ester storage disease, GM1 gangliosidosis (small vacuoles in late infantile (type 2) disease and larger vacuoles in infantile (type 1) disease) (see Fig 3.114), mannosidosis, Pompe disease, Tay–Sachs disease, juvenile Batten disease (but not other types of

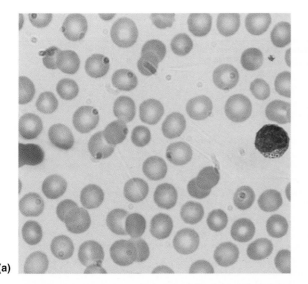

(a)

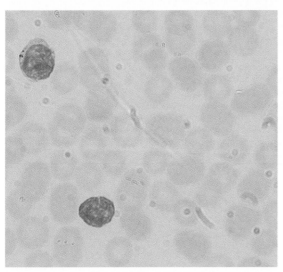

(b)

Fig. 3.124 Blood film of a patient with the Sanfilippo syndrome showing: (a) abnormal lymphocyte inclusions, which are surrounded by a halo; and (b) metachromatic staining of the lymphocyte inclusions when stained with toluidine blue. Courtesy of Mr Alan Dean.

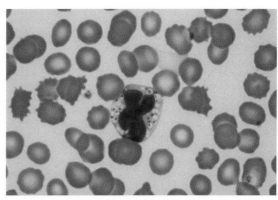

Fig. 3.125 Lymphocyte in a peripheral blood film in GM1 gangliosidosis (β galactosidase deficiency) showing vacuolation with abnormal granular material within the vacuoles. Courtesy of Dr Jiří Pavlů.

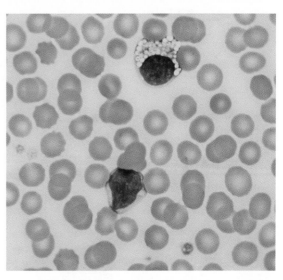

Fig. 3.126 Blood film of a child with I-cell disease. One of the two lymphocytes shows heavy cytoplasmic vacuolation.

Batten disease), galactosidaemia (see Fig. 3.143), galactosialidosis, sialic acid storage disease and several other rare congenital disorders of metabolism [75,258–264] (Table 3.11). In Tay–Sachs disease and Batten–Spielmeyer–Vogt disease, heterozygous carriers may also have lymphocyte vacuolation. The metabolic product responsible for vacuolation varies: it may be lipid, glycogen or mucopolysaccharide. In the mucopolysaccharidoses, vacuoles may result from dissolution of abnormal granules; there is variable metachromatic staining with toluidine blue, depending on the specific metabolic defect present.

Reactive changes in lymphocytes

Lymphocytes can respond to viral infections and other immunological stimuli by an increase in number and cytological alterations. B lymphocytes can differentiate into plasma cells (Fig. 3.127). Intermediate stages are also seen and are designated plasmacytoid lymphocytes (Fig. 3.128) or Türk cells. Plasmacytoid

Table 3.11 Characteristics of lymphocyte vacuoles and other peripheral blood features in inherited metabolic disorders; information is derived mainly from reference 264.

Inherited metabolic disorder	Characteristics of vacuoles and other haematological features
Pompe disease (type 2 glycogen storage disease)	1–6 small discrete PAS-positive vacuoles
Adult acid maltase deficiency	1–6 small discrete PAS-positive vacuoles but vacuoles less frequent than in Pompe disease
Salla disease (sialic acid storage disease)	Numerous small vacuoles
Sialidosis type 2 (neuraminidase deficiency)	Numerous large bold vacuoles
Neuraminidase and α galactosidase deficiency (galactosialidosis)	Numerous large bold vacuoles
I-cell disease (mucolipidosis II)	Numerous large bold vacuoles; vacuoles were reported to be PAS and Sudan black B positive in one patient but were negative in another [263]
GM1 ganglosidosis (β galactosidase deficiency)	Numerous large bold vacuoles; eosinophil granules are large, grey and sparse
Mucopolysaccharidosis 1H (Hurler syndrome); mucopolysaccharidosis 1S (Scheie syndrome); mucopolysaccharidosis 1HS (Hurler/Scheie syndrome)	Occasional vacuoles in occasional lymphocytes, some with basophilic inclusions; metachromatic inclusions with toluidine blue in < 5% of lymphocytes
Mucopolysaccharidosis 2 (Hunter syndrome)	Occasional vacuoles in occasional lymphocytes; pink-staining ring around cytoplasmic vacuoles [262]; metachromatic inclusions with toluidine blue in < 20% of lymphocytes
Mucopolysaccharidosis 3 (Sanfilippo syndrome)	Occasional vacuoles in occasional lymphocytes; metachromatic inclusions with toluidine blue in > 20% of lymphocytes
Mucopolysaccharidosis 4 (Morquio syndrome), type A	No vacuoles, no metachromasia
Mucopolysaccharidosis 4 (Morquio syndrome), type B	Small vacuoles in many lymphocytes, no metachromasia
Mucopolysaccharidosis 6 (Maroteaux–Lamy syndrome)	Small vacuoles in many lymphocytes, metachromatic inclusions with toluidine blue in lymphocytes, Alder–Reilly anomaly of neutrophils (basophilic, birefringent, metachromatic granules)
Mucopolysaccharidosis 7 (β glucuronidase deficiency)	Occasional lymphocytes with small vacuoles; Alder–Reilly anomaly of neutrophils (basophilic, birefringent, metachromatic granules)
Niemann–Pick disease	1–6 small vacuoles in most lymphocytes
Fucosidosis	Small discrete vacuoles in lymphocytes
Juvenile Batten disease	Numerous large bold vacuoles in many lymphocytes
Mannosidosis	Variable from numerous small to several large bold vacuoles
Wolman disease	1–6 small discrete vacuoles in most lymphocytes, which stain with oil red O and Sudan black B
Cholesteryl ester storage disease	Vacuoles stain with oil red O and Sudan black B

PAS, periodic acid–Schiff stain

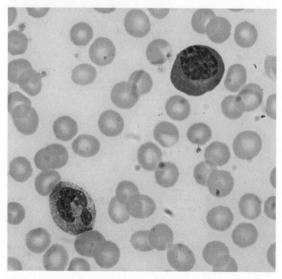

Fig. 3.127 Blood film of a post-operative patient showing a plasma cell and a neutrophil with toxic granulation and a drumstick.

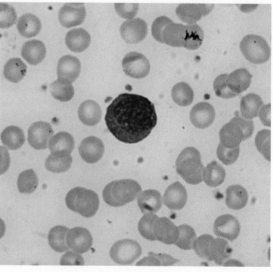

Fig. 3.128 The same peripheral blood film as shown in Fig. 3.127 showing a plasmacytoid lymphocyte.

lymphocytes may contain abundant globular inclusions (Fig. 3.129) composed of immunoglobulin. Such cells have been called 'Mott cells', 'morular cells' or 'grape cells' and the inclusions they contain are known as Russell bodies. Plasmacytoid lymphocytes may also contain crystals of immunoglobulin (Figs 3.130 & 3.131). Both T and B lymphocytes can also transform into immunoblasts – large cells with a central prominent nucleolus and abundant basophilic cytoplasm (Fig. 3.132). Cells showing other less specific changes in lymphocyte morphology are subsumed under the designation 'atypical lymphocytes' or 'atypical mononuclear cells' (Fig. 3.133). Abnormalities include increased size of the cell, immaturity of the nucleus including lack of chromatin condensation and the presence of a nucleolus, irregular nuclear outline or nuclear lobulation, cytoplasmic basophilia, cytoplasmic vacuolation, cytoplasmic granules and an irregular cellular outline. Mitotic figures may be observed (Fig. 3.134). The commonest cause of large numbers of atypical lymphocytes is infectious mononucleosis, due to infection by the Epstein–Barr virus (EBV), which is discussed, together with other causes of atypical lymphocytes, on p. 000. Cleft lymphocytes can be seen in pertussis and respiratory syncytial virus infection. Multilobated lymphocyte nuclei, often with a clover leaf–shaped nucleus, are characteristic of adult T-cell leukaemia/lymphoma (ATLL; see Chapter 9), but are also occasionally seen in carriers of the human T-cell lymphotropic virus 1 (HTLV-1) and in infectious mononucleosis, HIV

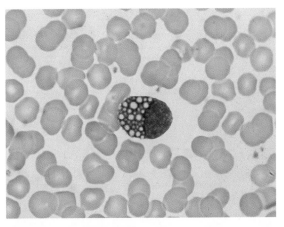

Fig. 3.129 A Mott cell in a peripheral blood film.

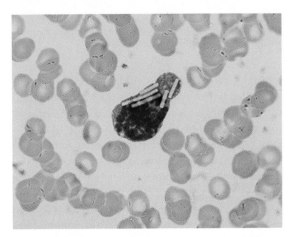

Fig. 3.130 A plasmacytoid lymphocyte containing crystals in the peripheral blood film of a patient with bacterial sepsis.

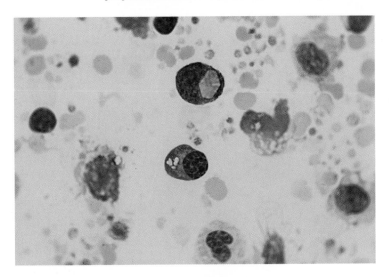

Fig. 3.131 A buffy coat film from the same patient whose peripheral blood film is shown in Fig. 3.130 showing one plasmacytoid lymphocyte containing globular inclusions and another containing a giant crystal.

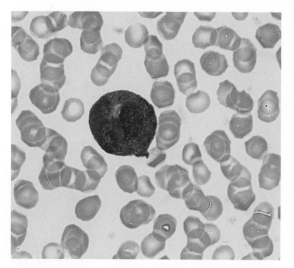

Fig. 3.132 An immunoblast in the peripheral blood film of a patient with infectious mononucleosis.

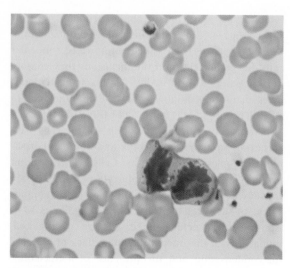

Fig. 3.134 A peripheral blood lymphocyte in mitosis.

infection, cytomegalovirus (CMV) infection, rickett-sial infection and toxoplasmosis [265,266]. Lymphocytes with convoluted nuclei, resembling Sézary cells, may occur in reactive conditions including HIV infection [267] and have been reported, together with skin infiltration, as an unusual reaction to hairy cell leukaemia [268]. Abnormal nuclear lobulation can be induced by hyperthermia [188]. Howell–Jolly body-like inclusions, likely to be drug-induced, have been reported in one patient [254]. Villous lymphocytes, resembling those of splenic lymphoma with villous

lymphocytes, can occur in hyper-reactive malarial sple-nomegaly [269]. Binucleated lymphocytes have been reported after low-dose irradiation and binucleated lymphocytes and lymphocytes with bilobed nuclei are characteristic of chronic polyclonal B-cell lymphocyto-sis of cigarette smokers (Fig. 3.135). Binucleated lymphocytes are induced by natalizumab therapy [270]. The number of large granular lymphocytes may also increase as a reactive phenomenon, e.g. in association with acute or chronic viral infection, such as EBV infection [271], CMV infection [272] or hepatitis.

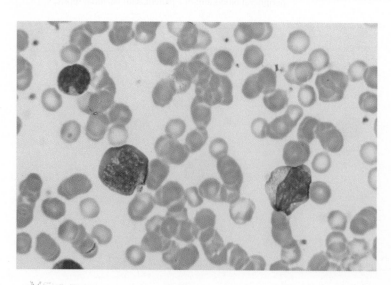

Fig. 3.133 Atypical lymphocytes in the peripheral blood film of a patient with cyto-megalovirus infection.

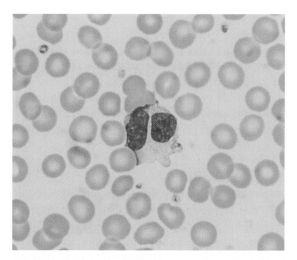

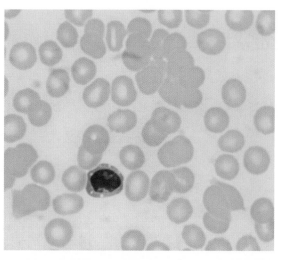

Fig. 3.135 A binucleated lymphocyte in the peripheral blood film of a female cigarette smoker with persistent polyclonal B-cell lymphocytosis.

Fig. 3.136 An apoptotic lymphocyte in the peripheral blood of a patient with infectious mononucleosis. There are also red cell agglutinates.

Apoptotic lymphoid cells

Increased numbers of apoptotic lymphocytes may be present in reactive conditions, particularly in viral infections including infectious mononucleosis, neonatal herpes simplex virus infection, rubella, measles and influenza A infection [244]. They are also increased, and correlate with disease severity, in invasive meningococcal disease [244]. They are recognised by peripheral condensation of the nucleus and a glassy appearance of the cytoplasm (Fig. 3.136).

Lymphocyte morphology in lymphoproliferative disorders

In most lymphoproliferative disorders the neoplastic cells are cytologically abnormal. Abnormalities show some overlap with those seen in reactive conditions, but the majority of lymphoid neoplasms can be recognised as such on cytology alone. Cytoplasmic inclusions are sometimes present. Lymphocytes in chronic lymphocytic leukaemia may contain vacuoles or crystalline or globular inclusions (Fig. 3.137). Rarely a ribosomal-lamella

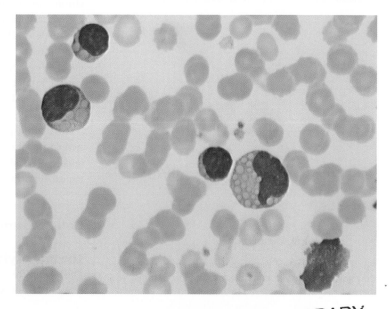

Fig. 3.137 Blood film in chronic lymphocytic leukaemia showing globular cytoplasmic inclusions. There is also a smear cell. Courtesy of Dr Jan Haskta and Professor Georgia Metzgeroth, Mannheim.

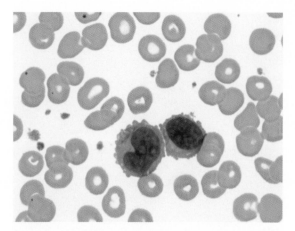

Fig. 3.138 Blood film in non-Hodgkin lymphoma showing Auer rod-like cytoplasmic inclusions. Courtesy of Lyndall Dial, Brisbane.

complex can be seen on light microscopy in hairy cell leukaemia. Rarely in non-Hodgkin lymphoma there are Auer rod–like cytoplasmic inclusions (Fig. 3.138). Round and rod-shaped inclusions representing parallel tubular arrays have been reported in a patient with T-lineage large granular lymphocyte leukaemia [273].

Typical features of different lymphoid neoplasms are described in Chapter 9.

Lymphocyte aggregates

Occasionally apparently normal lymphocytes appear in blood films in clumps (Fig. 3.139) [274]. The pres-

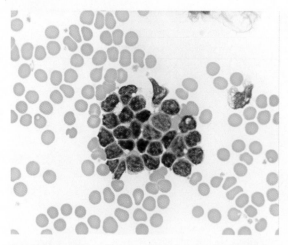

Fig. 3.139 Lymphocyte aggregation of uncertain significance (low power). There was no evidence of a clonal disorder. With thanks to Dr Jecko Thachil and Dr Anthony Carter, Liverpool.

ence of lymphocyte aggregates can also be an uncommon feature of lymphoproliferative disorders. It may represent an *in vitro* phenomenon [275] or, even more rarely, may indicate that the patient has an intravascular lymphoma [276]. As an *in vitro* artefact, this phenomenon has been associated particularly with splenic lymphoma with villous lymphocytes (splenic marginal zone lymphoma) [275,277] and has also been observed in mantle cell lymphoma [278].

The plasma cell

Plasma cells are usually tissue cells but, on occasion, they may be present in the peripheral blood, either as a feature of multiple myeloma or as a reactive phenomenon (see Figs 3.64 & 3.127). They are not seen in healthy subjects [279]. Reactive plasma cells are seen in the blood as a response to increased interleukin 6 secretion in infection, inflammation, following vaccination, in cirrhosis and in various neoplasms (e.g. AML, carcinoma, lymphoma and cardiac myxoma) [280,281]. Occasionally reactive plasma cells are present in large numbers, simulating plasma cell leukaemia. This has been reported following streptokinase therapy and in Castleman disease, bacterial sepsis [282], rubella, dengue fever [283] and angioimmunoblastic T-cell lymphoma [284]. Plasma cells range in size from somewhat larger than a small lymphocyte (8–10 μm) up to a diameter of about 20 μm and are oval in shape with an eccentric nucleus, coarsely clumped chromatin, a moderate amount of strongly basophilic cytoplasm and a less basophilic Golgi zone adjacent to the nucleus. The clock-face chromatin pattern that is seen in tissue sections stained with haematoxylin and eosin is less apparent in circulating plasma cells stained with a Romanowsky stain. Plasma cells may contain secretory products, which appear as round or globular inclusions or, less often, crystals.

Circulating plasma cells are also sometimes seen in neoplastic disorders (multiple myeloma, plasma cell leukaemia and related conditions). The range of cytological abnormalities in these conditions is very broad.

Cells of monocyte lineage

The monocyte

The monocyte (Fig. 3.140) is the largest normal peripheral blood cell with a diameter of about 12–20 μm. It

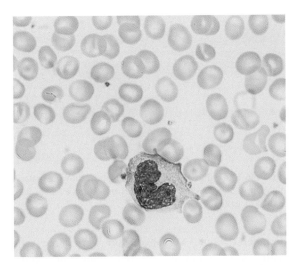

Fig. 3.140 A normal monocyte in the peripheral blood film of a healthy subject.

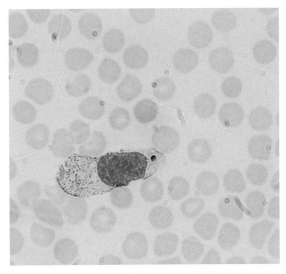

Fig. 3.141 Blood film of a patient with the Maroteaux–Lamy syndrome showing a monocyte with an abnormal cytoplasmic inclusion. Courtesy of Mr Alan Dean.

has an irregular, often lobulated nucleus and opaque greyish-blue cytoplasm with fine azurophilic granules. The cell outline is often irregular and the cytoplasm may be vacuolated. Sex chromatin may be seen condensed beneath the nuclear membrane [151].

Monocytes produced under conditions of bone marrow stimulation, e.g. infection or recovery from bone marrow suppression, show an increased nucleocytoplasmic ratio, a more delicate chromatin pattern, nucleoli and increased numbers of vacuoles [145]. Cytoplasmic basophilia and azurophilic granules may also be increased. The administration of G-CSF produces similar cytological changes [145]. Abnormal nuclear lobulation can be induced by hyperthermia [188]. Howell–Jolly body-like inclusions, likely to be drug induced, have been observed in one patient [254].

Monocytes may contain abnormal inclusions in various inherited conditions (Figs 3.141 and 3.142; see also Table 3.10). In some metabolic disorders they may be heavily vacuolated (Fig. 3.143). Since they are phagocytic they are occasionally found to have ingested red cells (Fig. 3.144), cryoglobulin (Fig. 3.145), micro-organisms, malaria pigment (Fig. 3.146) and, rarely, melanin [209] or bilirubin [210]. Erythrophagocytosis by monocytes may be the result of abnormal red cells (as in sickle cell disease) or antibody or complement binding to red cells (as in paroxysmal cold haemoglobinuria, autoimmune haemolytic anaemia or anti-D haemolytic disease of the newborn). Peripheral blood monocytes may

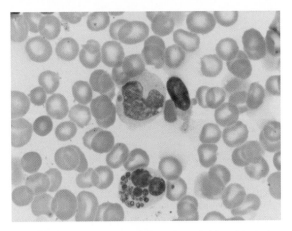

Fig. 3.142 A monocyte containing a large brick-red inclusion in Chédiak–Higashi syndrome. There is also an eosinophil with giant granules, some of which are more darkly staining than normal. With thanks to Dr Abbas Abdulsalam, Baghdad.

contain parasitised red cells in malaria [285]. Haemophagocytosis by peripheral blood monocytes has been observed in malaria [286]. In Hermansky–Pudlak syndrome monocytes may contain ceroid inclusions [287].

Monocyte precursors

Monocyte precursors, designated promonocytes and monoblasts, are not normally present in the

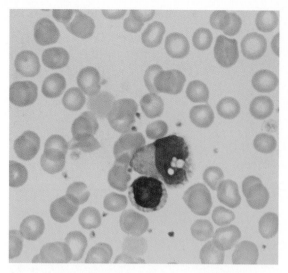

Fig. 3.143 An abnormally vacuolated monocyte and a very heavily vacuolated lymphocyte in the peripheral blood of a patient with galactosidaemia. By courtesy of Dr Guy Lucas.

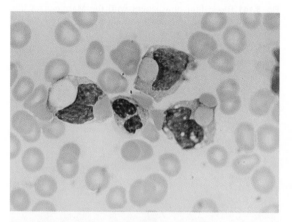

Fig. 3.144 Blood film of a patient with chronic renal failure taken during haemodialysis showing erythrocytes that have been phagocytosed by monocytes. The patient had a positive direct antiglobulin test but no overt haemolysis.

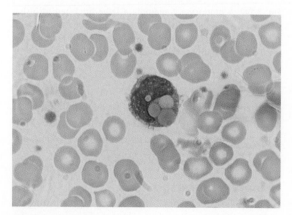

Fig. 3.145 Blood film of a patient with cryoglobulinaemia showing cryoglobulin within a monocyte. Courtesy of Mr Alan Dean.

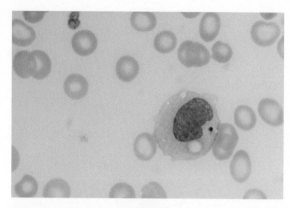

Fig. 3.146 Blood film of a patient with malaria showing malaria pigment within a monocyte. The film also shows a *Plasmodium falciparum* gametocyte.

peripheral blood. Monoblasts are very large cells with a large round nucleus and voluminous agranular or slightly granular cytoplasm, which is sometimes vacuolated (Fig. 3.147). They are only seen in the peripheral blood in acute leukaemia with monocytic differentiation. Promonocytes, as defined by the French–American–British (FAB) group and in the World Health Organization (WHO) classification of haematological neoplasms, are very primitive cells (in the WHO classification, equivalent to a monoblast in significance) with a diffuse chromatin pattern but with lobulation or other irregularity of the nucleus. They need to be distinguished from the immature or abnormal monocytes that are present in reactive conditions (see above) and in chronic myeloid neoplasms.

The macrophage

Monocytes usually develop into macrophages (also called histiocytes) in tissues rather than in the blood. However, occasionally circulating cells with the characteristics of macrophages are seen [288] (Fig. 3.148). They are associated with a variety of infective and inflammatory states (such as subacute bacterial endocarditis, tuberculosis, typhoid fever [289] and virus-associated haemophagocytic syndrome [290]), malignant disease and parasitic diseases. They may be a little larger than a monocyte or may be very large and multinucleated [201]. The cytoplasm may contain haemopoietic cells, recognisable cellular debris or amorphous debris. In certain inherited metabolic disorders foamy macrophages containing lipid are present in the peripheral blood [259]. Circulating phagocytic cells are also sometimes seen in malignant histiocytosis and acute monocytic

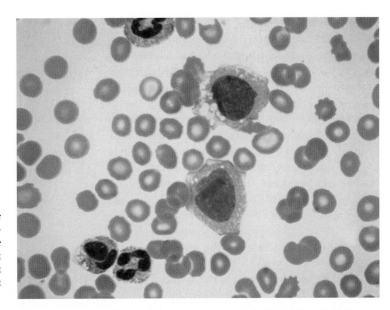

Fig. 3.147 Blood film of a patient with acute monocytic leukaemia showing a monoblast (left) and a promonocyte (right). The promonocyte has a lobulated nucleus but its chromatin pattern is as delicate as that of the monoblast. Both cells have abundant blue-grey vacuolated cytoplasm.

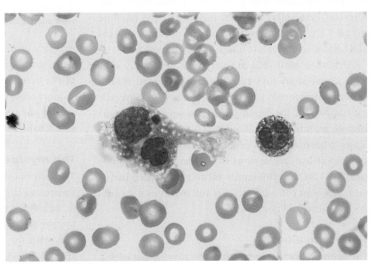

Fig. 3.148 A phagocytic macrophage in a peripheral blood film. Courtesy of Dr Z. Currimbhoy, Mumbai.

leukaemia. Very rarely Gaucher cells have been seen in the peripheral blood following splenectomy for Gaucher disease [291]. Foamy cells of monocyte/macrophage lineage may be seen in Niemann–Pick disease [291].

Granulocyte precursors

Granulocytes are generally produced in the bone marrow from myeloblasts, with the intervening stages being promyelocytes, myelocytes and metamyelocytes. On occasion, granulocyte precursors are seen in the blood. The appearance of appreciable numbers of such cells is designated a left shift. If NRBC are also present the blood film is described as leucoerythroblastic. The appearance in the peripheral blood of leucocytes of an earlier stage of development than the metamyelocyte is usually regarded as abnormal unless the blood is from a pregnant woman or a neonate. However, if buffy coat preparations are made, metamyelocytes and/or myelocytes are found in about 80% of healthy subjects with a frequency of about 1 in 1000 granulocytes [292].

The myeloblast

The myeloblast measures 12–20 μm and has a high nucleocytoplasmic ratio and a round or slightly oval nucleus (see Fig. 3.81). The cell is usually somewhat oval and the outline may be slightly irregular. The nucleus has a diffuse chromatin pattern and one to five (most often two or three) not very prominent nucleoli. The cytoplasm is pale blue. A myeloblast is often defined as a cell that has no granules visible by light microscopy, although ultrastructural examination and cytochemistry show that granules are actually present. It is now becoming usual for cells with a relatively small number of granules but without the other characteristics of promyelocytes (see below) also to be included in the myeloblast category, in accordance with the recommendations made by the FAB group in relation to the diagnosis of AML [293], and subsequently supported by the WHO classification. Although a myeloblast does have characteristic cytological features, it is not always possible to make the distinction between an agranular myeloblast and a lymphoblast on an MGG-stained film.

Circulating blast cells are very rare in healthy subjects; in one study they constituted, on average, 0.11% of mononuclear cells [279]. Small numbers of blast cells may appear in the blood during therapy with natulizumab, an integrin inhibitor [294]. Circulating myeloblasts in haematological neoplasms may show abnormal cytological features such as the presence of Auer rods (see Fig. 3.88) or cytoplasmic vacuoles. The presence of even one blast cell with an Auer rod indicates the existence of a myeloid neoplasm.

The promyelocyte

The promyelocyte is larger than the myeloblast with a diameter of 15–25 μm (Fig. 3.149). The cell is round or slightly oval. In comparison with the myeloblast, the nucleocytoplasmic ratio is lower and the cytoplasm is more basophilic. The nuclear chromatin shows only slight condensation and nucleoli are apparent. (Clumped or condensed chromatin, known as heterochromatin, is genetically inactive, whereas diffuse euchromatin is genetically active; cellular maturation is associated with progressive condensation of chromatin.) The promyelocyte nucleus is oval with an indentation in one side. The Golgi zone is apparent as a much less basophilic area adjacent to the nuclear indentation. The promyelocyte contains

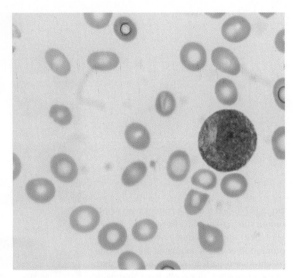

Fig. 3.149 A promyelocyte in the peripheral blood film of a patient with megaloblastic anaemia. The nucleolus and the Golgi zone are readily detectable. The film also shows anisocytosis and teardrop poikilocytes.

primary or azurophilic granules, which surround the Golgi zone and are scattered through the remainder of the cytoplasm.

Morphologically abnormal promyelocytes may be seen in the peripheral blood in several subtypes of AML (see Chapter 9).

The myelocyte

The myelocyte is smaller than the promyelocyte, measuring 10–20 μm in diameter. It can be identified as belonging to the neutrophil, eosinophil or basophil lineage by the presence of specific or secondary granules with the staining characteristics of these cell lines (Figs 3.150–3.152). Eosinophil myelocytes may have some pro-eosinophilic granules with basophilic staining characteristics. The myelocyte nucleus is oval and sometimes has a slight indentation in one side. Chromatin shows a moderate degree of coarse clumping and nucleoli are not apparent. The cytoplasm is more acidophilic than that of the promyelocyte and the Golgi zone is much less apparent. Neutrophil and eosinophil myelocytes may appear in the blood in reactive conditions and in leukaemias. The presence of basophil myelocytes in the peripheral blood is essentially confined to leukaemias. In acute leukaemias, circulating myelocytes may show morphological abnormalities such as hypogranularity or abnormally large granules.

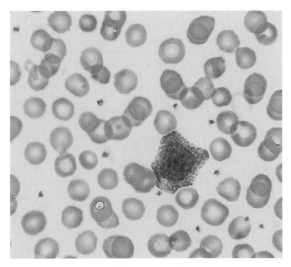

Fig. 3.150 A neutrophil myelocyte in the peripheral blood film of a healthy pregnant woman.

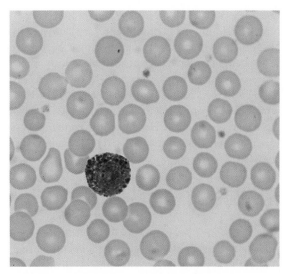

Fig. 3.152 A basophil myelocyte in the peripheral blood film of a patient with CML.

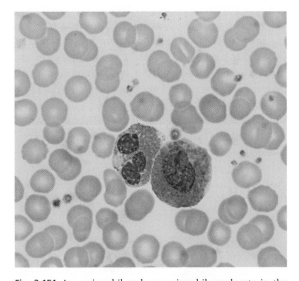

Fig. 3.151 An eosinophil and an eosinophil myelocyte in the peripheral blood film of a patient with CML.

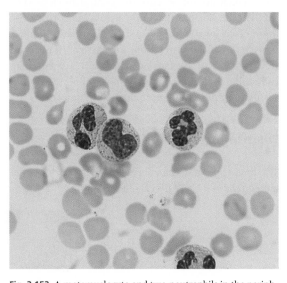

Fig. 3.153 A metamyelocyte and two neutrophils in the peripheral blood film of a patient with CML.

The metamyelocyte

The metamyelocyte measures 10–12 μm in diameter. Its chromatin is clumped and its nucleus is definitely indented or U-shaped (Fig. 3.153). Protein synthesis has stopped. A neutrophil metamyelocyte has acidophilic cytoplasm, while that of an eosinophil myelocyte is weakly basophilic. Small numbers of neutrophil metamyelocytes are occasionally seen in the blood in healthy subjects. They are commonly present in reactive conditions. Some eosinophil metamyelocytes may be seen in patients with eosinophilia.

Leucoerythroblastic blood films

A blood film is referred to as leucoerythroblastic if it contains NRBC and granulocyte precursors. This is normal in the fetus up to 28 weeks' gestation and can be seen late in pregnancy and in the postpartum period. In other circumstances a leucoerythroblastic film is abnormal. The change may be reactive (e.g. following trauma, shock or acute blood loss) or may indicate a bone marrow disease. A leucoerythroblastic blood film is particularly characteristic of primary myelofibrosis or bone marrow infiltration. In the first 24 hours of life, a leucoerythroblastic blood film may be the result of maternal sepsis/chorioamnionitis, severe birth asphyxia or Down syndrome [85].

The mast cell

Mast cells are essentially tissue cells. They are extremely rare in the peripheral blood of normal subjects. They are large cells with a diameter of 20–30 μm. The cellular outline is somewhat irregular. The cytoplasm is packed with basophilic granules, which do not obscure the central nucleus (Fig. 3.154). The nucleus is relatively small and round or, more often, oval with a dispersed chromatin pattern. In systemic mastocytosis and in mast cell leukaemia (see Chapter 9) circulating mast cells are cytologically quite abnormal and may have lobulated nuclei, scanty granules or a denser chromatin pattern.

Disintegrated cells

The finding of more than a small percentage of disintegrated cells in a blood film is of significance.

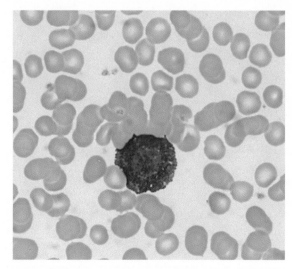

Fig. 3.154 A mast cell in the peripheral blood film of a patient having a health check for non-specific symptoms.

It may indicate that several days have elapsed since the blood was taken from the patient and that the specimen is unfit for testing. When disintegration of cells is due to prolonged storage the granulocytes are smeared preferentially and, if an attempt is made to perform a differential count, there will appear to be neutropenia.

If disintegration of cells occurs in films made from fresh blood it indicates that cells are abnormally fragile. Disintegrated lymphocytes, usually called 'smear cells' or 'smudge cells', are common in CLL (Fig. 3.155). Their presence is of some use in diagnosis since they

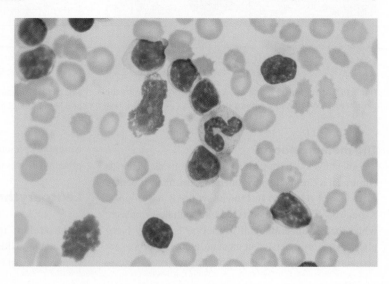

Fig. 3.155 Intact lymphocytes and several disintegrated cells (smear cells or smudge cells) in the peripheral blood film of a patient with CLL.

are not common in non-Hodgkin lymphoma, from which a distinction may have to be made. The fact that these cells are intact *in vivo* and are smeared during preparation of the film as a result of mechanical fragility is demonstrated by the fact that they are not present if a film of the same blood is made by centrifugation. Although smeared lymphocytes are characteristic of CLL they are not pathognomonic, being seen occasionally in non-Hodgkin lymphoma and even sometimes in reactive conditions such as whooping cough. Smear cell can also appear as a result of the effects of chemotherapy on neoplastic lymphoid cells [295]. Other abnormal cells, e.g. blast cells in AML, may also disintegrate on spreading the blood film. The term 'basket cell' has been applied to a very large, spread-out smear cell. Disintegrated cells, if at all frequent, should be included in the differential count. When the cell of origin is clear, e.g. as in CLL, they should be counted with intact cells of the same type.

Necrotic bone marrow cells

Necrotic bone marrow cells have been recognised in a venous blood sample from a patient with sickle cell crisis [296].

Platelets and circulating megakaryocytes

When platelets are examined in a blood film, an assessment should be made of their number (by relating them to the number of red cells), their size and their morphological features. The film should be examined for platelet aggregates, platelet satellitism and platelet phagocytosis. Megakaryocytes are seen, although rarely, in the blood of healthy people. Their number is increased in certain disease states.

Platelets

The normal platelet measures 1.5–3 μm in diameter. Platelets contain fine azurophilic granules, which may be dispersed throughout the cytoplasm or concentrated in the centre; in the latter case the central granule-containing cytoplasm is known as the granulomere and the peripheral, weakly basophilic agranular cytoplasm as the hyalomere (see Fig. 3.16). Platelets contain several different types of granules, of which the α granules

are the equivalent of the azurophilic granules seen on light microscopy. Occasionally proplatelets are seen in blood films. They are ribbon-like strands of megakaryocyte cytoplasm that have broken free in bone marrow sinusoids before fragmenting into platelets.

In EDTA-anticoagulated blood platelets generally remain separate from one another, whereas in native blood they show a tendency to aggregate (see Figs 1.6–1.8). In Glanzmann thrombasthenia, a severe inherited defect of platelet aggregation, the normal tendency of platelets to aggregate when films are made from native blood is completely absent.

Abnormalities of platelet size

Platelet size can be assessed by comparing the diameter of the platelets with the diameter of erythrocytes, or platelet diameter can be measured by means of an ocular micrometer.

Platelet size in healthy subjects varies inversely with the platelet count, but this variation is not sufficiently great to be detected when a blood film is examined by light microscopy. A sufficient size increase to be detectable microscopically occurs in certain congenital abnormalities of thrombopoiesis and in certain disease states (Table 3.12). Large platelets (i.e. those with a diameter greater than 4 μm) are designated macrothrombocytes. Particularly large platelets with diameters similar to those of red cells or lymphocytes are often referred to as giant platelets (Fig. 3.156). When platelet turnover is increased, platelets are usually large. The absence of large platelets in patients with thrombocytopenia is therefore of diagnostic significance; it suggests that there is a defect of platelet production. Decreased platelet size is less common than increased size but it is a feature of the Wiskott–Aldrich syndrome (Fig. 3.157).

Rarely platelets degranulate and swell in EDTA-anticoagulated blood, appearing both large and hypogranular on a blood film [303].

Other abnormalities of platelet morphology and distribution including platelet aggregation and satellism

Platelets that are lacking in α granules appear grey or pale blue. This occurs as a rare congenital defect known as the grey platelet syndrome resulting from an α granule deficiency [302] or a deficiency of both α and δ granules [304]. There may be a mixture of normal and abnormal platelets. In some families with the grey platelet syndrome, neutrophils are also

Table 3.12 Some causes of large platelets.

Congenital	Inheritance
Bernard–Soulier syndrome* [297]	AR
Heterozygous carriers of Bernard–Soulier syndrome* [124,297]	AD
Mediterranean stomatocytosis/macrothrombocytopenia (phytosterolaemia)	AR
MYH9-related disorders: May–Hegglin anomaly,* Epstein syndrome (associated with hereditary deafness and nephritis)* [230,298], Fechtner syndrome* [299], Sebastian syndrome* [299]	AD
Chédiak–Higashi anomaly*	AR
Associated with increased nuclear projections in neutrophils [165]	AD
Marfan syndrome and various other inherited connective tissue defects (in occasional families) [300]	
Type IIB von Willebrand disease* (and Montreal platelet syndrome* [299], which has now been shown to represent the same condition [301])	AD
Platelet-type von Willebrand syndrome* [299]	AD
Grey platelet syndrome* [302]	AR
Hereditary thrombocytopenia with giant platelets but without other morphological abnormality or associated disease*	AR or AD
Acquired	
Autoimmune thrombocytopenic purpura, primary and secondary*	
Thrombotic thrombocytopenic purpura*	
Disseminated intravascular coagulation*	
Myeloproliferative neoplasms: polycythaemia vera, chronic myelogenous leukaemia (chronic phase or in transformation),* primary myelofibrosis,* essential thrombocythaemia	
Myelodysplastic syndromes* and myelodysplastic/myeloproliferative neoplasms	
Megakaryoblastic leukaemia*	
Postsplenectomy and hyposplenic states (including sickle cell anaemia)	

*can also have thrombocytopenia

AR, autosomal recessive; AD, autosomal dominant

markedly hypogranular [192]. The grey platelet syndrome can occur as an isolated disorder but has also been reported in association with the Chédiak–Higashi syndrome, Hermansky–Pudlak syndrome, Griscelli syndrome, Wiskott–Aldrich syndrome, thrombocytopenia with absent radii and thrombocytopenia resulting from a *GATA1* mutation [304,305]. Grey platelets have also been identified as a feature of the

arthrogryposis renal dysfunction and cholestasis (ARC) syndrome of infants [306]. Inherited causes of agranular platelets are all uncommon. More commonly, apparently agranular platelets result from discharge of platelet granules *in vivo* or *in vitro* or from formation of defective platelets by dysplastic megakaryocytes (Fig. 3.158). If venepuncture is difficult, stimulation of platelets may cause granule release. This is

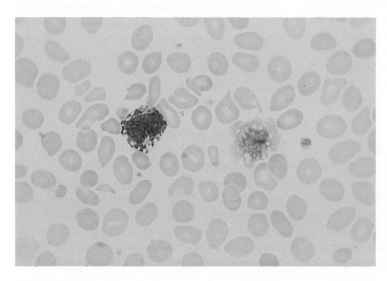

Fig. 3.156 A giant platelet, almost as large as the adjacent basophil, in the peripheral blood of a patient with primary myelofibrosis. The film also shows a platelet of normal size. The red cells show poikilocytosis.

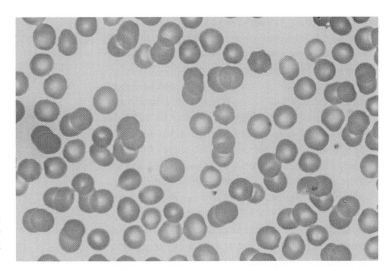

Fig. 3.157 The peripheral blood film of a patient with Wiskott–Aldrich syndrome showing thrombocytopenia and small platelets.

sometimes associated with platelet aggregation so that masses of agranular platelets may be seen. Rarely, a similar phenomenon is caused by a plasma factor causing *in vitro* platelet degranulation [303] or degranulation and aggregation [307]; in one patient the factor originated from a leiomyosarcoma [308]. Degranulation may be confined to platelets in blood anticoagulated with EDTA, platelet morphology being normal when either heparin or citrate is used as an anticoagulant [303,309]. Cardiopulmonary bypass can cause release of α granules with the agranular platelets continuing to circulate. In hairy cell leukaemia, agranular platelets probably result from degranulation within abnormal vascular channels (pseudosinuses lined by hairy cells), which are present in the spleen and other organs. Some agranular platelets are commonly present in MDS and are likely to indicate defec-

tive thrombopoiesis. Agranular platelets in the myeloproliferative neoplasms may result either from defective thrombopoiesis or from discharge of granules from hyperaggregable platelets. In both myelodysplastic and myeloproliferative conditions, platelets may be giant and of abnormal shape, features again indicative of abnormal thrombopoiesis. In the May–Hegglin anomaly, platelets may not only be larger than normal but also of unusual shape, e.g. cigar-shaped [310]. A population of platelets with one or more giant red granules on a Romanowsky-stained film has been reported in two members of a family with thrombocytopenia and an 11q23 deletion [311]; this syndrome has been referred to as the Jacobsen syndrome or as Paris–Trousseau thrombocytopenia.

Various particles, e.g. the parasites of *Plasmodium vivax* [312], may be found within platelets. This is unlikely

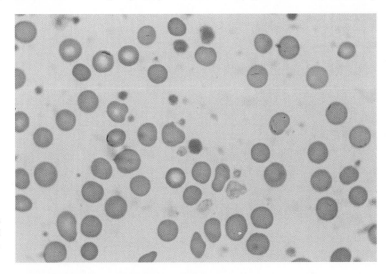

Fig. 3.158 The peripheral blood film of a patient with CML showing a mixture of normally granulated and agranular platelets. There is also platelet anisocytosis.

to represent phagocytosis; it is probably equivalent to emperipolesis, a phenomenon in which white cells and other particles enter the surface-connected membrane system of the megakaryocyte.

It is important to note the presence of platelet aggregates since they are often associated with a factitiously low platelet count. Platelet aggregation may be the result of platelet stimulation during skin prick or venepuncture, or be immunoglobulin mediated. When there is incipient clotting of blood the platelets may be partly degranulated and the blood film may, in addition, show fibrin strands. Platelet aggregation occurring *in vivo* has been reported, rarely, in type 2B von Willebrand disease, in addition to thrombocytopenia and some large platelets [313]. Platelet aggregation occurring as an *in vitro* phenomenon, particularly in EDTA-anticoagulated blood, is mediated by a cold antibody with specificity against platelet glycoprotein IIb/IIIa [314]. This antibody is not known to be of any clinical significance. The phenomenon may be observed transiently in neonates, being attributable to the transplacental passage of the causative antibody [315]. EDTA-related platelet aggregation may be induced by therapy with anti-glycoprotein IIb/IIIa monoclonal antibodies such as abciximab and can persist for several days after therapy [316].

Platelet satellitism (Fig. 3.159) is an *in vitro* phenomenon occurring particularly but not only in EDTA-anticoagulated blood. It is induced by a plasma factor, usually either immunoglobulin (Ig) G or IgM, which causes platelets to adhere to CD16 on neutrophils [317]. Platelets adhere to and encircle neutrophils and some may be

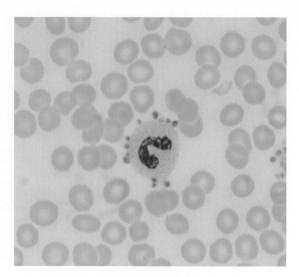

Fig. 3.159 Blood film showing platelet satellitism.

phagocytosed [318]. Neutrophils can be joined together by a layer of platelets. Sometimes satellitism is followed by phagocytosis of platelets [319] (Fig. 3.160). Occasionally satellitism involves other normal cells, e.g. lymphocytes [320], large granular lymphocytes [317], eosinophils [321], monocytes [321] or basophils. Reversal of this phenomenon after treatment of an autoimmune disease has been observed [322]. Platelet satellitism does not appear to be of any clinical significance, although it may lead to a factitiously low platelet count.

Platelet satellitism around lymphoma cells as a non-EDTA-dependent phenomenon has been reported in a

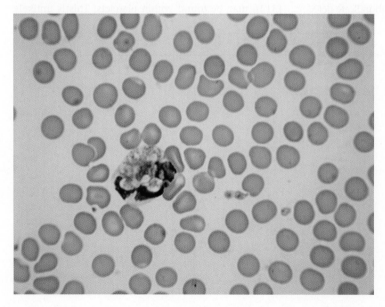

Fig. 3.160 Blood film showing phagocytosis of platelets.

single patient with mantle cell lymphoma [323] and as an EDTA-dependent phenomenon in a single patient with marginal zone lymphoma [324], in the latter instance associated with lympho-agglutination. Platelet satellitism has occasionally involved leukaemic basophils [320].

Platelet satellitism can interfere with the immunophenotyping of cells that are encircled.

Megakaryocytes

Megakaryocytes are rarely seen in the blood of healthy adults. They are released by the bone marrow but most are trapped in the pulmonary capillaries. However, the fact that they are detectable, albeit in low numbers, in venous blood arising from parts of the body lacking haemopoietic marrow indicates that some can pass through the pulmonary capillaries. Since their concentration is, on average, only between five and seven per millilitre they are more likely to be seen in buffy coat preparations or when special concentration procedures are carried out. In healthy subjects, 99% of the megakaryocytes in peripheral venous blood are almost bereft of cytoplasm (Fig. 3.161), but rare cells with copious cytoplasm are seen. The number of megakaryocytes is increased in the blood of neonates and young infants and also postpartum, postoperatively and in patients with infection, inflammation, malignancy, disseminated intravascular coagulation and myeloproliferative neoplasms [325–328]. In neonates there is a correlation with prematurity and with respiratory distress syndrome [329]. The

numbers of megakaryocytes in venous blood is increased during and after cardiopulmonary bypass [330]. The proportion of intact megakaryocytes with plentiful cytoplasm is increased in infants [326] and in patients with primary myelofibrosis and CML [328].

Abnormal megakaryocytes and megakaryoblasts

Abnormal megakaryocytes and megakaryoblasts may be seen in the blood in pathological conditions.

Micromegakaryocytes are seen in some patients with haematological neoplasms, e.g. primary myelofibrosis (Fig. 3.162) and CML, particularly CML in transformation. They are small diploid mononuclear cells with a diameter of 7–10 μm, which are not always immediately identifiable as megakaryocytes. The nucleus is round or slightly irregular with dense chromatin. Cytoplasm varies from scanty to moderate in amount; when scanty, the nucleus may appear 'bare', but electron microscopy shows that such cells usually have a thin rim of cytoplasm. Cytoplasm is weakly basophilic. There may be cytoplasmic vacuolation or a few or numerous cytoplasmic granules. Sometimes there are small cytoplasmic protrusions or 'blebs' and sometimes platelets appear to be 'budding' from the surface. Somewhat larger micromegakaryocytes with well-developed granular cytoplasm may be seen in acute megakaryoblastic leukaemia including transient abnormal myelopoiesis of Down syndrome (Fig. 3.163).

Megakaryoblasts (Fig. 3.164) vary from about 10 μm in diameter up to about 15–20 μm or larger.

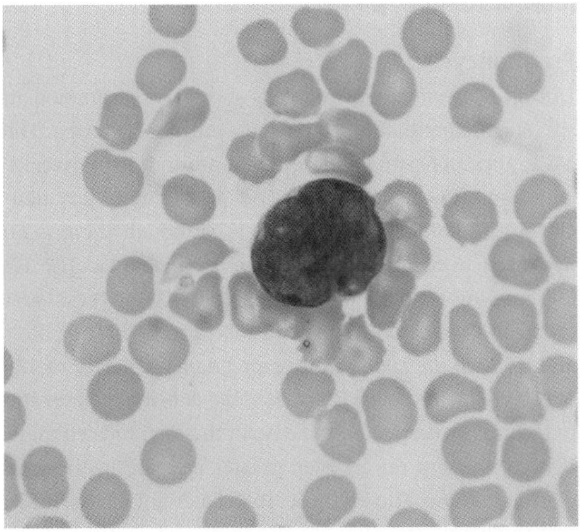

Fig. 3.161 A bare megakaryocyte nucleus in the peripheral blood film of a healthy subject; the size and lobulation of the nucleus indicate its origin from a polyploid megakaryocyte.

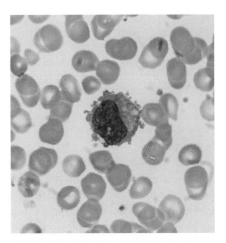

Fig. 3.162 A micromegakaryocyte in the peripheral blood film of a patient with primary myelofibrosis.

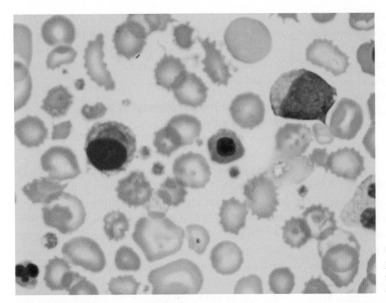

Fig. 3.163 Micromegakaryocyte in the peripheral blood film of a neonate with transient abnormal myelopoiesis of Down syndrome. There is also a blast cell and an NRBC.

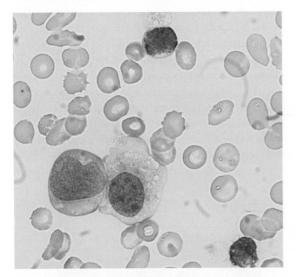

Fig. 3.164 Peripheral blood film of a patient with megakaryoblastic transformation of CML showing three megakaryoblasts. One of these is large with no distinguishing features, another shows some maturation and has cytoplasm that resembles that of a platelet, while the third resembles a lymphoblast. The lineage was confirmed by ultrastructural cytochemistry.

Smaller ones may resemble lymphoblasts and have no distinguishing features. Larger megakaryoblasts have a diffuse chromatin pattern and cytoplasmic basophilia varying from weak to moderately strong. Cytoplasm varies from scanty to moderate in amount and may form blebs. Megakaryoblasts are often not identifiable as such by cytology alone.

Blood film in healthy subjects

Healthy adult

The blood film in a normal adult shows only slight variation in size and shape of red cells (see Figs 3.16 & 3.66). White cells that are normally present are neutrophils, neutrophil band forms, eosinophils, basophils, lymphocytes and monocytes. Metamyelocytes and myelocytes are rare. Megakaryocytes, usually in the form of almost bare nuclei, are very rare. Platelets are present in such numbers that the ratio of red cells to platelets is of the order of 10–40:1.

Pregnancy

During pregnancy, the red cells show more variation in size and shape than is seen in non-pregnant women. The MCV also increases, being greatest around 30–35 weeks' gestation. This change occurs independently of any deficiency of vitamin B_{12} or folic acid, although there is an increased need for folic acid during pregnancy. The Hb falls, the lowest concentration being at 30–34 weeks' gestation. Although both iron and folic acid deficiency have an increased prevalence during pregnancy, this commonly observed fall in the Hb is not due to a deficiency state, and in fact occurs despite an increase in the total red cell mass. It is consequent on an even greater increase in the total plasma volume. The erythrocyte sedimentation rate (ESR) and rouleaux formation are also increased. Polychromatic cells are more numerous and the reticulocyte count is increased with peak levels of 6% at 25–30 weeks.

The WBC, neutrophil count and monocyte count rise, with neutrophils commonly showing toxic granulation and Döhle bodies. A left shift occurs: band forms, metamyelocytes and myelocytes are common, and occasional promyelocytes and even myeloblasts may be seen. Small numbers of NRBC may be seen, but it should be noted that small numbers of NRBC of fetal origin may also be present in the maternal circulation [331]. The WBC and neutrophil count continue to rise till term. The absolute lymphocyte and eosinophil counts fall. On Bayer H1 series instruments, the lobularity index (LI) and mean peroxidase index (MPXI) are increased.

The platelet count and platelet size do not usually change during normal pregnancy, but the platelet count may fall and the mean platelet volume (MPV) may rise if pregnancy is complicated by pregnancy-associated hypertension ('toxaemia'). Pregnancy-associated thrombocytopenia of unknown mechanism occurs in a small proportion of women with an uncomplicated pregnancy. Normal ranges for haematological parameters during pregnancy are given in Table 5.14.

Infancy and childhood

In normal infants and children, red blood cells are hypochromic and microcytic, in comparison with those of adults, and the MCV and mean cell haemoglobin (MCH) are lower. Iron deficiency is common in infancy and childhood, but the difference from adult norms is present even when there is no iron deficiency. The male–female difference in Hb, red blood cell count (RBC) and packed cell volume (PCV)/haematocrit (Hct) is not present before puberty.

The lymphocyte count of children is higher than that of adults and the lymphocyte percentage commonly exceeds the neutrophil percentage ('reversed differential'). A greater proportion of large lymphocytes is commonly observed and some of these may have visible nucleoli. Reactive changes in lymphocytes in response to infection and other immunological stimuli are far more common than in adults and even apparently completely healthy children may have a few 'atypical' lymphocytes.

Normal ranges for haematological parameters during infancy and childhood are given in Tables 5.10–5.13.

Neonate

The blood film of a healthy neonate may show hyposplenic features (see below), specifically Howell–Jolly bodies, acanthocytes and spherocytes. Spherocytes are, however, more numerous than in a hyposplenic adult. The WBC and the neutrophil, monocyte and lymphocyte counts are much higher in the neonate than in the older child or adult. NRBC are much more common and myelocytes are not uncommon. The number of circulating megakaryocytes is greater than in infants and children. The proportion of micromegakaryocytes is increased [332]. Hb, RBC and PCV are much higher than at any other time after birth and the resultant high viscosity of the blood leads to poor spreading so that the blood film appears 'packed'. This physiological polycythaemia also leads to a very low ESR. Red cell size is increased in comparison with that of infants, children and adults. The reticulocyte count is high during the first three days after birth [333].

Physiological changes in haematological variables occur in the first days and weeks of life. There is a rise, on average of about 60% of initial counts, in the WBC and the neutrophil count, with peak levels being reached at about 12 hours after birth [334]. By 72 hours the count has fallen back to below that observed at birth. The lymphocyte count falls to its lowest level at about 72 hours and then rises again [334]. By the end of the first week, the number of neutrophils has usually fallen below the number of lymphocytes. If there has been late clamping of the umbilical cord there are also rises in Hb, Hct and RBC due to 'autotransfusion' from the placenta followed by reduction of plasma volume. NRBC usually disappear from the blood by about the fourth day in healthy term babies and, by the end of the first week, most of the myelocytes and metamyelocytes have also disappeared. Band form are also more numerous during the first few days of life than thereafter, a plateau being reached by the fifth day.

Normal ranges for the neonatal period are given in Tables 5.8 and 5.9.

Premature neonate

Many haematological variables in premature babies differ from those of full-term babies (see above). Their blood films show greater numbers of NRBC, metamyelocytes, myelocytes, promyelocytes and myeloblasts. Hyposplenic features are much more marked than in term babies (Fig. 3.165) and may persist for the first few months of life. Premature babies often develop eosinophilia between the second and third weeks after birth [335].

Hyposplenism

Splenectomy in haematologically normal subjects produces characteristic abnormalities of the blood count and film. The same abnormalities are seen if the spleen is congenitally absent, suffers atrophy or extensive infarction, or becomes non-functional for any reason.

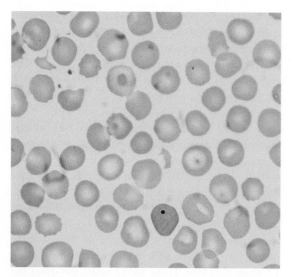

Fig. 3.165 Blood film from a premature but healthy infant, showing macrocytosis (relative to the film of an adult), a Howell–Jolly body in a polychromatic cell, target cells and a schistocyte.

Occasionally, if the spleen is heavily infiltrated by abnormal cells, features of hyposplenism are seen in the presence of splenomegaly. Immediately after splenectomy there is thrombocytosis and a marked neutrophil leucocytosis. If infection occurs post-splenectomy, the neutrophilia and left shift are very marked. After recovery from surgery, the neutrophil count falls to nearly normal levels and the platelet count falls to high normal or somewhat elevated levels – platelet counts of around 500–600×10^9/l may persist. A lymphocytosis and a monocytosis persist indefinitely; the lymphocytosis is usually moderate but counts up to 10×10^9/l are occasionally seen [336]. Characteristically large granular lymphocytes are increased (see Fig. 9.10); immunophenotypically these are natural killer cells [337,338]. T and B cells may also be increased [339]. In normal subjects the Hb does not change post-splenectomy but the red cell morphology is altered (see Figs 3.44 & 3.51). Abnormal features include target cells, acanthocytes, Howell–Jolly bodies, small numbers of Pappenheimer bodies (the presence of siderotic granules being confirmed on a stain for iron), occasional NRBC and small numbers of spherocytes. Small vacuoles may be seen in Romanowsky-stained films; on interference phase-contrast microscopy these appear as 'pits' or 'craters' but in fact they are autophagic vacuoles [340]. The reticulocyte count is increased. Special stains show small numbers of Heinz bodies. Some large platelets may be noted and the MPV is higher, in relation to the platelet count, than in non-splenectomised subjects.

In patients with underlying haematological disorders a greater degree of abnormality is often seen post-splenectomy. When there is anaemia that persists post-splenectomy a marked degree of thrombocytosis is usual. If Heinz bodies are being formed (e.g. because of an unstable haemoglobin or because an oxidant drug is administered) large numbers are seen when the pitting action of the spleen is lacking. If there is erythroblast iron overload (e.g. in sideroblastic anaemia or in thalassaemia major) Pappenheimer bodies are very numerous. If the bone marrow is megaloblastic or dyserythropoietic, Howell–Jolly bodies are particularly large and numerous.

Some of the causes of hyposplenism are given in Table 3.13.

Table 3.13 Some causes of hyposplenism.

Physiological
Neonatal period (particularly in premature babies and in those with intrauterine growth restriction), old age
Pathological
Congenital
Congenital absence or hypoplasia (may be hereditary [341]; may be associated with situs inversus and cardiac anomalies; may be associated with anophthalmia and agenesis of the corpus callosum [342]; occurs in reticular agenesis and Fanconi anaemia [343]; has been reported in Pearson syndrome; may be caused by maternal coumarin intake); associated with ATRX syndrome [344]
Inherited (AD) early involution of the spleen
Congenital polysplenism [345]
Acquired
Splenectomy
Splenic infarction (sickle cell anaemia, sickle cell/haemoglobin C disease and other sickling disorders; essential thrombocythaemia; polycythaemia vera; following splenic torsion; consequent on acute infection [346])
Splenic atrophy (associated with coeliac disease, dermatitis herpetiformis, ulcerative colitis [347], Crohn disease [347] and tropical sprue [348]; autoimmune splenic atrophy including that associated with autoimmune thyroid disease, systemic lupus erythematosus [349] and autoimmune polyglandular disease [350]; graft-versus-host disease [351]; following splenic irradiation [352] or Thorotrast administration [353])
Splenic infiltration or replacement (amyloidosis, sarcoidosis, leukaemia and lymphoma (occasionally); carcinoma [354] and sarcoma [355] (rarely), granulomas caused by atypical mycobacterial infection in AIDS [356])
Asbestos exposure (one case) [357]
Functional asplenia, e.g. caused by reticuloendothelial overload (early in the course of sickle cell disease and in severe haemolytic anaemia and immune-complex or autoimmune disease) [358]

AD, autosomal dominant; AIDS, acquired immune deficiency syndrome

Blood film evidence of hyposplenism should be deliberately sought when children present with pneumococcal sepsis [359] or if coeliac disease is suspected.

Non-haemopoietic cells

Non-haemopoietic cells may appear in a blood sample or in a blood film made from a skin-prick sample either because they are present in the circulating blood or because the sample has become contaminated during the process of obtaining it.

Endothelial cells

Endothelial cells (Figs 3.166 & 3.167) are most likely to be detected if blood films are made from the first drop of blood in a needle; this was particularly noted when needles were reused and were sometimes barbed [360]. Endothelial cells may appear singly or in clusters. They are large cells, often elongated, with diameters of 20–30 μm and a large amount of pale blue or blue-grey cytoplasm. The nucleus is round to oval with a diameter of 10–15 μm and one to three light blue nucleoli. Nuclei may appear grooved.

Increased numbers of endothelial cells are present in conditions with vascular injury (e.g. rickettsial infection, peripheral vascular disease, CMV infection, thrombotic thrombocytopenic purpura (TTP), sickle cell disease and following coronary angioplasty), but even in such circumstances they are very infrequent [361].

Virus-infected cells, interpreted as abnormal endothelial cells, have been detected in films of peripheral blood from patients with immunodeficiency and

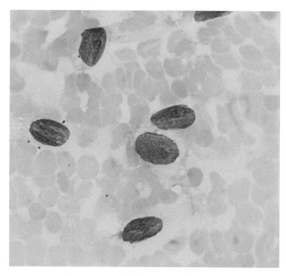

Fig. 3.166 Endothelial cells obtained by scraping the vena cava during post-mortem examination. Courtesy of Dr Marjorie Walker, Newcastle, Australia.

active CMV infection [362]. They were 50–60 μm in diameter with abundant basophilic cytoplasm and a central granular eosinophilic zone that appeared to displace the nucleus.

Epithelial cells

When blood is obtained by skin puncture, epithelial cells from the skin may occasionally be present in the blood film. They are large cells with a small nucleus and large amounts of sky-blue featureless cytoplasm (Fig. 3.168a). Some are anucleate (Fig. 3.168b).

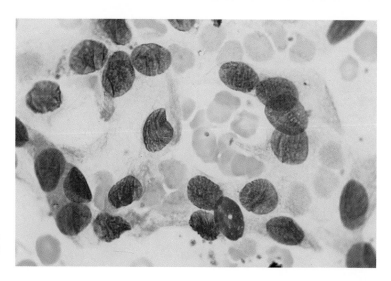

Fig. 3.167 Endothelial cells in a peripheral blood film made from a venous blood sample.

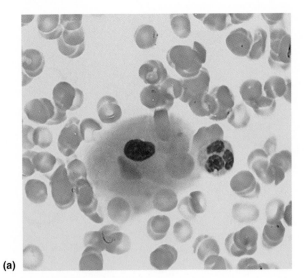 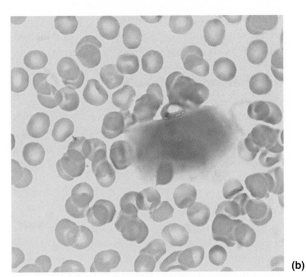

(a) (b)

Fig. 3.168 Epithelial cells in a peripheral blood film prepared from a drop of blood obtained by finger prick: (a) nucleated epithelial cell; and (b) anucleate epithelial cell.

Fat cells

Occasionally, recognisable fat cells are present in a blood film (Fig. 3.169). It is likely that they are derived from subcutaneous fat that is penetrated by the phlebotomy needle.

Mesothelial cells

Mesothelial cells have been reported in a blood film following multiple rib fractures [363].

Amniotic fluid cells

Amniotic fluid cells may be present if contamination occurs during fetal blood sampling.

Non-haemopoietic malignant cells and mucin

In various small cell tumours of childhood, tumour cells can circulate in the blood in appreciable numbers and be mistaken for the lymphoblasts of acute lymphoblastic leukaemia. Such circulating cells have been described in neuroblastoma, rhabdomyosarcoma and medulloblastoma [364–366]. In rhabdomyosarcoma, syncytial masses of tumour cells have been seen [367]. Rarely, circulating neuroblastoma cells are associated with neurofibrils [368]. Carcinoma cells can also circulate in the blood, but usually in such small numbers that they are

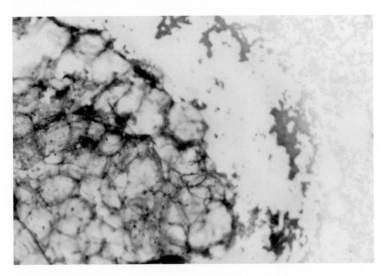

Fig. 3.169 A clump of fat cells, likely to represent subcutaneous fat, in a blood film prepared from EDTA-anticoagulated venous blood ($\times$ 40 objective).

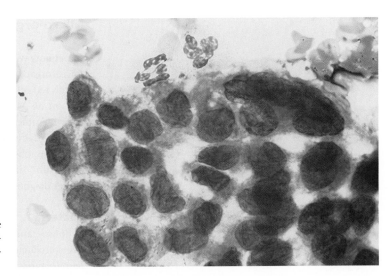

Fig. 3.170 Malignant cells in the routine peripheral blood film of a patient subsequently found to have widespread metastatic adenocarcinoma.

unlikely to be noted unless special concentration procedures are employed [369]. Rarely, they may be seen on routine blood films (Fig. 3.170). Even more rarely, a 'leukaemia' of carcinoma cells occurs. 'Carcinocythaemia' has been most often observed in carcinoma of the lung and breast [370] (Fig. 3.171). Malignant cells in the blood may be in clusters, sometimes large enough clusters to be visible macroscopically (see Fig. 3.4). Rarely, melanoma cells are present in large numbers in the circulation [371]; when they are amelanotic there is a potential for confusion with acute leukaemia. Circulating melanoma cells containing melanin are more readily identified [372] (Fig. 3.172).

Mucin has been reported within neutrophils or free in blood films in adenocarcinoma [7] and in Wilms tumour [373]. Free mucin can be stained with alcian blue, this being largely abolished by treatment with hyaluronidase [374].

In patients with advanced Hodgkin lymphoma small numbers of Reed–Sternberg cells and mononuclear Hodgkin cells have rarely been reported in the blood [375]. Even more rarely abnormal cells may be present in such numbers as to constitute a Reed–Sternberg cell leukaemia. In one such patient the total WBC was 140×10^9/l with 92% malignant cells [376]. These included typical Reed–Sternberg

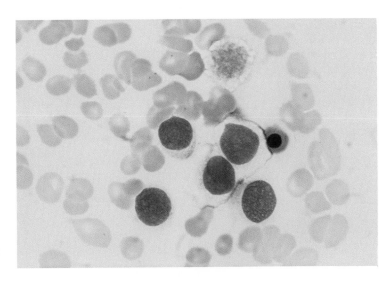

Fig. 3.171 Malignant cells in the peripheral blood of a patient with a past history of carcinoma of the breast, subsequently found to have widespread metastatic disease.

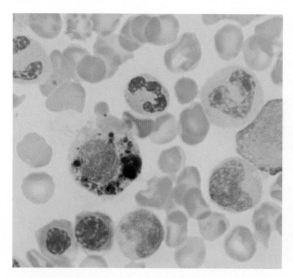

Fig. 3.172 Melanoma cell containing melanin in a buffy coat film from a patient with metastatic malignant melanoma and a leucoerythroblastic anaemia; the bone marrow was among the infiltrated tissues. By courtesy of Dr John Luckit and the late Dr David Swirsky.

cells (giant cells with a diameter of 12–40 µm with mirror-image nuclei and giant nucleoli) and multi-nucleated and mononuclear Hodgkin cells, also with giant nucleoli. However, it should be noted that there are no recent reports of circulating Reed–Sternberg or Hodgkin cells, even in patients with HIV infection who often present with widespread disease; descriptions of such cells pre-date the availability of immunophenotyping techniques.

Micro-organisms in blood films

In patients with bacterial, fungal or parasitic infections, micro-organisms may be observed free between cells or within red cells, neutrophils or monocytes. They are visible on an MGG-stained film but special stains aid in their identification. The only micro-organisms that are observed fairly frequently are malaria parasites, but the fortuitous observation of other micro-organisms in a blood film can also be diagnostically useful, leading to earlier diagnosis and treatment.

Bacteria

In louse- and tick-borne relapsing fevers the causative spirochetes, e.g. *Borrelia recurrentis*, *Borrelia duttoni*, *Borrelia turicata*, *Borrelia parkeri* or *Borrelia hermsii*, are observed free between cells (Fig. 3.173). Organisms can be detected in the peripheral blood film in 70% of cases of tick-borne relapsing fever [377]. When Borrelia species are being sought a thick film is useful.

It is quite uncommon for bacteria other than Borrelia to be noted in routine blood films. When present they are most often observed within neutrophils or, occasionally, free between cells. When they are being deliberately sought a buffy coat preparation makes detection more likely. Bacteria are most often seen in hyposplenic or immunosuppressed subjects and in those with indwelling intravenous lines or overwhelming infections. Bacteria that have been observed within neutrophils in routine peripheral blood films include streptococci, staphylococci, *Streptococcus pneumoniae*

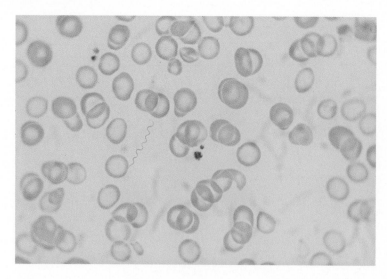

Fig. 3.173 Borrelia species in the peripheral blood of a febrile North African child.

(pneumococcus), *Neisseria meningitides* (meningococcus; Fig. 3.174), *Clostridium perfringens* (previously known as *Clostridium welchii*), *Yersinia pestis*, *Bacteroides distasonis* [378], corynebacterium species [378], *Capnocytophaga canimorsus* (Fig. 3.175) [379], *Escherichia coli* [380], *Klebsiella pneumoniae* [380], *Klebsiella oxytoca* [381], *Pseudomonas aeruginosa* [382], *Legionella pneumophila* [383] and *Citrobacter koseri* [384].

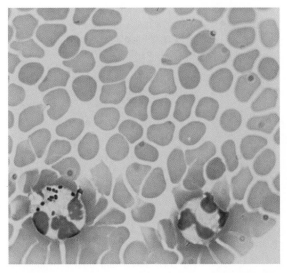

Fig. 3.174 A neutrophil containing diplococci from a patient with fatal *Neisseria meningitidis* septicaemia.

In bartonellosis or Oroya fever (Fig. 3.176), a disease confined to South America, the causative organism, a flagellated bacillus, is present on the surface of red cells and infection leads to spherocytosis and haemolytic anaemia. The organism, *Bartonella bacilliformis*, stains deep red or purple on an MGG stain [385]. *Bartonella quintana*, the causative organism of trench fever, has been detected in peripheral blood erythrocytes by immunofluorescence [386], so it seems possible that the bacilli could be detected in an MGG-stained film. Haemotropic bacilli, *Tropheryma whipplei* (previously *Tropheryma whippelii*), have also been reported in Whipple disease in hyposplenic subjects (Fig. 3.177) and have been recognised as PAS-positive inclusions in the monocytes of another patient [387]. Intraerythrocytic grahamella species have been reported in three Eastern European patients [388]. Rod-shaped structures, apparently associated with red cells and suspected of being bacterial in nature, have been reported in some patients with thrombotic thrombocytopenic purpura [389].

Micro-organisms are occasionally seen in monocytes and even in lymphocytes and platelets. *Tropheryma whipplei* has been detected in monocytes by means of immunocytochemical staining of a buffy coat preparation [390]. In HIV infection, the observation of rod-shaped negative images within monocytes or neutrophils suggests *Mycobacterium avium intracellulare* infection [391]. Ehrlichia and anaplasma may be detected in neutrophils, monocytes and, occasionally, lymphocytes. They may appear as small

(a)

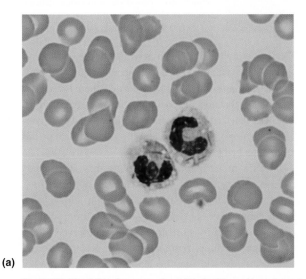

(b)

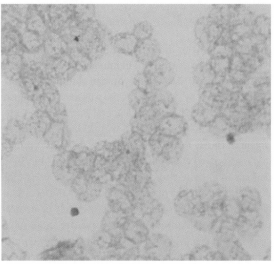

Fig. 3.175 Blood film from a patient who had been bitten by a dog showing *Capnocytophaga canimorsus*: (a) May–Grünwald–Giemsa (MGG) stain; (b) Gram stain. By courtesy of the late Dr Alan Mills.

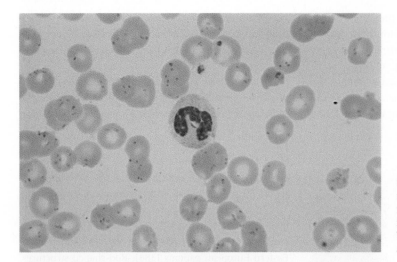

Fig. 3.176 Blood film showing multiple small rod-shaped bacilli associated with erythrocytes in a patient with bartonellosis. There is also a red cell containing a Howell–Jolly body. Courtesy of the late Dr David Swirsky and the late Professor Sir John Dacie.

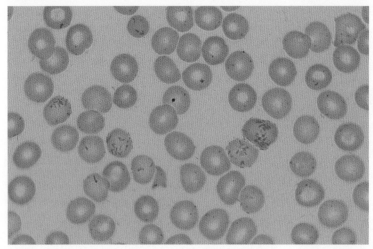

Fig. 3.177 Blood film from a hyposplenic patient with Whipple disease showing a red cell fragment, a red cell containing a Howell–Jolly body and several red cells with which are associated numerous delicate rod-shaped bacilli. Wright's stain. Courtesy of Dr B. J. Patterson, Toronto.

single organisms or as morulae containing a number of elemental bodies (Fig. 3.178). In human granulocytic anaplasmosis (previously known as human granulocytic ehrlichiosis), caused by *Anaplasma phagocytophilum* (previously known as *Ehrlichia phagocytophila* and *Ehrlichia equi*), the organisms are in granulocytes [392]. *Ehrlichia ewingii*, an organism closely related to *Ehrlichia canis*, also infects man and is associated with morulae in granulocytes [392,393]. Human monocytic ehrlichiosis, caused by *Ehrlichia chaffeensis*, has organisms mainly in monocytes but occasionally in lymphocytes (which may be atypical) or neutrophils [394,395]. Ehrlichia or anaplasma are more often seen in peripheral blood leucocytes in human granulocytic anaplasmosis than in human monocytic ehrlichiosis. Cases of ehrlichiosis and anaplasmosis have mainly been described in the USA but the disease also occurs in Europe

[396]. Anaplasma have been described in the neutrophils of a neonate with transplacentally acquired human granulocytic anaplasmosis [397]. In Venezuela there is a species of Ehrlichia that appears predominantly in platelets, which has been detected in individuals who have had close contact with dogs [398]; one clinically affected patient has been described [399].

Bacteria in peripheral blood films may have characteristic features that give a clue to their identity. They can be identified as cocci or bacilli and, following a Gram stain, as Gram negative or Gram positive. Spore formation by clostridia has been observed [400]. The plague bacillus, *Yersinia pestis* (Fig. 3.179), is found extracellularly and may be bipolar in a Romanowsky stain [401]. Ehrlichia and anaplasma are distinctive (see above). Bacteria that have colonised indwelling venous

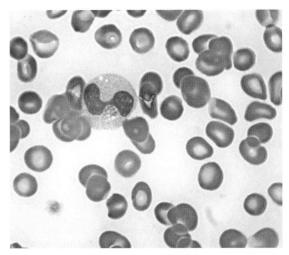

Fig. 3.178 Blood of a patient with human granulocytic anaplasmosis showing the morular form of the organism within a neutrophil. By courtesy of Dr Vandita Johari, Minneapolis.

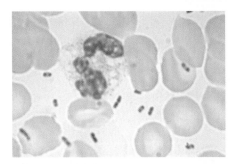

Fig. 3.179 Blood film from a patient with plague showing the bipolar bacilli of *Yersinia pestis*. By courtesy of the American Society of Hematology Slide Bank.

lines despite antibiotic therapy may be morphologically abnormal, appearing filamentous as a consequence of failure of septation (Fig. 3.180 & 3.181) [381].

The finding of bacteria in a blood film is usually highly significant. The exception is with cord blood samples, which are often collected in circumstances in which bacterial contamination is likely; if they are left at room temperature and delay occurs in delivery to the laboratory it is not uncommon to see bacteria in stained films.

Fungi

Fungi have also been observed in peripheral blood films, particularly in patients with indwelling central venous lines who are also neutropenic or have defective immunity. They may be observed free or within neutrophils or monocytes. Fungi that have been observed in neutrophils include *Candida albicans*, *Candida parapsilosis* [402] (Fig. 3.182), *Candida glabrata*, *Candida tropicalis* [403], *Candida krusei* [403], *Candida guilliermondii* [403], *Hansenula anomala* [404], *Histoplasma capsulatum* (Figs 3.183 & 3.184), *Cryptococcus neoformans* [405], *Penicillium marneffei* (Fig. 3.185) [406] and *Rhodotorula glutinis* [403], and in monocytes *Histoplasma capsulatum* and *Penicillium marneffei* [406]. *Malassezia furfur* has been observed extracellularly [407] and within neutrophils [408], characteristically in patients on intravenous lipid supplementation. *Rhodotorula rubra* has also been observed in blood films [403]. In *Candida albicans* infection, both yeast forms and pseudo-hyphae have been observed [409]. In febrile neutropenic patients a search

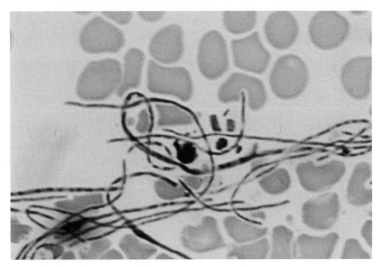

Fig. 3.180 *Klebsiella oxytoca* in a film of blood obtained from an indwelling venous line, showing failure of septation: (a) MGG stain. *Continued p. 152*

(a)

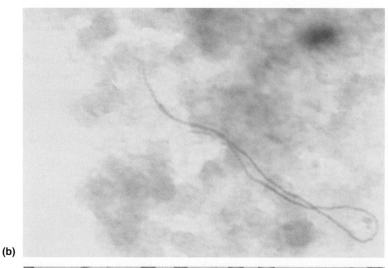

(b)

Fig. 3.180 *Continued* (b) Gram stain. Courtesy of Dr Carol Barton and Mr J. Kitaruth, Reading.

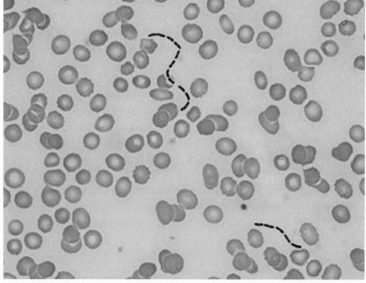

Fig. 3.181 Blood film of a patient with AML who developed *Escherichiae coli* infection. The patient was receiving prophylactic antifungal agents and it is postulated that this is the reason for the failure of the bacilli to separate from each other. By courtesy of Dr Catherine Bagot, Glasgow.

of the peripheral blood film can confirm a diagnosis of systemic fungal infection some days in advance of positive cultures in a significant proportion of patients [404].

Parasites

Some parasites, such as malaria parasites and babesiae, are predominantly blood parasites, while others, such as filariae, have part of their life cycle in the blood. Parasites that may be detected in the blood film are listed with their geographical distribution in Tables 3.14 and 3.15.

Malaria

Although malaria parasites may be detected in MGG-stained blood films, their detection and identification are facilitated by Leishman or Giemsa staining at a higher pH. A thick film is preferable for detection of parasites and a thin film for identification of the species. A thick film should be examined for at least 5–10 minutes (200 high power fields) before being considered negative. If only a thin film is available it should not be considered negative until it has been examined for 20–40 minutes or until 200 high power fields or the whole blood film have been examined. UK guidelines require all malaria films to be examined by two observers. Partially immune subjects are particularly likely to have a low parasite count so that a prolonged search may be required for parasite detection. Experienced observers may prefer to scan using a ×50 objective but otherwise a ×100 objective should be used. In patients

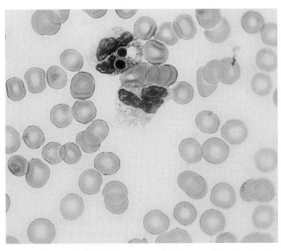
(a)

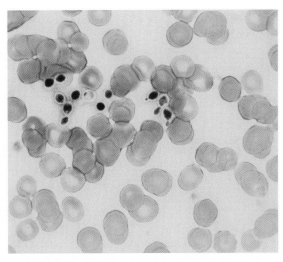
(b)

Fig. 3.182 *Candida parapsilosis* in a peripheral blood film: (a) within neutrophils; and (b) free between red cells. Several organisms are budding. Courtesy of Dr Bipin Vadher and Dr Marilyn Treacy, London.

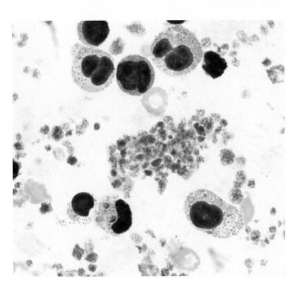

Fig. 3.183 A band neutrophil in a buffy coat film showing three *Histoplasma capsulatum*. By courtesy of Dr Sian Lewis, Oxford.

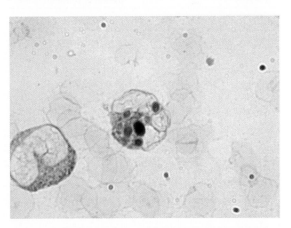

Fig. 3.184 Methenamine silver stain of *Histoplasma capsulatum* in the peripheral blood. Courtesy of Dr Hector Musa, Minneapolis.

with a strong suspicion of malaria whose initial films are negative, repeated blood examinations may be needed. *Plasmodium falciparum* is associated with the highest parasite counts with sometimes 10–40% of red cells being parasitised; paradoxically, patients may be seriously ill with no parasites being detectable on initial blood examination. This is the result of parasitised red cells being sequestered in tissues. When *P. falciparum* is detected, a count of the proportion of cells that are parasitised should be made to allow monitoring during therapy, gametocytes being excluded

from this count; a Miller graticule, as used for reticulocyte counts, facilitates this. A parasite count of more than 2% in an area of low transmission, or of more than 5% in an area of high and stable transmission, is indicative of severe malaria [413]. Alternatively, parasites can be counted in a thick film, their numbers being related to the number of leucocytes, to produce an absolute count. A failure of the parasite count to fall indicates a drug-resistant parasite. Exchange transfusion or erythrocytapheresis may be considered when the parasite count is very high, e.g. recommended by the US Centers for Disease Control when the proportion of parasitised cells is more than 10% [414]. Other haematological features indicative of severe malaria are an Hb of less than 50 g/l and haemoglobinuria [414].

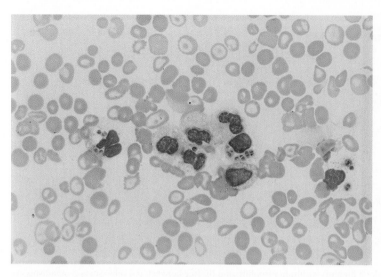

Fig. 3.185 *Penicillium marneffei* in the peripheral blood of a patient with AIDS. Courtesy of Dr K.F. Wong, Hong Kong.

Table 3.14 Protozoan parasites that may be detected in blood films.

Parasite	Disease or common name	Usual distribution
Sporozoans		
Plasmodium falciparum	Malignant tertian malaria	Widespread in tropics and sub-tropics, particularly in Africa
Plasmodium vivax	Benign tertian malaria	Widespread in tropics and occurs also in some temperate zones; quite uncommon in West and Central Africa
Plasmodium malariae	Quartan malaria	Scattered in the tropics
Plasmodium ovale	Benign tertian malaria	Tropical West Africa; scattered foci elsewhere including tropical Asia, New Guinea and the Western Pacific
Plasmodium knowlesi		Malaysian Borneo [410], peninsular Malaysia [411] and as far north as Burma; the Philippines, Singapore
Babesia microti	Babesiosis	North-Eastern coastal USA, West Coast and Mid-West
Babesia equi	Babesiosis	California
Babesia divergens	Babesiosis	Europe
Toxoplasma gondii [412]	Toxoplasmosis	
Haemoflagellates		
Trypanosoma brucei rhodesiense	Sleeping sickness	East Africa
Trypanosoma brucei gambiense	Sleeping sickness	Tropical West and Central Africa
Trypanosoma cruzi	South American trypanosomiasis or Chagas disease	Wide area of Central and South America
Trypanosoma rangeli	Non-pathogenic	Central and South America
Leishmania donovani	Visceral leishmaniasis or kala–azar	India, China, Central Asia, Central and Northern Africa, Portugal, the Mediterranean littoral, Central and South America

Table 3.15 Nematode (family filariidae) parasites that may be detected in blood films.

Parasite	Disease or common name	Usual distribution
Wuchereria bancrofti	Filariasis – end stage may be elephantiasis	Widespread in tropics and sub-tropics, particularly Asia, Polynesia, New Guinea, Africa and Central and South America
Brugia malayi	Filariasis – end stage may be elephantiasis	India, South-East Asia, China, Japan
Loa loa	Eye worm or Calabar swellings	African equatorial rainforest and its fringes
Mansonella perstans	Persistent filariasis, usually non-pathogenic	Tropical Africa, Central and South America
Mansonella ozzardi	Ozzard's filariasis, usually non-pathogenic	Central and South America, West Indies
Onchocerca volvulus	Onchocerciasis (river blindness)	Central and West Africa and Sudan, Central America

Useful features in distinguishing between the four major species are summarised in Fig. 3.186 and illustrated in Figs 3.187–3.191. *Plasmodium ovale* has recently been identified by molecular genetic analysis as two distinct species, *Plasmodium ovale curtisi* and *Plasmodium ovale wallikeri*, but these are morphologically indistinguishable [415]. The four major species are found in tropical and subtropical zones. *Plasmodium vivax* is particularly common in India, Sri Lanka and the Far East. *Plasmodium ovale* is prevalent in Africa, particularly West Africa, but also in the Philippines. In addition to these four species, human infection with the simian parasite, *Plasmodium knowlesi*, which was initially described in Malaysian Borneo (Sabah and Sarawak) and Indonesian Borneo, was later found to have extended to peninsular Malaysia and subsequently to Thailand, Vietnam, the Philippines, Singapore and Myanmar [410,416–420]. Morphologically this parasite can be difficult or impossible to distinguish from *Plasmodium malariae* and misidentification as *P. falciparum* also occurs. There may be small and medium-sized ring trophozoites, sometimes accolé forms, rings forms with the nucleus within the ring, double chromatin dots, compact band forms, ameboid trophozoites, schizonts (containing up to 16 merozoites) and, in some patients, gametocytes [421,422] (Fig. 3.191); mature parasites contain golden brown or dark brown pigment [421] and neutrophils may contain haemozoin [419]. Infection is asynchronous, multiple stages of the parasite generally being present. Red cells may contain multiple parasites, are not enlarged and may show fine dots (but fewer than in *P. vivax* or *P. ovale* infection) [421]. Associated thrombocytopenia is very common. *Plasmodium knowlesi* rather than *Plasmodium malariae* should be suspected in an infection acquired in Malaysia and particularly if there is a high parasite count and a seriously ill patient [416]. Molecular analysis is required for confirmation of the diagnosis (see below).

Specimens requiring examination for malaria parasites should be dealt with promptly, since storage can result in artefactual changes in the parasites and make determining the species more difficult. In *P. vivax* infection, mature schizonts may develop *in vitro* with reinvasion of red cells by merozoites; these may remain at the margin of the red cells, leading to possible confusion with accolé forms of *P. falciparum*. *P. falciparum* gametocytes can become rounded, leading to confusion with *P. malariae*. Male gametocytes can exflagellate on storage.

The percentage parasitaemia should be estimated for *P. knowlesi* as well as for *P. falciparum* infection. In *P. knowlesi* infection, 1% or more parasitaemia and a platelet count of 45×10^9/l or less are indicative of severe disease [419].

Associated abnormalities that may be noted in the films of patients with malaria are anaemia (the reticulocyte count being inappropriately low), thrombocytopenia, lymphopenia, lymphocytosis or atypical lymphocytes, eosinopenia (and suppression of pre-existing eosinophilia), early neutrophilia (with *P. falciparum*), neutropenia, monocytosis, occasionally phagocytosed merozoites and sometimes schizonts within neutrophils in *P. falciparum* infection with high parasitaemia [423,424], phagocytosis of parasitised and non-parasitised red cells by monocytes and malaria pigment (in monocytes and occasionally in neutrophils). Leucocytosis, neutrophilia, lymphocytosis and monocytosis correlate with severity of malaria [424]. In multivariate analysis leucocytosis, lymphocytosis and monocytopenia correlate with a higher rate of death [424]. Malaria pigment in monocytes is indicative of more chronic malaria than pigment in neutrophils and correlates with more severe disease and with mortality [425]. Thrombocytopenia can be a diagnostically useful feature, alerting the laboratory or the clinician to the likelihood of malaria. In one study of children presenting to an Accident and Emergency Department in London, one-quarter of patients with a platelet count of less than 150×10^9/l were found to have malaria [426]; thrombocytopenia was seen in association with both falciparum and vivax malaria and is characteristic of human *P. knowlesi* infection [416]. A study in India confirmed that a platelet count of less than 150×10^9/l was common in both vivax and falciparum malaria, as was a leucocyte count less than 4×10^9/l; the MPV was sometimes elevated [427]. Malaria pigment in leucocytes is mainly associated with *P. falciparum* malaria. The pigment is haemozoin, a degradation product of haemoglobin. It can be visualised readily in stained or unstained films and is birefringent when polarised light is used [428]. The pigment is released into the plasma during schizogony [423] and is then phagocytosed. The percentage of leucocytes containing pigment therefore reflects the sequestered parasite burden and has been found to be of prognostic significance [423]. Monocytes containing malaria pigment can often be found in the blood for many days after parasitised red cells have disappeared; this can be useful in making a retrospective diagnosis of malaria [429].

	General features and changes in red cells	Early trophozoite (ring form)	Mature trophozoite
Plasmodium vivax	Red cells much enlarged, irregular and pale with fine red stippling (Schüffner's dots); usually low or moderate parasitaemia; all stages of life cycle often present; sometimes multiple parasites per cell	Thick rings, $1/3$–$1/2$ the diameter of the red cell 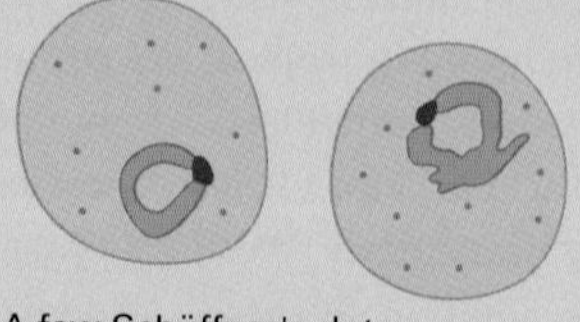 A few Schüffner's dots Accolé (shoulder) forms and double dots less common than with *P. falciparum*	Ameboid rings, $1/2$–$2/3$ the diameter of the red cell Pale blue or lilac parasite with prominent central valuole 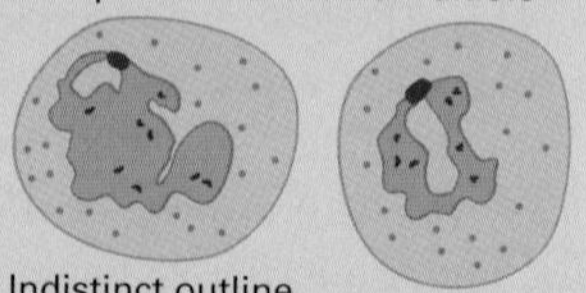 Indistinct outline Scattered fine yellowish-brown pigment granules or rods
Plasmodium ovale	Red cells enlarged but not as much as with *P. vivax*; cells pale and some are oval or pear-shaped; some are ragged (fimbriated) at one or both ends; fine to coarse red stippling (Schüffner's dots or James's dots; more than one parasite per cell is very unusual); low parasitaemia; often fewer stages present than with *P. vivax*	Thick, compact rings, $1/3$–$1/2$ the diameter of the red cell 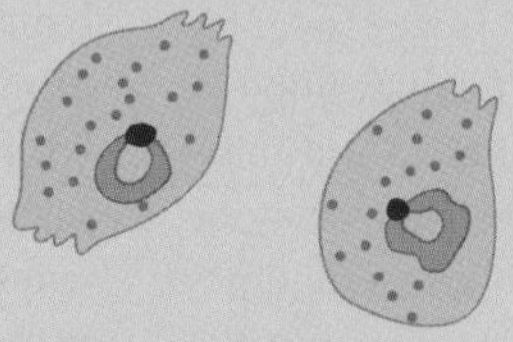 Numerous Schüffner's dots but paler than with *P. vivax*	Thick rings, less irregular than those of *P. vivax*, $1/3$–$1/2$ the diameter of the red cell 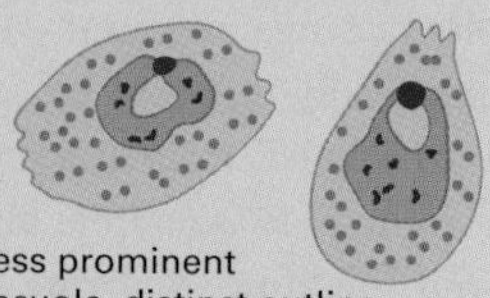 Less prominent vacuole, distinct outline Yellowish-brown pigment which is coarser and darker than that of *P. vivax* Schüffner's dots prominent
Plasmodium falciparum	Cells not enlarged; staining characteristics usually unaltered but sometimes there are some pale cells; sometimes multiple parasites per cell and heavy parasitaemia (10–40% of cells); often only ring forms are present	Delicate rings, $1/6$–$1/4$ the diameter of the red cell 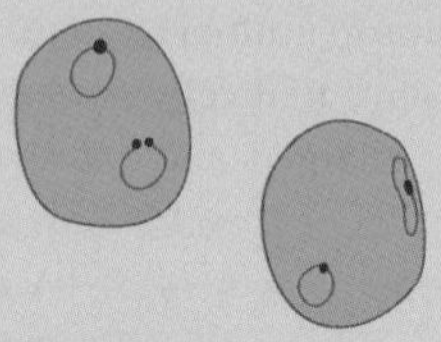 Double dots and accolé forms common	Fairly delicate rings, $1/3$–$1/2$ the diameter of the red cell 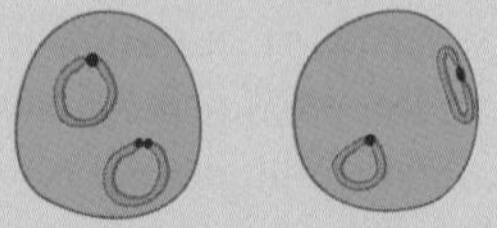 Red-mauve stippling (Maurer's dots or clefts) may be present Mature trophozoites are less often present in peripheral blood than ring forms Cytoplasm may be vacuolated
Plasmodium malariae	Cells not enlarged, sometimes contracted; staining characteristics not altered; lowest degree of parasitaemia; multiple parasites per cell rare; no stippling unless overstained; all stages usually present	Small, thick, compact rings Small chromatin dot which may be inside the ring 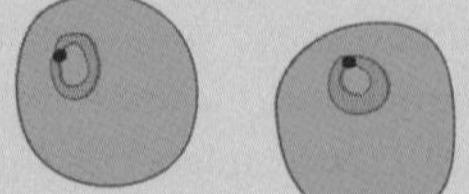 Double dots and accolé forms rare	Ameboid form more compact than *P. vivax* Sometimes angular or band forms 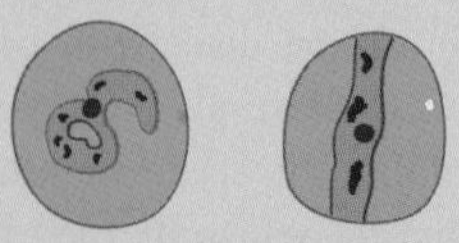 Heavy, dark yellow-brown pigment No stippling unless overstained

(a)

Fig. 3.186 Features that are useful in distinguishing between the different species of malaria parasites. *Continued p. 157*

Early schizont	Late schizont	Gametocyte	
		Macrogametocyte	Microgametocyte
Rounded or irregular Ameboid Loose central mass of fine yellowish-brown pigment 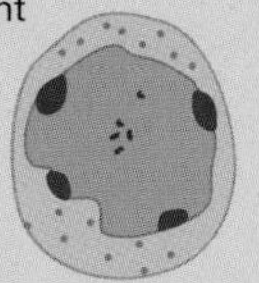 Schizont almost fills cell Schüffner's dots	12–24 (usually 16–24) medium-sized merozoites 1–2 clumps of peripheral pigment 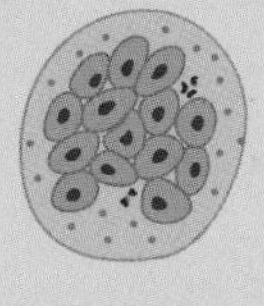 Schizont almost fills cell Schüffner's dots	Round or ovoid, almost fills enlarged cell Blue cytoplasm 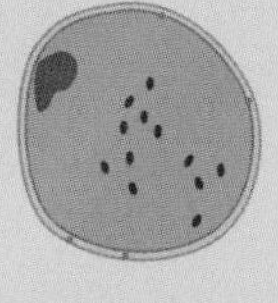 Eccentric compact red nucleus Scattered pigment	Round or ovoid, as large as a normal red cell but does not fill the enlarged red cell 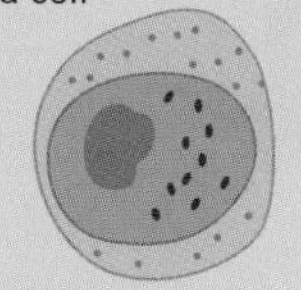 Faintly staining Larger, lighter red central or eccentric nucleus Fine, scattered pigment
Round, compact Darkish brown pigment, heavier and coarser than that of *P. vivax* 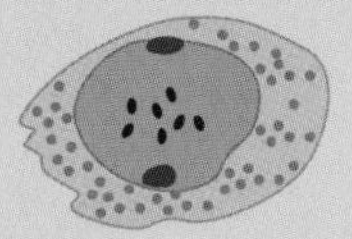 Schüffner's dots	6–12 (usually 8) large merozoites arranged irregularly like a bunch of grapes 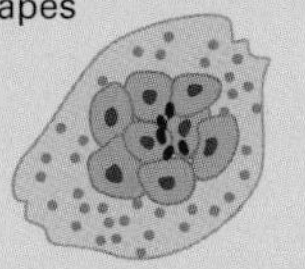 Central pigment Schüffner's dots	Similar to *P. vivax* but somewhat smaller 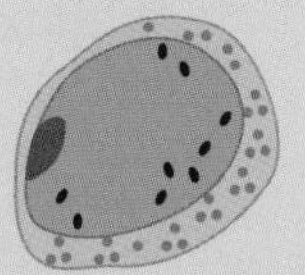 Pigment coarser and blacker, scattered but mainly near the periphery	Similar to *P. vivax* but smaller 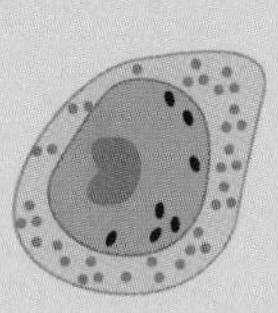
Not usually seen in blood Very small, ameboid Scattered light brown to black pigment	Not usually seen in blood 8–32 (usually few) very small merozoites; grouped irregularly Peripheral clump of coarse dark brown pigment	Sickle or crescent shaped Deforms cell which often appears empty of haemoglobin 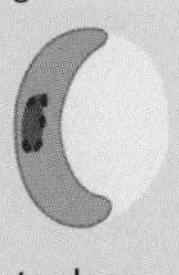 Blue cytoplasm Compact central nucleus with pigment aggregated around it	Oval or crescentic with blunted ends Pale blue or pink 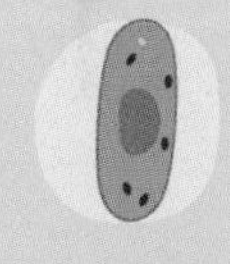 Large pale nucleus with pigment more scattered than in macrogametocyte
Compact, round, fills red cell 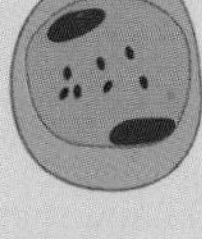 Coarse dark yellow-brown pigment	6–12 (usually 8–10) large merozoites, arranged symmetrically, often in a rosette or daisy head formation 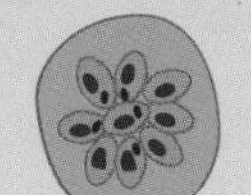 Central coarse dark yellowish-brown pigment	Similar to *P. vivax* but smaller, round or oval, almost fills cell, blue with a dark nucleus 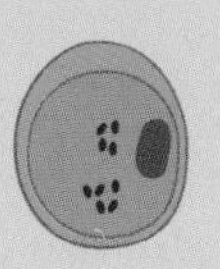 Prominent pigment concentrated at centre and periphery	Similar to *P. vivax* but smaller, pink or paler blue than macrogametocyte with a larger, paler nucleus 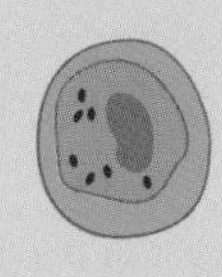 Prominent pigment

(b)

Fig. 3.186 *Continued*

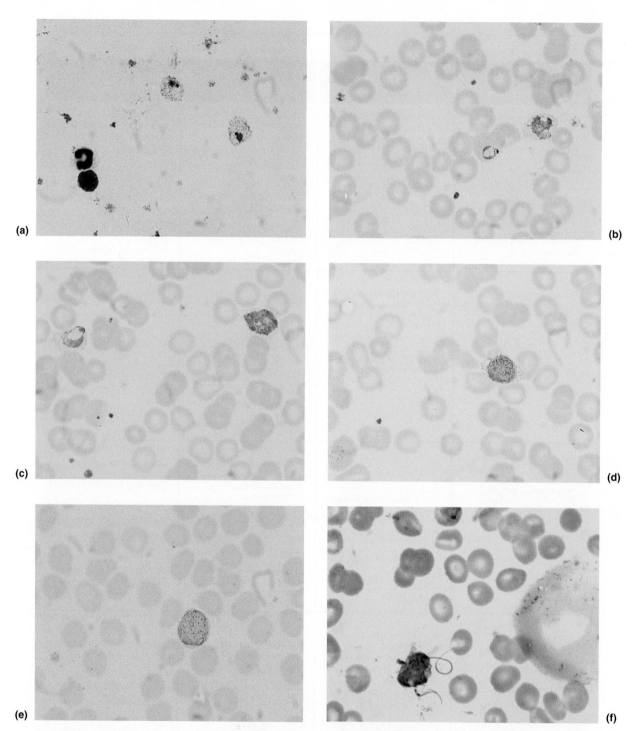

Fig. 3.187 Stages in the life cycle of *Plasmodium vivax* shown in Giemsa-stained peripheral blood thick (a) and thin (b–h) films: (a) two ring forms within red cell ghosts; (b) a ring form and an ameboid trophozoite – both the parasitised cells are enlarged and decolorised and contain faint Schüffner's dots; (c) a ring form and an early schizont containing two chromatin masses – both parasitised cells are decolorised and contain faint Schüffner's dots; (d) a microgametocyte – the pigment is fine and scattered and the parasite does not completely fill the cell; (e) a microgametocyte – the pigment is fine and scattered and the parasite completely fills the cell and is larger than the nonparasitised red cells; (f) exflagellation of microgametes from a gametocyte – this stage of the parasite life cycle usually occurs in the stomach of the mosquito. *Continued p. 159*

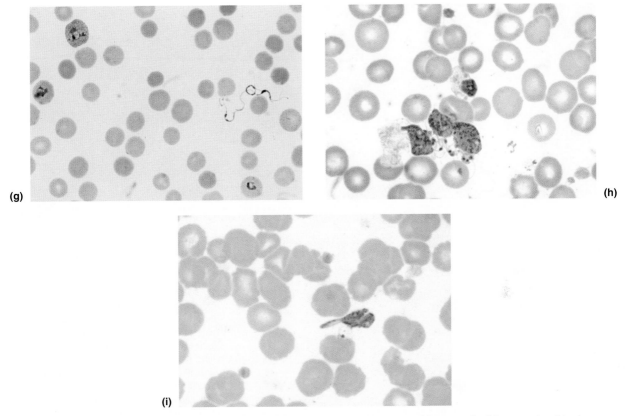

Fig. 3.187 *Continued* (g) microgametes – this stage of the parasite life cycle usually occurs in the stomach of the mosquito; (h) micro-gametes clustered around three macrogametes – it appears that one microgamete has fertilised a macrogamete since its nucleus appears to have penetrated the macrogamete – this stage of the parasite life cycle usually occurs in the stomach of the mosquito; (i) ookinete – this stage of the malaria parasite life cycle usually occurs in the stomach of the mosquito and is very rarely seen in the peripheral blood of man. By courtesy of Dr Wendi Bailey, Liverpool.

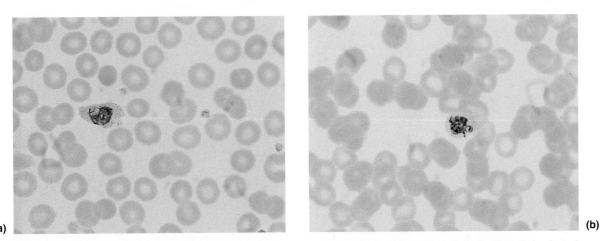

Fig. 3.188 Stages in the life cycle of *Plasmodium ovale* in Giemsa-stained thin films: (a) a late trophozoite in an enlarged, decolorised and oval red cell that has a fimbriated end – pigment is coarser and darker than in *Plasmodium vivax*, the parasite is more compact and Schüffner's dots are more prominent; (b) a schizont containing eight merozoites – coarse pigment is clustered centrally.

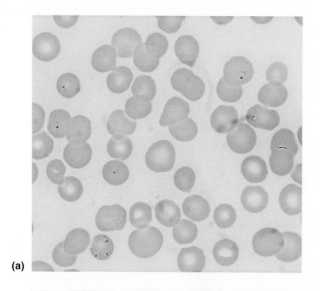

(a)

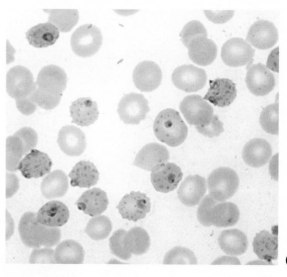

(b)

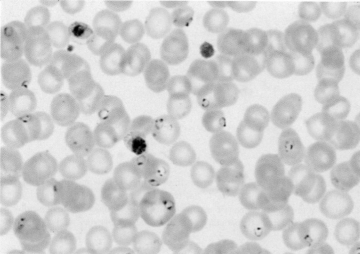

(c)

Fig. 3.189 Stages in the life cycle of *Plasmodium falciparum* in Giemsa-stained thin films; the cells are not enlarged or decolorised: (a) ring forms and one late trophozoite; (b) ring forms with prominent Maurer's clefts; (c) ring forms and early and late schizonts (schizonts are not commonly seen in the peripheral blood); (d) ring forms and an early gametocyte that has not yet assumed its banana shape; (e) a macrogametocyte – the parasite is sickle-shaped with a compact nucleus and pigment clustered centrally; (f) a microgametocyte that is broader and less curved than the macrogametocyte with a more diffuse nucleus and less concentrated pigment.

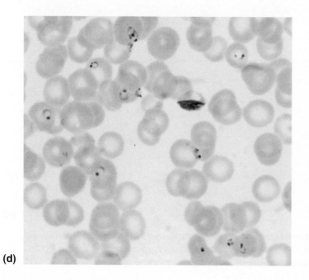

(d)

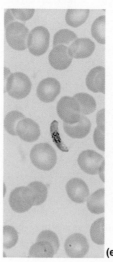

(e)

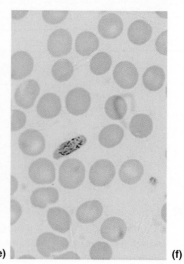

(f)

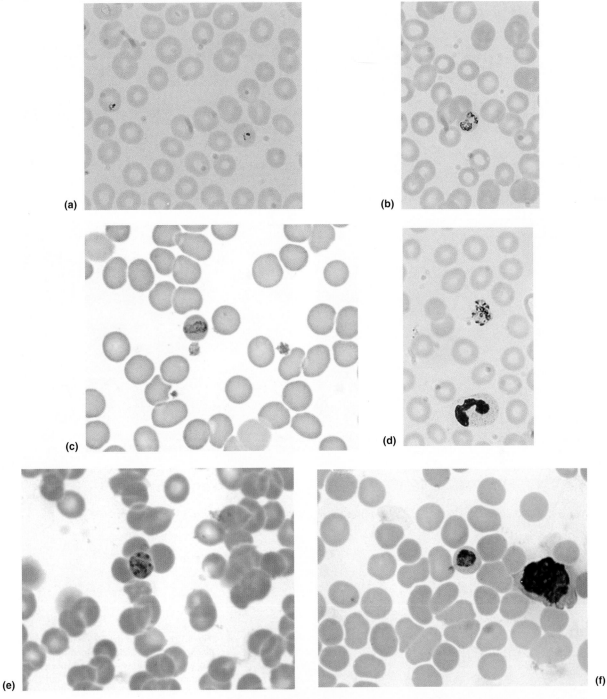

Fig. 3.190 Stages in the life cycle of *Plasmodium malariae* in Giemsa-stained thin films; red cells are not enlarged or decolorised: (a) early ring forms that are small but less delicate than those of *Plasmodium falciparum* – one parasite has a chromatin dot within the ring; (b) ameboid trophozoite with coarse dark-brown pigment; (c) band trophozoite; (d) schizont with about seven merozoites in a daisy-head arrangement with central coarse brown pigment; (e) schizont with merozoites grouped around the centrally placed pigment; (f) a gametocyte and a reactive lymphocyte.

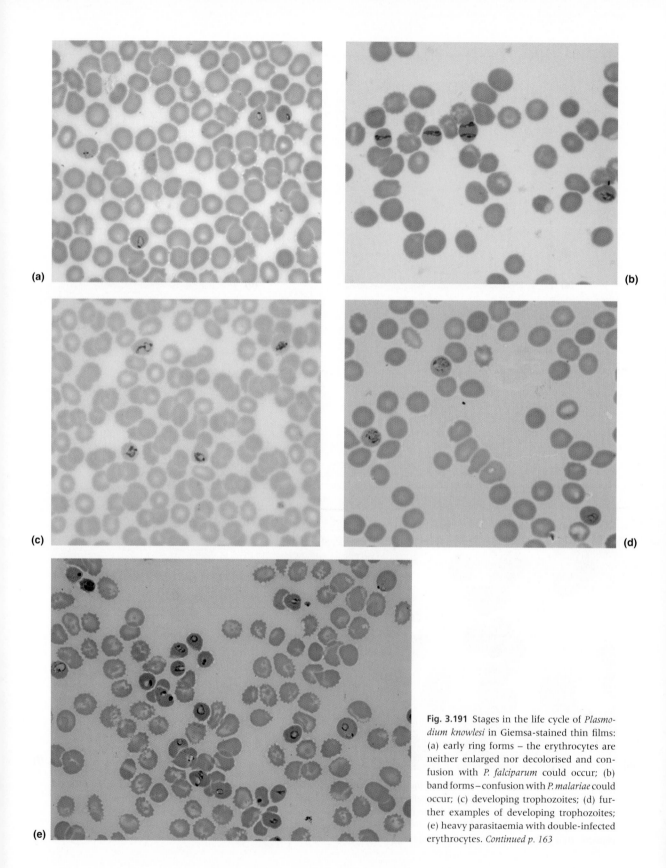

Fig. 3.191 Stages in the life cycle of *Plasmodium knowlesi* in Giemsa-stained thin films: (a) early ring forms – the erythrocytes are neither enlarged nor decolorised and confusion with *P. falciparum* could occur; (b) band forms – confusion with *P. malariae* could occur; (c) developing trophozoites; (d) further examples of developing trophozoites; (e) heavy parasitaemia with double-infected erythrocytes. *Continued p. 163*

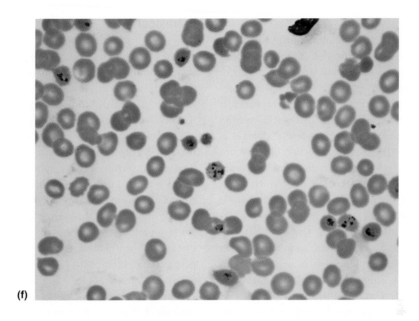

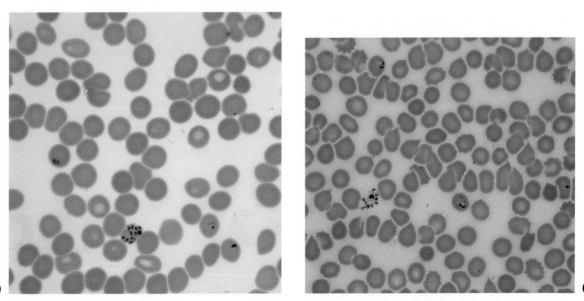

Fig. 3.191 *Continued* (f) heavy parasitaemia with double- and triple-infected erythrocytes; (g) a ring form and a ruptured schizont containing 10 merozoites and pigment; (h) a ring form and a ruptured schizont composed of 8 merozoites with pigment. By courtesy of Dr Janet Cox-Singh, St Andrews.

The histograms or scatter plots of automated full blood counters may be abnormal in the presence of malaria parasites. This has been noted with various Coulter, Sysmex, Cell-Dyn and Mindray instruments (see Chapter 2). Malaria parasites can cause pseusoe-osinophilia with Sysmex instruments because of the depolarisation of light by haemozoin.

Other tests

Malaria can be diagnosed immunologically using commercially available strips for immunochromatographic detection of either a *P. falciparum* antigen, histidine-rich protein-2, parasitic lactate dehydrogenase (pLDH) [430] or parasitic aldolase [431]. Parasitic LDH can be species-specific (identifying *P. falciparum* or *P. vivax*) or pan-specific [432]. Parasitic aldolase is pan-specific [432]. The strips for detection of pLDH are sensitive and specific for the detection of *P. falciparum* and are sensitive for the detection of *P. vivax*; however, only around half of cases of *P. ovale* or *P. malariae* infection are detected [433] and around three-quarters of *P. knowlesi* infections [431]. Only a quarter of *P. knowlesi* infections are detected using an aldoses test [431]. Tests for histidine-rich protein-2 remain positive for some time after an acute infection, whereas positivity for pLDH correlates with the presence of viable organisms and may give a clue to a drug-resistant infection. False positive tests may be observed in patients with rheumatoid arthritis with kits for detection of histidine-rich protein-2 and pLDH [434]. A large number of rapid diagnosis kits are commercially available. Individual kits have been assessed by the World Health Organization: http://www.wpro.who.int/sites/rdt and www.finddiagnostics.org/resource-centre/reports_brochures/malaria-diagnostic-test-report.html

P. knowlesi infection can be diagnosed by a nested polymerase chain reaction [416].

Babesiosis

Babesiosis is an uncommon tick-borne parasitic disease [435], which can easily be confused with malaria. *Babesia microti* is endemic in southern New England, southern New York state, Wisconsin and Minnesota. Healthy immunologically normal adults usually are asymptomatic [436]. Infection may persist for months or even years [436]. *Babesia duncani* occurs on the west coast of the USA [437]. *Babesia divergens* infection occurs sporadically in the USA [438] and in Europe (including Ireland) and Asia. About 30 human cases have been described in Europe, more than three-quarters of them in hyposplenic patients [439], but it is likely that milder disease in individuals with functioning spleens is going undetected [440]. *Babesia bovis* infection also occurs in Europe [441]. The trophozoites of babesia species are small rings, similar to those of *P. falciparum*, 1–5 μm in diameter with one, two or three chromatin dots and scanty cytoplasm. Sometimes they are pyriform (pear-shaped) and either paired (Fig. 3.192a) or have the pointed ends of four parasites being in contact to give a Maltese cross formation (Fig. 3.192b). Extracellular parasites are sometimes seen [442] and may form clusters [441]. *Babesia microti* and *Babesia duncani* are associated with Maltese cross and pleomorphic ring forms, the latter with small to large cytoplasmic vacuoles [430,437]. *Babesia divergens* and *Babesia venatorum* typically have

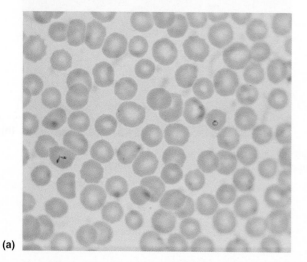
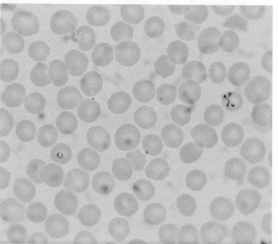

(a) (b)

Fig. 3.192 Blood film from a splenectomised monkey parasitised by *Babesia microti*: (a) a single ring form and a pair of pyriform parasites; (b) a single ring form and four pyriform parasites in a tetrad or Maltese cross formation. By courtesy of Mr John Williams, London.

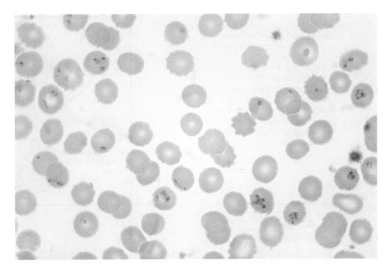

Fig. 3.193 Blood film from a hyposplenic patient with babesiosis caused by Babesia divergens, showing numerous parasites including a Maltese cross formation and paired pyriform parasites. By courtesy of Mr C. Murphy, Cork.

paired pyriform merozoites and rarely tetrads [430]. In *Babesia divergens* infection, the pyriform pairs are usually at the periphery of the erythrocyte [430]. The presence of multiple ring forms, up to four per cell, is said to be diagnostic of babesiosis [443]. The ring forms of *Babesia* species may be even smaller than those of *P. falciparum* (Fig. 3.193); this and the vacuolation of the parasite, the pleomorphism of the ring forms, the presence of extracellular trophozoites and the absence of haemozoin ('malaria pigment') can help in making the distinction. Babesiosis occurs particularly but not exclusively in hyposplenic subjects in whom 25% or more of cells may be parasitised. In those with a functioning spleen the level of parasitaemia is usually low, but in HIV-positive and immunosuppressed patients more severe infection occurs [442]. The method of detection is by thick and thin film examination, as for malaria. There is often associated thrombocytopenia and sometimes neutropenia [436].

Other tests

Babesiosis can be diagnosed serologically (although cross-reactivity with malaria can occur) and by a polymerase chain reaction (PCR) [442].

Toxoplasmosis

Rarely *Toxoplasma gondii* has been identified in the peripheral blood in patients with toxoplasmosis and underlying immune deficiency [444,445]. Organisms may be extracellular or within neutrophils [445].

Infection by haemoflagellates

The morphological features of haemoflagellates that may be found in the peripheral blood are summarised in Fig. 3.194. Trypanosomes may be detected in the peripheral blood as motile, extracellular parasites [446]. They have a slender body and move by means of a flagellum extending from the kinetoplast at the rear end of the parasite to the front end where the flagellum is free (Figs 3.195 & 3.196); the flagellum is joined to the body by an undulating membrane. The parasite may be seen moving in a wet preparation when a drop of anticoagulated blood is placed on a slide, beneath a coverslip, for microscopic examination. They may also be detected in fixed preparations such as thick or thin films or buffy coat films. Scanty parasites are more readily detected by examining the sediment of 10–20 ml of haemolysed blood. *Trypanosoma brucei rhodesiense* and *Trypanosoma brucei gambiense* (see Fig. 3.193) are morphologically identical but their geographical distributions differ (see Table 3.14). Examination of the peripheral blood is more likely to be useful in the case of *T. brucei rhodesiense*. Concentration techniques may be needed with *T. brucei gambiense*, or parasites may be undetectable in the blood, lymph node puncture being required for diagnosis. Patients with trypanosomiasis

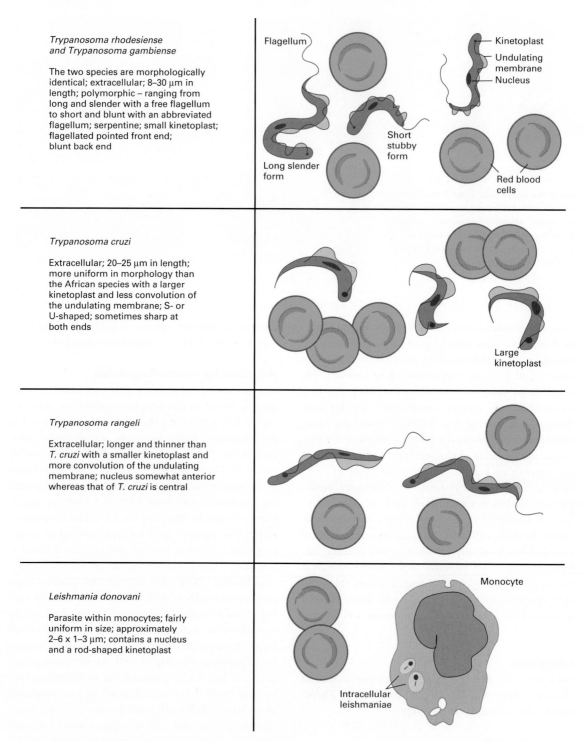

Trypanosoma rhodesiense and Trypanosoma gambiense

The two species are morphologically identical; extracellular; 8–30 μm in length; polymorphic – ranging from long and slender with a free flagellum to short and blunt with an abbreviated flagellum; serpentine; small kinetoplast; flagellated pointed front end; blunt back end

Trypanosoma cruzi

Extracellular; 20–25 μm in length; more uniform in morphology than the African species with a larger kinetoplast and less convolution of the undulating membrane; S- or U-shaped; sometimes sharp at both ends

Trypanosoma rangeli

Extracellular; longer and thinner than *T. cruzi* with a smaller kinetoplast and more convolution of the undulating membrane; nucleus somewhat anterior whereas that of *T. cruzi* is central

Leishmania donovani

Parasite within monocytes; fairly uniform in size; approximately 2–6 x 1–3 μm; contains a nucleus and a rod-shaped kinetoplast

Fig. 3.194 Summary of the morphological features of haemoflagellates.

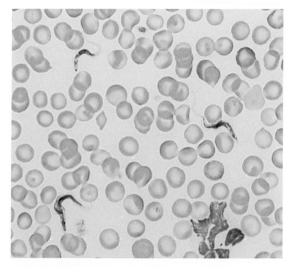

Fig. 3.195 *Trypanosoma brucei gambiense*; the parasites are serpentine with a small kinetoplast (× 40 objective).

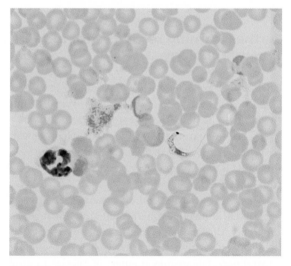

Fig. 3.196 *Trypanosoma cruzi*; the parasite is curved but not usually serpentine and has a large kinetoplast (× 40 objective).

often have a normocytic normochromic anaemia and thrombocytopenia [447].

Trypanosoma evansi, a parasite of domesticated mammals, has been reported in man in India, in a patient with a genetic susceptibility [448].

Trypanosoma cruzi (see Fig. 3.196), the causative agent of Chagas disease, differs morphologically from the African parasites. It is rarely detected by direct examination of the blood, concentration procedures usually being

required. Its distribution is manly in Latin America and in the southern USA, but it may occur in non-endemic areas, e.g. Spain and elsewhere in the USA, as a result of migration. Examining a wet preparation of buffy coat for motile parasites can be useful. *T. cruzi* can be distinguished on morphological grounds from the non-pathogenic *Trypanosoma rangeli*, which has a similar geographical distribution (see Fig. 3.169). Lymphocytosis and mild anaemia may be observed in the acute phase of Chagas disease.

Leishmania donovani, the causative organism of kala azar, may be detected in monocytes or neutrophils in the peripheral blood, in thick or thin films or in buffy coat preparations (Fig. 3.197). Examination of a peripheral blood film may avoid the need for a bone marrow or splenic aspiration, but these procedures are much more sensitive than peripheral blood examination. Both peripheral blood and bone marrow culture are more sensitive than microscopy. Associated features that may be noted in patients with kala azar are anaemia, leucopenia, neutropenia, thrombocytopenia and increased rouleaux formation. A cryoglobulin may be present and paraproteins can occur.

Other tests
Rapid immunological methods are available for the detection of *T. brucei gambiense* and *T. brucei rhodesiense* antigens [430]. Immunological techniques are also applicable to chronic *T. cruzi* infection. A variety of sensitive immunological tests are also available for the diagnosis of leishmaniasis.

Filariasis
In filariasis, adult worms reside in tissues and release microfilariae into the blood-stream. Microfilariae are detectable during the acute phase of the disease, but are not detectable in patients with chronic tissue damage but without active disease. As the microfilariae are motile, examination of a wet preparation is often useful; they can also be detected in thick and thin films. Repeated blood examinations may be needed and blood specimens must be obtained at an appropriate time for the species being sought: *Wuchereria bancrofti* and *Brugia malayi* release their microfilariae at night, whereas those of *Loa loa* are released during the day. *Mansonella ozzardi* is non-periodic. It lives in skin capillaries so may be more readily identified in capillary blood [449]. *Mansonella perstans* is usually non-periodic but release may be nocturnal or, less often, diurnal.

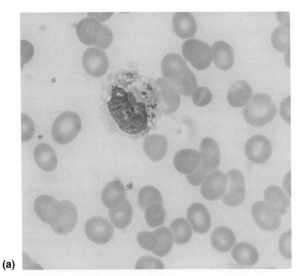

(a)

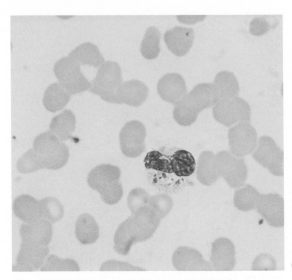

(b)

Fig. 3.197 *Leishmania donovani* in: (a) a monocyte; and (b) a neutrophil in the peripheral blood of a patient with AIDS.

Morphological features that are useful in distinguishing the various microfilariae are summarised in Fig. 3.198 and illustrated in Figs 3.199–3.202. In general, pathogenic filariae are sheathed and non-pathogenic are non-sheathed. However, *B. malayi* is sometimes seen unsheathed [449]. *Brugia timori*, which is confined to the Lesser Sunda Island of Indonesia, is similar to *B. malayi* but it is longer with fewer body kinks, a longer space at the head end, less dense nuclei and less intense staining [449]. *Onchocerca volvulus* is occasionally seen in the blood, especially in heavy infections and after therapy [449]; it is unsheathed and has a pointed tail without nuclei.

Microfilariae moving through tissues are responsible for the syndrome known as tropical eosinophilia in which respiratory symptoms are associated with eosinophilia, increased rouleaux formation and an elevated ESR. However, microfilariae are not usually detectable in the blood of patients with tropical eosinophilia.

Other tests

Rapid simple immunological tests for the detection of *Wuchereria bancrofti* antigens are available [449]. Tests for *Loa loa* are under development.

Further learning resources for blood film morphology

Lewis SM, Bain BJ and Swirsky DM (2001) *Bench Aids in the Morphological Diagnosis of Anaemia*. World Health Organization, Geneva. ISBN 92-4-154532-1.

Bain BJ (2005) Diagnosis from the blood smear. *N Engl J Med*, 353, 498–507.

Bain BJ (2014) *Interactive Haematology Imagebank*, 2nd edn, Wiley-Blackwell, Oxford.

For images of malaria and other parasites see www.med.cmu.ac.th/dept/parasite/default.htm (Chiang Mai University, Thailand) and then click on 'Image' or 'parasite web link' (both useful) or www.dpd.cdc.gov/dpdx/HTML/Image_Library.htm (Centers of Disease Control and Prevention, USA)

Tropical Health Technology, Doddington, Cambridgeshire, www.tht.ndirect.co.uk (low-cost books and bench aids for developing countries)

Learning Bench Aid No 1. Malaria

Learning Bench Aid No 2. African and S. American Trypanosomiasis – Leishmaniasis

Learning Bench Aid No 3. Microscopical Diagnosis of Lymphatic Filariasis, Loiasis, Onchocerciasis.

Learning Bench Aid No 7. Blood: Normal cells – Anaemias – Infections – Leukaemias

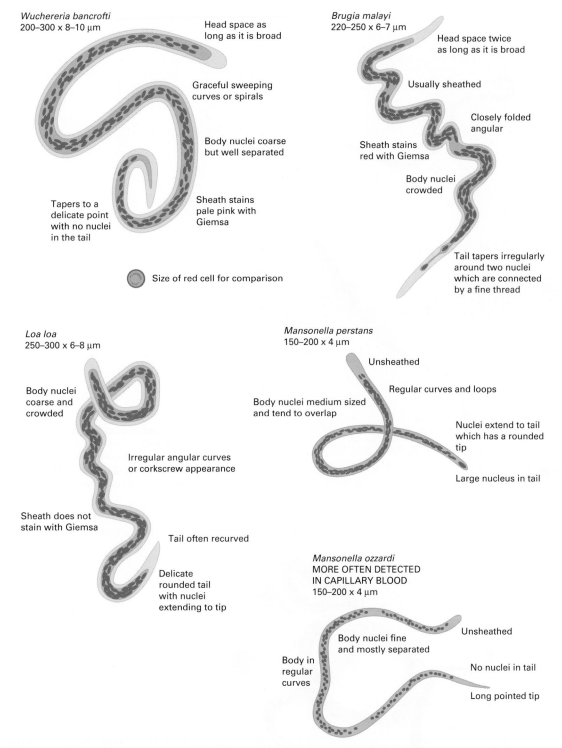

Wuchereria bancrofti
200–300 x 8–10 μm

Head space as long as it is broad

Graceful sweeping curves or spirals

Body nuclei coarse but well separated

Tapers to a delicate point with no nuclei in the tail

Sheath stains pale pink with Giemsa

Size of red cell for comparison

Brugia malayi
220–250 x 6–7 μm

Head space twice as long as it is broad

Usually sheathed

Closely folded angular

Sheath stains red with Giemsa

Body nuclei crowded

Tail tapers irregularly around two nuclei which are connected by a fine thread

Loa loa
250–300 x 6–8 μm

Body nuclei coarse and crowded

Irregular angular curves or corkscrew appearance

Sheath does not stain with Giemsa

Tail often recurved

Delicate rounded tail with nuclei extending to tip

Mansonella perstans
150–200 x 4 μm

Unsheathed

Regular curves and loops

Body nuclei medium sized and tend to overlap

Nuclei extend to tail which has a rounded tip

Large nucleus in tail

Mansonella ozzardi
MORE OFTEN DETECTED IN CAPILLARY BLOOD
150–200 x 4 μm

Body nuclei fine and mostly separated

Unsheathed

No nuclei in tail

Body in regular curves

Long pointed tip

Fig. 3.198 Morphological features that are useful in distinguishing between the microfilariae of different species of filaria.

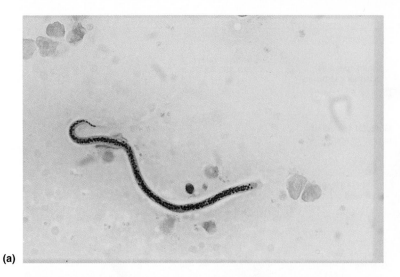

(a)

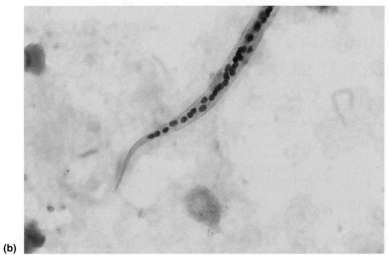

(b)

Fig. 3.199 Microfilariae of *Wuchereria bancrofti* in thick films: (a) microfilaria showing the negative impression of the sheath (× 40 objective); (b) tail of a microfilaria showing that the nuclei do not extend into the tail.

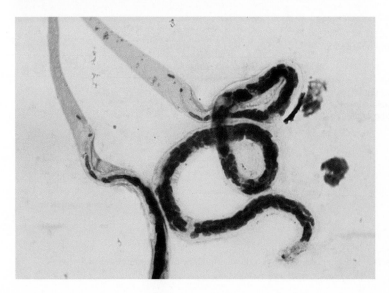

Fig. 3.200 Microfilariae of *Brugia malayi* in thick film showing the widely separated tail nuclei. By courtesy of Dr Saad Abdalla, London.

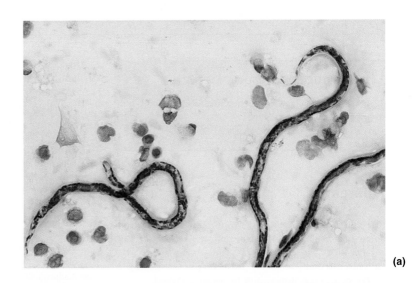

(a)

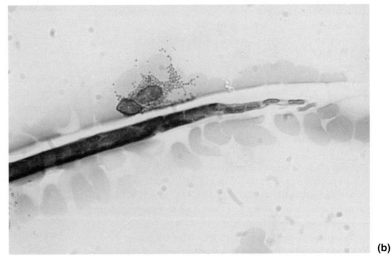

Fig. 3.201 Microfilariae of *Loa loa*: (a) a thick film showing the head and tail of microfilariae – nuclei extend to the tail (× 40 objective); (b) the tail of a microfilaria in a thin film showing the negative impression of the sheath – the nuclei extend to the tail.

(b)

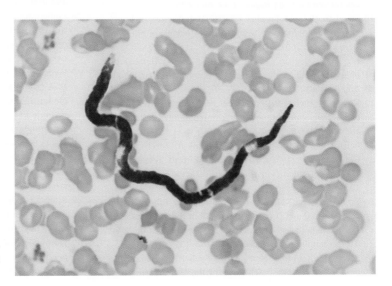

Fig. 3.202 Microfilaria of *Mansonella perstans* in a thin film. By courtesy of Dr Saad Abdalla.

References

1 Le Coz C and Goosens A (1998) Contact dermatitis from an immersion oil for microscopy. *N Engl J Med*, **339**, 406–407.

2 Nguyen D and Diamond L (2000) *Diagnostic Hematology: a Pattern Approach*. Butterworth-Heinemann, Oxford.

3 Bain BJ and Liesner R (1996) Pseudopyropoikilocytosis: a striking artefact. *J Clin Pathol*, **49**, 772–773.

4 Anonymous (2009) Chemical-associated artifacts. *Blood*, **113**, 4487.

5 Shirato K, Reid C, Ibbetson JS, Hissaria P and Shireen S (2009) Diagnosis of type I cryoglobulinaemia made through identifying crystals in the blood smear. *Australas J Dermatol*, **50**, 281–284.

6 Zaini WSM, Hamour S, Swamy R and Kumar P (2013) Type 1 cryoglobulinaemia with precipitated crystals. *Br J Haematol*, **161**, 301.

7 Nosanchuk J, Terzian J and Posso M (1987) Circulating mucopolysaccharide (mucin) in two adults with metastatic adenocarcinoma. *Arch Pathol Lab Med*, **111**, 545–548.

8 Hoffbrand AV and Pettit JE (1988) *Sandoz Atlas of Clinical Haematology*. Gower, London.

9 Mohandas N and Gascard P (2000) What do mouse gene knockouts tell us about the structure and function of the red cell membrane? *Clin Haematol*, **12**, 605–620.

10 Sheehan RG and Frenkel EP (1983) Influence of hemoglobin phenotype on the mean erythrocyte volume. *Acta Haematol*, **69**, 260–265.

11 Maggio A, Gagliano F and Siciliano S (1984) Hemoglobin phenotype and mean erythrocyte volume in Sicilian people. *Acta Haematol*, **71**, 214.

12 Kaplan E, Zuelzer WW and Neel JV (1953) Further studies on haemoglobin C alone and in combination with sickle cell anemia. *Blood*, **8**, 735–746.

13 Fairbanks VF, Gilchrist GS, Brimhall B, Jereb JA and Goldston EC (1979) Hemoglobin E trait reexamined: a cause of microcytosis and erythrocytosis. *Blood*, **53**, 109–115.

14 Bird AR, Wood K, Leisegang F, Mathew CG, Ellis P, Hartley PS and Karabus CD (1984) Hemoglobin E variants: a clinical, haematological and biosynthetic study of four South African families. *Acta Haematol*, **72**, 135–137.

15 Stavem P, Romslo I, Hovig T, Rootwelt K and Emblem R (1985) Ferrochelatase deficiency of the bone marrow in a syndrome of congenital microcytic anaemia with iron overload of the liver and hyperferraemia. *Scand J Haematol*, **34**, 204–206.

16 Horina JH and Wolf P (2000) Epoetin for severe anemia in hepatoerythropoietic porphyria. *N Engl J Med*, **342**, 1294–1295.

17 Shahidi NT, Nathan DE and Diamond LK (1945) Iron deficiency anemia associated with an error of iron metabolism. *J Clin Invest*, **43**, 510–521.

18 Cooley TB (1945) A severe form of hereditary anemia with elliptocytosis: interesting sequence of splenectomy. *Am J Med Sci*, **209**, 561–568.

19 Hartman KR and Barker JA (1996) Microcytic anemia with iron malabsorption: an inherited disorder of iron metabolism. *Am J Hematol*, **51**, 269–275.

20 Andrews NC (1998) Disorders of iron metabolism. *N Engl J Med*, **341**, 1986–1995.

21 Miyoshi I, Saito T and Iwahara Y (2004) Copper deficiency anaemia. *Br J Haematol*, **125**, 106.

22 Yachie A, Niida Y, Toma T, Shimura S, Ohta K, Fujimoto K *et al.* (2000) What did we learn from the first case of human heme oxygenase deficiency? *Acta Haematol*, **103**, Suppl. 1, 82.

23 Priwitzerova M, Pospisilova D, Prchal JT, Hlobilkova A, Mihal V, Indrak K *et al.* (2003) The first human mutation of DMT1 (Nramp2) causes severe defect of erythropoiesis that can be rescued in vitro by Fe-SIH. *Blood*, **102**, 156a.

24 Iolascon A, d'Apolito M, Servedio V, Cimmino F, Piga A and Camaschella C (2006) Microcytic anemia and hepatic iron overload in a child with compound heterozygous mutations in *DMT1 (SCL11A2)*. *Blood*, **107**, 349–354.

25 Camaschella C, Campanella A, De Falco L, Boschetto L, Merlini R, Silvestri L *et al.* (2007) The human counterpart of zebrafish *shiraz* shows sideroblastic-like microcytic anemia and iron overload. *Blood*, **110**, 1353–1358.

26 Finberg KE, Heeney MM, Campagna DR, Aydinok Y, Pearson HA, Hartman KR *et al.* (2008) Mutations in TMPRSS6 cause iron-refractory iron deficiency anemia (IRIDA). *Nat Genet*, **40**, 569–571.

27 Ferguson PJ, Chen S, Tayeh MK, Ochoa L, Leal SM, Pelet A *et al.* (2005) Homozygous mutations in *LPIN2* are responsible for the syndrome of chronic recurrent multifocal osteomyelitis and congenital dyserythropoietic anaemia (Majeed syndrome). *J Med Genet*, **42**, 551–557.

28 Tulliez M, Testa U, Rochant H, Henri A, Vainchenker W, Toubol J *et al.* (1982) Reticulocytosis, hypochromia, and microcytosis: an unusual presentation of the preleukemic syndrome. *Blood*, **59**, 293–299.

29 Ruocco L, Baldi A, Cecconi N, Marini A, Azzarà A, Ambrogi F and Grassi B (1986) Severe pancytopenia due to copper deficiency. *Acta Haematol*, **76**, 224–226.

30 Simon SR, Branda RF, Tindle BF and Burns SL (1988) Copper deficiency and sideroblastic anemia associated with zinc ingestion. *Am J Hematol*, **28**, 181–183.

31 Ramadurai J, Shapiro C, Kozloff M and Telfer M (1993) Zinc abuse and sideroblastic anemia. *Am J Hematol*, **42**, 227–228.

32 Kumar A and Jazieh AR (2001) Case report of sideroblastic anemia caused by ingestion of coins. *Am J Hematol*, **66**, 126–129.

33 Sampson B, Fagerhol MK, Sunderkötter C, Golden BE, Richmond P, Klein N *et al.* (2003) Hyperzincaemia with hypercalprotectinaemia: a new disorder of zinc metabolism. *Lancet*, **360**, 1742–1745.

34 How J, Davidson RJL and Bewsher PD (1979) Red cell changes in hyperthyroidism. *Scand J Haematol*, **23**, 323–328.

35 Ural AU (1997) Anemia related to ascorbic acid deficiency. *Am J Hematol*, **56**, 69.

36 Hillman RS and Finch CA (1985) *Red Cell Manual*, 5th edn. FA Davis, Philadelphia.

37 Larrick JW and Hyman ES (1984) Acquired iron deficiency anemia caused by an antibody against the transferrin receptor. *N Engl J Med*, **311**, 214–218.

38 Cauchi MN and Smith MB (1981) Quantitative aspects of red cell size variation during pregnancy. *Clin Lab Haematol*, **4**, 149–154.

39 Helman N and Rubenstein LS (1975) The effects of age, sex, and smoking on erythrocytes and leukocytes. *Am J Clin Pathol*, **63**, 35–44.

40 Sallah S, Hanrahan LR and Phillips DL (1999) Intrathecal methotrexate–induced megaloblastic anemia in patients with acute leukemia. *Arch Pathol Lab Med*, **123**, 774–777.

41 Au WY, Tsang J, Cheng TS, Chow WS, Woo YC, Ma SK and Tam S (2003) Cough mixture abuse as a novel cause of megaloblastic anaemia and peripheral neuropathy. *Br J Haematol*, **123**, 956–957.

42 Billemont B, Izzedine H and Rixe O (2007) Macrocytosis due to treatment with sunitinib. *N Engl J Med*, **357**, 1351–1352.

43 Gillessen S, Graf L, Korte W and Cerny T (2007) Macrocytosis and cobalamin deficiency in patients treated with sunitinib. *N Engl J Med*, **356**, 2330–2331.

44 Horstman AL, Serk SL and Go RS (2005) Macrocytosis associated with monoclonal gammopathy. *Eur J Haematol*, **75**, 146–149.

45 Porter KG, McMaster D, Elmes ME and Love AHG (1977) Anaemia and low serum copper during zinc therapy. *Lancet*, **ii**, 774.

46 Heaven R, Duncan M and Vukelja SJ (1994) Arsenic intoxication presenting with macrocytosis and peripheral neuropathy, without anaemia. *Acta Haematol*, **92**, 142–143.

47 Sechi LA, De Carli S, Catena C, Zingaro L and Bartoli E (1996) Benign familial macrocytosis. *Clin Lab Haematol*, **18**, 41–43.

48 Willig T-N, Draptchinskaia N, Dianzani I, Ball S, Niemeyer C, Ramenghi U *et al.* (1999) Mutations in ribosomal protein S19 gene and Diamond–Blackfan anemia: wide variations in phenotypic expression. *Blood*, **94**, 4294–4306.

49 Tuckfield A, Ratnaike S, Hussein S and Metz J (1997) A novel form of hereditary sideroblastic anaemia with macrocytosis. *Br J Haematol*, **97**, 279–285.

50 Mehler PS and Howe SE (1995) Serous fat atrophy with leukopenia in severe anorexia nervosa. *Am J Hematol*, **49**, 171–172.

51 Barton JC, Bertoli LF and Rothenberg BE (2000) Peripheral blood erythrocyte parameters in hemochromatosis: evidence for increased erythrocyte hemoglobin content. *J Lab Clin Med*, **135**, 96–104.

52 Papakonstantinou G, Loeffler H, Haferlach T and Brugger W (2010) Severe idiopathic erythroblastic synartesis: successful treatment with the anti-CD20 monoclonal antibody rituximab. *Eur J Haematol*, **84**, 547–549.

53 Sipes SL, Weiner CP, Wenstrom KD, Williamson RA and Grant SS (1991) The association between fetal karyotype and mean corpuscular volume. *Am J Obstet Gynecol*, **165**, 1371–1376.

54 Eastham RD and Jancar J (1970) Macrocytosis in Down's syndrome and during long term anticonvulsant therapy. *J Clin Pathol*, **23**, 296–298.

55 Pai GS, Grush OC and Shuman C (1982) Hematological abnormalities in triploidy. *Am J Dis Child*, **136**, 367–369.

56 Bader-Meunier B, Rieux-Laucat F, Croisille L, Yvart J, Mielot F, Dommergues JP *et al.* (2000) Dyserythropoiesis associated with a fas-deficient condition in childhood. *Br J Haematol*, **108**, 300–304.

57 Li J, Yang C, Xia Y, Bertino A, Glaspy J, Roberts M and Kuter DJ (2001) Thrombocytopenia caused by the development of antibodies to thrombopoietin. *Blood*, **98**, 3241–3248.

58 Stewart GW and Turner EJH (2000) The hereditary stomatocytoses and allied disorders of erythrocyte membrane permeability to Na and K. *Baillière's Clin Haematol*, **12**, 707–727.

59 Rees MI, Worwood M, Thompson PW, Gilbertson C and May A (1994) Red cell dimorphism in a young man with a constitutional chromosomal translocation t(11;22) (p15.5;q11.21). *Br J Haematol*, **87**, 386–395.

60 Perrotta AL and Finch CA (1972) The polychromatophilic erythrocyte. *Am J Clin Pathol*, **57**, 471–477.

61 Escobar MC, Rappaport ES, Tipton P, Balentine P and Riggs MW (2002) Reticulocyte estimate from peripheral blood smear: a simple, fast, and economical method for evaluation of anemia. *Lab Med*, **33**, 703–705.

62 Rowles PM and Williams ES (1983) Abnormal red cell morphology in venous blood of men climbing at high altitude. *BMJ*, **286**, 1396.

63 Franco M, Collec E, Connes P, van den Akker E, Billette de Villemeur T, Belmatoug N *et al.* (2013) Abnormal properties of red blood cells suggest a role in the pathophysiology of Gaucher disease. *Blood*, **121**, 546–555.

64 Bessis M (1973) *Living Blood Cells and Their Ultrastructure*, trans. Weed RI. Springer-Verlag, Berlin.

65 Wolf PL and Koett J (1980) Hemolytic anemia in hepatic disease with decreased erythrocyte adenosine triphosphate. *Am J Clin Pathol*, **73**, 785–788.

66 Shilo S, Werner D and Hershko C (1985) Acute hemolytic anemia caused by severe hypophosphatemia in diabetic ketoacidosis. *Acta Haematol*, **73**, 55–57.

67 Polizzotto MN, Shortt J, Opat SS and Cole-Sinclair MF (2008) A drop of vitriol: microspherocytosis following sulphuric acid exposure. *Br J Haematol*, **140**, 596.

68 McGrath KM, Zalcberg JR, Slonin J and Wiley JS (1982) Intralipid induced haemolysis. *Br J Haematol*, **50**, 376–378.

69 Bianchi P, Fermo E, Alfinito F, Vercellati C, Baserga M, Ferraro F *et al.* (2003) Molecular characterization of six unrelated Italian patients affected by pyrimidine 5′-nucleotidase deficiency. *Br J Haematol*, **122**, 847–851.

70 Austin RF and Desforges JF (1969) Hereditary elliptocytosis: an unusual presentation of hemolysis in the newborn associated with transient morphologic abnormalities. *Pediatrics*, **44**, 196–200.

71 Melvin JD and Watts RG (2002) Severe hypophosphatemia: a rare cause of intravascular hemolysis. *Am J Hematol*, **69**, 223–224.

72 Chan TK, Chan WC and Weed RI (1982) Erythrocyte hemighosts: a hallmark of severe oxidative injury *in vivo*. *Br J Haematol*, **50**, 573–582.

73 Bain BJ (1999) Images in haematology: Heinz body haemolytic anaemia in Wilson's disease. *Br J Haematol*, **104**, 647.

74 Wickramasinghe SN (1998) Congenital dyserythropoietic anaemias: clinical features, haematological morphology and new biochemical data. *Blood Rev*, **12**, 178–200.

75 Nurse GT, Coetzer TL and Palek J (1992) The elliptocytoses, ovalocytoses and related disorders. *Baillière's Clin Haematol*, **5**, 187–207.

76 Hur M, Lee KM, Cho HC, Park YI, Kim SH, Chang YM *et al.* (2004) Protein 4.1 deficiency and deletion of chromosome 20q are associated with acquired elliptocytosis in myelodysplastic syndrome. *Clin Lab Haematol*, **26**, 69–72.

77 Patel SS, Mehlotra RK, Kastens W, Mgone CS, Kazura JW and Zimmerman PA (2001) The association of the glycophorin C exon 3 deletion with ovalocytosis and malaria susceptibility in the Wosera, Papua New Guinea. *Blood*, **98**, 3489–3491.

78 Khositseth S, Sirikanaerat A, Khoprasert S, Opastirakul S, Kingwatanakul P, Thongnoppakhum W and Yenchitsomasus PT (2008) Hematological abnormalities in patients with distal renal tubular acidosis and hemoglobinopathies. *Am J Hematol*, **83**, 465–471.

79 Farolino DL, Rustagi PK, Currie MS, Doeblin TD and Logue GL (1986) Teardrop-shaped cells in autoimmune hemolytic anemia. *Am J Hematol*, **21**, 415–418.

80 Domingo-Claros A, Larriba I, Rozman M, Irriguible D, Vallespi T, Aventin A *et al.* (2002) Acute erythroid neoplastic proliferations. A biological study based on 62 patients. *Haematologica*, **87**, 148–153.

81 Miwa S, Fujii H, Tani K, Takahashi K, Takegawa S, Fujinami N *et al.* (1981) Two cases of red cell aldolase deficiency associated with hereditary hemolytic anemia in a Japanese family. *Am J Hematol*, **11**, 425–437.

82 Carlyle RF, Nichols G and Rowles PM (1979) Abnormal red cells in blood of men subjected to simulated dives. *Lancet*, **i**, 1114–1116.

83 Altomare I, Desman G and Aledort LM (2006) Echinocytosis – an unusual manifestation of hemangioma. *Am J Hematol*, **81**, 532–534.

84 Feo CT, Tchernia G, Subtil E and Leblond PF (1978) Observations of echinocytosis in eight patients: a phase contrast and SEM study. *Br J Haematol*, **40**, 519–526.

85 Roberts I (2011) Personal communication.

86 Weber YG, Storch A, Wuttke TV, Brockmann K, Kempfle J, Maljevic S *et al.* (2008) GLUT1 mutations are a cause of paroxysmal exertion-induced dyskinesias and induce hemolytic anemia by a cation leak. *J Clin Invest*, **118**, 2157–2168.

87 Kho AN, Hui S, Kesterson JG and McDonald CJ (2007) Which observations from the complete blood cell count predict mortality for hospitalized patients? *J Hosp Med*, **2**, 5–12.

88 Bain BJ and Bain PG (2013) Choreo-acanthocytosis. *Am J Hematol*, **88**, 712.

89 Higgins JJ, Patterson MC, Papadopoulos NM, Brady RO, Pentchev PG and Barton NW (1992) Hypoprebetalipoproteinemia, acanthocytosis, retinitis pigmentosa, and pallidal degeneration (HARP syndrome). *Neurology*, **42**, 194–198.

90 Udden MM, Umeda M, Hirano Y and Marcus DM (1987) New abnormalities in the morphology, cell surface receptors, and electrolyte metabolism of In(Lu) erythrocytes. *Blood*, **69**, 52–57.

91 Bruce LJ, Kay MM, Lawrence C and Tanner MJ (1993) Band 3HT, a human red-cell variant associated with acanthocytosis and increased anion transport carries the mutation Pro-868–Leu in the membrane domain of band 3. *Biochem J*, **293**, 317–320.

92 Fawaz NA, Beshlawi IO, Al Zadjali S, Al Ghaithi HK, Elnaggari MA, Elnour I *et al.* (2012) dRTA and hemolytic anemia: first detailed description of *SLC4A1* A858D mutation in homozygous state. *Eur J Haematol*, **88**, 350–355.

93 Sinha R, Agarwal I, Bawazir WM and Bruce LJ (2013) Renal tubular acidosis with hereditary spherocytosis. *Indian Pediatr*, **50**, 693-695.

94 Lainey E, Ogier H and Fenneteau O (2008) Vacuolation of neutrophils and acanthocytosis in a child with medium chain acyl-CoA dehydrogenase deficiency. *Br J Haematol*, **140**, 595.

95 Yawata Y, Kanzaki A, Yawata A, Kaku M, Takezono M, Sugihara T *et al.* (1997) Hereditary xerocytosis is a phenotypically different entity from hereditary high red cell membrane phosphatidyl choline hemolytic anemia. *Blood*, **90**, Suppl. 1, 5a.

96 Doll DC, Lest AF, Dayhoff DA, Loy TS, Ringenberg QS and Yarbro JW (1989) Acanthocytosis associated with myelodysplasia. *J Clin Oncol*, **7**, 1569–1572.

97 Freson K, Devriendt K, Matthijs G, Van Hoof A, De Vos R, Thys C *et al.* (2001) Platelet characteristics in patients with X-linked macrothrombocytopenia because of a novel *GATA1* mutation. *Blood*, **98**, 85–92.

98 Lesesve JF, Perrin J, Georges A and Morali A (2009) Acanthocytosis in Anderson's disease. *Br J Haematol*, **145**, 1.

99 Palek J and Jarolim P (1993) Clinical expression and laboratory detection of red blood cell membrane protein mutations. *Semin Hematol*, **30**, 249–283.

100 Bassen FA and Kornzweig AL (1950) Malformation of the erythrocytes in a case of atypical retinitis pigmentosa. *Blood*, **5**, 381–387.

101 Estes JW, Morley TJ, Levine IM and Emerson CF (1967) A new hereditary acanthocytosis syndrome. *Am J Med*, **42**, 868–881.

102 Sakai T, Mawatari S, Iwashita H, Goto I and Kuroiwa Y (1981)Choreoacanthocytosis. *Arch Neurol*, **38**, 335.

103 Chowdhury F, Saward R and Erber W (2005) Neuroacanthocytosis. *Br J Haematol*, **131**, 285.

104 Rampoldi L, Dobson-Stone C, Rubio JP, Danek A, Chalmers RM, Wood NW *et al.* (2001) A conserved sorting-associated protein is mutant in chorea-acanthocytosis. *Nat Genet*, **28**, 119–120.

105 Walker RH, Rasmussen A, Rudnicki D, Holmes SE, Alonso E, Matsuura T *et al.* (2003) Huntington's disease-like 2 can present as chorea-acanthocytosis. *Neurology*, **61**, 1002–1004.

106 Udden MM, Umeda M, Hirano Y and Marcus DM (1987) New abnormalities in the morphology, cell surface receptors and electrolyte balance in In(lu) erythrocytes. *Blood*, **69**, 52–57.

107 Amare M, Lawson B and Larsen WE (1972) Active extrusion of Heinz bodies in drug-induced haemolytic anaemia. *Br J Haematol*, **23**, 215–219.

108 Harrington AM, Ward PCJ and Kroft SH (2008) Iron deficiency anemia, β-thalassemia minor, and anemia of chronic disease. *Am J Clin Pathol*, **129**, 466–471.

109 Zini G, d'Onofrio G, Briggs C, Erber W, Jou JM, Lee SH *et al.*; International Council for Standardization in Haematology (ICSH) (2012) ICSH recommendations for identification, diagnostic value, and quantitation of schistocytes. *Int J Lab Hematol*, **34**, 107–116.

110 Ward PC, Smith CM and White JG (1979) Erythrocytic ecdysis. An unusual morphologic finding in a case of sickle cell anemia with intercurrent cold-agglutinin syndrome. *Am J Clin Pathol*, **72**, 479–485.

111 Samson RE, Abdalla DH and Bain BJ (1998) Teaching cases from the Royal Marsden and St Mary's Hospitals. Case 18. Severe anaemia and thrombocytopenia with red cell fragmentation. *Leuk Lymphoma*, **31**, 433–435.

112 Crook M, Williams A and Schey S (1998) Target cells and stomatocytes in heterozygous familial hypobetalipoproteinaemia. *Eur J Haematol*, **60**, 68–69.

113 McGrath KM, Collecutt MF, Gordon A, Sawers RJ and Faragher BS (1984) Dehydrated hereditary stomatocytosis – a report of two families and a review of the literature. *Pathology*, **16**, 146–150.

114 Reinhardt WH, Gössi U, Bütikofer P, Ott P, Sigrist H, Schatzmann H-J *et al.* (1989) Haemolytic anaemia in analpha-lipoproteinaemia (Tangier disease): morphological, biochemical, and biophysical properties of the red blood cell. *Br J Haematol*, **72**, 272–277.

115 Godin DV, Garnett ME, Hoag G, Wadsworth LD and Frohlich J (1988) Erythrocyte abnormalities in hypoalphalipoproteinemia syndrome resembling fish eye disease. *Eur J Haematol*, **41**, 176–181.

116 Clayton PT, Bowron A, Mills KA, Massoud A, Casteels M and Milla PJ (1993) Phytosterolaemia in children with parenteral nutrition-associated cholestatic liver disease. *Gastroenterology*, **105**, 1806–1813.

117 Exner M and Schwarzinger I (2001) Targeting the dust. *Br J Haematol*, **114**, 739.

118 Lesesve JF, Garçon L and Lecompte T (2010) Transient red-blood-cell morphological anomalies after acute liver dysfunction. *Eur J Haematol*, **84**, 92–93.

119 Miller DR, Rickles FR, Lichtman MA, La Celle PL, Bates J and Weed R (1971) A new variant of hereditary hemolytic anemia with stomatocytosis and erythrocyte cation abnormality. *Blood*, **38**, 184–204.

120 Davidson RJ, How J and Lessels S (1977) Acquired stomatocytosis: its prevalence and significance in routine haematology. *Scand J Haematol*, **19**, 47–53.

121 Wislöff F and Boman D (1979) Acquired stomatocytosis in alcoholic liver disease. *Scand J Haematol*, **23**, 43–50.

122 Mallory DM, Rosenfield RE, Wong KY, Heller C, Rubinstein P, Allen FH *et al.* (1976) Rh_{mod}, a second kindred (Craig). *Vox Sang*, **30**, 430–440.

123 Gallagher PG and Lux SE (2003) Disorders of the erythrocyte membrane. In: Nathan DG, Orkin SH, Ginsburg D and Look AT, *Nathan and Oski's Hematology of Infancy and Childhood*, 6th edn. Saunders, Philadelphia.

124 von Behrens WE (1975) Splenomegaly, macrothrombocytopenia and stomatocytosis in healthy Mediterranean subjects. *Scand J Haematol*, **14**, 258–267.

125 Rees DC, Iolascon A, Carella M, O'Marcaigh AS, Kendra JR, Jowitt SN *et al.* (2005) Stomatocytic haemolysis and macrothrombocytopenia (Mediterranean stomatocytosis/macrothrombocytopenia) is the haematological presentation of phytosterolaemia. *Br J Haematol*, **130**, 297–309.

126 Mowafy N (2005) Hematomorphology. *Hematology*, **10**, Suppl. 1, 182–185.

127 Corazza GR, Ginaldi L, Zoli G, Frisoni M, Lalli G, Gasbarrini G and Quaglino D (1990) Howell–Jolly body counting as a measure of splenic function. A reassessment. *Clin Lab Haematol*, **12**, 269–275.

128 Valentine WN (1979) Hemolytic anemia and inborn errors of metabolism. *Blood*, **54**, 549–559.

129 Paglia DE, Valentine WN, Nakatani M and Rauth BJ (1983) Selective accumulation of cytosol CDP-choline as an isolated erythrocyte defect in chronic hemolysis. *Proc Natl Acad Sci USA*, **80**, 3081-3085.

130 Hapgood G and Roy S (2013) A mysterious case of Dr Cabot. *Br J Haematol*, **162**, 719.

131 Merino A, To-Figueras J and Herrero C (2006) Atypical red cell inclusions in congenital erythropoietic porphyria. *Br J Haematol*, **132**, 124.

132 Green DW, Hendon B and Mimouni FR (1995) Nucleated erythrocytes and intraventricular hemorrhage in preterm neonates. *Pediatrics*, **96**, 475–478.

133 Stachon A, Segbers E, Holland-Letz T, Kempf R, Hering S and Krieg M (2007) Nucleated red blood cells in the blood of medical intensive care patients indicate increased mortality risk: a prospective cohort study. *Crit Care*, **11**, R62.

134 Eichner ER (1984) Erythroid karyorrhexis in the peripheral blood smear in severe arsenic poisoning: a comparison with lead poisoning. *Am J Clin Pathol*, **81**, 533–537.

135 Pettit JE, Scott J and Hussein S (1976) EDTA dependent red cell neutrophil rosetting in autoimmune haemolytic anaemia. *J Clin Pathol*, **29**, 345–346.

136 Gregory GP, Opat S, Quach H, Shortt J and Tran H (2011) Failure of eculizumab to correct paroxysmal cold hemoglobinuria. *Ann Hematol*, **90**, 989–990.

137 Mathy KA and Koepke JA (1974) The clinical usefulness of segmented vs. stab neutrophil criteria for differential leukocyte counts. *Am J Clin Pathol*, **61**, 947–958.

138 Akenzua GI, Hui YT, Milner R and Zipursky A (1974) Neutrophil and band counts in the diagnosis of neonatal infections. *Pediatrics*, **54**, 38–42.

139 Christensen RD and Rothstein G (1978) Pitfalls in the interpretation of leukocyte counts of newborn infants. *Am J Clin Pathol*, **72**, 608–611.

140 Christensen RD, Rothstein G, Anstall HB and Bybee B (1981) Granulocyte transfusions in neonates with bacterial infection, neutropenia, and depletion of mature bone marrow neutrophils. *Pediatrics*, **70**, 1–6.

141 Alvarado A (1986) A practical score for the early diagnosis of acute appendicitis. *Ann Emerg Med*, **15**, 557–564.

142 Chanarin I (1979) *Megaloblastic Anaemias*, 2nd edn. CV Mosby, St Louis.

143 Edwin E (1967) The segmentation of polymorphonuclear neutrophils. *Acta Med Scand*, **182**, 401–410.

144 Westerman DA, Evans D and Metz J (1999) Neutrophil hypersegmentation in iron deficiency anaemia: a case-control study. *Br J Haematol*, **107**, 512–515.

145 Kerrigan DP, Castillo A, Foucar K, Townsend K and Neidhart J (1989) Peripheral blood morphologic changes after high-dose antineoplastic chemotherapy and recombinant human granulocyte colony-stimulating factor administration. *Am J Clin Pathol*, **92**, 280–285.

146 Wickramasinghe SN (1999) The wide spectrum and unresolved issues of megaloblastic anemia. *Semin Hematol*, **36**, 3–18.

147 Davidson WM (1968) Inherited variations in leukocytes. *Semin Haematol*, **5**, 255–274.

148 Hess U, Ganser A, Schnürch H-G, Seipelt G, Ottman OG, Falk S *et al.* (1992) Myelokathexis treated with recombinant human granulocyte-macrophage colony-stimulating factor (rhGM-CSF). *Br J Haematol*, **80**, 254–256.

149 Gorlin RJ, Gelb B, Diaz GA, Lofsness KG, Pittelkow MR and Fenyk JR (2000) WHIM syndrome, an autosomal dominant disorder: clinical, hematological, and molecular studies. *Am J Med Genet*, **91**, 368–376.

150 Davidson WM and Smith DR (1954) A morphological sex difference in the polymorphonuclear neutrophil leucocytes. *BMJ*, **ii**, 6–7.

151 Murthy MSN and von Emmerich H (1958) The occurrence of the sex chromatin in white blood cells of young adults. *Am J Clin Pathol*, **30**, 216–227.

152 Davidson WM, Fowler JF and Smith DR (1958) Sexing the neutrophil leucocytes in natural and artificial chimaeras. *Br J Haematol*, **4**, 231–238.

153 Mittwoch U (1963) The incidence of drumsticks in patients with three X chromosomes. *Cytogenetics*, **2**, 24–33.

154 Pai GS, Grush OC and Shuman C (1982) Hematological abnormalities in triploidy. *Am J Dis Child*, **136**, 367–369.

155 Tomonaga M, Matsuura G, Watanabe B, Kamochi Y and Ozono N (1961) Leukocyte drumsticks in chronic granulocytic leukaemia and related disorders. *Blood*, **18**, 581–590.

156 Archer RK, Engisch HJC, Gaha T and Ruxton J (1971) The eosinophil leucocyte in the blood and bone marrow of patients with Down's anomaly. *Br J Haematol*, **21**, 271–276.

157 Goasguen JE, Bennett JM, Bain BJ, Brunning R, Vallespi MT, Tomonaga M *et al.*; International Working Group on Morphology of MDS (IWGM-MDS) (2014) Proposal for refining the definition of dysgranulopoiesis in acute myeloid leukemia and myelodysplastic syndromes. *Leuk Res*, **38**, 447–453.

158 Huehns ER, Lutzner M and Hecht F (1964) Nuclear abnormalities of the neutrophils in $D_1(13–15)$-trisomy syndrome. *Lancet*, **i**, 589–590.

159 Salama ME, Shah V, Lebel RR and VanDyke DL (2004) Aberrant nuclear projections of neutrophils in Trisomy 13. *Arch Pathol Lab Med*, **128**, 243–244.

160 Davey FR, Erber WN, Gatter KC and Mason DY (1988) Abnormal neutrophil morphology in acute myeloid

leukaemia and myelodysplastic syndrome. *Hum Pathol*, **19**, 454–459.

161 Strauss RG, Bove KE, Jones JF, Mauer AM and Fulginiti VA (1974) An anomaly of neutrophil morphology with impaired function. *N Engl J Med*, **290**, 478–484.

162 Vilboux T, Lev A, Malicdan MC, Simon AJ, Järvinen P, Racek T *et al.* (2013) A congenital neutrophil defect syndrome associated with mutations in VPS45. *N Engl J Med*, **369**, 54–65.

163 Plum CM, Warburg M and Danielsen J (1978) Defective maturation of granulocytes, retinal cysts and multiple skeletal malformations in a mentally retarded girl. *Acta Haematol*, **59**, 53–63.

164 Banerjee R, Halil O, Bain BJ, Cummins D and Banner N (2001) Neutrophil dysplasia caused by mycophenolate mofetil. *Transplantation*, **77**, 1608–1610.

165 Girolami A, Fabris F, Caronato A and Randi ML (1980) Increased numbers of pseudodrumsticks in neutrophils and large platelets. A 'new' congenital leukocyte and platelet morphological abnormality. *Acta Haematol*, **64**, 324–330.

166 Moore CM and Weinger RS (1980) Pseudo-drumsticks in granulocytes of a male with a Yqh+ polymorphism. *Am J Hematol*, **8**, 411–414.

167 Gibson BES (1991) Inherited disorders. In: Hann IM, Gibson BES and Letsky EA, eds. *Fetal and Neonatal Haematology*. Baillière Tindall, London.

168 Seman G (1959) Sur une anomalie constitutionnelle héréditaire du noyau des polynucléaires neutrophiles. *Rev Hématol*, **14**, 409–412.

169 Langenhuijsen MMAC (1984) Neutrophils with ring shaped nuclei in myeloproliferative disorders. *Br J Haematol*, **58**, 227–230.

170 Stavem P, Hjort PF, Vogt E and Van der Hagen CB (1969) Ring-shaped nuclei of granulocytes in a patient with acute erythroleukaemia. *Scand J Haematol*, **6**, 31–32.

171 Kabob T, Saigo K and Yamagishi M (1986) Neutrophils with ring-shaped nuclei in chronic neutrophilic leukaemia. *Am J Clin Pathol*, **86**, 748–751.

172 Craig A (1988) Ring neutrophils in megaloblastic anaemia. *Br J Haematol*, **67**, 247–248.

173 Hernandez JA, Aldred SW, Bruce JR, Vanatta PR, Mattingly TL and Sheehan WW (1980) 'Botryoid' nuclei in neutrophils of patients with heat stroke. *Lancet*, **ii**, 642–643.

174 Neftel KA and Müller OM (1981) Heat-induced radial segmentation of leucocyte nuclei: a non-specific phenomenon accompanying inflammatory and necrotizing diseases. *Br J Haematol*, **48**, 377–382.

175 Gustke SS, Becker GA, Garancis JC, Geimer NF and Pisciotta AV (1970) Chromatin clumping in mature leukocytes: a hitherto unrecognized abnormality. *Blood*, **35**, 637–658.

176 Ozanne C, Bain B and Catovsky D (1996) Teaching cases from the Royal Marsden and St Mary's Hospitals. Case 11: Dysplastic neutrophils in an African woman. *Leuk Lymphoma*, **18**, 351–352.

177 Bain BJ (1989) *Blood Cells: a Practical Guide*. Gower Medical Publishing, London.

178 Brunning RD (1970) Morphologic alterations in nucleated blood and marrow cells in genetic disorders. *Hum Pathol*, **1**, 99–124.

179 Skendzel LP and Hoffman GC (1962) The Pelger anomaly of leukocytes: forty cases in seven families. *Am J Clin Pathol*, **37**, 294–301.

180 Hoffmann K, Dreger CK, Olins AL, Olins DE, Shultz LD, Lucke B *et al.* (2002) Mutations in the gene encoding the lamin B receptor produce an altered nuclear morphology in granulocytes (Pelger–Huët anomaly). *Nat Genet*, **31**, 410-414.

181 Klein A, Hussar AE and Bornstein S (1955) Pelger–Huët anomaly of leukocytes. *N Engl J Med*, **253**, 1057–1062.

182 Erice JG, Pérez JM and Pericás FS (1999) Homozygous form of the Pelger–Huet anomaly. *Haematologica*, **84**, 748.

183 Ardeman S, Chanarin I and Frankland AW (1963) The Pelger–Huët anomaly and megaloblastic anemia. *Blood*, **22**, 472–476.

184 Parmley RT, Tzeng DY, Baehner R and Boxer LA (1983) Abnormal distribution of complex carbohydrates in neutrophils of a patient with lactoferrin deficiency. *Blood*, **62**, 538–548.

185 Deutsch PH and Mandell GL (1985) Reversible Pelger–Huët anomaly associated with ibuprofen therapy. *Arch Intern Med*, **145**, 166.

186 Juneja SK, Matthews JP, Luzinat R, Fan Y, Michael M, Rischin D *et al.* (1996) Association of acquired Pelger–Huët anomaly with taxoid therapy. *Br J Haematol*, **93**, 139–141.

187 May RB and Sunder TR (2005) Hematologic manifestations of long-term valproate therapy. *Epilepsia*, **34**, 1098–1101.

188 Chew E and Juneja S (2013) Botryoid white-cell nuclei. *N Engl J Med*, **368**, e22.

189 Schmitz LL, McClure JS, Letz CE, Dayton V, Weisdorf DJ, Parkin IL and Brunning RD (1994) Morphologic and quantitative changes in blood and marrow cells following growth factor therapy. *Am J Clin Pathol*, **101**, 67–75.

190 Dickinson M and Juneja S (2009) Haematological toxicity of colchicine. *Br J Haematol*, **146**, 465.

191 Lach-Szyrma V and Brito-Babapulle F (1997) The significance of apoptotic cells in peripheral blood smears. *Br J Haematol*, **97**, Suppl. 1, 70.

192 Drouin A, Favier R, Massé J-M, Debili N, Schmitt A, Elbin C *et al.* (2001) Newly recognized cellular abnormalities in the gray platelet syndrome. *Blood*, **98**, 1382–1391.

193 Campbell LJ, Maher DW, Tay DLM, Boyd AW, Rockmart S, McGrath K *et al.* (1992) Marrow proliferation and the

appearance of giant neutrophils in response to recombinant human granulocyte colony stimulating factor (rhG-CSF). *Br J Haematol*, **80**, 298–304.

194 Ryder JW, Lazarus HM and Farhi DC (1992) Bone marrow and blood findings after marrow transplantation and rhGM-CSF therapy. *Am J Clin Pathol*, **97**, 631–637.

195 Ghandi MK, Howard MR and Hamilton PJ (1996) The Alder–Reilly anomaly in association with the myelodysplastic syndrome. *Clin Lab Haematol*, **18**, 39–40.

196 Gale PF, Parkin JL, Quie PG, Pettitt RE, Nelson RP and Brunning RD (1986) Leukocyte granulation abnormality associated with normal neutrophil function and neurological abnormality. *Am J Clin Pathol*, **86**, 33–49.

197 Newburger PE, Robinson JM, Pryzwansky KB, Rosoff PM, Greenberger JS and Tauber AI (1983) Human neutrophil dysfunction with giant granules and defective activation of the respiratory burst. *Blood*, **61**, 1247–1257.

198 Van Slyck EJ and Rebuck JW (1974) Pseudo-Chediak–Higashi anomaly in acute leukemia. *Am J Clin Pathol*, **62**, 673–678.

199 Merino A and Esteve J (2005) Acute myeloid leukaemia with peculiar blast cell inclusions and pseudo-eosinophilia. *Br J Haematol*, **131**, 286.

200 Davidson RJ and McPhie JL (1980) Cytoplasmic vacuolation of peripheral blood cells in acute alcoholism. *J Clin Pathol*, **33**, 1193–1196.

201 Chetty-Raju N, Cook R and Erber W (2005) Vacuolated neutrophils in ethanol toxicity. *Br J Haematol*, **127**, 478.

202 Jordans GHW (1953) The familial occurrence of fat containing vacuoles in the leucocytes diagnosed in two brothers suffering from dystrophic musculorum progressiva. *Acta Med Scand*, **145**, 419–423.

203 Schopfer K and Douglas SD (1976) Fine structural studies of peripheral blood leucocytes from children with kwashiorkor: morphological and functional studies. *Br J Haematol*, **32**, 573–577.

204 Aprikyan AAG, Liles WC, Park JR, Jonas M, Chi EY and Dale DC (2000) Myelokathexis, a congenital disorder of severe neutropenia characterized by accelerated apoptosis and defective expression of *bcl-x* in neutrophil precursors. *Blood*, **95**, 320–327.

205 Peterson LC, Rao KV, Crosson JT and White JG (1985) Fechtner syndrome – a variant of Alport's syndrome with leukocyte inclusions and macrothrombocytopenia. *Blood*, **65**, 397–406.

206 Ribeiro RC, Howard TH, Brandalise S, Behm FG, Parham DM, Wang WC *et al.* (1994) Giant actin inclusions in hematopoietic cells associated with transfusion-dependent anemia and grey skin coloration. *Blood*, **83**, 3717–3726.

207 Yu PH and Wong KF (1996) Circulating leukocytes with ingested mucin in a child with Hirschsprung's disease. *Am J Hematol*, **52**, 240.

208 Chomet B, Kirshen MM, Schaefer G and Mudrik P (1953) The finding of the LE (lupus erythematosus) cells in smears of untreated, freshly drawn peripheral blood. *Blood*, **8**, 1107–1109.

209 Weil SC, Holt S, Hrisinko MA, Little L and De Backer N (1985) Melanin inclusions in peripheral blood leukocytes of a patient with malignant melanoma. *Am J Clin Pathol*, **84**, 679–681.

210 Sen Gupta PC, Ghosal SP, Mukherjee AK and Maity TR (1983) Bilirubin crystals in neutrophils of jaundiced neonates and infants. *Acta Haematol*, **70**, 69–70.

211 Smith H (1967) Unidentified inclusions in haemopoietic cells, congenital atresia of the bile ducts and livedo rcticularis in an infant. A new syndrome? *Br J Haematol*, **13**, 695–705.

212 Miale JB (1982) *Laboratory Medicine: Hematology*, 6th edn. CV Mosby, St Louis.

213 Roberts GT, Perry JL, Al-Jefri A and Scott CS (2005) Intra-leukocytic hemosiderin inclusions detected as pseudoeosinophils by automated depolarization analysis in a patient with beta-thalassaemia major and immune hemolysis. *Blood Cells Mol Dis*, **34**, 162–165.

214 Hernandez JA and Steane SM (1984) Erythrophagocytosis by segmented neutrophils in paroxysmal cold hemoglobinuria. *Am J Clin Pathol*, **81**, 787–789.

215 Jaber A, Nong M and Thiagarajan P (2006) Transient neutrophilic thrombophagocytosis associated with citrobacter freundii septicemia. *Arch Pathol Lab Med*, **130**, 1754–1755.

216 Campbell V, Fosbury E and Bain BJ (2009) Platelet phagocytosis as a case of pseudothrombocytopenia. *Am J Hematol*, **84**, 362.

217 Wang J, Fan L, Ma C, Zhang Y and Xu D (2013) Effects of parenteral lipid emulsions on leukocyte numerical and morphological parameters determined by LH750 hematology analyzer. *Int J Lab Hematol*, **35**, e4–e7.

218 Schofield KP, Stone PCW, Beddall AC and Stuart J (1983) Quantitative cytochemistry of the toxic granulation blood neutrophil. *Br J Haematol*, **53**, 15–22.

219 Nevsímalová S, Elleder M, Smíd F and Zemánkova M (1984) Multiple sulphatase deficiency in homozygotic twins. *J Inherit Metab Dis*, **7**, 38–40.

220 Presentey B (1986) Alder anomaly accompanied by a mutation of the myeloperoxidase structural gene. *Acta Haematol*, **75**, 157–159.

221 Doocey R, Thula R and Jackson S (2002) Giant actin inclusions in hematopoietic cells: a variant of Brandalise syndrome. *J Pediatr Hematol Oncol*, **24**, 781–782.

222 Rosenszajn L, Klajman A, Yaffe D and Efrati P (1966) Jordans anomaly in white blood cells. *Blood*, **28**, 258–265.

223 Markesbery WR, McQuillen MP, Procopis PG, Harrison AR and Engel AG (1974) Muscle carnitine deficiency:

association with lipid myopathy, vacuolar neuropathy, and vacuolated leukocytes. *Arch Neurol*, **31**, 320–324.

224 Dorfman ML, Hershko C, Eisenberg S and Sagher F (1974) Ichthyosiform dermatosis with systemic lipidosis. *Arch Dermatol*, **110**, 261–266.

225 Chanarin I, Patel A, Slavin G, Wills EJ, Andrews TM and Stewart G (1975) Neutral-lipid storage disease: a new disorder of lipid metabolism. *BMJ*, **i**, 553–555.

226 Cawley JC and Hayhoe FGJ (1972) The inclusions of the May–Hegglin anomaly and Döhle bodies of infection: an ultrastructural comparison. *Br J Haematol*, **22**, 491–496.

227 Abernathy MR (1966) Döhle bodies associated with uncomplicated pregnancy. *Blood*, **27**, 380–385.

228 Itoga T and Laszlo J (1962) Döhle bodies and other granulocytic alterations during chemotherapy with cyclophosphamide. *Blood*, **20**, 668–674.

229 Jenis EH, Takeuchi A, Dillon DE, Ruymann FB and Rivkin S (1971) The May–Hegglin anomaly: ultrastructure of the granulocyte inclusion. *Am J Clin Pathol*, **55**, 187–196.

230 Drachman JG (2004) Inherited thrombocytopenia: when a low platelet count does not mean ITP. *Blood*, **103**, 390–398.

231 Volpé R and Ogryzlo MA (1955) The cryoglobulin inclusion cell. *Blood*, **10**, 493–496.

232 Dennis R, Cummins D and Amin S (1995) Peripheral blood film deposits in a patient with lymphoproliferative disorder. *Clin Onc*, **7**, 65.

233 Powell HC and Wolf PL (1976) Neutrophilic leukocyte inclusions in colchicine intoxication. *Arch Pathol Lab Med*, **100**, 136–138.

234 Williams ST, Khare VK, Johnston GA and Blackall DP (1995) Severe intravascular hemolysis associated with brown recluse spider envenomation. *Am J Clin Pathol*, **104**, 463–467.

235 Lewandowski K, Homenda W, Mital A, Complak A and Hellmann A (2011) Erythrophagocytosis by neutrophils – a rare morphological phenomenon resulting in acquired haemolytic anaemia? *Int J Lab Hematol*, **33**, 447–450.

236 Au WY and Kwong YL (1999) Haemophagocytosis in the peripheral blood. *Br J Haematol*, **105**, 321.

237 Etzell J, Lu CM, Browne LW and Wang E (2005) Erythrophagocytosis by dysplastic neutrophils in chronic myelomonocytic leukemia and subsequent transformation to acute myeloid leukemia. *Am J Hematol*, **79**, 340–342.

238 Sen Gupta PC, Ghosal SP, Mukherjee AK and Maity TR (1983) Bilirubin crystals in neutrophils of jaundiced neonates and infants. *Acta Haematol*, **70**, 69–70.

239 Harris VN, Malysz J and Smith MD (2009) Green neutrophilic inclusions in liver disease. *J Clin Pathol*, **62**, 853–854.

240 Davison WM, Milner RDG and Lawler SD (1960) Giant neutrophil leucocytes: an inherited anomaly. *Br J Haematol*, **6**, 339–343.

241 Özbek N, Derbent M, Olcay L, Yilmaz Z and Tokel K (2004) Dysplastic changes in the peripheral blood in children with microdeletion 22q11.2. *Am J Hematol*, **77**, 126–131.

242 Cooke WE (1927) The macropolycyte. *BMJ*, i, 12–13.

243 Shidham VB and Swami VK (2000) Evaluation of apoptotic leukocytes in peripheral blood smears. *Arch Pathol Lab Med*, **124**, 1291–1294.

244 Smith H, Rogers SL, Smith HV, Gillis D, Siskind V and Smith JA (2013) Virus-associated apoptosis of blood neutrophils as a risk factor for invasive meningococcal disease. *J Clin Pathol*, **66**, 976–981.

245 Guibaud S, Plumet-Leger A and Frobert Y (1971) Transient neutrophil aggregation in a patient with infectious mononucleosis. *Am J Clin Pathol*, **80**, 883–884.

246 Foucar K (2001) *Bone Marrow Pathology*, 2nd edn. ASCP Press, Chicago.

247 Nand S, Bansal VK, Kozeny G, Vertuno L, Remlinger KA and Jordan JV (1985) Red cell fragmentation syndrome with the use of subclavian hemodialysis catheters. *Arch Intern Med*, **145**, 1421–1423.

248 Tracey R and Smith H (1978) An inherited anomaly of human eosinophils and basophils. *Blood Cells*, **4**, 291–300.

249 Presentey BZ (1968) A new anomaly of eosinophilic granulocytes. *Am J Clin Pathol*, **49**, 887–890.

250 Archer RK, Engisch HJC, Gaha T and Ruxton J (1971) The eosinophil leucocytes in the blood and bone marrow of patients with Down's anomaly. *Br J Haematol*, **21**, 271–276.

251 Kay NE, Nelson DA and Gottlieb AJ (1973) Eosinophilic Pelger–Huët anomaly with myeloproliferative disorder. *Am J Clin Pathol*, **60**, 663–668.

252 Catovsky D, Bernasconi C, Verdonck PJ, Postma A, Hows J, ven der Does-van den Berg A *et al.* (1980) The association of eosinophilia with lymphoblastic leukaemia or lymphoma: a study of seven patients. *Br J Haematol*, **45**, 523–534.

253 Bain BJ (1989) The significance of ring eosinophils in humans. *Br J Haematol*, **73**, 580–581.

254 Andre E, Chevalier C and Scheiff JM (2011) Howell–Jolly-like bodies in leucocytes: first description in leucocytes other than neutrophils. *Eur J Haematol*, **86**, 182–183.

255 Chevalier C and Detry G (2012) Vacuolated lymphocytes and abnormal eosinophils in GM gangliosidosis, type 1. *Br J Haematol*, **156**, 293.

256 Weil SC and Hrisinko MA (1987) A hybrid eosinophilic–basophilic granulocyte in chronic granulocytic leukaemia. *Am J Clin Pathol*, **87**, 66–70.

257 Douglas SD, Blume RS and Wolff SM (1969) Fine structural studies of leukocytes from patients and heterozygotes with the Chediak–Higashi syndrome. *Blood*, **33**, 527–540.

258 Groover RV, Burke EC, Gordon H and Berdon WE (1972) The genetic mucopolysaccharidoses. *Semin Haematol*, **9**, 371–402.

259 Kolodny EH (1972) Clinical and biochemical genetics of the lipidoses. *Semin Haematol*, **9**, 251–271.

260 Forestier F, Hohlfeld P, Vial Y, Olin V, Andreux J-P and Tissot J-D (1996) Blood smears and prenatal diagnosis. *Br J Haematol*, **95**, 278–280.

261 Patel MS, Callahan JW, Zhang S, Chan AKJ, Unger S, Levin AV *et al.* (1999) Early-infantile galactosialidosis: prenatal presentation and postnatal follow-up. *Am J Med Genet*, **85**, 38–47.

262 Maier-Redelsperger M, Stern M-H and Maroteaux P (1988) Pink rings lymphocyte: a new cytologic abnormality characteristic of mucopolysaccharidosis type II Hunter disease. *Pediatrics*, **82**, 286–287.

263 van der Meer W, Jakobs BS, Bocca G, Smeitink JAM, Schuurmans Steckhoven JH and de Keijzer MH (2001) Peripheral blood lymphocyte appearance in a case of I cell disease. *J Clin Pathol*, **54**, 724–726.

264 Anderson G, Smith VV, Malone M and Sebire NJ (2005) Blood film examination for vacuolated lymphocytes in the diagnosis of metabolic disorders: retrospective experience of more than 2500 cases from a single centre. *J Clin Pathol*, **58**, 1305–1310.

265 Iwasaki H, Ueda T, Uchida M, Nakamura T, Takada N and Mahara F (1991) Atypical lymphocytes with a multilobated nucleus from a patient with tsutsugamushi disease (scrub typhus) in Japan. *Am J Hematol*, **36**, 150–151.

266 Huhn KM, Dalal BI, Naiman SC and Buskard NA (1995) Case of chronic B-lymphocytic leukemia with clover leaf nuclei. *Am J Hematol*, **49**, 360–361.

267 Bachelez H, Hadida F and Gorochov G (1996) Massive infiltration of the skin by HIV-specific cytotoxic CD8-positive T cells. *N Engl J Med*, **335**, 61–62.

268 Wulf GG, Schulz H, Hallermann C, Kunze E and Wörmann B (2001) Reactive polyclonal T-cell lymphocytosis mimicking Sezary syndrome in a patient with hairy cell leukemia. *Haematologica*, **86**, E27.

269 Bates I, Bedu-Addo G, Bevan D and Rutherford T (1996) Circulating villous lymphocytes – the link between reactive malarial splenomegaly and splenic lymphoma. *Br J Haematol*, **93**, Suppl. 1, 69.

270 Lesesve J-F, Debouverie M, Decarvalho Bittencourt M and Béné M-C (2011) CD49d blockade by natalizumab therapy in patients with multiple sclerosis increases immature B-lymphocytes. *Bone Marrow Transplantation*, **46**, 1489–1491.

271 Kanegane H, Wado T, Nunogami K, Seki H, Taniguchi N and Tosato G (1996) Chronic persistent Epstein–Barr virus infection of natural killer cells and B cells associated with granular lymphocyte expansion. *Br J Haematol*, **95**, 116–122.

272 Prokocimer M and Potasman I (2008) The added value of peripheral blood cell morphology in the diagnosis and management of infectious diseases – part 2: illustrative cases. *Postgrad Med J*, **84**, 586–589.

273 Ross DM and Stirling J (2013) Giant parallel tubular arrays in T lymphocytes. *Blood*, **121**, 422.

274 Lesesve J-F and Troussard X (2001) EDTA-dependent lymphoagglutination. *Br J Haematol*, **115**, 237.

275 Shelton JB and Frank IN (2000) Splenic B cell lymphoma with lymphocyte clusters in peripheral blood smears. *J Clin Pathol*, **53**, 228–230.

276 Cobcroft R (1999) Diagnosis of angiotropic large B-cell lymphoma from a peripheral blood film. *Br J Haematol*, **104**, 429.

277 Imbing F, Kumar D, Kumar S, Yuoh G and Gardner F (1995) Splenic lymphoma with circulating villous lymphocytes. *J Clin Pathol*, **48**, 584–587.

278 Wenburg JJ and Go RS (2003) EDTA-dependent lymphocyte clumping. *Haematologica*, **88**, EIM09.

279 Oertel J, Oertel B, Schleicher J and Huhn D (1998) Detection of small numbers of immature cells in the blood of healthy subjects. *J Clin Pathol*, **51**, 886–890.

280 Pellat-Deceunynck C, Jego G, Robilard N, Accard F, Amiot M and Bataille R (2000) Reactive plasmacytoses, a model for studying the biology of human plasma cell progenitors and precursors. *Hematol J*, **1**, 362–366.

281 Blanchard-Rohner G, Pulickal AS, Jol-van der Zijde CM, Snape MD and Pollard AJ (2009) Appearance of peripheral blood plasma cells and memory B cells in a primary and secondary immune response in humans. *Blood*, **114**, 4998–5002.

282 Shtalrid M, Shvidel L and Vorst E (2003) Polyclonal reactive peripheral blood lymphocytosis mimicking plasma cell leukemia in a patient with staphylococcal sepsis. *Leuk Lymphoma*, **44**, 379–380.

283 Gawoski JM and Ooi WW (2003) Dengue fever mimicking plasma cell leukemia. *Arch Pathol Lab Med*, **127**, 1026–1027.

284 Yamane A, Awaya N, Shimizu T, Ikeda Y and Okamoto S (2007) Angioimmunoblastic T-cell lymphoma with polyclonal proliferation of plasma cells in peripheral blood and marrow. *Acta Haematol*, **117**, 74–77.

285 La Raja M (2002) Erythrophagocytosis by peripheral monocytes in Plasmodium falciparum malaria. *Haematologica*, **87**, EIM14.

286 Klein E and Ronez E (2012) Peripheral hemophagocytosis in malaria infection. *Blood*, **119**, 910.

287 White JG, Witkop CJ and Gerritsen SM (1973) The Hermansky–Pudlak syndrome: inclusions in circulating leucocytes. *Br J Haematol*, **24**, 761–765.

288 Currimbhoy Z (1991) An outbreak of an infection associated with circulating activated monocytes and haemophagocytes in children in Bombay, India. *Am J Pediatr Hematol Oncol*, **13**, 274–279.

289 Piankijagum A, Visudhiphan S, Aswapokee P, Suwanagool S, Kruatrachue M and Na-Nakorn S (1977) Hematological changes in typhoid fever. *J Med Assoc Thai*, **60**, 828–838.

290 Tsuda H (1997) The use of cyclosporin-A in the treatment of virus–associated haemophagocytic syndrome in adults. *Leuk Lymphoma*, **28**, 73-82.

291 Sheehan AM (2011) Peripheral blood and bone marrow manifestations in metabolic storage disease.

In: Proytcheva MA (ed.) *Diagnostic Pediatric Hematopathology*, Cambridge University Press, Cambridge.

292 Efrati P and Rozenszajn L (1960) The morphology of buffy coats in normal human adults. *Blood*, **15**, 1012–1019.

293 Bennett IM, Catovsky D, Daniel MT, Flandrin G, Galton DAG, Gralnick HR and Sultan C (1982) Proposals for the classification of the myelodysplastic syndromes. *Br J Haematol*, **51**, 189–199.

294 Meteesatien P, Plevy SE, Fender JD and Fedoriw Y (2010) Circulating blasts in a Crohn's patient treated with natalizumab. *Lab Med*, **43**, 453–456.

295 Yun HD and Waller EK (2013) Smudge cells following treatment with pentostatin in a patient with B-cell prolymphocytic leukemia. *Blood*, **122**, 474.

296 van Hoeven KH, Wanner JL and Ballas SK (1997) Cytologic diagnosis of fat emboli in peripheral blood during sickle cell infarctive crisis. *Diagn Cytopathol*, **17**, 54–56.

297 Hicsönmez G and Ozkaynak F (1984) Diagnosis of heterozygous state for Bernard–Soulier disease. *Acta Haematol*, **71**, 285–286.

298 Epstein CJ, Sahud MA, Piel CF, Goodman JR, Bernfield MR, Kushner JH and Ablin AR (1972) Hereditary macrothrombocytopathia, nephritis and deafness. *Am J Med*, **52**, 299–310.

299 Bellucci S (1997) Megakaryocytes and inherited thrombocytopenias. *Baillière's Clin Haematol*, **10**, 149–162.

300 Estes JW (1968) Platelet size and function in the hereditable disorders of connective tissues. *Ann Intern Med*, **68**, 1237–1249.

301 Jackson SC, Sinclair GD, Cloutier GD, Duab Z, Rand ML and Poon MC (2009) The Montreal platelet syndrome kindred has type 2B von Willebrand disease with the VWF V1316M mutation. *Blood*, **113**, 3348–3351.

302 Raccuglia G (1971) Gray platelet syndrome. A variety of qualitative platelet disorder. *Am J Med*, **51**, 818–827.

303 Lesesve J-F, Latger-Cannard V and Lecompte T (2005) Pseudo-storage pool disease due to platelet degranulation in EDTA-collected peripheral blood: a rare artifact. *Clin Lab Haematol*, **27**, 336–342.

304 Biddle DA, Neto TG and Nguyen AND (2001) Platelet storage pool deficiency of α and δ granules. *Arch Pathol Lab Med*, **125**, 1125–1126.

305 Geddis AE (2005) Congenital cytopenias. The molecular basis of congenital thrombocytopenias: insights into megakaryopoiesis. *Hematology*, **10**, Suppl. 1, 299–305.

306 Kim SM, Chang HK, Song JW, Koh H and Han SJ; Severance Pediatric Liver Disease Research Group (2010) Agranular platelets as a cardinal feature of ARC syndrome. *J Pediatr Hematol Oncol*, **32**, 253–258.

307 Mant MJ, Doery JCG, Gauldie J and Sims H (1975) Pseudothrombocytopenia due to platelet aggregation and degranulation in blood collected in EDTA. *Scand J Haematol*, **15**, 161–170.

308 Stavem P and Kjaerheim A (1977) *In vitro* platelet stain preventing (degranulating) effect of various substances. *Scand J Haematol*, **18**, 170–176.

309 Cockbill SR, Burmester HB and Heptinstall S (1988) Pseudo grey platelet syndrome – grey platelets due to degranulation of platelets in blood collected into EDTA. *Eur J Haematol*, **41**, 326–333.

310 Hamilton RW, Shaikh BS, Ottic JN, Storch AE, Saleem A and White JG (1980) Platelet function, ultrastructure and survival in the May–Hegglin anomaly. *Am J Clin Pathol*, **74**, 663–668.

311 Breton-Gorius J, Favier R, Guichard J, Cherif D, Berger R, Debili N *et al.* (1995) A new congenital dysmegakaryopoietic thrombocytopenia (Paris–Trousseau) associated with giant platelet α-granules and chromosome 11 deletion at 11q23. *Blood*, **85**, 1805–1814.

312 Fajardo LF and Tallent C (1974) Malaria parasites within human platelets. *JAMA*, **229**, 1205–1207.

313 Nurden P, Debili N, Vainchenker W, Bobe R, Bredoux R, Corvazier E *et al.* (2006) Impaired megakaryocytopoiesis in type 2B von Willebrand disease with severe thrombocytopenia. *Blood*, **108**, 2587–2595.

314 Casonato A, Bertomoro A, Pontara E, Dannhauser D, Lazzaro AR and Girolami A (1994) EDTA dependent pseudothrombocytopenia caused by antibodies against the cytoadhesive receptor of platelet gpIIB/IIIA. *J Clin Pathol*, **47**, 625–630.

315 Chiurazzi F, Villa MR and Rotoli B (1999) Transplacental transmission of EDTA-dependent pseudothrombocytopenia. *Haematologica*, **84**, 664.

316 Stiegler HM, Fischer Y and Steiner S (1999) Thrombocytopenia and glycoprotein IIb-IIIa receptor antagonists. *Lancet*, **353**, 1185.

317 Español I, Muñiz-Diaz E and Domingo-Clarós A (2000) The irreplaceable image: platelet satellitism to granulated lymphocytes. *Haematologica*, **85**, 1322.

318 Yoo D, Weems H and Lessin LS (1982) Platelet to leukocyte adherence phenomenon. *Acta Haematol*, **68**, 142–148.

319 Campbell V, Fosbury E and Bain BJ (2009) Platelet phagocytosis as a case of pseudothrombocytopenia. *Am J Hematol*, **84**, 362.

320 Zandecki M, Genevieve F, Gerard J and Godon A (2007) Spurious counts and spurious results on haematology analysers: a review. Part I: platelets. *Int J Lab Hematol*, **1**, 4–20.

321 Lazo-Langner A, Piedras J, Romero-Lagarza P, Lome-Maldonado C, Sánchez-Guerrero J and López-Karpovitch X (2002) Platelet satellitism, spurious neutropenia, and cutaneous vasculitis: casual or causal association? *Am J Hematol*, **70**, 246–249.

322 Hosseinzadeh M, Kumar PV and Rahemi M (2006) Platelet satellitism in lupus erythematosus resolving after treatment. *Acta Haematol*, **115**, 131–132.

323 Cesca C, Ben-Ezra J and Riley RS (2001) Platelet satellitism as presenting finding in mantle cell lymphoma. *Am J Clin Pathol*, **115**, 567–570.

324 Latger-Cannard V, Debourgogne A, Montagne K, Plénat F and Lecompte T (2009) Platelet satellitism and lymphoagglutination as presenting finding in marginal zone B-cell lymphoma. *Eur J Haematol*, **83**, 81–82.

325 Hansen M and Pedersen NT (1979) Circulating megakar-yocytes in patients with pulmonary inflammation and in patients subjected to cholecystectomy. *Scand J Haematol*, **23**, 211–216.

326 Pederson NT and Petersen S (1980) Megakaryocytes in the foetal circulation and in cubital venous blood in the mother before and after delivery. *Scand J Haematol*, **25**, 5–11.

327 Pederson NT and Cohn J (1981) Intact megakaryocytes in the venous blood as a marker for thrombopoiesis. *Scand J Haematol*, **27**, 57–63.

328 Pederson NT and Laursen B (1983) Megakaryocytes in cubital venous blood in patients with chronic myeloprolif-erative disorders. *Scand J Haematol*, **30**, 50–58.

329 Swami VK, Solomon-Pestcoe F and Chen X (1996) Significance of circulating megakaryocytes in neonates: a prospective study of 68 cases. *Am J Clin Pathol*, **105**, 513–514.

330 Wilde NT, Burgess R, Keenan DJM and Lucas GS (1997) The effect of cardiopulmonary bypass on circulating mega-karyocytes. *Br J Haematol*, **98**, 322–327.

331 Bianchi DW (1999) Fetal cells in the maternal circulation: feasibility in prenatal diagnosis. *Br J Haematol*, **105**, 574–583.

332 Levine RF, Olson TA, Shoff PK, Miller MK and Weisman LE (1996) Mature micromegakaryocytes: an unusual develop-mental pattern in term infants. *Br J Haematol*, **94**, 391–399.

333 Lowenstein ML (1959) The mammalian reticulocyte. *Int Rev Cytol*, **9**, 135–174.

334 Xanthou M (1970) Leucocyte blood picture in full-term and premature babies during neonatal period. *Arch Dis Child*, **45**, 242–249.

335 Gibson EL, Vaucher Y and Corrigan JJ (1984) Eosinophilia in premature infants: relationship to weight gain. *J Pediatr*, **95**, 99–101.

336 Wilkinson LS, Tang A and Gjedsted A (1983) Marked lymphocytosis suggesting chronic lymphocytic leukemia in three patients with hyposplenism. *Am J Med*, **75**, 1053–1056.

337 Kelemen E, Gergely P, Lehoczky D, Triska E, Demeter J and Vargha P (1986) Permanent large granular lymphocytosis in the blood of splenectomized individuals without con-comitant increase of *in vitro* natural killer cell cytotoxicity. *Clin Exp Immunol*, **163**, 696–702.

338 Demeter J (1995) Persistent lymphocytosis of natural killer cells after splenectomy. *Br J Haematol*, **91**, 253–254.

339 Millard RE and Banerjee DK (1979) Changes in T and B blood lymphocytes after splenectomy. *J Clin Pathol*, **32**, 1045–1049.

340 Holyroyde CP and Gardner FH (1970) Acquisition of autophagic vacuoles by human erythrocytes: physiological role of the spleen. *Blood*, **36**, 566–575.

341 Kevy SV, Tefft M, Vawter GF and Rosen FS (1968) Heredi-tary splenic hypoplasia. *Pediatrics*, **42**, 752–757.

342 Devriendt K, Naulaers G, Matthijs G, Van Houdt K, Dev-lieger H, Gewillig M and Fryns JP (1997) Agenesis of corpus callosum and anophthalmia in the asplenia syn-drome. A recognisable association? *Ann Genet*, **40**, 14–17.

343 Garriga S and Crosby WH (1959) The incidence of leuke-mia in families of patients with hypoplasia of the marrow. *Blood*, **14**, 1008–1114.

344 Leahy RT, Philip RK, Gibbons RJ, Fisher C, Suri M and Reardon W (2005) Asplenia in ATR-X syndrome: a second report. *Am J Med Genet A*, **139**, 37–39.

345 Rodin AE, Sloan JA and Nghiem QX (1972) Polysplenia with severe congenital heart disease and Howell–Jolly bod-ies. *Am J Clin Pathol*, **58**, 127–134.

346 Eshel Y, Sarova-Pinhas I, Lampl Y and Jedwab M (1991) Autosplenectomy complicating pneumococcal meningitis in an adult. *Arch Intern Med*, **151**, 998–999.

347 Ryan FP, Smart RC, Holdsworth CD and Preston FE (1978) Hyposplenism in inflammatory bowel disease. *Gut*, **19**, 50–55.

348 Corazza GR and Gasbarrini G (1983) Defective spleen function and its relation to bowel disease. *Clin Gastroenterol*, **12**, 651–669.

349 Dillon AM, Stein HB and English RA (1982) Splenic atro-phy in systemic lupus erythematosus. *Ann Intern Med*, **96**, 40–43.

350 Friedman TC, Thomas PM, Fleisher TA, Feuillan P, Parker RI, Cassorla F and Chrousos GP (1991) Frequent occurrence of asplenia and cholelithiasis in patients with autoimmune pol-yglandular disease type 1. *Am J Med*, **91**, 625–630.

351 Kahls P, Panzer S, Kletter K, Minar E, Stain-Kos M, Walter R *et al.* (1988) Functional asplenia after bone marrow transplantation: a late complication related to extensive chronic graft-versus-host disease. *Ann Intern Med*, **109**, 461–464.

352 Dailey MO, Coleman CN and Fajardo LF (1981) Splenic injury caused by therapeutic irradiation. *Am J Surg Pathol*, **5**, 325–331.

353 Bensinger TA, Keller AR, Merrell LF and O'Leary DS (1971) Thorotrast-induced reticuloendothelial blockade in man. *Am J Med*, **51**, 663–668.

354 Kurth D, Deiss A and Cartwright GE (1969) Circulating siderocytes in human subjects. *Blood*, **34**, 754–764.

355 Steinberg MH, Gatling RR and Tavassoli M (1983) Evi-dence of hyposplenism, in the presence of splenomegaly. *Scand J Haematol*, **31**, 437–439.

356 Khan AM, Harrington RD, Nadel M and Greenberg BR (1998) Hyposplenism from *Mycobacterium avium* complex infection in a patient with AIDS and immune thrombocy-topenia. *Acta Haematol*, **99**, 44–48.

357 William BM (2009) Hyposplenism associating long-term asbestos exposure. *Rom J Intern Med*, **47**, 415–416.

358 Sunder-Plassmann G, Geissler K and Penner E (1992) Functional asplenia and vasculitis associated with antineu-trophil cytoplasmic antibodies. *N Engl J Med*, **327**, 437–438.

359 Fadel M, Luyt D, Pandya H, Nichani S and Jenkins D (2004) Pneumococcal sepsis: should we look for asplenia? *J R Soc Med*, **97**, 582–583.

360 Shanberge IN (1954) Accidental occurrence of endothelial cells in peripheral blood smears. *Am J Clin Pathol*, **25**, 460–464.

361 George F, Brouqui P, Bofta M-C, Mutin M, Drancourt M, Brisson C et al. (1993) Demonstration of *Rickettsia conorii*-induced endothelial injury *in vivo* by measuring circulating endothelial cells, thrombomodulin, and von Willebrand factor in patients with Mediterranean spotted fever. *Blood*, **82**, 2109–2116.

362 Pooley R, Peterson L, Finn W and Kroft S (1998) Cytomegalovirus-infected cells in routinely prepared peripheral blood films of immunosuppressed patients. *Am J Clin Pathol*, **112**, 108–112.

363 Alabdulaali MK, Alayed KM and Baltow BA (2010) Circulating mesothelial cells following multiple ribs fractures. *Br J Haematol*, **149**, 1.

364 Christensen WN, Ultmann JE and Mohos SC (1956) Disseminated neuroblastoma in an adult presenting with the picture of thrombocytopenic purpura. *Blood*, **11**, 273–278.

365 Nunez C, Abboud SL, Leman NC and Kemp JA (1983) Ovarian rhabdomyosarcoma presenting as leukemia. *Cancer*, **52**, 297–300.

366 Pollak ER, Miller HJ and Vye MV (1981) Medulloblastoma presenting as leukemia. *Am J Clin Pathol*, **76**, 98–103.

367 Krause JR (1979) Carcinocythemia. *Arch Pathol Lab Med*, **103**, 98.

368 Moodley V and Pool R (2003) Circulating neuroblastoma cells in peripheral blood. *Br J Haematol*, **123**, 2.

369 Melamed MR, Cliffton EE and Seal SH (1962) Cancer cells in the peripheral venous blood. A quantitative study of cells of problematic origin. *Am J Clin Pathol*, **37**, 381–388.

370 Brace W, Bain B, Walker M and Catovsky D (1995) Teaching cases from the Royal Marsden Hospital. Case 9: an elderly patient with unusual circulating cells. *Leuk Lymphoma*, **18**, 529–530.

371 Trefzer U, Schlegel C, Sterry W, Späth-Schwalbe E, Possinger K and Denkert C (1999) Fulminant intravascular malignant melanoma mimicking acute leukemia. *Blood*, **94**, 1483–1484.

372 Swirsky D and Luckit J (1999) Images in haematology: the peripheral blood in metastatic melanoma. *Br J Haematol*, **107**, 219.

373 Millar AJ, Sinclair-Smith C, Mills AE, Rode H, Hartley P and Cywes S (1990) Mucin-secreting Wilms' tumor. Report of two cases. *Am J Pediatr Hematol Oncol*, **12**, 201–204.

374 Schaub CR and Farhi DC (1988) Circulating mucin in Wilms' tumor and nephroblastomatosis. Effect on leukocyte counts. *Arch Pathol Lab Med*, **112**, 656–657.

375 Bouroncle BA (1966) Sternberg–Reed cells in the peripheral blood of patients with Hodgkin's disease. *Blood*, **27**, 544–556.

376 Sinks LF and Clein GP (1966) The cytogenetics and cell metabolism of circulating Reed–Sternberg cells. *Br J Haematol*, **12**, 447–453.

377 Le CT (1980) Tick-borne relapsing fever in children. *Pediatrics*, **66**, 963–966.

378 Lawrence C, Brown ST and Freundlich LF (1988) Peripheral blood smear bacillemia. *Am J Med*, **85**, 111–113.

379 Yu RK, Shepherd LE and Rapson DA (2000) *Capnocytophaga canimorsus*, a potential emerging microorganism in splenectomized patients. *Br J Haematol*, **109**, 679.

380 Gloster ES, Strauss RA, Jimenez JF, Neuberg RW, Berry DH and Turner EJ (1985) Spurious elevated platelet counts associated with bacteremia. *Am J Hematol*, **18**, 329–332.

381 Fife A, Hill D, Barton C and Burden P (1993) Gram negative septicaemia diagnosed on peripheral blood smear appearances. *J Clin Pathol*, **47**, 82–84.

382 Torlakovic E, Hibbs JR, Miller JS and Litz CE (1996) Intracellular bacteria in blood smears in patients with central venous catheters. *Arch Intern Med*, **155**, 1547–1550.

383 Babe KS and Reinhardt JF (1994) Diagnosis of legionella sepsis by examination of a peripheral blood smear. *Clin Inf Dis*, **19**, 1164.

384 Fernando SL and Lehmann P (2011) Bugs on film: the presence of bacterial rods (*Citrobacter koseri*) on a routine blood film in a septic immunocompromised patient with a femoral vein line. *Ind J Pathol Bacteriol*, **54**, 840–841.

385 Dooley JR (1980) Haemotropic bacteria in man. *Lancet*, **ii**, 1237–1239.

386 Rolain J-M, Foucault C, Guieu R, La Scola B, Brouqui P and Raoult D (2002) *Bartonella quintana* in human erythrocytes. *Lancet*, **360**, 226–228.

387 Invernizzi R, Travaglino E and Perfetti V (2003) PAS positive monocytes in Whipple's disease. *Haematologica*, **88**, EIM16.

388 Puntarić V, Borčič D, Bejuk D, Vrhovec B, Madić J, Busch K and Richter B (1994) Haemotropic bacteria in man, *Lancet*, **343**, 359–360.

389 Tarantolo SR, Landmark JD, Iwen PC, Kessinger A, Chan WC and Hinrichs SH (1997) *Bartonella*-like erythrocyte inclusions in thrombotic thrombocytopenic purpura. *Lancet*, **350**, 1602.

390 Raoult D, Lepidi H and Harle JR (2001) *Tropheryma whipplei* circulating in blood monocytes. *N Engl J Med*, **345**, 548.

391 Godwin JH, Stopeck A, Chang VT and Godwin TA (1991) Mycobacteremia in acquired immune deficiency syndrome. Rapid diagnosis based on inclusions in the peripheral blood smear. *Am J Clin Pathol*, **95**, 369–375.

392 Buller RS, Areno M, Hmiel SP, Paddock CD, Sumner JW, Rikihisa Y et al. (1999) *Ehrlichia ewingii*, a newly recognized agent of human ehrlichiosis. *N Engl J Med*, **341**, 148–155.

393 Chen S-M, Dumler JS, Bakken JS and Walker DH (1994) Identification of a granulocytotropic Ehrlichia species as the etiologic-agent of human disease. *J Clin Microbiol*, **32**, 589–595.

394 Rynkiewicz DL and Liu LX (1994) Human ehrlichiosis in New England. *N Engl J Med*, **330**, 292–293.

395 McDade JE (1990) Ehrlichiosis – a disease of animals and humans. *J Infect Dis*, **161**, 609–617.

396 Morais JD, Dawson JE, Greene C, Filipe AP, Galhardas LC and Bacellar F (1991) First European case of ehrlichiosis. *Lancet*, **338**, 633–634.

397 Horowitz HW, Kilchevsky E, Haber S, Aguero-Rosenfeld M, Kranwinkel R, James EK *et al.* (1998) Perinatal transmission of the agent of human granulocytic ehrlichiosis. *N Engl J Med*, **339**, 375–378.

398 Tamí I, Martinez JI, Tamí M, Redondo MC, Finol H and Simonovis N (1966) Identification of *Ehrlichia* species in blood smear. *Inf Dis Clin Practice*, **5**, 555–557.

399 Arraga-Alvarado C, Montero-Ojeda M, Bernardoni A, Anderson BE and Parra O (1996) [Human ehrlichiosis: report of the 1st case in Venezuela] (Article in Spanish). *Invest Clin*, **37**, 35–49.

400 Kuberski TT (1977) Intraleukocytic spore formation and leukocytic vacuolization during *Clostridium perfringens* septicemia. *Am J Clin Pathol*, **68**, 794–796.

401 Mann JM, Hull HF, Schmid GP and Droke WE (1984) Plague and the peripheral smear. *JAMA*, **251**, 953.

402 Monihan JM, Jewell TW and Weir GT (1986) Candida parapsilosis diagnosed by peripheral blood smear. *Arch Pathol Lab Med*, **110**, 1180–1181.

403 Yera H, Poulain D, Lefebvre A, Camus D and Sendid B (2004) Polymicrobial candidaemia revealed by the peripheral blood smear and chromogenic medium. *J Clin Pathol*, **57**, 196–198.

404 Girmenia C and Jaalouk G (1994) Detection of Candida in blood smears of patients with hematologic malignancies. *Eur J Haematol*, **52**, 124–125.

405 Yao YDC, Arkin CF, Doweiko JP and Hammer SM (1990) Disseminated cryptococcosis diagnosed on peripheral blood smear in a patient with acquired immunodeficiency syndrome. *Am J Med*, **89**, 100–102.

406 Wong KF, Tsang DNC and Chan JKC (1994) Bone marrow diagnosis of penicilliosis. *N Engl J Med*, **330**, 717–718.

407 Nayar R, Marley EF, Laban NLC and Campos JM (1995) Clinical pathology rounds: early diagnosis of fungemia in children. *Lab Med*, **26**, 381–383.

408 Bhargava P and Longhi LP (2007) Peripheral smear with *Malassezia furfur*. *N Engl J Med*, **356**, e25.

409 Berrouane Y, Bisiau H, Le Baron F, Cattoen C, Duthilleul P and Dei Cas E (1998) *Candida albicans* blastoconidia in peripheral blood smears from non-neutropenic surgical patients. *J Clin Pathol*, **51**, 537–538.

410 Singh B, Kim Sung L, Matusop A, Radhakrishnan A, Shamsul SS, Cox-Singh J *et al.* (2004) A large focus of naturally acquired Plasmodium knowlesi infections in human beings. *Lancet*, **363**, 1017–1024.

411 Singh B and Daneshvar C (2010) *Plasmodium knowlesi* Malaria in Malaysia. *Med J Malaysia*, **65**, 166–172.

412 Albrecht H, Sobottka I, Stellbrink HJ, van Lunzen J and Greten H (1996) Diagnosis of disseminated toxoplasmosis using a peripheral blood smear. *AIDS*, **10**, 799–800.

413 Willcox ML, Mant J and O'Dempsey T (2013) Imported malaria. *BMJ*, **347**, 34–35.

414 Griffith KS, Lewis LS, Mali S and Parise ME (2007) Treatment of malaria in the United States: a systematic review. *JAMA*, **297**, 2264–2277.

415 Sutherland CJ, Tanomsing N, Nolder D, Oguike M, Jennison C, Pukrittayakamee S *et al.* (2010) Two nonrecombining sympatric forms of the human malaria parasite *Plasmodium ovale* occur globally. *J Infect Dis*, **201**, 1544–1550.

416 Cox-Singh J, Davis TM, Lee KS, Shamsul SS, Matusop A, Ratnam S *et al.* (2008) Plasmodium knowlesi malaria in humans is widely distributed and potentially life threatening. *Clin Infect Dis*, **46**, 165–171.

417 Daneshvar C, Davis TM, Cox-Singh J, Rafàee MZ, Zakaria SK, Divis PC and Singh B (2009) *Plasmodium knowlesi* malaria in humans is widely distributed and potentially life threatening. *Clin Infect Dis*, **49**, 852–860.

418 Figtree M, Lee R, Bain L, Kennedy T, Mackertich S, Urban M *et al.* (2010) *Plasmodium knowlesi* in human, Indonesian Borneo. *Emerg Infect Dis*, **16**, 672–674.

419 Willmann M, Ahmed A, Siner A, Wong IT, Woon LC, Singh B *et al.* (2012) Laboratory markers of disease severity in Plasmodium knowlesi infection: a case control study. *Malar J*, **11**, 363.

420 Singh B and Daneshvar C (2013) Human infections and detection of Plasmodium knowlesi. *Clin Microbiol Rev*, **26**, 165–184.

421 Lee KS, Cox-Singh J and Singh B (2009) Morphological features and differential counts of Plasmodium knowlesi parasites in naturally acquired human infections. *Malar J*, **8**, 73.

422 Lee WC, Chin PW, Lau YL, Chin LC, Fong MY, Yap CJ *et al.* (2013) Hyperparasitaemic human *Plasmodium knowlesi* infection with atypical morphology in peninsular Malaysia. *Malar J*, **12**, 88.

423 Wickramasinghe SN and Abdalla SH (2000) Blood and bone marrow changes in malaria. *Baillière's Clin Haematol*, **13**, 277–299.

424 Ladhani S, Lowe B, Cole AO, Kowuondo K and Newton CRJC (2003) Changes in white blood cells and platelets in children with falciparum malaria: relationship to disease outcome. *Br J Haematol*, **119**, 839–847.

425 Shankar AH and Fawzi WW (2010) Moving toward hematological predictors of disease severity in malaria: going with the flow. *Am J Hematol*, **85**, 225–226.

426 Ladhani S, Khatri P, El-Bashir H and Shingadia D (2005) Imported malaria is a major cause of thrombocytopenia in children presenting to the emergency department in east London. *Br J Haematol*, **129**, 707–709.

427 Chandra S and Chandra H (2013) Role of haematological parameters as an indicator of acute malarial infection in Uttarakhand State of India. *Mediter J Hematol Infect Dis*, **5**, e2013009.

428 Lawrence C (1999) Laveran remembered: malaria haemozoin in leucocytes. *Lancet*, **353**, 1852.

429 Day NPJ, Diep PT, Ly PT, Sinh DX, Chuong LV, Chau TTH *et al.* (1996) Clearance kinetics of parasites and pigment-containing leukocytes in severe malaria. *Blood*, **88**, 4694–4700.

430 Moody AH and Chiodini PL (2000) Methods for the detection of blood parasites. *Clin Lab Haematol*, **22**, 189–202.

431 Bailey JW, Williams J, Bain BJ, Parker-Williams J, Chiodini PL, General Haematology Task Force of the British Committee for Standards in Haematology. (2013) Guideline: the laboratory diagnosis of malaria. *Br J Haematol*, **163**, 573–580.

432 Wilson ML (2013) Laboratory diagnosis of malaria: conventional and rapid diagnostic methods. *Arch Pathol Lab Med*, **137**, 805–811.

433 Moody A, Hunt-Cooke A, Gabbett E and Chiodini P (2000) Performance of the OptiMAL malaria antigen capture dipstick for malaria diagnosis and treatment monitoring at the Hospital for Tropical Diseases, London. *Br J Haematol*, **109**, 891–894.

434 Grobusch MP, Alpermann U, Schwenke S, Jelinek T and Warhurst DC (1999) False-positive rapid tests for malaria in patients with rheumatoid factor. *Lancet*, **353**, 297.

435 Spach DH, Liles WC, Campbell GL, Quick RE, Anderson DE and Fritsche TR (1993) Tick-borne diseases in the United States. *N Engl J Med*, **329**, 936–947.

436 Yager PH, Luginbuhl LM and Dekker JP (2014) Case records of the Massachusetts General Hospital. Case 6-2014: a 35-day-old boy with fever, vomiting, mottled skin, and severe anemia. *N Engl J Med*, **370**, 753–762.

437 Vannier E and Krause PJ (2012) Human babesiosis. *N Engl J Med*, **366**, 2397–2407.

438 Beattie JF, Michelson ML and Holman PJ (2002) Acute babesiosis caused by *Babesia divergens* in a resident of Kentucky. *N Engl J Med*, **347**, 697–698.

439 Rajpal DR, Murray DR, Morrell DR and O'Dwyer DR (2005) Human babesiosis: an unusual cause of haemolytic anaemia. *Br J Haematol*, **129**, Suppl. 1, 51.

440 Martinot M, Zadeh MM and De Briel D (2012) Human babesiosis, *N Engl J Med*, **367**, 1070.

441 Setty S, Khalil Z, Schori P, Azar M and Ferrieri P (2003) Babesiosis: two atypical cases from Minnesota and a review. *Am J Clin Pathol*, **120**, 554–559.

442 Pantanowitz L, Ballesteros E and de Girolami P (2001) Laboratory diagnosis of babesiosis. *Lab Med*, **32**, 184–188.

443 Stowell CP, Gelfand JA, Shepard J-AO and Kratz A (2007) Case 17-2007: a 25-year-old woman with relapsing fevers and recent onset dyspnea. *N Engl J Med*, **356**, 2313–2319.

444 Albrecht H, Sobottka I, Stellbrink H-J, van Lunzen J and Greten H (1996) Diagnosis of disseminated toxoplasmosis using a peripheral blood smear. *AIDS*, **10**, 799–800.

445 Arnold SJ, Kinney MC, McCormick MS, Dunmer S and Scott MA (1997) Disseminated toxoplasmosis: unusual presentations in the immunocompromised host. *Arch Pathol Lab Med*, **121**, 869–873.

446 http://www.dpd.cdc.gov/dpdx/html/trypanosomiasisafrican.htm (accessed April 2014).

447 Moore AC, Ryan ET and Waldron MA (2002) A 37-year-old man with fever, hepatosplenomegaly and a cutaneous foot lesion after a trip to Africa. *N Engl J Med*, **346**, 2069–2077.

448 Vanhollebeke B, Truc P, Poelvoorde P, Pays A, Joshi PP, Katti R *et al.* (2006) Human *Trypanosoma evansi* infection linked to a lack of apolipoprotein L-I. *N Engl J Med*, **355**, 2752–2756.

449 Learning Bench Aid No 3 (n.d.) *Microscopical Diagnosis of Lymphatic Filariasis, Loiasis, Onchocerciasis.* Tropical Health Technology, Doddington, Cambridgeshire.

CHAPTER 4
Detecting erroneous blood counts

The sources of errors in blood counts

Errors in blood counts may be pre-analytical, analytical or post-analytical. Pre-analytical errors are those that precede the analysis of the sample and include errors in producing a request form, errors during venesection and errors in transport and storage of the specimen (Table 4.1). Pre-analytical errors include those resulting from storage of blood specimens at room temperature. For example, with the Sysmex 2100 there is a rise in the mean cell volume (MCV) and haematocrit (Hct) and a fall in the mean cell haemoglobin concentration (MCHC) from 6 hours, and from 48 hours there is a rise in the neutrophil count and a fall in the monocyte count [4]. Siemens instruments show similar changes in red cell variables. It is essential that all laboratories that receive specimens from outlying clinics are aware of the adverse effects of prolonged transport or storage at room temperature. Analytical errors are those that occur during the analysis of the sample (Table 4.2). Post-analytical errors are those that occur after analysis is completed and involve mishandling of data (Table 4.3). Sometimes an error at one stage of the process gives rise to an error at another. Thus, incomplete or erroneous patient identification details or clinical information may lead to a result being issued with a wrong reference range or to interpretative comments being misleading.

The detection of errors in automated blood counts

Since automated blood counts may be inaccurate, it is the responsibility of the laboratory staff performing a count or authorising a report to detect inaccuracies whenever possible.

The validation of an automated count requires: (i) knowledge that an instrument is capable of measuring all variables accurately, that it has been correctly calibrated and that quality control procedures indicate normal functioning; and (ii) assessment of each individual count as to whether it is likely to be correct or that, alternatively, it requires further review. If the first set of conditions has been met then it may be possible to validate counts by means of a computer program, either built into the automated counter or developed to fit the specifications of an individual laboratory. Counts can be computer-validated if: (i) all measurements fall within predetermined limits (which may be somewhat wider than the reference limits for that measurement) and there are no 'flags'; or (ii) measurements fall outside predetermined limits but nevertheless have not changed significantly in comparison with previous measurements on that individual. When results do not meet either set of criteria they should be individually assessed in relation to the clinical details and, if necessary, further steps should be taken to validate the results. These further steps may include: (i) examination of the histograms produced by an automated instrument to establish the likely reason for anomalous results or flags; (ii) examination of the blood specimen, e.g. to check the date and time when venesection was performed, to confirm that the specimen was of adequate volume and to detect clots, fibrin strands, hyperlipidaemia or haemolysis; (iii) examination of a blood film; or (iv) various combinations of these procedures. Which procedures are necessary depends on the nature of the abnormality shown on the automated count and the safeguards that are already built into the instrumentation, e.g. to confirm the identity of the patient and detect specimens of inadequate volume or containing clots. Opinions differ as to whether blood films should always be examined in conjunction with the initial blood count from a patient or whether an automated count with no flags can be accepted as valid evidence that there is no significant haematological abnormality. The latter policy will miss some

Blood Cells A Practical Guide, Fifth Edition. By Barbara J. Bain © 2015 John Wiley & Sons, Ltd. Published 2015 by John Wiley & Sons, Ltd.
Companion Website: www.wiley.com/go/bain/bloodcells

Table 4.1 Some pre-analytical sources of errors in blood counts.

Type of error	Examples
Clerical errors	Patient's name, age or gender missing from request form
	Ethnic origin not supplied when it is essential for interpretation of a test result
	Information that the patient is pregnant not given
	Location of patient or relevant clinician details missing
Unannounced blood transfusion	Previous blood transfusion, unknown to laboratory staff
Fault during patient identification or phlebotomy	Blood from wrong patient; blood specimen and request form relate to different patients
	Maternal and neonatal samples confused
	Specimen diluted (e.g. taken from above intravenous infusion or excess liquid EDTA relative to volume of blood)
	Specimen taken into wrong anticoagulant
	Specimen taken into too high a concentration of EDTA
	Specimen haemoconcentrated due to prolonged application of tourniquet
	Specimen partly clotted
	Specimen haemolysed
	Specimen too small leading to 'short sample'
	Specimen contaminated with subcutaneous fat [1]
Fault during fetal blood sampling	Contamination with amniotic fluid [2]
Fault during specimen transport or storage	Specimen inadvertently heated [3] or frozen
	Aged blood

EDTA, ethylenediaminetetra-acetic acid

Table 4.2 Some analytical sources of errors in blood counts.

Type of error	Examples
Faulty sampling	Failure to prime instrument
	Inadequate mixing
	Aspiration probe blocked, e.g. by clot from previous sample
	'Short sample' or clotted sample not detected
	Carryover from preceding very abnormal specimen (minor with modern instruments)
Faulty calibration	Use of control material as calibrant or error in assigning values to calibrant
Faulty maintenance, other instrument malfunction, reagent failure	
Inaccuracy inherent in specific methodologies	Underestimation of MCV by impedance counters in the presence of hypochromia
	Failure of identification of cells caused by peroxidase deficiency
Inaccuracy due to unusual characteristics of specimen	Error in Hb or red cell indices caused by presence of cold agglutinins, cryoglobulinaemia, hyperlipidaemia or (rarely) rosetting of red cells around neutrophils
	Error in platelet count caused by platelet aggregation or satellitism
	Factitious 'neutropenia' or other cytopenia caused by peroxidase deficiency

MCV, mean cell volume; Hb, haemoglobin concentration

Table 4.3 Some post-analytical sources of errors in blood counts.

Type of error
Transcription error in laboratory
Transcription error in ward or outpatient department when results are telephoned
Results not issued in a timely manner
Results never reach intended destination
Results filed in wrong patient's notes and so applied to wrong patient
Results issued with incorrect reference range or no reference range
Results issued with inappropriate interpretation

abnormalities of clinical significance but not many and it has now become the usual procedure. Validation of a count before it is released also includes ensuring that results have been produced for all tests required, i.e. that no result has been 'voted out' because of poor replicate counts or because it is beyond the linearity limits of the instrument.

Blood count results should be assessed as to probability in the light of the clinical details. For example, cytopenia could be accepted without further review in a patient known to have had recent chemotherapy. Similarly, an increased white blood cell count (WBC) with a 'left shift' flag could be accepted in a postpartum or postoperative patient. Counts that have flags indicating the presence of blast cells or atypical lymphocytes require microscopic review. Whether flags for 'left shift' or 'immature granulocytes' or nucleated red blood cells (NRBC) always require review is a matter of individual laboratory policy. Blood count results that are unexpected or that fall a long way outside reference limits generally require further attention. A very abnormal MCHC is a useful indicator of factitious results since it is derived from all measured red cell variables, i.e. haemoglobin concentration (Hb), red blood cell count (RBC) and MCV or Hct. It is thus sensitive to erroneous measurements in any of these three variables caused, for example, by hyperlipidaemia, intravascular haemolysis, non-lysis of red cells in the Hb channel and red cell agglutination. A markedly elevated MCV is also often factitious. Some types of factitious result occur with all instruments while others are specific to a methodology. Laboratory workers should be familiar with the factitious results that are

likely with the particular instrument they are operating. The rest of this chapter will deal with factitious results other than those consequent on technical errors or instrument and reagent malfunction.

When contamination with amniotic fluid leads to an inaccurate fetal blood count, two mechanisms are operating. One is simple dilution, which affects all variables. The other is activation of coagulation in the sample, which has a disproportionate effect on the platelet count. A related blood film may show platelet aggregates and amniotic fluid cells [2].

It should be noted that factitious results are more likely to have been reported for instruments that have been in use for a long time or have been studied in detail. The lack of reported factitious results for other instruments does not indicate that they do not occur.

Poorly mixed specimens can produce pseudopolycythaemia, pseudoanaemia and inaccurate WBCs and platelet counts. This should be avoided by following a standard operating procedure. Such errors have led to unnecessary blood transfusion and bone marrow examination.

Errors in automated WBC

Errors that may occur in automated WBCs are summarised in Tables 4.4 and 4.5 and instrument printouts from a sample producing an erroneous count because of contamination with subcutaneous fat are shown in Fig. 4.1 [1]. The only common causes of erroneous counts are factitiously high counts caused by NRBC, platelet aggregates or non-lysis of red cells. Factitiously low counts are uncommon, unless the blood has taken many days to reach the laboratory. When a low WBC is the result of neutrophil aggregation it may be ethylenediaminetetra-acetic acid (EDTA)-dependent, temperature-dependent or dependent on both [15]. Aggregation is antibody-mediated and may be reversed by addition of kanamycin in a final concentration of 30 mg/ml [15]. Neutrophil–platelet aggregation, which may represent an exaggerated form of platelet satellitism, will similarly lower the WBC. A quite uncommon phenomenon that may lower the WBC is aggregation of lymphoma cells or of the cells of chronic lymphocytic leukaemia (CLL) or aggregation of all types of leucocyte [12].

Table 4.4 Some causes of a falsely high WBC.

Cause	Instruments on which fault can occur
Presence of NRBC	All instruments unless NRBC are specifically enumerated and excluded from the WBC
Non-lysis of red cells	
uraemia	Bayer H.1 series*
fetal and neonatal specimens	Bayer H.1 series,* Cell-Dyn instruments (optical channels), some Sysmex instruments, Coulter STKS
abnormal haemoglobins (e.g. AS, SS, AC, AE, AD, AO-Arab)	Bayer H.1 series,* some Sysmex instruments
Liver disease	Coulter and some Sysmex instruments
Cold agglutinins	Coulter instruments
Myelodysplastic syndromes	Coulter STKS
Megaloblastic anaemia	Coulter instruments
Post-splenectomy	Coulter instruments
Numerous giant platelets or megakaryocyte fragments	All instruments
Platelet aggregates	Coulter, Bayer and Horiba instruments
Platelet phagocytosis by neutrophils	Abbott Cell-Dyn 3500 (impedance count accurate, optical count inaccurate) [5]
Cryoglobulinaemia and cryofibrinogenaemia	Coulter, Sysmex and Bayer instruments [6]
Precipitation of mucin (in adenocarcinoma and Wilms tumour)	Ortho ELT-8 [7]
Paraproteinaemia	Coulter and Sysmex instruments
Fibrin strands	Coulter instruments
Hyperlipidaemia	Coulter instruments
Exogenous lipid following chemoembolisation with Lipiodol	Sysmex XE-2100 [8]
Contamination of specimen with subcutaneous fat	Bayer H.1 series [1]
Malarial parasites	Coulter and Sysmex instruments
Candida glabrata	Basophil channel of Siemens Advia 120 and DIFF channel of Sysmex XE2000i [9]
Candida glabrata, *Candida parapsilosis* and *Candida albicans* (mainly misidentified as lymphocytes)	Siemens Advia series [10]
Candida albicans, *Candida tropicalis*, *Candida krusei* and *Candida dubliniensis*	Sysmex XE-2100 (classified as basophils), Siemens Advia series (classified as lymphocytes and LUC) and Coulter LH 750 (classified as eosinophils) [11]
Candida glabrata and *Candida parapsilosis*	Sysmex XE-2100 but not Siemens Advia series or Coulter LH 750 [11]
Micro-organisms, if clumped	[12]
Unstable haemoglobin	Coulter instruments

LUC, large unstained cells; NRBC, nucleated red blood cells; WBC, white blood cell count
*basophil channel gives accurate WBC but differential counts are erroneous

Table 4.5 Some causes of a falsely low WBC.

Cause	Instruments on which abnormality can occur
Cell lysis caused when blood is more than 3 days old	Coulter instruments, Cobas Argos 5 Diff and probably other instruments
Storage at room temperature for 24 hours or more	Cell-Dyn 3500 (fall in optical WBC, impedance WBC stable) [13]
Storage at 4°C for more than 24 hours	Horiba instruments
Leucocyte or leucocyte and platelet aggregation due to an antibody or to alteration of the cell membrane or to the presence of neoplastic cells with abnormal characteristics (e.g. antibody-mediated aggregation of neutrophils, mucin-induced aggregation in adenocarcinoma, aggregation of lymphoma cells or neoplastic plasma cells) – depending on the cause, may be aggregation of neutrophils or of all leucocytes; leucocyte rosetting around other cells [14]	Coulter instruments, Sysmex instruments, Bayer H.1 series instruments
Potent cold agglutinin	Coulter instruments

WBC, white blood cell count

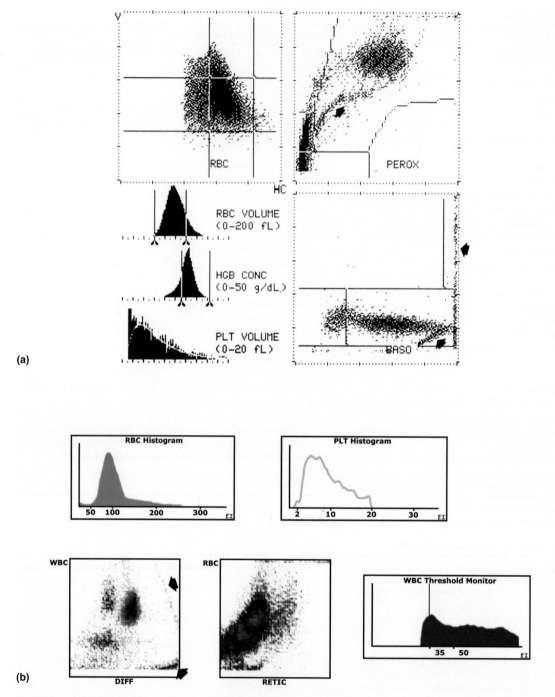

Fig. 4.1 Instrument printout from: (a) Bayer H.2; and (b) Beckman–Coulter Gen S counters from a specimen accidentally contaminated with subcutaneous fat [1]. The signals generated by the fat are arrowed. The H.2 count was inaccurate whereas the Gen S count was accurate.

Erroneous WBCs are usually detected because of instrument flags and improbable results for the WBC or other measurements, or by abnormalities detectable on instrument scatter plots or histograms. For example, an erroneous WBC resulting from the presence of a cold agglutinin would usually be accompanied by an improbably high MCV and MCHC. Neutrophil aggregation may be indicated by an abnormal cloud at the top of the neutrophil area of the Coulter STKS or Bayer H.1 series instruments.

For older instruments, if significant numbers of NRBC are present and an accurate WBC is needed, it is necessary to correct the total nucleated cell count (TNCC) for the number of NRBC by counting their percentage on a blood film. However, it is also possible to accept the total nucleated cell count as a definitive measurement and calculate the absolute count of NRBC and each leucocyte type from the manual differential count. Later instruments often correct the TNCC for the presence of NRBC. Non-lysis of red cells is mainly a problem when the WBC is measured by light-scattering technology. Impedance counters usually produce an accurate result. The observation of factitious elevation of the WBC caused by non-lysis of red cells can be clinically useful since it may be indicative of a previously undiagnosed haemoglobinopathy. This has been noted with H.1 series instruments and on the differential count channel of Sysmex instruments. Drugs administered to patients can also lead to non-lysis of red cells, e.g. noted with a CELL-DYN Sapphire because of the presence of polyoxyethylated castor oil, which is used to solubilise paclixatel [16].

Factitious counts caused by aggregation of platelets can usually be prevented by taking the blood specimen into citrate rather than into EDTA (necessitating a correction for dilution), by collecting capillary blood into ammonium oxalate (previously Unopette, Becton Dickinson, now Thrombo-TIC, Bioanalytic GmbH), or by adding aminoglycosides to disaggregate platelet clumps [17]. Erroneous counts caused by cryoproteins and cold agglutinins can be rectified by keeping the specimen warm. Aggregation of leucocytes is often time-dependent [18] and is sometimes caused by a cold antibody, so that keeping the specimen warm and performing the blood count rapidly after phlebotomy can produce an accurate count. When erroneous counts are due to causes other than white cell clumping, haemocytometer counts will be accurate.

Failure to discover that a low white cell count is factitious has led to unnecessary bone marrow examination and antibiotic and granulocyte colony-stimulating factor (G-CSF) therapy [19].

Errors in haemoglobin concentration and red cell indices

Haemoglobin concentration

Errors that can occur in automated measurements of the Hb and red cell indices are shown in Tables 4.6–4.8. Such erroneous results are usually suspected from a markedly elevated MCV, a markedly abnormal MCHC or a discrepancy between MCHC and cellular haemoglobin concentration mean (CHCM).

Table 4.6 Some causes of a falsely high Hb estimate.

Cause	Instruments on which fault can occur	Detection
Poorly mixed specimen	All	Unexpected result
High WBC	All, but to a variable extent	Check whenever WBC is very high
Hyperlipidaemia, endogenous or due to parenteral nutrition	Coulter and Bayer instruments, Cell-Dyn instruments but error eliminated by modified reagent [20]	Improbable results for MCH and MCHC or flagging of MCHC/CHCM discrepancy; fuzzy red cell outlines on blood films
Paraprotein or hypergammaglobulinaemia	Coulter instruments, Sysmex NE 8000, Bayer instruments	MCH and MCHC slightly elevated [21] MCHC/CHCM discrepancy
Cryoglobulinaemia	Coulter instruments	MCH and MCHC slightly elevated
High concentration of carboxyhaemoglobin [14]		
Turbidity resulting from non-lysis of red cells [14]		

CHCM, cellular haemoglobin concentration mean; Hb, haemoglobin concentration; MCH, mean cell haemoglobin; MCHC, mean cell haemoglobin concentration; WBC, white blood cell count

Table 4.7 Some causes of inaccurate estimates of RBC, MCV and Hct estimations.

Fault	Cause	Instruments on which fault can occur
Falsely high RBC	WBC very high	Coulter and Bayer instruments
	Numerous large platelets	Coulter instruments
	Hyperlipidaemia (not consistently)	Coulter instruments, Bayer- instruments (if concentration very high)
	Cryoglobulinaemia	Coulter instruments
	Cryofibrinogenaemia	Coulter instruments
Falsely low RBC	Cold agglutinins	Coulter and Bayer instruments
	Rarely warm autoantibodies	Coulter S Plus II [22]
	EDTA-dependent panagglutination	Coulter instruments [23]
	In vitro red cell lysis due to mishandling of specimen or very abnormal red cells	All instruments
	Extreme microcytosis or fragmentation causing red cells to fall below the lower threshold	Coulter (and probably other) instruments
Falsely high MCV	Storage of blood at room temperature	Most instruments, to a varying extent but particularly Bayer instruments (see text)
	Cold agglutinins and EDTA- dependent red cell panagglutinins [23]	Coulter and Bayer instruments
	Rarely warm autoantibodies	Coulter S Plus II [22]
	WBC very high	Coulter instruments
	Hyperosmolar states (e.g. hypernatraemia, hyperglycaemia or blood taken from near a glucose infusion)	Coulter instruments, Bayer- instruments [12]
	Excess K_2EDTA	Bayer H.1 series
Falsely low MCV	Hypochromic red cells	Some impedance instruments (Coulter STKR and earlier Coulter instruments, K-1000 to a lesser extent but not Sysmex NE-8000) [24]
	Increase in ambient temperature	Coulter instruments
	Hypo-osmolar states (e.g. hyponatraemia)	Coulter instruments
	Repeated mixing of sample leading to increased oxygenation	Sysmex instruments [25] and probably also other impedance counters
Falsely high Hct	Factitious elevation of MCV (except when due to a cold agglutinin)	See above
	Factitious reduction of RBC	See above
Falsely low Hct	Factitious reduction of MCV	See above
	Factitious reduction of RBC by extreme microcytosis or in vitro red cell lysis	See above
	Cold agglutinin	Coulter instruments
	Repeated mixing of sample leading to increased oxygenation	Sysmex instruments [25] and probably also other impedance counters

EDTA, ethylenediametetra-acetic acid; Hct, haematocrit; MCV, mean cell volume; RBC, red blood cell count; WBC, white blood cell count

Erroneous estimations of Hb (see Table 4.6) most often result from turbidity caused by a high WBC or lipid in the plasma, either endogenous lipid [27,28] or that consequent on parenteral nutrition [29]. The degree of elevation of the WBC that causes an erroneous Hb varies greatly between instruments since it is dependent on the strength of the lytic agent that is employed in the WBC/Hb channel. The problem can be circumvented if separate channels are used for the WBC and the Hb, as in later Sysmex instruments, since a more powerful lytic agent can then be used. The instrument operator should be aware of the degree of leucocytosis that is likely to make the Hb erroneous on a specific instrument and results should then be checked by manual techniques. The haemolysate is centrifuged before absorbance is read so that turbidity caused by the presence of cellular

Table 4.8 Some causes of inaccurate MCH and MCHC estimations.

Fault	Cause	Instruments on which fault can occur
MCH falsely high	Factitious elevation of Hb	See Table 4.6
	Factitious reduction of RBC	See Table 4.7
	Intravascular haemolysis with free haemoglobin in plasma (e.g. in *Clostridium perfringens* sepsis)	All instruments
	Administration of haemoglobin-based oxygen carriers [26]	All instruments
		Probably all
	Red cell panagglutinin [23]	Coulter
MCHC falsely high or true fall of MCHC masked	Factitious elevation of Hb	See Table 4.6
	Intravascular haemolysis with free haemoglobin in plasma or *in vitro* lysis of red cells	All instruments
	Factitious reduction in Hct or the product of the MCV and RBC	See Table 4.7
	Hypo-osmolar states	Coulter instruments
	Administration of haemoglobin- based oxygen carriers [26]	All instruments
	Red cell panagglutinin [23]	Coulter
MCHC falsely low	Factitious elevation of MCV (except when caused by cold agglutinins)	See Table 4.7
	Factitious elevation of RBC by numerous giant platelets	All instruments
	Hyperosmolar states	Coulter instruments
	Falsely low Hb caused by extreme leucocytosis	Bayer H1 series [6]

Hb, haemoglobin concentration; Hct, haematocrit; MCH, mean cell haemoglobin; MCHC, mean cell haemoglobin concentration; MCV, mean cell volume; RBC, red blood cell count

debris does not affect the reading. Erroneous results from hyperlipidaemia may be suspected when red cell indices are improbable or red cells on stained blood films have fuzzy outlines. This error can be confirmed by examining the plasma, after either centrifugation or red cell sedimentation, and noting the milky appearance. The problem can be dealt with by performing a microhaematocrit and a 'blank' measurement using the patient's plasma. A correction is then as follows:

$$\text{true Hb} = \text{measured Hb} - ['Hb' \text{ of lipaemic plasma} \times (1 - \text{Hct})]$$

Alternatively, the plasma can be carefully removed and replaced by an equal volume of isotonic fluid before repeating the automated count. Similarly, the use of a plasma blank permits the correction of errors caused by the presence of a paraprotein or polyclonal hyper-gammaglobulinaemia (Table 4.9). With the Bayer H.1 series and Advia 120 instruments, a correct Hb can be calculated from the CHCM and a microhaematocrit when there is lipid or other interfering substance in the plasma. The errors introduced into the Hb estimation by

marked hyperbilirubinaemia and the presence of high levels of carboxyhaemoglobin are not of such magnitude as to be of practical importance and can therefore be ignored.

A falsely low Hb is a much less frequent observation than a falsely high estimate, but has been reported with a Bayer H.2 instrument in three patients with a very

Table 4.9 Erroneous estimates of haemoglobin on Coulter Gen S counter caused by a paraprotein.

	FBC on whole blood	'FBC' of EDTA-plasma	FBC on washed and resuspended red cells
RBC ($\times 10^{-12}$/l)	2.68	0.02	2.62
Hb (g/l)	101	17	82
MCV (fl)	94.3	88.2	95.5
MCH (pg)	37.6	++++	31.4
MCHC (g/l)	399	++++	329

EDTA, ethylenediaminetetra-acetic acid; FBC, full blood count; Hb, haemoglobin concentration; MCH, mean cell haemoglobin; MCHC, mean cell haemoglobin concentration; MCV, mean cell volume; RBC, red blood cell count; ++++, no result produced high WBC (243, 348 and 850×10^9/l) [30]. There was an associated factitious reduction of the MCHC leading to a discrepancy between the MCHC (calculated from the Hb) and the CHCM (measured directly). An unstable colour reaction was postulated as the cause of this observation. Sulphaemoglobinaemia has been reported to lower the estimate of Hb [12]. Increased blood viscosity, e.g. due to the presence of a cold agglutinin or a cryoglobulin, can lead to incomplete aspiration and some reduction of the Hb and RBC [12].

RBC, MCV and Hct

Errors in the RBC, MCV and Hct are summarised in Table 4.7. Impedance and earlier light-scattering instruments have an intrinsic error that leads to the MCV of hypochromic cells being underestimated and their MCHC being overestimated. This can also lead to two apparent populations on a red cell size histogram with blood samples that, on Bayer H.1 and Advia series instruments, show a single population of cells on a histogram of red cell size but two populations on a histogram of red cell haemoglobinisation.

Storage of blood at room temperature may cause errors in the MCV and Hct. Coulter instruments usually give stable measurements unless blood has been stored for several days, but a 6 fl rise by 24 hours has been observed with another impedance counter, the Sysmex NE-8000 [31]. With the Abbott Cell-Dyn 2500 a rise of 2–3 fl by 24 hours was observed [13]. The MCV on the Cobas Argos 5 Diff rises by about 2 fl by 24 hours [32]. Marked changes are seen with Bayer H.1 series instruments (and it is likely that they also occur with the Advia series); a rise in the MCV starts after about 8 hours and by 24 hours the average rise varies between 4–5 and 7–8 fl, depending on the ambient temperature. A low MCHC, without any corresponding hypochromia being detectable on a blood film, can indicate that an elevation in the MCV is caused by red cell swelling as a result of storage. A factitious rise in the Hct occurs in parallel with the rise in the MCV.

When blood samples are processed without delay, errors in the RBC, MCV and Hct (excluding those that are intrinsic to the methodology) are most often caused by cold agglutinins. Impedance counters are prone to more major errors for this reason than are current Siemens light-scattering instruments. The factitious elevation of MCV is consequent on the doublets and triplets that pass through the aperture being counted and sized as if they were single cells. The RBC is factitiously low both for this reason and because, with some counters, larger agglutinates are above the upper threshold for red cells and are excluded from the count. The size of doublets and triplets is also underestimated. For these reasons, although MCV (Hct × 1000/RBC) is overestimated, Hct is underestimated. The underestimation of Hct means that there is a factitious elevation of mean cell haemoglobin (MCH) and MCHC. Erroneous counts can generally be eliminated by warming the sample before processing. When the cold agglutinin is very potent, it may be necessary both to warm the blood specimen and to predilute the sample for analysis in warmed diluent.

Other causes of factitious errors in the RBC, MCV and Hct are uncommon. Various changes in plasma osmolality lead to artefacts in MCV measurement by impedance counters. If a cell is in a hyperosmolar environment *in vivo* due, for example, to severe hypernatraemia or severe hyperglycaemia, then the cytoplasm of the cell will also be hyperosmolar. When the blood is diluted within the automated counter in a medium of much lower osmolality, the more rapid movement of water than of electrolytes, glucose or urea across the cell membrane will lead to acute swelling of the cell, which will be reflected in the measured MCV. Since the Hct is calculated from the MCV it will also be increased, whereas the MCHC will be correspondingly reduced. This phenomenon may occur in hypernatraemic dehydration [33], severe uraemia [26] and hyperglycaemia, e.g. due to uncontrolled diabetes mellitus [34]. Not only may factitious macrocytosis be produced, but true microcytosis may be masked. The converse error of a falsely low MCV and Hct with elevation of the MCHC may be seen in patients with hyponatraemia [33] such as may be seen in chronic alcoholics and patients with inappropriate secretion of antidiuretic hormone. The factitious reduction of MCV in hypo-osmolar states can lead to masking of a true macrocytosis as well as factitious microcytosis. This error can be eliminated in instruments with a predilute mode by diluting the sample and allowing time for equilibration of solutes across the red cell membrane. A control sample should be prediluted and tested in parallel since, although the osmolality of the recommended diluent differs between instruments, it is often somewhat hypertonic so that the MCV of cells from normal subjects may also alter on predilution.

With the Bayer H.1 series of instruments, factitious macrocytosis can result from cell swelling that is induced by taking a small volume of blood into excess K_2EDTA. A hypochromia 'flag' also occurs [35].

If microcytosis is severe, some red cells may fall below the lower threshold of the instrument and, as these cells are excluded from the measurements, the MCV is overestimated. In the case of impedance counters this is usually more than counteracted by the fact that the cells are likely to be hypochromic and the inherent error of the methodology leads to the size of those cells that fall above the threshold being underestimated. If there are normochromic red cell fragments falling below the lower threshold, the MCV will be overestimated without any counterbalancing effect being expected. Neither of these artefacts is of practical importance.

Inaccuracies in the Hct are those expected from inaccuracies in the RBC and MCV.

MCH, MCHC and RDW

Errors that may occur in the MCH and MCHC are summarised in Table 4.8. Errors in these variables are consequent on errors in the primary measurements from which they are derived. Mechanisms have been explained above. The inherent error of impedance counting leads to the MCHC being a very stable variable that fails to reflect the true changes occurring in red cells. This is paradoxically useful, since abnormalities of the MCHC are commonly factitious and therefore serve to alert the laboratory scientist to the possibility of an erroneous result. In the case of Bayer/Siemens instruments, true abnormality of the MCHC is more common, but so is a factitious

reduction resulting from swelling of cells as blood ages. A discrepancy between MCHC and CHCM serves as a flag since the latter variable is measured directly and thus is not affected by errors in Hb estimation.

With Coulter instruments, and probably with others, the RDW (red cell distribution width) rises with room-temperature storage. In the case of the Coulter Gen S, the rise starts from day 2 [36].

Errors in platelet counts

The causes of erroneous platelet counts are summarised in Tables 4.10 and 4.11. Many instruments are inaccurate in the measurement of low platelet counts. A small inaccuracy can be clinically significant when a platelet count of $10 \times 10^9/l$ is used as a trigger for platelet transfusion, e.g. in patients with acute leukaemia. In one study, one immunological method (Cell-Dyn) and one optical method (XE-2100) were accurate, whereas another impedance method (LH750) and four optical methods (H.3, Advia, Cell-Dyn and XE-2100) overestimated by $2-5 \times 10^9/l$ [53]. The Pentra 120 impedance method underestimated by about $4 \times 10^9/l$. Impedance counts (manufacturer not specified) have been found to underestimate platelet counts in comparison with flow cytometry immunofluorescence counts in patients with autoimmune thrombocytopenia purpura [54], whereas in patients with leukaemia and lymphoma it is possible that there is overestimation. A comparison of four instru-

Table 4.10 Some causes of falsely low automated platelet counts.

Cause	Instrument on which observed
Partial clotting of specimen	All instruments
Activation of platelets during venepuncture with consequent aggregation	All instruments
Activation of platelets during cardiopulmonary bypass [37]	All instruments
EDTA-induced platelet aggregation (appears to be more common in viral infections, particularly hepatitis A, but also cytomegalovirus and influenza A) [38]	All instruments
EDTA-induced platelet degranulation and swelling	Coulter STKS [39]
Lipiodol-induced platelet clumping following chemoembolisation	Reported for Sysmex XE-2100 but likely with all instruments [8]
Platelet satellitism	All instruments
Platelet phagocytosis by neutrophils and monocytes	Observed with Cell-Dyn 3500 but would be expected to occur with all instruments [5]
Storage of blood at 4°C for more than 24 hours	Horiba instruments
Giant platelets falling above upper threshold for platelet count	All instruments
Heparin addition to blood sample in patient with antibodies to heparin-platelet factor 4 [40]	

EDTA, ethylenediaminetetra-acetic acid

Table 4.11 Some causes of falsely high automated platelet counts.

Cause	Instrument on which observed
Microcytic red cells or red cell fragments falling below upper threshold for the platelet count	All instruments
Microspherocytes in hereditary spherocytosis	Coulter MAXM [41]
Microspherocytes in burns	Coulter instruments [42,43]
Inadvertent heating of blood sample	Bayer H.1 series [3]
White cell fragments counted as platelets (fragments of leukaemic blast cells, hairy cells or lymphoma cells)	All instruments
Haemoglobin H disease	Coulter instruments
Cryoglobulin*	Coulter instruments, Bayer H.1 series, Cell-Dyn 4000 (impedance count inaccurate; optical count accurate) [44]
Hypertriglyceridaemia or hyperlipidaemia	Sysmex NE-8000, Bayer H.1 series [20,45], impedance counters
Use of perfluorocarbon emulsions (blood substitute)	Cell-Dyn 3200 and 3500 (both optical and impedance counts affected) [46]
Bacteria in blood sample, either in patients with bacteraemia [47,48] or due to delay in processing in a hot climate [49]	Ortho ELT8 [47], Cell-Dyn 4000 [48]
Fungi such as candida species in blood sample, often from fungal growth on indwelling intravenous line	Bayer H.1 [50] and Advia series, Sysmex XT 2000i [9]
Candida glabrata and *Candida parapsilosis* (but not *Candida albicans*)	Siemens Advia series [10]
Parasitised red cells in malaria	Cell-Dyn 4000, optical and impedance channels [51]
Non-platelet particles in platelet concentrates	Sysmex XE-2100 and Advia 120 optical counts but not Sysmex impedance counts [52]

*Platelet count and histograms of platelet size became normal on warming the blood

ments in patients with acute leukaemia or suspected disseminated intravascular coagulation found a good correlation with the international reference method, but the Cell-Dyn Sapphire, Sysmex XE-2100 and Beckman-Coulter LH 750 all tended to underestimate the counts; only the Advia 2120 did not [55]. Erroneous counts were found to be more common when there was evidence of platelet activation, which causes loss of granules and sphering of platelets [55]. In addition to these errors, intrinsic to the technology, major errors in the platelet count can result from characteristics of the blood sample. Factitiously low platelet counts are quite common as a result either of partial clotting of the specimen or of platelet aggregation or satellitism. Platelet aggregation may be due to activation of platelets during a difficult venepuncture or may be mediated by an antibody, which is either an immunoglobulin (Ig) G or IgM EDTA-dependent antibody or an EDTA-independent antibody. IgG-dependent platelet antibodies are directed at a crypto-antigen on platelet glycoprotein IIb [56]. EDTA-dependent platelet aggregation can be a transient phenomenon, e.g. occurring during infectious mononucleosis [57]. Platelet aggregation often leads to

instrument flags, abnormal histograms of platelet distribution and abnormal white cell scatter plots. Abnormal white cell scatter plots can lead to the flagging of erroneous platelet counts that are not detected in the platelet channel; instruments that incorporate an automated differential count are more likely to flag erroneous platelet counts than instruments without this capacity. Platelet satellitism is also an antibody-mediated EDTA-dependent phenomenon, which may be followed by phagocytosis of platelets [58]. Neither *in vitro* aggregation nor platelet satellitism is of any significance *in vivo*, but the detection of all factitiously low platelet counts is very important in order to avoid unnecessary investigation and treatment of the patient. There have been instances in which a factitiously low platelet count has led to a mistaken diagnosis of 'idiopathic' (i.e. autoimmune) thrombocytopenic purpura (ITP) and consequent corticosteroid treatment and even splenectomy. Accurate platelet counts in subjects with EDTA-dependent platelet aggregation can be achieved by adding 20 mg of kanamycin either to the EDTA into which blood is taken or to the EDTA-anticoagulated blood sample [59], by adding excess EDTA to cause disaggregation or by using $MgSO_4$ as an anticoagulant [60].

Alternatively, blood can be taken into sodium citrate or a finger-prick sample can be collected using an alternative anticoagulant, e.g. ammonium oxalate.

The accuracy of any unexpectedly low platelet counts must always be confirmed. The specimen should be examined with an orange stick to detect any small clots or fibrin strands and the instrument histograms and scatter plots should be assessed. Some instruments are able to detect fibrin strands or small clots and flag their presence. The presence of platelet aggregates may also be flagged and an abnormal cluster or band of particles may be apparent in scattergrams. The presence of an abnormal cluster along the top of the neutrophil box with the Bayer H.1 series instruments may indicate the occurrence of platelet satellitism. However, not all falsely low platelet counts are flagged or associated with abnormal scattergrams. For example, platelet aggregates may be so large that they are the same size as white cells and are thus not identified. It is therefore important to examine a blood film for the presence of fibrin strands, platelet aggregates, platelet satellitism and giant platelets whenever a platelet count is unexpectedly low. Falsely low counts should be deleted from reports, since clinical staff often do not realise that a comment such as 'platelet aggregates' is likely to mean that the platelet count is wrong; ill-advised platelet transfusions have been given for this reason. When platelet aggregation is antibody-mediated, accurate counts can usually be obtained on specimens taken into citrate or heparin rather than EDTA (but the effect of dilution must be allowed for). Some such antibodies are cold antibodies, so performing a count rapidly on a specimen that has been kept warm can also produce a valid count. Alternatively, if the platelet count is clearly normal, the comment 'platelet count normal on film' may be acceptable and obviate the need to obtain a further blood specimen. However, when platelet aggregation occurs in patients being managed for essential thrombocythaemia, appropriate measures must be taken to achieve an accurate count and permit monitoring [61]. Laboratories should be alert to platelet aggregation induced by therapy with monoclonal antibodies, such as abciximab, directed at platelet antigens, since these agents may also cause true thrombocytopenia [62,63].

It may be impossible to obtain an accurate automated platelet count in the presence of numerous giant platelets, in which case a haemocytometer count is required. Alternatively, the platelet:red cell ratio can be determined from a blood film and the platelet count can be calculated from the RBC. If a low platelet count is supported by the blood film, but is nevertheless unexpected, a repeat specimen should be obtained with careful attention to venepuncture technique before the count is regarded as a valid result on which management decisions should be based.

Falsely elevated platelet counts are much less common than falsely reduced counts. They are usually due to the presence of marked microcytosis (e.g. in haemoglobin H disease) or to the presence of red cell fragments (e.g. in microangiopathic haemolytic anaemia, severe burns or hereditary pyropoikilocytosis), so that a significant number of red cells fall below the upper threshold for platelets. Factitious elevation of the platelet count can also be produced by red cell fragmentation produced *in vitro* by inadvertent heating of a blood sample [3]. Even with variable thresholds and fitted curves, it may not be possible to separate very small red cells or fragments from platelets. An accurate platelet count despite the presence of red cell fragments or microcytes can be produced by a Sysmex R-1000 Reticulocyte Analyzer. The ribonucleic acid (RNA) of both platelets and reticulocytes is stained with the fluorescent dye auramine, and the two populations are then separated by gating [64]. Microcytic red cells do not take up the dye since they do not contain RNA.

Occasionally, falsely elevated platelet counts are caused by other particles of a similar size to platelets. The counting of fragments of white cell cytoplasm as platelets has been described in acute myeloid leukaemia [65,66] (Fig. 4.2), acute lymphoblastic leukaemia [66], hairy cell leukaemia [67] and lymphoma [68]. In patients with acute leukaemia this phenomenon is actually quite common [66]. The counting of red and white cell fragments [69] or extraneous particles such as fungi [50] (Fig. 4.3) as platelets may have serious implications in acute leukaemia as a severe thrombocytopenia may be masked and left untreated.

When platelets are distributed evenly in a blood film, the platelet count can be validated by counting the ratio of platelets to red cells and calculating the platelet count indirectly from the RBC.

With Coulter instruments, and probably with others, the MPV rises with room-temperature storage of the blood sample. In the case of the Coulter Gen S, the rise starts from day 2 of storage [36]. With the Coulter STKS and the Sysmex SE-9000, an artefactually elevated MPV has been observed as a result of platelet swelling and degranulation in EDTA-anticoagulated blood [39].

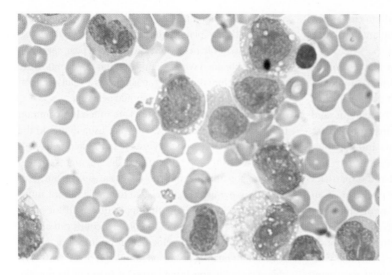

Fig. 4.2 Peripheral blood film of a patient with acute monoblastic leukaemia. Despite only a slight reduction of the 'platelet' count the patient had major bleeding. Inspection of the film showed that there were many fragments of cytoplasm derived from leukaemic cells that were of similar size to platelets and accounted for an erroneous Beckman–Coulter Gen S platelet count.

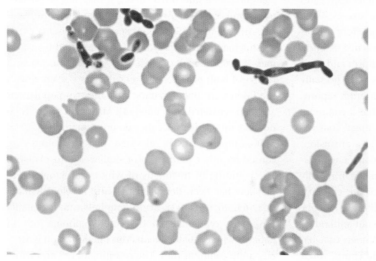

Fig. 4.3 Peripheral blood film of a patient with persistent pancytopenia after intensive chemotherapy for acute myeloid leukaemia. After many weeks of platelet dependency the 'platelet' count suddenly rose. Inspection of the film showed that platelets continued to be very sparse; the particles that were counted as platelets were fungi, subsequently identified as *Candida glabrata*, originating from the patient's indwelling central intravenous line [50].

Errors in automated differential counts

Automated differential counts should be regarded as a means of screening blood samples for an abnormality and producing a differential count when there are only numerical abnormalities. Instruments may show systematic inaccuracies or may be inaccurate only with abnormal specimens of various types.

When mean automated counts for different leucocyte categories are compared with mean manual counts, it is not uncommon for automated instruments to show inaccuracies that are statistically significant but too small to be of practical importance. Even when a discrepancy is larger, it is not necessarily a practical problem as long as

differential counts on patient samples are compared with a carefully derived reference range for the same instrument.

It is often not possible to obtain an accurate automated count on blood specimens with abnormal characteristics, e.g. if there are cells present for which the instrument does not have recognition criteria. The philosophy differs between instrument manufacturers as to whether counts on such samples are usually rejected (STKS and Sysmex NE-8000) or whether a count is usually produced but is flagged (Bayer H.1 series and Cell-Dyn 3000) [70]. A possible disadvantage of the latter policy is that there are some laboratory scientists with an inclination to believe any figure produced by a laboratory instrument, even if it is flagged. However, of more concern is the occurrence of inaccurate counts that are not flagged. All instruments fail to flag some samples containing NRBC, immature granulocytes, atypical lymphocytes and even, occasionally, blast cells.

Storage of blood at room temperature, e.g. during transport from outlying clinics or satellite hospitals, leads to inaccurate measurements, but the time taken for such inaccuracy to occur differs according to the instruments and the cell type. Storage effects are generally greater with impedance counters than with cytochemical light-scattering instruments. The effect of storage is a great deal less if the specimen can be stored at 4°C when any delay in analysis is anticipated.

Two-part and three-part differential counts on impedance-based automated full blood counters

Inevitably, two-part and three-part differential counts do not identify an increase of eosinophils or basophils and two-part differential counts do not identify monocytosis. The loss of clinically useful information is not great since most differential counts are performed to detect abnormalities of neutrophil or lymphocyte counts. The 'monocyte' or 'mononuclear cell' count is also not very accurate since

some eosinophils, basophils and neutrophils are counted in this category [71]. Automated three-part differential counts on Coulter counters and other impedance instruments may be inaccurate within 30 minutes of venesection and become inaccurate again when the blood has been stored at room temperature for more than 6 hours. There is then a fall in the neutrophil count and a rise in the 'mononuclear cell' count, which is progressive with time.

The majority of (but not all) specimens containing NRBC, blast cells, immature granulocytes and atypical lymphocytes are flagged by impedance-based three-part automated differential counters.

Five-to-seven part differential counts
Differential count of Bayer H.1 and Advia series instruments

Since the Bayer H.1 series and Advia series instruments base the differential WBC on peroxidase cytochemistry in addition to light scattering, they can produce erroneous counts as a result of inherited or acquired deficiency of peroxidase in neutrophils, eosinophils or monocytes. Some of the factitious results that have been observed with these instruments are shown in Table 4.12 and illustrated in Figs 4.4–4.11. A systematic underestimation of

Table 4.12 Some causes of inaccurate differential white cell counts on Bayer H.1 series and Siemens Advia series instruments.

Mechanism	Nature of factitious result
Non-lysis of red cells	Elevation of 'lymphocyte' count and reduction of neutrophil count (Fig. 4.4)
Neutrophil peroxidase deficiency; rarely in healthy people, affects only a proportion of the neutrophils [72]	Reduction of neutrophil count; increase of monocyte and LUC counts (Fig. 4.5)
Eosinophil peroxidase deficiency	Reduction of eosinophil count; increase of neutrophil, monocyte or LUC count (Fig. 4.6)
Monocyte peroxidase deficiency	Reduction of monocyte count and increase of LUC count (Fig. 4.7)
Dysplastic monocytes misidentified as neutrophils	Reduction of monocyte count and increase of neutrophil count [73]
Neutrophil cluster misidentified as eosinophils	Reduction of neutrophil count and elevation of eosinophil count (Fig. 4.8)
Leukaemic blasts or maturing cells with strong peroxidase activity misidentified as eosinophils	Increase in eosinophil count [74]
Hypergranular promyelocytes misclassified as eosinophils	Increase in eosinophil count
Eosinophil cluster not recognised, sometimes but not always caused by reduced numbers of granules in eosinophils	Reduction of eosinophil count and elevation of neutrophil count [75]
Large cell residues in basophil channel due to presence of NRBC, blast cells, lymphoma cells, myeloma cells [73] or other abnormal cells or caused by coincidence, presence of heparin or storage of the sample at 4°C [76]	Elevation of 'basophil' count (Figs 4.9 and 4.10)
Contamination of specimen with subcutaneous fat	Elevation of lymphocyte, monocyte and neutrophil counts [1]
Ageing of sample (more than 24 h)	'Left shift' flag

LUC, large unstained cells; NRBC, nucleated red blood cells

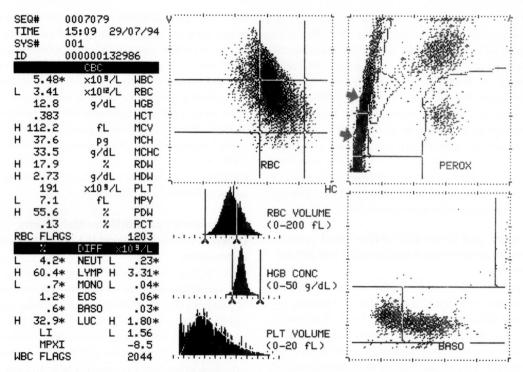

SEQ#	0007079		
TIME	15:09 29/07/94		
SYS#	001		
ID	000000132986		

CBC		
	5.48*	×10⁹/L WBC

Fig. 4.4 Bayer H.2 histograms and scatter plots showing an erroneous differential count caused by failure of lysis of neonatal red cells (green arrows). The peroxidase channel white blood cell count (WBC) of $75.8 \times 10^9/1$ has been rejected in favour of the basophil channel WBC of $5.48 \times 10^9/1$, but the differential count has been derived from the peroxidase channel where many of the non-lysed red cells have been counted as lymphocytes or large unstained cells (LUC). This has led to a factitious neutropenia. The erroneous differential count was flagged. The plots also illustrate the increased size of fetal red cells.

the monocyte count, in comparison with that obtained by flow cytometry with anti-CD14/CD45 monoclonal antibodies, was observed in one study [77]. Storage effects are relatively minor with Bayer H.1 series and Siemens Advia series automated differential counts. On average there is no more than 1–2% change in any category of leucocyte by 72 hours.

Five-part differential counts on Coulter, Sysmex and other instruments

Some systematic inaccuracies in counts have been reported. One study of the Coulter STKS five-part differential [70] found an overestimation of lymphocyte numbers and an underestimation of monocyte numbers. In another study, the STKS gave less accurate granulocyte

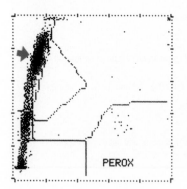

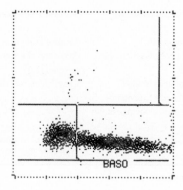

Fig. 4.5 Bayer H.2 white cell scatter plots from a patient with severe neutrophil peroxidase deficiency leading to an erroneous neutrophil count. Virtually all the neutrophils have been classified as large unstained (i.e. peroxidase-negative) cells (green arrow) and the neutrophil count was zero. The basophil lobularity channel, however, shows a normal number of granulocytes.

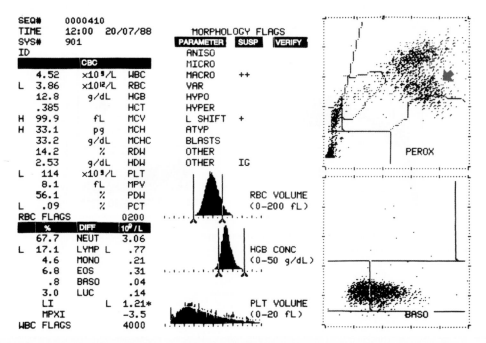

```
SEQ#      0000410
TIME      12:00  20/07/88        MORPHOLOGY FLAGS
SYS#      901              PARAMETER  SUSP  VERIFY
ID                               ANISO
            CBC                  MICRO
     4.52  x10⁹/L   WBC          MACRO      ++
L    3.86  x10¹²/L  RBC          VAR
    12.8   g/dL     HGB          HYPO
     .385           HCT          HYPER
H   99.9   fL       MCV          L SHIFT    +
H   33.1   pg       MCH          ATYP
    33.2   g/dL     MCHC         BLASTS
    14.2   %        RDW          OTHER
     2.53  g/dL     HDW          OTHER      IG
L    114   x10⁹/L   PLT
     8.1   fL       MPV
    56.1   %        PDW
L    .09   %        PCT
RBC FLAGS          0200
      %      DIFF   10⁹/L
    67.7   NEUT     3.06
L   17.1   LYMP  L  .77
     4.6   MONO     .21
     6.8   EOS      .31
      .8   BASO     .04
     3.0   LUC      .14
    LI          L  1.21*
    MPXI          -3.5
WBC FLAGS          4000
```

RBC VOLUME
(0–200 fL)

HGB CONC
(0–50 g/dL)

PLT VOLUME
(0–20 fL)

PEROX

BASO

Fig. 4.6 Bayer H.2 white cell scatter plots from a patient with partial eosinophil peroxidase deficiency showing an eosinophil cluster (green arrow) that has not been recognised. About two-thirds of the eosinophils have been classified as neutrophils.

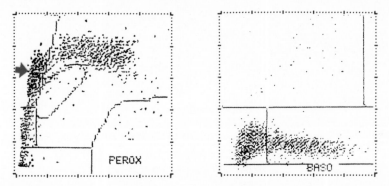

Fig. 4.7 Bayer H.2 white cell scatter plots from a healthy subject with monocyte peroxidase deficiency causing an erroneous monocyte count. Almost all the monocytes have been counted as LUC (green arrow). The automated monocyte count was $0.09 \times 10^9/l$ while the manual count was $0.5 \times 10^9/l$.

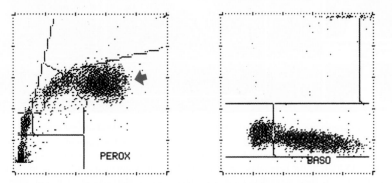

Fig. 4.8 Bayer H.1 white cell scatter plots showing neutrophils that have caused less forward light scatter than normal (green arrow) and have been misclassified as eosinophils.

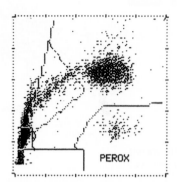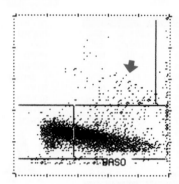

Fig. 4.9 Bayer H.2 white cell scatter plots from a patient with follicular lymphoma showing pseudobasophilia as a consequence of lymphoma cells (green arrow) being misclassified as basophils.

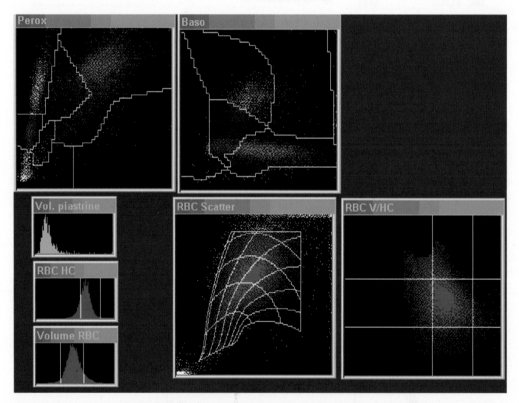

Fig. 4.10 Scatter plots and histograms produced by the Siemens Advia 120 on a blood sample from a patient with diffuse large B-cell lymphoma showing pseudobasophilia as a result of circulating lymphoma cells. The basophil/lobularity channel (centre top) shows an abnormal compact cluster of signals that extends from the mononuclear area (blue) to the basophil area (yellow); the 'basophil' count was 0.95×10^9/l (15.9%). In the peroxidase channel (top left) the lymphoma cells appear in the LUC area (turquoise); the count was 1.41×10^9/l (23.5%). There were flags for atypical lymphocytes, blast cells and left shift. Other abnormalities shown by the red cell histograms and cytograms are an increase of hypochromic cells and of macrocytes, including hypochromic macrocytes. By courtesy of Professor Gina Zini, Rome.

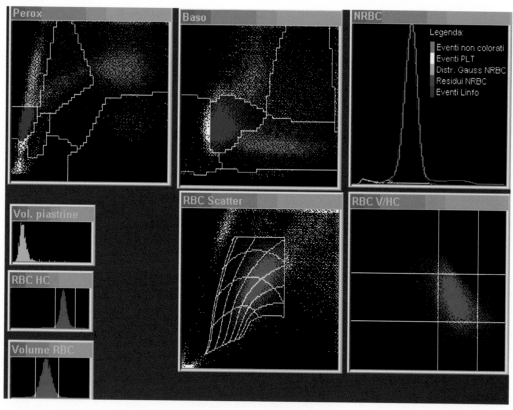

Fig. 4.11 Siemens Advia series cytograms and histograms from a patient with T-lineage non-Hodgkin lymphoma. The full blood count (FBC) showed WBC 74.6 × 10⁹/l, neutrophils 7.23 × 10⁹/l, lymphocytes 58.4 × 10⁹/l, monocytes 1.35 × 10⁹/l, eosinophils 0.2 × 10⁹/l, basophils 2.7 × 10⁹/l, large unstained (i.e. peroxidase-negative) cells 4.7 × 10⁹/l. There were flags for blast cells (+) and atypical lymphocytes (+). The Perox scattergrams show that there is an abnormal population extending from the lymphocyte box into the LUC box. This is a clue to the fact that the basophilia is factitious. The abnormal population can be seen in the Baso scattergram to be extending from the lymphocyte box into the basophil box. By courtesy of Professor Gina Zini.

and lymphocyte counts in patients infected with the human immunodeficiency virus (HIV) than in other subjects [78]; some granulocyte counts were falsely low and lymphocyte counts were more scattered than with a Coulter S Plus IV three-part differential. Cobas instruments have been observed to overestimate monocyte counts [79], whereas the Beckman–Coulter LH750 showed good agreement with the count obtained by flow cytometry with anti-CD14/CD45 monoclonal antibodies [77].

Storage effects differ between instruments. The accuracy of the Coulter STKS differential count shows some deterioration after 6–8 hours of room-temperature storage with a significant fall in the monocyte and eosinophil counts and a rise in the lymphocyte count [80], whereas, as noted above, counts on Bayer instruments are relatively stable. With the Coulter Gen S, there is

a rise in the neutrophil, lymphocyte and eosinophil counts and a fall in the monocyte count, the inaccuracies appearing from days 1 to 2 of room temperature storage [36]. Some Sysmex instruments, e.g. the NE-8000, have shown a marked rise in the monocyte count after 8 hours of room-temperature storage and a rise in the neutrophil count after 24 hours [81]. The Cobas Argos 5 Diff shows a significant rise in the lymphocyte count and a fall in the counts of other types of leucocyte between 6 and 24 hours [82]. The effects of storage may differ for certain types of specimen. A study with the Sysmex NE-8000 counter found that in HIV-positive patients the lymphocyte count fell after 24 hours of room-temperature storage [83].

Blood specimens with abnormal characteristics can give rise to inaccurate counts, as shown in Table 4.13.

Table 4.13 Some causes of inaccurate automated differential white cell counts on impedance and impedance/light-scattering instruments.*

Fault	Effect	Instrument on which observed
Some or many neutrophils counted as monocytes, particularly after 24 h storage of blood	Falsely high monocyte count and falsely low neutrophil count	Sysmex NE-1500 and NE-8000 [84,85]
Storage effects at room temperature	Falsely low neutrophil and monocyte counts, falsely high lymphocyte counts after 24 h at room temperature	Abbott Cell-Dyn 3500 [13]
	Falsely low neutrophil count and falsely high lymphocyte count after more than 18 h storage	Coulter STKS [86]
		Sysmex NE 1500 and NE 8000 (see above)
	Falsely low neutrophil count and falsely high monocyte count	
	Lymphocyte count rises significantly with less than 24 h storage and eosinophil count falls	Cobas Argos 5 Diff [82]
Neutrophil aggregation	Falsely low WBC and neutrophil percentage, falsely high lymphocyte percentage	All instruments
Lymphocyte aggregation	Falsely high neutrophil percentage	Coulter STKS [87]
Non-lysis of red cells	Falsely high WBC and lymphocyte count	
Neonatal red cells		Coulter STKS [88]
Hyperlipidaemia		Coulter STKS
Abnormal haemoglobins (e.g. C, S, D, G)		Sysmex NE-8000
Obstructive jaundice		Sysmex NE-8000
Myelodysplastic syndrome		Coulter STKS
Malaria parasites	Falsely high lymphocyte and monocyte counts	Sysmex NE-8000
Malaria (*P. vivax* more often than *P. falciparum*)	Pseudoeosinophilia	Sysmex XE-2100 [89]
Malaria (neutrophils containing malaria pigment counted as eosinophils; rarely pigment-containing parasites in non-lysed red cells similarly counted)	Falsely high eosinophil count and falsely low neutrophil counts as malarial pigment polarises light	Cell-Dyn 3500 [90,91]
Plasma interference	Falsely high eosinophil count	Coulter STKS [80]
Neutrophils containing haemosiderin counted as eosinophils	Falsely high eosinophil count and falsely low neutrophil count	Cell-Dyn CD3700 [92]
Hypogranular eosinophils counted as neutrophils	Falsely low eosinophil count; falsely high neutrophil count	Sysmex NE-8000 [75]
		Coulter STKS [93]
Hypogranular or hypolobated neutrophils counted as lymphocytes	Falsely low neutrophil count	Horiba instruments
Hypogranular neutrophils counted as monocytes	Falsely low neutrophil count and falsely high monocyte count	Sysmex XE-2100 [94]
Other cells counted as basophils	Falsely high basophil count (pseudobasophilia)	
Abnormal lymphocytes in HIV-infected subjects		Coulter STKS [95]
Type of cell not specified		Coulter STKS [80]
Myeloblasts		Sysmex NE-8000 [96]
Promyelocytes in acute promyelocytic leukaemia		Sysmex NE-8000 [97]
Various abnormal cells		Cell-Dyn 3000 [98]
Lymphoblasts and myeloblasts		Coulter STKS [99]
Dysplastic neutrophils		Coulter STKS [73]
Atypical lymphocytes, lymphoma cells, myeloblasts, leukaemic promyelocytes		Horiba instruments
Atypical lymphocytes		Sysmex XE-2100 and XE-2100D [100]
Maroteaux–Lamy syndrome neutrophils		Sysmex XE-2100 [101]

Fault	Effect	Instrument on which observed
Fault	**Effect**	**Instrument on which observed**
Basophils counted as lymphocytes in some cases of CML	Falsely low basophil count	Coulter STKS [80]
Various abnormal cells counted as monocytes–lymphocytes in chronic lymphocytic leukaemia, lymphoma cells, myeloblasts, lymphoblasts and hypergranular promyelocytes	Falsely high monocyte count	Horiba instruments
Lymphocytes of infectious mononucleosis		Coulter STKS and Sysmex NE-8000 [102]
Myeloma cells		Sysmex SE-9000 [73]
Neutrophils in patients with left shift		Horiba instruments
Poor separation of leucocyte clusters	Some eosinophils sometimes counted as neutrophils, some neutrophils sometimes counted as monocytes, pseudobasophilia	Coulter STKS [82,103]
Giant platelets counted as lymphocytes	Falsely high lymphocyte count	Coulter STKS [103]
Nucleated red blood cells counted as lymphocytes	Falsely high lymphocyte count	Horiba instruments
Intravenous lipid infusion causing alterations in cells	Neutrophil count reduced, monocyte count increased	Coulter LH 750 [104]

* This list of errors should not be regarded as exhaustive.

CML, chronic myelogenous leukaemia; HIV, human immunodeficiency virus; WBC, white blood cell count

Errors in automated reticulocyte counts and other reticulocyte measurements

Automated reticulocyte counts may be falsely elevated when there is autofluorescence or when fluorescence is produced by binding of the fluorochrome to something other than the RNA of reticulocytes, usually deoxyribonucleic acid (DNA) or RNA in other cells. Less information is available on erroneous counts with non-fluorescent nucleic acid stains. However, a tendency to underestimate the reticulocyte count with technology based on New Methylene Blue staining has been noted in haemoglobin H disease [105] and a factitious elevation was found in the presence of a high NRBC count, using an oxazine 750 method [106]. With the New Methylene Blue method, factitiously elevated counts were also observed in some samples, but only when a longer than recommended period of incubation was used [105]. Some known causes of falsely elevated reticulocyte counts are shown in Table 4.14. Inaccuracy of reticulocyte counts in the presence of nucleated red cells is method dependent, in one study being more likely with the XE-2100 than with the Pentra 120 Retic

Table 4.14 Some causes of falsely elevated automated reticulocyte counts.

Increased autofluorescence
Neonatal samples and post-splenectomy [107]
Heinz bodies [108]
Binding of fluorescent dye to something other than RNA of reticulocytes
High WBC or NRBC count and/or abnormal leucocytes, e.g. in chronic lymphocytic leukaemia [109], acute myeloid leukaemia [110], acute biphenotypic leukaemia [110] and chronic myelogenous leukaemia (chronic phase or blast crisis) [110]
Howell–Jolly bodies [111]
Irreversibly sickled cells [104]
Cold agglutinins [107]
Large platelets [107]
Malaria parasites [112]
Babesia parasites
Heinz bodies [113]
Autofluorescence due to porphyria or drugs [12]
Binding of non-fluorescent dye to something other than RNA of reticulocytes
NRBC [106]
Microcytic red cells [114]

NRBC, nucleated red blood cells; RNA, ribonucleic acid; WBC, white blood cell count

[115]. Malarial parasites within red cells may lead to a bimodal reticulocyte histogram, suggesting this diagnosis [116,117]. In the presence of malaria parasites there is also a factitious elevation of the immature reticulocyte fraction [117].

Erroneously low reticulocyte counts have been observed if blood is obtained from a patient after fluorescent retinal angiography has been performed [118].

Quantification of high fluorescence reticulocytes is affected by the presence of white cells and is likely to be erroneous when the white cell count is elevated [119].

Reticulocyte indices may be inaccurate when large platelets are present [120].

A factitiously elevated reticulocyte count may be associated with a factitiously elevated immature reticulocyte fraction [110].

TEST YOUR KNOWLEDGE

Visit the companion website for MCQs and EMQs on this topic:
www.wiley.com/go/bain/bloodcells

References

1 Whiteway A and Bain BJ (1999) Artefactual elevation of an automated white cell count following femoral vein puncture. *Clin Lab Haematol*, **21**, 65–68.

2 Hohlfeld P, Forestier F, Kaplan C, Tissot JD and Daffos F (1994) Fetal thrombocytopenia: a retrospective survey of 5,194 fetal blood samplings. *Blood*, **84**, 1851–1856.

3 Bain BJ and Liesner R (1996) Pseudopyropoikilocytosis: a striking artefact. *J Clin Pathol*, **49**, 772–773.

4 Cornet E, Behier C and Troussard X (2012) Guidance for storing blood samples in laboratories performing complete blood count with differential. *Int J Lab Hematol*, **34**, 655–660.

5 Criswell KA, Breider MA and Bleavins MR (2001) EDTA-dependent platelet phagocytosis: a cytochemical, ultrastructural, and functional characterization. *Am J Clin Pathol*, **115**, 376–384.

6 Fohlen-Walter A, Jacob C, Lecompte T and Lesesve J-F (2002) Laboratory identification of cryoglobulinemia from automated blood cell counts, fresh blood samples, and blood films. *Am J Clin Pathol*, **117**, 606–614.

7 Machicao CN, Schaub CR and Farhi DC (1988) Circulating mucin in breast carcinoma and automated leukocyte counts. *Hematol Pathol*, **2**, 159–161.

8 Todd A, Pardoe L and O'Brian R (2010) Unexpected blood abnormalities following chemoembolisation. *Br J Haematol*, **150**, 500.

9 Lesesve JF, Khalifa MA, Denoyes R and Braun F (2009) Peripheral blood candidosis infection leading to spurious platelet and white blood cell counts. *Int J Lab Hematol*, **31**, 572–576.

10 Branda JA and Kratz A (2006) Effects of yeast on automated cell counting. *Am J Clin Pathol*, **126**, 248–254.

11 Kim HR, Park BRG and Lee MK (2008) Effects of bacteria and yeast on WBC counting in three automated hematology counters. *Ann Hematol*, **87**, 557–562.

12 Zandecki M, Genevieve F, Gerard J and Godon A (2007) Spurious counts and spurious results on haematology analysers: a review. Part II: white blood cells, red blood cells, haemoglobin, red cell indices and reticulocytes. *Int J Lab Hematol*, **1**, 21–41.

13 Wood BL, Andrews J, Miller S and Sabath DE (1999) Refrigerated storage improves the stability of the complete blood count and automated differential. *Am J Clin Pathol*, **112**, 687–695.

14 Brigden Ml and Dalal BI (1999) Cell counter-related abnormalities. *Lab Med*, **30**, 325–334.

15 Hoffmann EDTA-induced pseudo-neutropenia resolved with kanamycin. *Clin Lab Haematol*, **23**, 193–196.

16 Anonymous (2009) Chemical-associated artifacts. *Blood*, **113**, 4487.

17 Zandecki M, Genevieve F, Gerard J and Godon A (2007) Spurious counts and spurious results on haematology analysers: a review. Part I: platelets. *Int J Lab Hematol*, **1**, 4–20.

18 Bizzaro N (1993) Granulocyte aggregation is edetic acid and temperature dependent. *Arch Pathol Lab Med*, **117**, 528–530.

19 Glasser L (2005) Pseudo-neutropenia secondary to leukoagglutination. *Am J Hematol*, **80**, 147.

20 Grimaldi E and Scopacasa F (2000) Evaluation of the Abbott CELL-DYN 4000 hematology analyzer. *Am J Clin Pathol*, **113**, 497–505.

21 McMullin MF, Wilkin HJ and Elder E (1999) Inaccurate haemoglobin estimation in Waldenström's macroglobulinaemia. *J Clin Pathol*, **48**, 787.

22 Weiss GB and Besman JD (1984) Spurious automated red cell values in warm autoimmune hemolytic anemia. *Am J Hematol*, **17**, 433–435.

23 Vagace JM, Rodriguez MÁ, de la Maya MD and Gervasini G (2013) Ethylenediaminetetraacetic acid-dependent pseudomacrocytosis. *J Clin Pathol*, **66**, 811–814.

24 Paterakis GS, Laoutaris NP, Alexia SV, Siourounis PV, Stamulakatou AK, Premitis EE *et al.* (1993) The effect of red cell shape on the measurement of red cell volume. A proposed method for the comparative assessment of this effect among various haematology analysers. *Clin Lab Haematol*, **16**, 235–245.

25 Bryner MA, Houwen B, Westengard J and Klein O (1997) The spun micro-haematocrit and mean red cell volume are

affected by changes in the oxygenation state of red blood cells. *Clin Lab Haematol*, **19**, 99–103.

26 Ali CYA (2000) Blood substitutes — clinical applications and impact of the laboratory. Paper presented at 24th World Congress of Medical Technology, Vancouver, Canada.

27 Nosanchuk JS, Roark MF and Wanser C (1974) Anemia masked by triglyceridemia. *Am J Clin Pathol*, **62**, 838–839.

28 Miller CE, Hirani B and Bain BJ (2013) Hyperlipidaemia revealed by erythrocyte morphology. *Am J Hematol*, **88**, 625.

29 Nicholls PD (1977) The erroneous haemoglobin-hyperlipidaemia relationship. *J Clin Pathol*, **30**, 638–640.

30 Fohlen-Walter A, Goupil JJ, Lecompte T and Lesesve J-F (2002) Underestimation of haemoglobin concentration in blood samples with high hyperleukocytosis: case report and alternative method for determination on blood cells automated analysers. *Haematologica*, **87**, ELT40.

31 Brigden ML, Page NE and Graydon C (1993) Evaluation of the Sysmex NE-8000 automated hematology analyzer in a high-volume outpatient laboratory. *Am J Clin Pathol*, **100**, 618–625.

32 Lewis SM, Bainbridge I, McTaggart P, Garvey BJ, England JM and Perry TE (1992) *MDD Evaluation Report: Cobas Argos 5 Diff Automated Hematology Analyser*. London: Medical Devices Directorate.

33 Beautyman W and Bills T (1974) Osmotic error in measurements of red cell volume. *Lancet*, **ii**, 905–906.

34 Strauchen JA, Alston W, Anderson J, Gustafson Z and Fajardo LF (1981) Inaccuracy in automated measurement of hematocrit and corpuscular indices in the presence of severe hyperglycemia. *Blood*, **57**, 1065–1067.

35 Hinchliffe RF, Bellamy GJ and Lilleyman JS (1992) Use of the Technicon Hl hypochromia flag in detecting spurious macrocytosis induced by excessive K_2EDTA concentration. *Clin Lab Haematol*, **14**, 268–269.

36 Gulati GL, Hyland LJ, Kocher W and Schwarting R (2002) Changes in automated complete blood cell count and differential leukocyte count results induced by storage of blood at room temperature. *Arch Pathol Lab Med*, **126**, 336–342.

37 Bannister N, Bannister E and Besser M (2011) High incident [sic] of pseudothrombocytopenia after cardio-pulmonary bypass. *Br J Haematol*, **153**, Suppl. 1, 85.

38 Choe W-H, Cho Y-U, Chae J-D and Kim S-H (2013) Pseudothrombocytopenia or platelet clumping as a possible cause of low platelet count in patients with viral infection: a case series from single institution focusing on hepatitis A virus infection. *Int J Lab Hematol*, **35**, 70–76.

39 Lesesve J-F, Latger-Cannard V and Lecompte T (2005) Pseudo-storage pool disease due to platelet degranulation in EDTA-collected peripheral blood: a rare artifact. *Clin Lab Haematol*, **27**, 336–342.

40 Nomoto Y, Hirose Y, Tanaka T, Kinoshita H and Yamazaki Y (2007) Heparin-induced thrombocytopenia, anomalous laboratory findings lead to the correct diagnosis. *Am J Hematol*, **82**, 499–500.

41 Bonifazi F, Stanzani M and Bandini G (1999) A case of pseudothrombocytosis. *Haematologica*, **84**, 275.

42 Savage DG and Kolevska T. Microspherocytosis and pseudothrombocytosis after severe burns. http://www.bloodmed.com/home/slide-popup.asp?id=118 (accessed April 2014).

43 Akwari AM, Ross DW and Stass SA (1982) Spuriously elevated platelet counts due to microspherocytosis. *Am J Clin Pathol*, **77**, 220–221.

44 Delgado J, Jiminez C, Larrocha C and Viloria A (2002) Cryoglobulinemia detected as a PIC/POC discrepancy of the automated complete blood count. *Eur J Haematol*, **69**, 65–66.

45 Kabutomori O, Iwatani Y and Kabutomori M (1999) Effects of hypertriglyceridemia on platelet counts in automated hematologic analysis. *Ann Intern Med*, **130**, 1152.

46 Cuignet OY, Wood BL, Chandler WL and Spiess BD (2000) A second-generation blood substitute (Perfluorodichlorooctane emulsion) generates spurious elevations in platelet counts from automated hematology analyzers. *Anesth Analg*, **90**, 517–522.

47 Gloster ES, Strauss RA, Jimenez JF, Neuberg RW, Berry DH and Turner EJ (1985) Spurious elevated platelet counts associated with bacteremia. *Am J Hematol*, **18**, 329–332.

48 Latif S, Veillon DM, Brown D, Kaltenbach J, Curry S, Linscott AJ *et al.* (2003) Spurious automated platelet count: enumeration of yeast forms as platelets by the Cell-DYN 4000. *Am J Clin Pathol*, **120**, 882–885.

49 Kakkar N (2004) Spurious rise in the automated platelet count because of bacteraemia. *J Clin Pathol*, **57**, 1096–1097.

50 Arnold JA, Jowzi Z and Bain BJ (1999) Images in haematology: *Candida glabrata* in a blood film. *Br J Haematol*, **104**, 1.

51 Crabbe G, van Poucke M and Cantineaux B (2002) Artefactually-normal automated platelet counts due to malaria-infected RBC. *Clin Lab Haematol*, **24**, 179–182.

52 Maurer-Spurej E, Pittendreigh C, Yakimec J, De Badyn MH and Chipperfield K (2010) Erroneous automated optical platelet counts in 1-hour post-transfusion blood samples. *Int J Lab Hematol*, **32**, e1–8.

53 Segal HC, Briggs C, Kunka S, Casbard A, Harrison P, Machin SJ and Murphy MF (2005) Accuracy of platelet counting haematology analysers in severe thrombocytopenia and potential impact on platelet transfusion. *Br J Haematol*, **128**, 520–525.

54 Bowles KM, Bloxham DM, Perry DJ and Baglin TP (2006) Discrepancy between impedance and immunofluorescence platelet counting has implications for clinical decision making in patients with idiopathic thrombocytopenia purpura. *Br J Haematol*, **134**, 320–322.

55 Kim SY, Kim JE, Kim HK, Han KS and Toh CH (2010) Accuracy of platelet counting by automated hematologic analyzers in acute leukemia and disseminated intravascular coagulation: potential effects of platelet activation. *Am J Clin Pathol*, **134**, 634–647.

56 Fiorin F, Steffan A, Pradella P, Bizzaro N, Potenza R and de Angelis V (1998) IgG platelet antibodies in EDTA-dependent pseudothrombocytopenia bind to membrane glycoprotein IIb. *Am J Clin Pathol*, **110**, 178–183.

57 Hsieh AT, Chao TY and Chen YC (2003) Pseudothrombocytopenia associated with infectious mononucleosis. *Arch Pathol Lab Med*, **127**, e17–e18.

58 Campbell V, Fosbury E and Bain BJ (2009) Platelet phagocytosis as a case of pseudothrombocytopenia. *Am J Hematol*, **84**, 362.

59 Sakurai S, Shiojima I, Tanigawa T and Nakahara K (19977) Aminoglycosides prevent and dissociate the aggregation of platelets in patients with EDTA-dependent pseudothrombocytopenia. *Br J Haematol*, **99**, 817–823.

60 Schuff-Werner P, Steiner M, Fenger S, Gross HJ, Bierlich A, Dreissiger K *et al.* (2013) Effective estimation of correct platelet counts in pseudothrombocytopenia using an alternative anticoagulant based on magnesium salt. *Br J Haematol*, **162**, 684–692.

61 Braester A (2003) Pseudothrombocytopenia as a pitfall in the treatment of essential thrombocythemia. *Eur J Haematol*, **70**, 251–252.

62 Stiegler HM, Fischer Y and Steiner S (1999) Thrombocytopenia and glycoprotein IIb-IIIa receptor antagonists. *Lancet*, **353**, 1185.

63 Jubelirer SJ, Koenig BA and Bates MC (1999) Acute profound thrombocytopenia following C7E3 Fab (Abciximab) therapy: case reports, review of the literature and implications for therapy. *Am J Hematol*, **61**, 205–208.

64 Paterakis G, Konstantopoulos K and Loukopoulos D (1994) Spuriously increased platelet count due to microcyte interference: value of the R-1000 (Sysmex) Reticulocyte Analyzer. *Am J Hematol*, **45**, 57–58.

65 Shulman G and Yapit MK (1980) Whole blood platelet counts with impedance type particle counter. *Am J Clin Pathol*, **73**, 104–106.

66 van der Meer W, MacKenzie MA, Dinnissen JWB and de Keijzer MH (2003) Pseudoplatelets: a retrospective study of their incidence and interference with platelet counting. *J Clin Pathol*, **56**, 772–774.

67 Stass SA, Holloway ML, Slease RB and Schumacher HR (1977) Spurious platelet counts in hairy cell leukemia. *Am J Clin Pathol*, **68**, 530–531.

68 Stass SA, Holloway ML, Peterson V, Creegan WJ, Gallivan M and Schumacher HR (1979) Cytoplasmic fragments causing spurious platelet counts in the leukemic phase of poorly differentiated lymphocytic lymphoma. *Am J Clin Pathol*, **71**, 125–128.

69 Hammerstrom J (1992) Spurious platelet counts in acute leukaemia with DIC due to cell fragmentation. *Clin Lab Haematol*, **14**, 239–243.

70 Bentley SA, Johnson A and Bishop CA (1993) A parallel evaluation of four automated hematology analyzers. *Am J Clin Pathol*, **100**, 626–632.

71 Bain BJ (1986) An assessment of the three-population differential count on the Coulter Counter Model S Plus IV. *Clin Lab Haematol*, **8**, 347–359.

72 Hinchliffe R and Vora A (2006) A subject with populations of both peroxidase-positive and -negative neutrophils. *Br J Haematol*, **135**, 421.

73 Hur M, Lee YK, Lee KM, Kim HJ and Cho HI (2004) Pseudobasophilia as an erroneous white blood cell differential count with a discrepancy between automated cell counters: report of two cases. *Clin Lab Haematol*, **26**, 287–290.

74 Merino A and Esteve J (2005) Acute myeloid leukaemia with peculiar blast cell inclusions and pseudo-eosinophilia. *Br J Haematol*, **131**, 286.

75 Kabutomori O and Iwatani Y (1997) Unusual eosinophilia not detected by an automated analyser in a patient with liver cirrhosis. *J Clin Pathol*, **50**, 967–968.

76 Bizzaro N (1996) Pseudobasophilia in the Technicon automated cell counters. *Clin Lab Haematol*, **18**, 298–299.

77 Grimaldi E, Carandente P, Scopacasa F, Romano MF, Pellegrino M, Bisogni R and de Caterina M (2005) Evaluation of the monocyte counting by two automated haematology analysers compared with flow cytometry. *Clin Lab Haematol*, **27**, 91–97.

78 Cohen AI, Peerschkc EIB and Steigbigel RT (1993) A comparison of the Coulter STKS, Coulter S+IV, and manual analysis of white cell differential counts in a human immunodeficiency virus-infected population. *Am J Clin Pathol*, **100**, 611–617.

79 Bentley SA, Johnson TS, Sohier CH and Bishop CA (1994) Flow cytometric differential leucocyte analysis with quantification of neutrophil left shift: an evaluation of the Cobas-Helios Analyzer. *Am J Clin Pathol*, **102**, 223–230.

80 Robertson EP, Lai HW and Wei DCC (1992) An evaluation of leucocyte analysis on the Coulter STKS. *Clin Lab Haematol*, **14**, 53–68.

81 Hu C-Y, Wang C-H, Chuang H-M and Shen M-C (1993) Evaluation of performance for automated differential leucocyte counting on Sysmex NE-8000 by NCCLS recommended protocol H20-T. *Clin Lab Haematol*, **15**, 287–299.

82 Sheridan BL, Lollo M, Howe S and Bergeron N (1994) Evaluation of the Roche Cobas Argos 5 Diff automated haematology analyser with comparison with Coulter STKS. *Clin Lab Haematol*, **16**, 117–130.

83 Koepke JA and Smith-Jones M (1992) Lymphocyte counting in HIV-positive individuals. *Sysmex J Int*, **2**, 71–74.

84 Theodorsen L (1995) Evaluation of monocyte counting with two automated instruments by the use of CD14-specific immunomagnetic Dynabeads. *Clin Lab Haematol*, **17**, 225–229.

85 Bartels PCM and Schoorl M (1998) Time dependent increase of differential monocyte count on the Sysmex NE-2000. *Clin Lab Haematol*, **20**, 165–168.

86 Warner BA and Reardon DM (1991) Field evaluation of the Coulter STKS. *Am J Clin Pathol*, **95**, 207–217.

87 Shelton JB and Frank IN (2000) Splenic B lymphoma with lymphocyte clusters in peripheral blood smears. *J Clin Pathol*, **53**, 228–230.

88 Fournier M, Adenis C, Fontaine H, Camaille B and Goudemand J (1994) Evaluation and use of the white blood cell differential provided by the Coulter STKS in a children's hospital. *Clin Lab Haematol*, **16**, 33–42.

89 Jain M, Gupta S, Jain J and Grover RK (2012) Usefulness of automated cell counter in detection of malaria in a cancer set up—our experience. *Indian J Pathol Microbiol*, **55**, 467–473.

90 Mendelow BV, Lyons C, Nhlangothi P, Tana M, Munster M, Wypkema E *et al.* (1997) Automated malaria ascertainment by depolarization of laser light. *Proceedings of the 37th Annual Congress of the Federation of South African Societies of Pathology*, 145.

91 Hanscheid T, Pinto BG, Cristino JM and Grobusch MP (2000) Malaria diagnosis with the haematology analyser Cell-Dyn 3500™: what does the instrument detect? *Clin Lab Haematol*, **22**, 259–261.

92 Roberts GT, Perry JL, Al-Jefri A and Scott CS (2005) Intraleukocytic hemosiderin inclusions detected as pseudoeosinophils by automated depolarization analysis in a patient with beta-thalassaemia major and immune hemolysis. *Blood Cells Mol Dis*, **34**, 162–165.

93 Kim HJ, Lee YJ, Lee DS and Cho HI (1999) A case of idiopathic hypereosinophilic syndrome with hypersegmented and hypogranular eosinophils. *Clin Lab Haematol*, **21**, 428–430.

94 McIlwaine L, Parker A, Sandilands G, Gallipoli P and Leach M (2013) Neutrophil-specific granule deficiency. *Br J Haematol*, **160**, 735.

95 Germain PR and Lammers DB (1994) False basophil counts on the Coulter STKS. *Lab Med*, **25**, 376–379.

96 Sivakumaran M, Allen B and Wood JK (1994) Automated differential leucocyte counting on the Sysmex NE8000 analyser. *Clin Lab Haematol*, **16**, 206–207.

97 Meyepa LC, Tsoi G and Gan TE (1995) A new approach to the study of the blast suspect flag of the Sysmex NE 8000. *Aust NZ J Med*, **25**, 74.

98 Cornbleet PJ, Myrick D, Judkins S and Levy R (1992) Evaluation of the CELL-DYN 3000 differential. *Am J Clin Pathol*, **98**, 603–614.

99 Pettit AR, Grace P and Chu P (1995) An assessment of the Coulter VCS automated differential counter scatterplots in the recognition of specific acute leukaemia variants. *Clin Lab Haematol*, **17**, 125–129.

100 Jácomo RH, Lozano VF, Gastao da Cunha Neto J and Costa SS (2011) What's the meaning of basophilia in Sysmex XE-2100? *Arch Pathol Lab Med*, **135**, 415.

101 Piva E, Pelloso M, Ciubotaru D, Penello L, Burlina A and Plebani M (2013) The role of automated analyzers in detecting abnormal granulation of leucocytes in lysosomal storage diseases: Maroteaux-Lamy disease. *Am J Hematol*, **88**, 527.

102 Brigden ML, Au S, Thompson S, Brigden S, Doyle P and Tsaparas Y (1999) Infectious mononucleosis in an outpatient population: diagnostic utility of 2 automated hematology analyzers and the sensitivity and specificity of Hoagland's criteria in heterophile-positive patients. *Arch Pathol Lab Med*, **123**, 875–881.

103 Cornbleet PJ, Myrick D and Levy R (1993) Evaluation of the Coulter STKS five-part differential. *Am J Clin Pathol*, **99**, 72–81.

104 Wang J, Fan L, Ma C, Zhang Y and Xu D (2013) Effects of parenteral lipid emulsions on leukocyte numerical and morphological parameters determined by LH750 hematology analyzer. *Int J Lab Hematol*, **35**, e4–e7.

105 Lai SK, Yow CMN and Benzil IFF (1999) Interference of Hb-H disease in automated reticulocyte counting. *Clin Lab Haematol*, **21**, 261–264.

106 Brugnara C, Hipps MJ, Irving PJ, Lathrop H, Lee PA, Minchello EM and Winkelman J (1994) Automated reticulocyte counting and measurement of reticulocyte cellular indices: evaluation of the Miles H3 blood analyzer. *Am J Clin Pathol*, **102**, 623–632.

107 Chin-Yee I, Keeney M and Lohmann RC (1991) Flow cytometric reticulocyte analysis using thiazole orange; clinical experience and technical limitations. *Clin Lab Haematol*, **13**, 177–188.

108 Hinchliffe RF (1993) Error in automated reticulocyte counts due to Heinz bodies. *J Clin Pathol*, **46**, 878–879.

109 Ferguson DJ, Lee S-F and Gordon PA (1990) Evaluation of reticulocyte counts by flow cytometry in a routine laboratory. *Am J Hematol*, **33**, 13–17.

110 Kim A, Park J, Kim M, Lim J, Oh E-J, Kim Y *et al.* (2012) Correction of pseudoreticulocytosis in leukocytosis samples using the Sysmex XE-2100 analyzer depends on the type and number of white blood cells. *Ann Lab Med*, **32**, 392–398.

111 Lofsness KG, Kohnke ML and Geier NA (1994) Evaluation of automated reticulocyte counts and their reliability in the presence of Howell–Jolly bodies. *Am J Clin Pathol*, **101**, 85–90.

112 Hoffman JJML and Pennings JMA (1999) Pseudo-reticulocytosis as a result of malaria parasites. *Clin Lab Haematol*, **21**, 257–260.

113 Español I, Pedro C and Remache AF (1999) Heinz bodies interfere with automated reticulocyte counts. *Haematologica*, **84**, 373–374.

114 Buttarello M, Bulian P, Farina G, Temporin V, Toffolo L, Trabuio E and Rizzotti P (2000) Flow cytometric reticulocyte counting: parallel evaluation of five fully automated analyzers: an NCCLS-ICSH approach. *Am J Clin Pathol*, **115**, 100–111.

115 Briggs C, Grant D and Machin SJ (2001) Comparison of the automated reticulocyte counts and immature reticulocyte fraction measurements obtained with the ABX Pentra 120 Retic blood cell analyzer and the Sysmex XE-2100 automated haematology analyzer. *Lab Haematol*, **7**, 1–6.

116 Mellors I, Hardy J, Lambert J, Kendall R and McArdle B (2001) Detection of intra-erythrocyte malarial parasites by an automated haematology analyser — a case study. *Br J Haematol*, **113**, Suppl. 1, 50.

117 Scott CS, van Zyl D, Ho E, Ruivo L, Kunz D and Coetzer TL (2002) Patterns of pseudo-reticulocytosis in malaria: fluorescent analysis with the Cell-Dyn® CD4000. *Clin Lab Haematol*, **24**, 15–20.

118 Hirata R, Morita Y, Hirai N, Seki M, Imanishi A, Toriumi J *et al.* (1992) The effects of fluorescent substances on the measurement of reticulocytes—using automated reticulocyte analyzers R-1000 and R-3000. *Sysmex J Int*, **2**, 10–15.

119 Villamor N, Kirsch A, Huhn D, Vives-Corrons JL and Serke S (1996) Interference of blood leucocytes in the measurements of immature red cells (reticulocytes) by two different (semi-) automated flow-cytometry technologies. *Clin Lab Haematol*, **18**, 89–94.

120 Bowen D, Williams K, Phillips I and Cavill I (1996) Cytometric analysis and maturation characteristics of reticulocytes from myelodysplastic patients. *Clin Lab Haematol*, **18**, 155–160.

CHAPTER 5

Normal ranges

The interpretation of any laboratory test result requires assessment as to whether or not the result is normal. 'Normal' means that the results are those expected in that individual when in a state of optimal health (assuming that the person does not have any inherited disorder affecting the blood). Since one rarely has the information to make this assessment, it is necessary instead to consider whether the result is what would be expected in a healthy subject as biologically similar to the particular individual as possible. Test results are conventionally compared with normal ranges, such ranges often being derived from textbooks and sometimes being of obscure origin. More recently, test results have been compared with reference ranges. The concepts underlying the derivation of a reference range are as follows.

A reference individual is one selected using defined criteria and coming from a population that includes all individuals who meet those criteria. A reference sample is a number of reference individuals chosen to represent the reference population. Reference values are test results derived from the reference individuals and can be analysed and statistically described: they will fall within certain limits; and they will have a certain distribution with a mean, a median and a mode. The usual method of describing a collection of reference values is in terms of the reference limits that exclude 2.5% of the values at either end of the observed range, i.e. the reference interval represents the central 95% of the observed values. Such a reference interval derived from the sample individuals will be representative of the reference interval of the population from which it is derived; the closeness of fit of the two intervals can be represented by the confidence limits of the mean and each of the reference limits. Closeness of fit is determined by the size of the sample and by whether the reference individuals have been chosen from the reference population in a way that is free of bias. Reference individuals can be derived from the reference population by random sampling or carefully selected to reflect the mix of age, gender, social class and other variables in the reference population. Reference intervals are commonly referred to as 'reference ranges', a readily understandable term although it is not officially recommended.

A reference individual is not necessarily healthy, but if a good state of health is included as a criterion for selection, then it is clear that the reference interval may be very similar to a traditional 'normal range', although more carefully defined.

If reference ranges are to be useful in assessing haematology results, they should take account of whether test results are influenced by age, gender or ethnic origin and separate ranges should be derived when necessary. Pregnant women would normally be excluded unless one is deriving a range for application during pregnancy. Reference ranges are often derived from test results obtained in carefully controlled conditions with fasting and rested subjects who have abstained from alcohol, cigarettes and drugs and whose blood specimens are taken at a defined time of day. Such conditions are not often met by patient populations and it may be more useful to use ambulant, non-fasting individuals whose habits reflect those of the population from which they and the patients are drawn. The site of blood sampling and other variations in the technique of obtaining a blood sample affect results of haematological tests (Table 5.1). For this reason, blood specimens should be taken in the same manner and using the same anticoagulant (dry or liquid) as in the patient population.

Establishing reference ranges on a population sample is a difficult and expensive procedure, which is often beyond the resources of an individual laboratory. Nevertheless, laboratories should, whenever possible, establish their own ranges using their own techniques and instrumentation. Normal ranges can be derived from healthy volunteers, from subjects attending health screening clinics or having annual medical examinations, or from staff having pre-employment testing. Hospital staff may not be ideal because their average age is likely to be considerably lower than that of the patient population. First-time blood donors are satisfactory, but

Blood Cells A Practical Guide, Fifth Edition. By Barbara J. Bain © 2015 John Wiley & Sons, Ltd. Published 2015 by John Wiley & Sons, Ltd.
Companion Website: www.wiley.com/go/bain/bloodcells

Table 5.1 Some effects of the method of obtaining a blood specimen on haematological variables.[*]

Site of obtaining blood specimen

During the first week of life, the Hb, PCV/Hct and RBC are approximately 15% higher in heel-prick than in venous specimens[†]; the difference may be greater in babies with sepsis with poor peripheral circulation [3]; the MCV, MCH and RDW do not differ but the MCHC is higher [3]; the WBC is about 20% higher in capillary blood [4]; in older infants, children and adults no consistent differences have been observed between finger-prick and venous specimens, but ear-lobe capillary specimens have Hb, Hct/PCV and RBC values 6–17% higher than finger-prick or venous specimens.

In neonates, heel-prick specimens have WBC, neutrophil and lymphocyte counts about 20% higher than arterial or venous samples; counts are most likely to approximate to those of venous blood if there is a free flow of blood and if early drops, excluding the first, are used for the count; in adults, the WBC and the neutrophil count are significantly higher in finger-prick samples than in venous samples with a progressive fall occurring with successive drops [5]. In adults, the platelet count is lower in capillary samples and the Hb is higher [6].

In neonates the platelet count and MPV are lower in capillary samples than in venous samples [3].

Position of the arm

Hb, Hct/PCV and RBC are 2–3% higher if the arm is hanging down than if it is at the level of the atrium of the heart.

Use of tourniquet

Hb, Hct/PCV and RBC are increased by 2–3% by prolonged application of a tourniquet.

Nature of anticoagulant

The dilution caused by using a liquid anticoagulant causes a slight reduction of cell counts, Hb and Hct/PCV.

Oxygenation of the blood

Oxygenation of the blood lowers the Hct/PCV and MCV and raises the MCHC [7].

Prior rest

The Hb, Hct/PCV and RBC fall by 5–8% after as little as half an hour's bed rest; rest lowers the lymphocyte count [8].

Hb, haemoglobin concentration; Hct, haematocrit; MCH, mean cell haemoglobin; MCHC, mean cell haemoglobin concentration; MCV mean cell volume; MPV, mean platelet volume; PCV, packed cell volume; RBC, red blood cell count; RDW, red cell distribution width; WBC, white blood cell count.

[*]For other relevant references the reader is referred to the first edition of this book [1].

[†]It has been reported that, at birth, capillary Hb is higher than that of cord blood Hb [2], but it appears likely that this observation was the result of the 20–60 minutes' delay that occurred before the capillary sample was obtained.

those who have donated regularly in the past may have depleted iron stores, which will affect haematological test results. It is also possible to derive normal ranges from data on patients, based on the assumption that the test results for any measurement will represent a normal and an abnormal population with some overlap. Large numbers are necessary and the statistics are fairly complex [9].

Particular problems exist in deriving ranges for elderly people because of the high prevalence of known and occult disease. It is desirable, if possible, to separate the effects of the increasing incidence of disease from the effects of the ageing process itself. Similarly, it may be difficult in a developing country to select an adequate population sample that is not adversely affected by malnutrition and subclinical disease. In such circumstances it may be necessary to derive normal ranges from 'elite' individuals such as the army, police force, medical students, doctors, nurses and laboratory work-

ers; such individuals will not be typical of the communities from which they are drawn, but their test results will more closely approximate to those that would be expected in an optimal state of health. Problems also occur in populations with a high prevalence of genetic disease. In deriving ranges for red cell variables it is necessary to exclude subjects with haemoglobinopathies and α and β thalassaemia trait. Exclusion of β thalassaemia trait and haemoglobinopathies is not difficult since diagnosis is usually easy, but exclusion of α thalassaemia trait requires deoxyribonucleic acid (DNA) analysis. However, unless this is done it is not possible to distinguish genuine ethnic differences from differences caused by a high prevalence of a genetic abnormality. Thus, subtle differences in haemoglobin concentration (Hb) and red cell indices between African Americans and Caucasian Americans are attributable in part to the 25–30% prevalence of α thalassaemia trait among African Americans; however, when the effects of α thalassaemia and iron deficiency are excluded, haemoglobin concentration is about 3.4 g/l lower in African American men and about 3.2 g/l lower in African American women that in Caucasians [10]; this residual difference is not explained by sickle cell trait or by socio-economic differences or differences in renal function. These differences are sufficient to lead to 6% of African American women and 8% of African American men being classified as anaemic if Caucasian reference ranges are used [10]. Similar differences are seen in African American children who have an Hb 2–7 g/l lower than age-matched non-Hispanic Caucasian controls [11]. Italian studies of genetically isolated populations have found strong evidence within genetic isolates that Hb is a hereditable feature [12], these results supporting previous evidence of heritability from two Australian twin studies [13]. In addition, two southern Italian genetic isolates had lower Hbs than a northern Italian genetic isolate [12]. In deriving reference ranges for children, it is desirable to exclude subclinical iron deficiency. Even in adults, subtle differences in iron status may affect population means. For example, heterozygosity for mutations associated with genetic haemochromatosis is common among Northern European populations (around 12%) and has been found to be associated with a slightly but significantly higher Hb, the difference between carriers and non-carriers being of the order of 4 to 6 g/l [14]. Hb, haematocrit (Hct), mean cell volume (MCV), mean cell haemoglobin (MCH) and mean cell haemoglobin concentration (MCHC) have all been found to be higher in patients with untreated haemochromatosis, probably as a result of enhanced delivery of iron to erythroblasts [15].

Once test results are available they must be dealt with by statistical techniques that are appropriate for the distribution of the data. If data have a normal (Gaussian) distribution, then a mean and standard deviation (SD) can be estimated and the mean ±1.96 SD will represent the central 95% of the data. The commonly used mean ±2 SD represents 95.4% of the data. The Hb and the other red cell variables can be treated as if they have a Gaussian distribution, although they are not strictly Gaussian [16]. Various other haematological variables have a skewed distribution with a tail of higher values; this is true for the white blood cell count (WBC) and the absolute counts of various types of leucocyte. If data with this type of distribution are treated inappropriately, as if they were Gaussian, the estimates for

both the upper and lower limits will be too low and the lower limit will often be negative. A logarithmic transformation may be appropriate or a more complex transformation may be necessary [17]. If a Gaussian distribution cannot be produced by transformation of the data, a non-parametric analysis must be carried out, i.e. one that makes no assumptions about the distribution. The advantages of using transformation to a Gaussian distribution is that a smaller sample size is adequate, of the order of 36 samples in contrast with the 120 samples that is the smallest adequate sample size for non-parametric analysis [18].

Use of the central 95% range is arbitrary, but gives a reasonable balance between missing a clinically significant abnormality and misclassifying a normal subject as abnormal. However, comparison of an observed value in a patient with a laboratory's normal range should be done with the constant awareness that, for each test, 5% of values of healthy subjects will fall outside the 'normal' range. Conversely, an individual may, as a result of a pathological process, have an alteration in a test result away from his or her own normal value while still remaining within the 'normal' range. When a patient's previous results are available, some attention should be paid to any change as well as to whether a result falls outside the laboratory's normal range.

If a laboratory does not derive its own normal ranges but adopts those of others, it is incumbent on it to be certain not only that the type of population is similar and the appropriate statistical techniques have been applied, but also that the blood sampling techniques and laboratory methods, including the methods of calibrating instruments, are identical.

Haematological variables are affected not only by age, gender, ethnic origin and altitude, but also by a number of other biological factors and extraneous influences (Tables 5.2 & 5.3).

The effects of age are complex and consistent results have not always been observed. The gender difference in the Hb and related variables lessens after the menopause but, at any given ferritin concentration or transferrin saturation, values continue to differ by about 10 g/l [33]. The Hb in men falls by about 10 g/l between youth and old age, particularly after the age of 60 years, whereas the Hb in women is fairly stable [33]. In a longitudinal population study in Sweden, Hb rose in women and fell in men between the

Table 5.2 Some demographic factors affecting haematological variables.[*]

Gender

RBC, Hb and Hct/PCV are higher in men than in women.

Women in the reproductive age range have a higher WBC and neutrophil count than men, whereas in postmenopausal women the WBC is lower than in men.

The platelet count is higher in women than in men.

Age

Normal values of neonates, infants and children differ widely from those of adults (see Tables 5.8–5.12).

In most studies the Hb rises in women and falls in men after the age of 40–50 years and in both men and women it falls in old age.

The lymphocyte counts fall in old age.

Ethnic origin

The WBC and neutrophil counts are lower in Black people than in Caucasians, are lower in Africans than in Afro-Caribbeans or African Americans (see Table 5.7) and are also lower in Yemenite Jews than in other Caucasians. The lower WBC in Black people is not apparent at birth but has appeared by the age of 1 year. The absolute lymphocyte count of African Americans is slightly but significantly higher than that of Caucasian Americans [10]. WBC and differential counts of Indians, Chinese and South-East Asian populations are the same as those of Northern European Caucasians. Eosinophil counts do not differ between healthy subjects of different ethnic groups.

Black people have lower platelet counts than Caucasians.

African Americans have a lower Hb than Caucasian Americans by about 3.2 g/l in women and 3.4 g/l in men, when iron deficiency and α thalassaemia trait have been eliminated [10].

Geographical location

RBC, Hb and Hct/PCV are increased at higher altitude; in one study the response to moderate altitude was a rise in RBC alone with the MCV being lower, whereas at a greater altitude Hb and Hct also rose [19]. In another study of the acute effects of changing altitude, the rise in RBC and Hb at 14 days was proportionately greater than the rise in Hct [20]; during this time the mean MCV had risen from 85 to 93 fl. The platelet count is significantly higher at altitude [20,21]. Babies born at a high altitude have a higher WBC and neutrophil count [22].

Season

Overall, Hb and Hct are somewhat lower in summer [23]. In non-smokers, Hb and PCV are lower in summer, due to an increase in plasma volume [24]; in smokers the MCHC is lower and the Hct and RBC are higher in summer; the plasma volume is unchanged [24].

Hb, haemoglobin concentration; Hct, haematocrit; MCHC, mean cell haemoglobin concentration; MCV, mean cell volume; PCV, packed cell volume; RBC, red blood cell count; WBC, white blood cell count.

[*]For further relevant references the reader is referred to the first edition of this book [1].

ages of 40–50 and 70–80 years [34]. In a very large cross-sectional French study, Hb was higher in women over the age of 50 years, probably due to a lower prevalence of iron deficiency since MCV and MCH also rose [35]. Healthy men showed a mean decline in Hb from 152 to 141 g/l between the ages of 70 and 88 years ($p < 0.05$), whereas in healthy women there was no significant change (mean values 140 and 138 g/l, $p > 0.05$) [34], so that after the age of 85 years there was no gender difference. Lower limits of normal for Hb had been defined previously as 133 g/l for healthy elderly men and 120 g/l for healthy elderly women [36]. In an Italian study, Hb was significantly higher in postmenopausal Italian women than in premenopausal, whereas men over the age of 60 years have a significantly lower mean Hb than younger men [12]. In the USA, results for men were similar but a decline in Hb was seen in women from the age of 50 years [13]. Above the age

of 80 years, mean Hb is lower in both genders, but the influence of occult ill-health cannot be excluded [12]. In a Japanese study, men showed a decline in Hb from the fourth decade, whereas women showed a peak in the sixth and seventh decades and a decline only thereafter [37]; this decline with age was seen in the absence of any apparent anaemia-related disease [37].

Locally derived reference ranges are needed for red cell variables for populations living at high altitude. Above 2000 m the Hb is elevated by 10–15 g/l and red blood cell count (RBC) and Hct/packed cell volume (PCV) are also elevated [19]. Cities at a high enough altitude that altitude-adjusted normal ranges are needed include Mexico City and Puebla (Mexico), La Paz (Bolivia), Quito (Ecuador), Bogota (Columbia), Johannesburg (South Africa), Tehran (Iran) and, in the USA, Santa Fe, Denver, Albuquerque, Reno, Salt Lake City, El Paso and Billings [38].

Table 5.3 Some biological factors and common extraneous influences affecting haematological variables.*

Diurnal variation

The Hb and Hct/PCV are higher in the morning than the evening.

The WBC and neutrophil counts are higher in the afternoon than in the morning. The eosinophil count is lowest at 10 a.m. to midday, and up to twice as high between midnight and 4 a.m. The lymphocyte count is lowest in the morning and highest in the evening [25].

The platelet count is higher in the afternoon and evening.

Pregnancy (see Table 5.14)

RBC, Hb and Hct/PCV fall; MCV rises, on average about 6 fl.

The WBC, neutrophil count and monocyte count rise during pregnancy; a left shift occurs; lymphocyte, eosinophil and basophil counts fall.

The neutrophil alkaline phosphatase score rises.

The platelet count has been observed to fall during pregnancy, but if subjects with pregnancy-related hypertension are excluded there is usually no fall.

The ESR rises.

Labour

During labour there is a further marked rise in the WBC and the neutrophil count together with a steep fall in the eosinophil count and a slight further fall of the lymphocyte count.

Postpartum

RBC, Hb and Hct/PCV fall to the lowest level at 3–4 days postpartum.

WBC and neutrophil count remain markedly elevated for some days postpartum then fall gradually over 4–6 weeks.

Menstruation

WBC, neutrophil count and monocyte count fall steeply during menstruation; a reciprocal change is seen in the eosinophil count; the basophil count falls mid-cycle.

Menopause

The Hb rises postmenopausally.

The WBC and the neutrophil count fall.

Exercise

The WBC and absolute counts of all leucocyte types rise as a response to vigorous exercise; the absolute rise in the WBC and neutrophil count is less in Black people than in Caucasians [26]; in babies, vigorous crying similarly causes an increase in the WBC, with recently circumcised babies showing a left shift [4].

The RBC, Hb and PCV rise as a response to vigorous exercise.

Intensive training leads to a fall in the lymphocyte count [27].

Cigarette smoking [28]

The RBC, Hb, Hct/PCV, MCV and MCH are higher in smokers.

The WBC, neutrophil count and monocyte count are higher.

The platelet count is higher.

The ESR is higher.

Alcohol intake

Alcohol consumption may be associated with an increased Hb [29], but heavy alcohol intake can cause anaemia, leucopenia and thrombocytopenia.

The MCV and MCH are higher and RBC is lower.

Obesity

WBC correlates with body fat [30] and is increased in morbid obesity [31].

WBC, neutrophil count, lymphocyte count and RBC increase with obesity; MCV and MCH decrease [32].

ESR, erythrocyte sedimentation rate; Hb, haemoglobin concentration; Hct, haematocrit; MCH, mean cell haemoglobin; MCV, mean cell volume; PCV, packed cell volume; RBC, red blood cell count; WBC, white blood cell count.

*For further relevant references the reader is referred to the first edition of this book [1].

Normal ranges for adults

Some reference ranges for red cell variables for Caucasian adults are shown in Table 5.4 and some data for Black adults in Table 5.5. It should be explained that if a table shows the RBC $\times 10^{-12}$/l to be e.g. 4.32, then the RBC is 4.32×10^{12}/l (and similarly for the WBC). Data are also available derived from more than 30 000 mainly Caucasian French subjects, but iron deficiency and haemoglobinopathies were not specifically excluded [35]. Ranges for Caucasian adults can also be applied to Indian, Chinese and South-East Asian populations. Indigenous Greenlanders have been found to have a lower Hb than Danish subjects, the difference not being explicable on the basis of diet, cigarette smoking or the prevalence of iron deficiency [29].

White cell variables for Caucasian adults are shown in Table 5.6. For leucocyte counts, particularly neutro-

Table 5.5 Haemoglobin concentration and MCV in Afro-Americans in whom iron deficiency and alpha thalassaemia trait were excluded [10]; 95% range and mean are shown.*

	Male (n = 172)	Females (n = 42)
Hb g/l	127–167	113–149
MCV fl	80–99	81.5–99

Hb, haemoglobin concentration; MCV mean cell volume

*Hb was significantly lower than that of Caucasians, whereas MCV was not; sickle cell trait did not have any influence on the Hb or MCV.

phil counts, it is necessary to have specific reference ranges applicable to Africans and Afro-Caribbeans (Table 5.7). The lower WBC and neutrophil counts observed in these ethnic groups may be partly explicable on the basis of diet and other extraneous influences, but there is also a true biological difference [26,27,55]. Ethnic neutropenia in individuals of African origin is

Table 5.4 95% ranges for red cell variables in Caucasian adults in five large series of subjects.

	Male					Female				
RBC × 10⁻¹²/l	4.32–5.66*				4.5–5.6†	3.88–4.99*				3.9–5.1†
Hb g/l‡	133–167*	133–176§	132–180¶	132–169**	137–172†	118–148*	120–158§	122–150¶	115–154**	120–152†
Hct l/l	0.39–0.50*		0.39–0.51¶		0.40–0.50†	0.36–0.44*		0.36–0.48¶		0.37–0.46†
MCV fl	82–98††			82–99**	83–98†	82–98††			81–99**	85–98†
MCH pg	27.3–32.6				28–32†	27.3–32.6				28–32†
MCHC g/l	316–349				320–360†	316–3.9				320–360†
RDW (SD or %)	9.9–15.5†† (SD)					9.9–15.5††				
	11.6–13.9‡‡ (%)			11.6–14.1 (%)†		11.6–13.9‡‡				12–14.7 (%)†
HDW g/dl	1.82–2.64‡‡					1.82–2.64‡‡				

*based on 700 healthy subjects, aged between 18 and 60 years, studied by the author: 350 were male and 350 female; half were studied on Coulter instruments (S and S Plus IV) and half on Bayer-Technicon instruments (Hemalog 8 and H.2); except where indicated, the ranges are derived from all 750 subjects.

†Sysmex XE 2100, 159 males, 91 females, aged 30–65 [39].

‡2.5 centile 134 g/l for men aged 20–59 (n = 6709), 128 g/l for men aged 60 years or more (n = 5615), 119 g/l for women (n = 11 286) [40].

§based on 1379 iron-replete Danish males and 1003 iron-replete Danish females [29].

¶ based on 1382 males and 1837 females for Hb and 1368 males and 1818 females for Hct [41].

**6240 males and 5780 females having health screening, iron deficiency was excluded [10]; MCV is very dependent on the technology used and the method of instrument calibration so that derivation of normal ranges for individual laboratories is important.

††Coulter S Plus IV, n = 200.

‡‡Bayer H.2, n = 200.

Hb, haemoglobin concentration; Hct, haematocrit; HDW, haemoglobin distribution width; MCH, mean cell haemoglobin; MCHC, mean cell haemoglobin concentration; MCV, mean cell volume; PCV, packed cell volume; RBC, red blood cell count; RDW, red cell distribution width; SD, standard deviation.

Table 5.6 95% ranges for automated and manual leucocyte counts in Caucasian adults, derived by the author, using data from 750 healthy subjects aged between 18 and 60 years.

	Male	Female	Method and number of Subjects (n)
WBC × 10⁻⁹/l	3.7–9.5	3.9–11.1	Various methods, n = 750
Neutrophils × 10⁻⁹/l	1.7–6.1	1.7–7.5	Automated counts, Bayer H.2, n = 200
Lymphocytes × 10⁻⁹/l	1.0–3.2		
Monocytes × 10⁻⁹/l	0.2–0.6		
Eosinophils × 10⁻⁹/l	0.03–0.46		
Basophils × 10⁻⁹/l	0.02–0.09		
LUC × 10⁻⁹/l	0.09–0.29		
Granulocytes × 10⁻⁹/l	1.8–7.5	2.1–8.9	Automated counts, Coulter S Plus IV, n = 200
Lymphocytes × 10⁻⁹/l	1.15–3.25		
Mononuclear cells × 10⁻⁹/l	0.18–0.86		
Neutrophils × 10⁻⁹/l	1.5–6.5	1.8–7.4	WBC on Coulter S or S IV; 500-cell manual differential count, n = 400
Lymphocytes × 10⁻⁹/l	1.1–3.5		
Monocytes × 10⁻⁹/l	0.21–0.92		
Eosinophils × 10⁻⁹/l	0.02–0.67		
Basophils × 10⁻⁹/l	0.00–0.13		

LUC, large unstained (peroxidase-negative) cells; WBC, white blood cell count.

Table 5.7 95% ranges for leucocyte counts in adult Africans, Afro-Caribbeans and Black Americans.

Ethnic origin	Male WBC	Female WBC	Male neutrophils	Female neutrophils	Comment
African	2.8–7.2	3.0–7.4	0.9–4.2	1.3–3.7	n = 57 M, 29 F*
Afro-Caribbean	3.1–9.4	3.2–10.6	1.2–5.6	1.3–7.1	n = 38 M, 39 F*
Ugandan (Kampala)	1.9–8.3	—	0.32–3.6	—	n = 250 [42]
Ugandan (Makerere)	2.2–8.9	—	0.55–3.7	—	n = 160 [42]
Ugandan†	3.4–8.7		0.84–3.37		n = 845, HIV negative [43]
Ugandan (Kampala)	2.8–8.2	3.2–9.0	0.9–3.8	1.1–4.4	n = 520 M, 140 F, negative for HIV and hepatitis B and C [44]
Tanzanian	3.2–8.0	3.0–7.9	1.1–4.8	1.2–5.4	n = 150 M, 126 F, HIV negative [45]
Ethiopian‡	3–9.8	3–12.2	1.05–7.2	0.75–5.5	n = 280 M, 205 F, HIV negative [46]
Gambian	3.3–8.2	3.5–8.4	—	—	90% rather than 95% range, HIV negative [47]
Rwandan, Kenyan, Ugandan, Zambian	3.1–9.1		1.0–5.3		n = M 1083, F 1022, negative for HIV and hepatitis B and C [48]
Kenyan	2.5–7.4	3.3–9.7	0.8–3.9	1.3–3.8	n = M 77, F 83, HIV negative [49]
Nigerian	3.0–10.0		2.4–7.2		n = 49, aged 14 to 17 [50]
Black American	3.6–10.2	1.3–7.4	—	—	n = 65 [51]
Black American	3.5–9.6	3.4–11.2	1.1–6.7	1.5–8.1	n = 172 M, 525 F [52]
Black American	3.2–10.2¶	—	1.1–6.8¶	—	n = 493 [53]
Black American aged 12–18	3.2–9.3		1.0–6.2		n = 401 [54]
Black American aged > 18 years	3.1–9.9		1.3–6.6		

F, female; HIV, human immunodeficiency virus; M, male; WBC, white blood cell count
*Derived by the author.
†Lymphocyte count was 1.4–4.2.
‡Lymphocyte count was 1.0–3.5 in men and 1.1–3.5 in women.
§Lymphocyte count was 1.0–3.5 for men and 1.3–3.8 for women; the gender difference in the WBC and neutrophil counts was statistically very significant.
¶Read from graph.

associated with a Duffy-null phenotype and is the result of a variant of the Duffy antigen receptor for chemokines [56]. The lower WBC and neutrophil count relate to a difference in bone marrow production of neutrophils [55] rather than to any difference in margination; the response to brief exercise [26], sustained exercise [27] and administration of granulocyte colony-stimulating factor [57] is less than in Caucasians, although the absolute response to corticosteroids is similar to that of Caucasians [57]. Monocyte counts are also somewhat lower in those of African origin than in Caucasians [53]. The higher eosinophil counts previously reported in Africans and Indians do not represent a biological difference from Caucasians; eosinophilia observed was explicable on the basis of subclinical disease, particularly parasitic infection. Leucocyte and neutrophil counts have been reported to be significantly higher in Mexican Americans than in Caucasian Americans [58] and in Latin Americans than in Caucasian, Black or Asian Americans [52]. Because of superior precision, reference ranges for automated differential leucocyte counts are narrower than those for manual differential counts (see Table 5.6). They are also dependent on methodology and thus need to

be derived specifically for individual models of instrument. Not even all instruments operating on the same principles give identical results.

Normal ranges for neonates and fetuses

Some normal ranges for haematological variables in neonates are shown in Tables 5.8 and 5.9. A higher WBC and neutrophil count are seen in female babies [70,75]. Published ranges for red cell variables in Indian babies [76] and in Jamaican babies in whom haemoglobinopathies and β thalassaemia trait had been excluded [65] are similar to those for European neonates, whereas Nigerian babies have been observed to have lower RBCs, Hbs and PCVs [66]. Since haemoglobinopathies and thalassaemia trait were not excluded in the latter group, it may be more appropriate to apply ranges for red cell variables derived for Caucasian babies to all ethnic groups, including Africans. The lower neutrophil count that is noted in Africans and Afro-Caribbeans later in life is not apparent in the neonatal period, so that the same reference ranges for leucocyte counts can be applied to neonates

Table 5.8 95% ranges for red cell variables in healthy full-term babies during the first month of life.

	RBC × 10⁻¹²/l	Hb g/l	Hct or PCV l/l	MCV fl
Caucasian				
Cord blood (early cord clamping) [59]	3.5–6.7	137–201	0.47–0.59	90–118
Cord blood (time of cord clamping not specified)* [60]	3.13–4.85	113–176		99–115
Birth – 96 h (early cord clamping) [61,62]	3.8–6.5	142–240	0.46–0.75	101–137
(late cord clamping) [62]		161–240		
'newborn' [63]	4.1–6.7	150–240	0.44–0.70	102–115
1–2 weeks (early cord clamping) [61]	3.2–6.4	128–218	0.38–0.70	75–149
3–4 weeks (early cord clamping) [61,64]	2.8–5.3	101–183	0.32–0.55	90–120
Jamaican				
1 day [65]	4.6–7.6	157–275		90–118
1 week [65]	4.0–6.9	134–224		88–116
4 weeks [65]	3.1–5.9	95–181		83–107
Nigerian				
1 day [66]	2.7–5.3	116–196	0.32–0.58	113 (mean)
2 weeks [66]	2.35–4.55	94–168	0.31–0.47	113 (mean)
4 weeks [66]	2.1–3.95	75–136	0.24–0.41	108 (mean)
1–7 days [50]		135–180	0.40–0.53	
8–14 days [50]		130–160	0.38–0.51	

*Brazilian, from Porto Alegre, so likely to be essentially Caucasian.

Hb, haemoglobin concentration; Hct, haematocrit; MCV, mean cell volume; PCV, packed cell volume; RBC, red blood cell count.

Table 5.9 90% or 95% ranges for white cell and NRBC counts for full-term Caucasian babies during the first month of life.[*]

Age	WBC × 10⁻⁹/l	Neutrophils × 10⁻⁹/l	Lymphocytes × 10⁻⁹/l	Monocytes × 10⁻⁹/l	Eosinophils × 10⁻⁹/l	NRBC × 10⁻⁹/l
Cord blood [59,60,67,71]	5–23	1.7–19	1–11	0.1–3.7	0.05–2.0	0.03–5.4
Half hour [69,72]		1.9–5.8				
12 hours [67,69]		6.6–23.5				
24 hours [67,69]		4.8–17.1				
'newborn' [63]	9.1–34	6–23.5	2.5–10	< 3.5	< 2.0	< 0.4
48 hours [67,69]		3.8–13.4				
0–60 hours [68]			2–7.3	0–1.9	0–0.8	
72 hours [67,69]		2.0–9.4				
4 days [67,69,72]		1.3–8.0	2.2–7.1	0.2–1.8	0.2–1.9	
60 hours–5 days [68,69]		2.0–6.0	1.9–6.6	0–1.7	0–0.8	
7–8 days [67,69,73]	9–18.4	1.8–8	3–9	0.03–0.98	0.16–0.94	0.03–0.11
2 weeks [67,69]		1.7–6				
5 days–4 weeks [68,69]		1.8–5.4	2.8–9.1	0.09–1.7	0–0.8	
3–4 weeks [68.69]		1.6–5.8				
4 weeks [74]	5–19.5	1–9	4–13.5			

NRBC, nucleated red blood cells; WBC, white blood cell count.

[*]Data from different series have been amalgamated to include the lowest and highest limits found in different studies. The ranges of Gregory and Hey [67] and Weinberg *et al.* [68] are 90% rather than 95% ranges, while the scatter plots of Manroe *et al.* [69] show the full range of counts. It should be noted that Schmutz *et al.* [70], in a study carried out at an altitude of about 4800 feet, found a similar pattern of changes in WBC and neutrophil count with time, but absolute counts were much higher than those of Manroe *et al.* [69].

of all ethnic groups [69–71,77]. The lymphocyte count in the neonatal period is of considerable importance in suggesting the possibility of congenital immunodeficiency. In severe combined immunodeficiency the count is almost invariably less than 2.8×10^9/l and it has been suggested that investigation is mandatory if the lymphocyte count is less than 1.0×10^9/l.

The Hb, Hct/PCV and RBC in the neonate are considerably influenced by the time of umbilical cord clamping (see Table 5.8), since inflow from the placenta increases the blood volume of the neonate by up to 50–60% during the first few minutes after birth. The rate of transfer of placental blood to the neonate is increased if oxytocin is administered to the mother to stimulate uterine contraction and is decreased if the baby is held above the level of the mother immediately after delivery. During the first few hours of life, plasma volume decreases so that the Hb, Hct/PCV and RBC rise appreciably, particularly when late clamping has been practised. Nucleated red blood cells (NRBC) may be present in appreciable numbers at birth, but the count falls rapidly in the first 24 hours. By 4 days they are infrequent. NRBC are more numerous in the cord blood of premature infants and the infants of diabetic mothers [78]. They are also increased when there has been fetal blood loss, haemolysis or intra-uterine hypoxia. The reticulocyte count at birth is higher than at any other time of life, but it drops markedly after birth. There is a steady decline in the RBC, Hb and Hct/PCV but, as shown in Table 5.8, an Hb of less than 140 g/l in the first week of life is indicative of anaemia. The WBC at birth is influenced by the mode of delivery, being lower after an elective caesarean section than after vaginal delivery or when a caesarean section has been performed after labour has commenced [70,79]. The WBC and neutrophil counts rise after birth to a peak level at about 12 hours and thereafter fall sharply [69,70]. The lymphocyte count falls in the first few days of life [72]. The neutrophil count is initially higher than the lymphocyte count. This is reversed between the fourth and seventh days of life.

Maternal smoking causes a small increase in the neonatal Hb, Hct/PCV and MCV and a more substantial decrease in the neutrophil count, which persists for at least the first few days after birth [80]. Healthy babies with low birth weight for gestational age differ from normal birth weight babies: RBC, Hb, Hct and MCV are higher while MCH and MCHC are lower; erythroblasts and granulocyte precursors are more numerous; neutrophil and platelet counts may be lower [81,82]. Other maternal and fetal factors influencing the neutrophil count in the neonate are shown in Tables 6.5 and 6.23 and causes of polycythaemia and anaemia in the neonatal period in Tables 6.2 and 6.20. Increased circulating NRBC on the first day of life have been found predictive of intraventricular haemorrhage in premature neonates [83].

Ranges applicable to the fetus from 8 weeks' gestation onwards have also been published and a graphical representation is shown in Fig. 5.1 [84–87]. In another study of Thai fetuses of between 18 and 22 weeks' gestation, who did not have any α thalassaemia mutation, 95% ranges were: Hb 96.8–130 g/l, MCV 107–138 fl, MCH 34.7–48.1 pg and MCHC 308–360 g/l [88]. The platelet count in the fetus has a mean value of around 250×10^9/l and does not change between 17 weeks' gestation and term [89]; in this study of 5194 fetuses, the 95% range was $138–344 \times 10^9$/l, but fetuses with significant abnormalities causing thrombocytopenia were not excluded from the analysis. An unexpectedly high eosinophil count is sometimes observed in healthy fetuses [90].

Premature babies have a lower WBC and lower neutrophil and lymphocyte counts than term babies; NRBC and immature myeloid cells are more numerous and the reticulocyte count is higher [72,91]. At birth, the Hb and Hct/PCV are similar to those of term babies but the RBC is lower and the MCV higher [92]. Neutrophil and lymphocyte counts reach the levels of term babies by about 1 week [72,91]. In premature babies the eosinophil count often becomes elevated 2–3 weeks after birth.

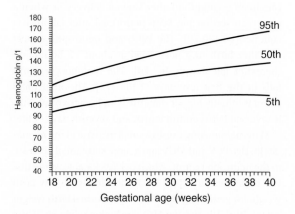

Fig. 5.1 Haemoglobin concentrations in 265 healthy fetuses and reference range derived from the data, modified from Mari *et al.* [87].

Normal ranges in infants and children

Normal ranges applicable to Caucasian infants and children are shown in Tables 5.10 and 5.11 and for African American children and adolescents in Table 5.12. The steady decline in RBC, Hb and Hct/PCV that follows the early peak continues to a nadir around 2 months of age. There is a simultaneous rapid fall in MCV and MCH. In premature babies the postnatal decline in Hb is more rapid and continues for longer, 8 to 12 weeks rather than 4 to 8 weeks; the nadir is lower (Table 5.13). In populations where iron deficiency is uncommon, early clamping of the umbilical cord is not associated with any lowering of the Hb or the MCV at 4 months of age, although serum ferritin and transferrin saturation are lower than in babies in whom cord clamping was delayed [110].

The exclusion of children with iron deficiency is important in deriving paediatric normal ranges, since one of the purposes of such ranges is to facilitate the diagnosis of iron deficiency. The iron stores of the neonate are adequate to sustain erythropoiesis for 3–5 months, depending on whether the infant was full term or premature and on whether the cord was clamped early or late. Thereafter, iron deficiency is common. Iron deficiency can be excluded by requiring a normal serum ferritin or transferrin saturation, or a normal red cell protoporphyrin concentration, or by administering iron supplements before testing. Population studies often show a lower limit of normal that is lower than figures appearing in textbooks. For example, Emond *et al.* carried out a study on 1075 infants in Bristol (of whom only 1.2% had a serum ferritin concentration less than 12 µg/l) and found the 5th percentile for Hb to be as low as 97 g/l [98]. In another UK study in which iron deficiency was not excluded, 83 infants aged 9 months had a mean Hb of 98 g/l (95% range approximately 72–123 g/l) [100].

Girls have a higher neutrophil count than boys from puberty onwards [103]. The lower WBC and neutrophil counts noted in Black adults have been observed in children between the ages of 1 and 5 years [111] and in infants by 9–12 months of age [112]. Published reference ranges for Melanesian children show lower Hbs and MCVs than for Caucasians, even though α and β thalassaemia traits were excluded and iron deficiency was uncommon [113]; this probably reflects a high prevalence of malnutrition and malaria in the population studied.

Table 5.10 95% (or 90%) ranges for red cell variables for Caucasian infants and children*; for one study differences according to the diet of the infants is shown.

	RBC × 10⁻¹²/l	Hb g/l	Hct/ PCV l/l	MCV fl	MCH pg
2 months [64,69,95]	2.6–4.3	89–132	0.26–0.40	75–125† [69] 84–106‡ [64]	
	2.95–4.09 [95]	91–125 [95]	0.27–0.38 [95]	84.7–98.1 [95]	28.6–33.1 [95]
3 months [69,97]	3.1–4.3	93–138	0.27–0.39	73–103	
4 months [64]	3.5–5.1	103–141	0.32–0.44	76–97	
5 months [95]	3.79–4.87	101–129	0.30–0.38	73.3–84.1	24.5–28.7
6 months [64,97]	3.9–5.5	99–141	0.31–0.41	68–85	
8 months [98]		97–136§			
1 year [64,97]	4.1–5.3	98–141	0.33–0.41	71–84	
1 year [99]		100–134§			
13 months [95]	3.92–5.10	105–133	0.31–0.39	72.8–83.6	24.3–28.7
18 months [97]		97–151			
18 months [99]		102–130§			
18 months [100]		91–147 (cow's milk); 98–147 (unfortified formula), 91–147 (iron-fortified formula)			
1–23 months [63]	3.8–5.4	105–140	0.32–0.42	72–88	
1–2 years [94]		107–133			
1–4 years¶ [101]	3.5–5.3	107–151	0.31–0.45	72–100	23.8–34.2
3–5 years [94]		109–137			
2–5/6 years [64,74,93]	4.23–5.03	96–148	0.34–0.40	73–86	
2–9 years [63]	4–5.3	115–145	0.30–0.43	76–90	
5–8 years¶ [101]	3.45–5.49	103–151	0.31–0.44	71–99	24.6–33.4
5/6–9 years [74,102,103]	3.93–5.11	107–146	0.33–0.42	75–89.5	
6–11 years [94]		115–145			
8–12 years [104]	4.34–5.74	121–145	0.366–0.452	76.5–92.1	
9–12 years [74,102,103]	4.08–5.11	115–154	0.34–0.42	76–91	
9–12 years¶ [101]	4.11–5.49	113–153	0.34–0.44	72–99.6	24–34
12–14/15 years					
Males	4.19–5.54	115–158	0.36–0.46	76–92	
Females	4.00–5.09	115–153	0.35–0.44	77–92.5	
[74,93,94,103]					
13/14–18 years					
Males	4.34–5.88	127–170	0.37–0.49	77–95.6	
Females	3.90–5.42	113–154	0.35–0.46	75–93.8	
[74,102,103,104]					

Hb, haemoglobin concentration; Hct, haematocrit; MCH, mean cell haemoglobin; MCV, mean cell volume; PCV, packed cell volume; RBC, red blood cell count.

*Some data have been amalgamated to include the highest and lowest limits in different series. Iron deficiency was largely excluded in most series [64,74,93–95]. Others have reported that the Hb is rarely less than 110 g/l in children who are not iron deficient [96] and the data of Castriota-Scanderberg et al. [93] and early data of Dallman and Siimes [74] support this. In more recent investigations the Hb was sometimes below 110 g/l in children of less than 5 years of age [94].

†MCV calculated from microhaematocrit and RBC [69].

‡MCV measured by impedance counter [64].

§90% rather than 95% range, low prevalence of iron deficiency, Hb measured by HemoCue on a heel-prick sample; at 18 months of age girls had a significantly higher Hb than boys, but the magnitude of the difference was trivial (1.41 g/l).

¶Central America, altitude 0 to 750 m, Hb by haemoglobinometry, microhaematocrit and RBC on Coulter Counter Model B [101].

Table 5.11 94% or 95% ranges for total and differential white cell counts for Caucasian infants, children and adolescents.

Age	9 days–1 year*	2 months†	5 months†	1 year*	1 year‡	13 months†
WBC × 10⁻⁹/l	7.3–16.6	5.1–15.4	5.9–16.6	5.6–17	6.0–17.5	5.9–16.1
Neutrophils × 10⁻⁹/l	1.5–6.9	0.7–4.7	1.1–5.6	1.5–6.9	1.5–8.5	1.0–7.6
Lymphocytes × 10⁻⁹/l	3.4–9.4	3.0–9.9	3.2–10.6	2.5–8.6	4.0–10.5	3.1–9.6
		(3.3–10.5)	(3.4–11.3)			(3.5–10.4)
Monocytes × 10⁻⁹/l	0.21–1.64	0.36–1.2	0.25–1.2	0.15–1.28		0.25–0.91
Eosinophils × 10⁻⁹/l	0.06–0.62	0.09–0.84	0.1–1.0	0.06–0.62		0.05–0.88
Basophils × 10⁻⁹/l	0.02–0.17	0.02–0.13	0.02–0.18	0.02–0.12		0.02–0.13
Large unstained cells × 10⁻⁹/l	0.09–0.61	0.17–0.91	0.17–1.00	0.13–0.72		0.20–1.1

Age	2 years*	2 years‡	3 years*	4 years*	4 years‡	5 years*
WBC × 10⁻⁹/l	5.6–17.0	6.0–17.0	4.9–12.9	4.9–12.9	5.5–15.5	4.9–12.9
Neutrophils × 10⁻⁹/l	1.5–6.9	1.5–8.5	1.5–6.9	1.8–7.7	1.5–8.5	1.8–7.7
Lymphocytes × 10⁻⁹/l	2.2–7.7	3.0–9.5	1.7–5.5	1.7–5.5	2.0–8.0	1.6–4.3
Monocytes × 10⁻⁹/l	0.15–1.28		0.15–1.28	0.15–1.28		0.15–1.28
Eosinophils × 10⁻⁹/l	0.04–1.19		0.04–1.19	0.9–1.40		0.9–1.40
Basophils × 10⁻⁹/l	0.02–0.12		0.02–0.12	0.03–0.12		0.03–0.12
Large unstained cells × 10⁻⁹/l	0.11–0.68		0.09–0.48	0.09–0.38		0.08–0.32

Age	6 years*	6 years‡	4–6 years§	4–7 years¶	7 years*	7–8 years§
WBC × 10⁻⁹/l	4.4–10.6	5.0–14.5	4.8–12.1	6.3–16.2	4.4–10.6	4.5–11.7
Neutrophils × 10⁻⁹/l	1.5–5.9	1.5–8.9	1.7–7.6	1.6–9.0	1.5–5.9	1.7–7.4
Lymphocytes × 10⁻⁹/l	1.6–4.3	1.5–7.0	1.6–4.2	2.2–9.8	1.6–4.3	1.7–4.3
Monocytes × 10⁻⁹/l	0.15–1.28		0.33–1.16	0.06–1.00	0.15–1.28	0.32–1.21
Eosinophils × 10⁻⁹/l	0.08–1.10		0.06–0.95	0–1.4	0.08–1.01	0.08–1.00
Basophils × 10⁻⁹/l	0.02–0.12		0–0.73	0–0.026	0.02–0.12	0.02–0.51
Large unstained cells × 10⁻⁹/l	0.07–0.26				0.07–0.26	

Age	8 years*	8 years‡	9–10 years*	9–10 years§	10 years‡	
WBC × 10⁻⁹/l	3.9–9.9	4.5–13.5	3.9–9.9	4.4–10.6	4.5–13.5	
Neutrophils × 10⁻⁹/l	1.5–5.9	1.5–8.0	1.5–5.9	1.7–6.4	1.8–8.0	
Lymphocytes × 10⁻⁹/l	1.4–3.8	1.5–6.8	1.4–3.8	1.7–3.9	1.5–6.5	
Monocytes × 10⁻⁹/l	0.15–1.28		0.15–1.28	0.33–0.99		
Eosinophils × 10⁻⁹/l	0.08–1.01		0.08–1.01	0.06–1.03		
Basophils × 10⁻⁹/l	0.02–0.12		0.02–0.12	0.01–0.54		
Large unstained cells × 10⁻⁹/l	0.07–0.26		0.07–0.26			

Age	11 years*	11–12 years§	12–13 years*	13–14 years§	14 years*	15–16 years*
WBC × 10⁻⁹/l	3.9–9.9	4.0–10.4	3.9–9.9	4.2–10.7	3.9–9.9	3.9–9.9
Neutrophils × 10⁻⁹/l	1.5–5.9	1.6–6.2	1.5–5.9	1.7–7.2	1.4–5.6	1.7–5.7
Lymphocytes × 10⁻⁹/l	1.4–3.8	1.5–3.7	1.4–3.8	1.4–3.6	1.4–3.8	1.4–3.8
Monocytes × 10⁻⁹/l	0.15–1.28	0.31–1.00	0.15–1.28	0.26–1.0	0.15–1.28	0.15–1.28
Eosinophils × 10⁻⁹/l	0.04–0.76	0.06–1.12	0.04–0.76	0.05–0.61	0.04–0.76	0.04–0.76
Basophils × 10⁻⁹/l	0.02–0.12	0.01–0.38	0.02–0.1	0.01–0.43	0.07–0.1	0.02–0.10
Large unstained cells × 10⁻⁹/l	0.07–0.26		0.02–0.1		0.07–0.26	0.07–0.26

WBC, white blood cell count

*Differential count performed on a Hemalog D automated differential counter [73]; 'large unstained cells' are large peroxidase-negative cells, in healthy infants and children representing mainly large lymphocytes.

†Differential count performed on a Bayer H.1 analyser [105]; 'large unstained cells' are large peroxidase-negative cells, in healthy infants and children, representing mainly large lymphocytes; for the lymphocyte count the figures in parentheses represent lymphocytes plus large unstained cells.

‡100-cell manual differential count [106].

§Differential count performed on Coulter STKS; figures for males and females have been amalgamated [103].

¶200-cell manual differential count, recalculated to make allowance for skewed distribution [107,108].

Table 5.12 95% ranges (mean) derived from 5039 African American children and adolescents (iron deficiency, β thalassaemia and 'suspected α thalassaemia trait' excluded) [11].

Age (years) and gender	Hb (g/l)	Hct (l/l)*	MCV (fl)*
2–5	104–135 (119.4)	0.315–0.40 (0.36)	74.65–85 (79.8)
6–10	103–146 (124.4)	0.33–0.42 (0.37)	76.45–86.4 (81.44)
11–15, male	110–154 (132)	0.33–0.42 (0.39)	78–88.4 (83.2)
11–15, female	101–152 (126.7)	0.33–0.43 (0.38)	78–89.2 (83.6)
16–18, male	113–174 (143.5)	0.38–0.49 (0.435)	80.8–91.2 (86)
16–18, female	103–148 (125.5)	0.32–0.43 (0.37)	79.4–91.1 (85.3)

Hb, haemoglobin concentration; Hct, haematocrit; MCV, mean cell volume

*Upper limit of normal calculated from mean + 2 standard deviations (after correcting an apparent error in the published figures for MCV).

Table 5.13 95% ranges for haemoglobin concentration (g/l) in pre-term but iron-replete babies in the first 6 months of life [109].

	Birthweight 1000– 1500 g	Birthweight 1501– 2000 g
2 weeks	117–184	118–196
4 weeks	87–152	82–150
2 months	71–115	80–114
3 months	89–112	93–118
4 months	91–131	91–131
6 months	94–138	107–126

Normal ranges for Coulter instruments Red cell Size factor (RSf) for children have been derived, being 82–102 fl for children aged 6 months to 6 years and 83.7–103.1 fl for ages 6–18 years [114].

Normal ranges in pregnancy

The changes in haematological variables that occur during pregnancy are shown in Table 5.3. Normal ranges are given in Table 5.14. The Hb usually remains above 100 g/l unless there is iron deficiency or some other complication.

Table 5.14 95% ranges for haematological variables during pregnancy.

Period of gestation	18 weeks		32 weeks	39 weeks
WBC × 10⁻⁹/l	5.6–13.8*		6.0–15.7*	5.8–15.2*
Period of gestation	**7–14 weeks**	**15–22 weeks**	**23–30 weeks**	**31–38 weeks**
Hb g/l	128–136†	114–138†	109–138†	111–136†
Period of gestation	**First trimester**		**Second trimester**	**Third trimester**
RBC × 10⁻¹²/l	3.52–4.52		3.2–4.41	3.1–4.44
Hb g/l	110–143		100–137	98–137
PCV/Hct l/l	0.31–0.41		0.30–0.38	0.28–0.39
MCV fl	81–96		82–97	81–99
WBC × 10⁻⁹/l	5.7–13.6		6.2–14.8	5.9–16.9, 5.9–13.7‡
Neutrophil count × 10⁻⁹/l	3.6–10.1		3.8–12.3	3.9–13.1, 3.7–10.8‡
Lymphocyte count × 10⁻⁹/l	1.1–3.5		0.9–3.9	1–3.6, 1–3.1‡
Monocyte count × 10⁻⁹/l	0–1		0.1–1.1	0.1–1.1, 0.3–1.1‡
Eosinophil count × 10⁻⁹/l	0–0.6		0–0.6	0–0.6, 0.02–0.33‡
Basophil count × 10⁻⁹/l	0–0.1		0–0.1	0–0.1, 0–0.09‡
Platelet count × 10⁻⁹/l	174–391		171–409	155–429
Period of gestation	**18 weeks**		**32 weeks**	**39 weeks**
Platelet count × 10⁻⁹/l	155–359		146–361	139–364

Hb, haemoglobin concentration; Hct, haematocrit; MCV, mean cell volume; PCV, packed cell volume; RBC, red blood cell count; WBC, white blood cell count.

*data derived from Milman *et al.* [115]; this reference also gives normal ranges for MCV and for Hb and MCHC based on haemoglobin expressed in mmol/l.

†data derived from Cruikshank [116].

‡data derived from England and Bain [117].

Other data from Balloch *et al.* [113].

Normal ranges for platelet counts and other platelet variables

The manual platelet count is imprecise and both manual and automated platelet counts are prone to inaccuracy.

As a consequence, there are considerable discrepancies in published ranges (Table 5.15). It is therefore important for laboratories to establish their own reference ranges for their own methodologies. Platelet counts are higher in women than men and the plateletcrit

Table 5.15 95% ranges for platelet counts ($\times 10^{-9}$/l) in healthy adults of differing ethnic origins.

Method	Male	Female	Reference
Caucasians			
Microscopy	140–440		[118]
	127–351	165–359	[119]
	140–340		[119]
	145–375		[120]
Impedance counting in platelet-rich plasma	143–179	156–417	[121]
Impedance counting in whole blood	170–430		[122]
	168–411	188–445	[123]
	184–370	196–451	[124]
	157–365	164–384	[125]
	140–320	180–380	[39]
Light-scattering in whole blood	162–346*		
Hemalog 8	143–332*	169–358*	
H.1	144–328	137–347	[126]
H2			
Advia 120	159–376 (aged 18–45 years)		[127]
Advia 120	156–300 (aged 45–65 years)	156–351 (aged 45–65 years)	[127]
Advia 120	139–363 (aged > 65 years)		[127]
Advia 2120	172–398 (France)	185–445 (France)	[35]
	139–332 (Iran)	152–371 (Iran)	[128]
Japanese			
Light-scattering in whole blood	130–350		[129]
Africans and Afro-Caribbeans			
Microscopy (Nigeria)	95–278		[130]
	114–322		[130]
	100–430		[50]
Impedance counting (Zambia)	36–258		[131]
Impedance counting (Ethiopia)	97–324	98–352	[46]
Impedance counting (Uganda)	80–288	100–297	[43]
Impedance counting (Uganda)	106–362	138–457	[44]
Sysmex KX-21N (Tanzanians)	147–356	152–425	[45]
Impedance counting (Gambia)	124–367 (90% range)	140–397 (90% range)	[47]
Impedance counting (Kenya)	102–307	88–439	[49]
Impedance counting (Rwanda, Kenya, Uganda, Zambia)	126–438		[48]
Impedance counting			
(Africans in London)	128–365	166–377	[123]
(Afro-Caribbeans in London)	210–351	160–411	[123]
Light-scattering			
(Africans in London)	118–297*	149–332*	
(Afro-Caribbeans in London)	134–332*	165–368*	

*Unpublished observations of the author.

(Pct) is similarly higher [52,132–134]. Platelet counts in Africans have been observed to be lower than those of Caucasians [130,131], but this is less true of Afro-Caribbeans and of Africans living in Britain [123] and no such difference was observed between Black and Caucasian Americans [52]. This suggests that the low platelet counts observed in Africa are in part genetic but in part caused by dietary factors or subclinical disease. Genetic factors are also operative within Caucasian populations. A study of five isolated communities in Italy found significant differences between groups; there was also a significant steady decline with age [133].

The platelet count correlates with body weight, being higher in obese subjects [135].

In early studies, infants and children were reported to have similar platelet counts to adults [85,136]. Likewise, neonates, both premature and full term, were reported to have similar platelet counts to older children and adults [81,85,136], although babies that were small for gestational age [81] and many sick babies had lower counts. However, in more recent studies children have been observed to have higher counts than adults (Table 5.16). By adolescence, counts are similar to those of adults.

Many automated instruments measure the mean platelet volume (MPV). This is an inherited characteristic, which varies inversely with the platelet count [137]. The reference ranges are very instrument/method dependent. Reported ranges for five instruments are shown in Table 5.17. The

Table 5.16 94% ranges for platelet counts ($\times 10^{-9}$/l) in healthy Caucasian children and adolescents.

Age	Male	Female
Cord blood[*] [60]	180–428	
2 months[†] [95]	216–658	
5 months[†] [95]	241–591	
13 months[†] [95]	209–455	
4–6 years[‡]	213–429	220–443
7–8 years[‡]	211–422	218–396
9–10 years[‡]	166–429	197–406
1–10 years[†] [127]	220–422	
11–12 years[‡]	175–375	174–374
13–14 years[‡]	166–360	192–439
15–19 years[‡]	171–370	171–356
8–14 years[‡]	193–445	183–410
15–18 years[‡]	145–330	163–361
10–18 years[†] [127]	165–396	

[*]Brazilian, from Porto Alegre, so likely to be essentially Caucasian; Abbott Cell-Dyn 4000.

[†]Bayer H.1 [95] or Advia 120 [127].

[‡]Coulter STKS [103,104].

Table 5.17 Mean platelet volume (MPV) in normal subjects [134,138–141].

Instrument	Principle	MPV
Coulter STKS [139]	Impedance	7.9 (5.6–10.9)
Coulter LH 750 [138]	Impedance	8.86 (6.36–11.36)
Sysmex XE-2100 [140]	Impedance	10.50 (25th–75th centile, 10.20–11.20)
Sysmex XE-2100D [138]	Impedance	10.76 (8.26–13.26)
Siemens Advia 2120 [140]	Light-scattering	8.20 (25th–75th centile, 7.80–8.70)
Siemens Advia 2120 [138]	Light-scattering	8.81 (5.45–12.17)
Siemens Advia 2120 [134]	Light-scattering	7.8 (6.7–9.6)
Abbott Cell-Dyn [141]	Impedance	(6.9–10.4)

Table 5.18 Comparison of mean platelet volume and platelet distribution width when the same samples are evaluated on different instruments [142].

Instrument	Reference range for mean platelet volume (MPV) (fl)	Reference range for platelet distribution width (PDW) (%)
Cell-Dyn 4000	7.6–11	15–17.2
Sysmex XE-2100	9.8–12.6	11.0–16.9
Advia 120	7.1–10.4	46.4–68.0
ABX Pentra 120	7.7–10.3	12.5–20.0
Coulter LH750	7.9–11.3	15.6–17.5

platelet distribution width (PDW) may also be measured. Results for MPV and PDW on the same series of samples measured on five different instruments are shown in Table 5.18. Higher MPVs may be predictive of thrombotic risk, both venous and arterial [143].

Reference ranges for a wider range of platelet variables are available for the Advia 2020 [134], the Cell-Dyn Sapphire [141] and the XE-2100 [144].

Normal ranges for reticulocyte counts

When reticulocyte counts are expressed as a percentage, reported normal ranges have been between 0.4 and 2% in one study [145] and 0.8–2.5% and 0.8–4.1% for males and females respectively in another [146]. Later studies with automated reticulocyte counts have not generally found any gender difference in the percentage of reticulocytes. Reticulocyte counts are more meaningfully expressed as absolute numbers. In one study, a mean of 88×10^9/l and a range of $18–158 \times 10^9$/l were found

Table 5.19 Reported reference ranges for manual and automated reticulocyte counts.

Method	95% range (median) of percentage reticulocytes	95% range (median) or [mean] of absolute reticulocyte count ($\times 10^{-9}$/l)	Reference
Manual		18–158 (88)	147
Manual	0.8–2.5 (males)		146
	0.8–4.1 (females)		
Manual	0.4–2.0		145
Manual	0.4–2.3 (1.0)	19–111 (46)	150
		19–59	148
		40–140	149
Bayer Advia 120	0.6–2.5 (1.2)	27–125 (58)	150
		16–72 [44]	151
Abbott Cell Dyn 4000	0.4–2.2 (1.3)	25–108 (57)	150
		19–97 [58]	151
Coulter Gen S	0.5–1.8 (1.0)	20–85 (43)	150
Coulter General S		16–79 [47.5]	151
Sysmex SE 9500 RET	0.5–1.9 (0.9)	23–95 (44)	150
		9–72 [44]	151
Sysmex XE 2100		27–93 (males)	39
		22–76 (females)	
VEGA RETIC/ABX	0.6–2.6 (1.3)	30–30 (60)	150
Pentra 120 Retic		16–100 [58]	151

[147]. Reference ranges reported for automated reticulocyte counts have varied considerably, from 19–59×10^9/l [148] to 40–140×10^9/l [149]. The higher values reported by Chin-Yee *et at.* [149] appear more acceptable since, in this study, automated and manual counts were similar. These and other reported reference ranges for reticulocyte counts are summarised in Tables 5.19 and 5.20. Table 5.20 also shows reference ranges for the mean reticulocyte volume and the immature reticulocyte fraction on various instruments. A higher range, approximately 94–222×10^9/l, has been reported in the neonatal period [60]; these were automated counts using an Abbott Cell-Dyn 4000 instrument. Data applicable to infants are shown in Table 5.21 [95].

Table 5.20 Reference ranges for reticulocyte count, immature reticulocyte fraction and mean reticulocyte volume derived on the same specimens on different instruments.

Instrument	Reference range ($\times 10^{-9}$/l) for reticulocyte count [142]	Reference range for Immature Reticulocyte Fraction [142]	Reference range for mean reticulocyte volume (fl) [152]
Cell-Dyn 4000	28–119	0.20–0.40	
Sysmex XE-2100	27–99	0.02–0.11	
Advia 120	33–104	0.06–0.20	100–114
ABX Pentra 30–105	30–105	0.09–0.17	
ABX Pentra 120			91–111
Coulter LH750	18–114	0.22–0.40	98–120
Reference method	29–129		

Table 5.21 Reported reference ranges for reticulocyte counts in infants using Advia H1 [95].

Age	Absolute reticulocyte count ($\times 10^{-9}$/l)
2 months	63–235
3 months	41–124
13 months	36–142

TEST YOUR KNOWLEDGE

Visit the companion website for MCQs and EMQs on this topic:
www.wiley.com/go/bain/bloodcells

References

1 Bain BJ (1989) *Blood Cells: a Practical Guide*. Gower, London.
2 Moe PJ (1967) Umbilical cord blood and capillary blood in the evaluation of anaemia in erythroblastosis foetalis. *Acta Pediatr Scand*, **56**, 391–394.
3 Özbek N, Gürakan B and Kayiran SM (2000) Complete blood cell counts in capillary and venous blood of healthy term newborns. *Acta Haematol*, **103**, 226–228.
4 Christensen RD and Rothstein G (1979) Pitfalls in the interpretation of leukocyte counts of newborn infants. *Clin Lab Haematol*, **72**, 608–611.
5 Yang Z-W, Yang S-H, Chen L, Qu J, Zhu J and Tang Z (2001) Comparison of blood counts in venous, fingertip and arterial blood and their measurement variation. *Clin Lab Haematol*, **23**, 155–159.
6 Leppänen EA (1988) Experimental basis of standardized specimen collection: the effect of site of venipuncture on the blood picture, the white blood cell differential count, and the serum albumin concentration. *Eur J Haematol*, **41**, 445–448.
7 Bryner MA, Houwen B, Westengard J and Klein O (1997) The spun micro-haematocrit and mean red cell volume are affected by changes in the oxygenation state of red blood cells. *Clin Lab Haematol*, **19**, 99–103.
8 Campbell PJ, Aurelius S, Blowees G and Harvey J (1995) Decrease in CD4 counts with rest; implications for the monitoring of HIV infection. *Br J Haematol*, **89**, 73.
9 Balloch Al and Cauchi MN (1993) Reference ranges for haematology parameters in pregnancy derived from patient populations. *Clin Lab Haematol*, **15**, 7–14.
10 Beutler E and West C (2005) Hematologic differences between African-Americans and whites; the role of iron deficiency and α-thalassemia on hemoglobin levels and mean corpuscular volume. *Blood*, **106**, 740–745.
11 Robins EB and Blum S (2007) Hematologic reference values for African American children and adolescents. *Am J Hematol*, **82**, 611–614.
12 Sala C, Ciullo M, Lanzara C, Nutile T, Bione S, Massacane R et al. (2008) Variation of hemoglobin levels in normal Italian populations from genetic isolates. *Haematologica*, **93**, 1372–1375.
13 Patel KV (2008) Variability and heritability of hemoglobin concentration: an opportunity to improve understanding of anemia in older adults. *Haematologica*, **93**, 1281–1283.
14 Beutler E, Felitti V, Gelbart T and Waalen J (2003) Haematological effects of the C282Y *HFE* mutation in homozygous and heterozygous states among subjects of northern and southern European ancestry. *Br J Haematol*, **120**, 887–893.
15 Barton JC, Bertoli LF and Rothenberg BE (2000) Peripheral blood erythrocyte parameters in hemochromatosis: evidence for increased erythrocyte hemoglobin content. *J Lab Clin Med*, **135**, 96–104.
16 Giorno R, Clifford JH, Beverly S and Rossing RG (1980) Hematology reference ranges. Analysis by different statistical technics and variations with age and sex. *Am J Clin Pathol*, **74**, 765–770.
17 Solberg EK (1981) Statistical treatment of collected reference values and determination of reference limits. In: Grasbeck R and Alstrom W, eds. *Reference Values in Laboratory Medicine*. John Wiley, Chichester.
18 Amador E (1975) Health and normality. *JAMA*, **232**, 953–955.
19 Ruiz-Argüelles GJ, Sanchez-Medal L, Loria A, Piedras J and Córdova MS (1980) Red cell indices in normal adults residing at altitude from sea level to 2670 meters. *Am J Hematol*, **8**, 265–271.
20 Bonfichi M, Balduini A, Arcaini L, Lorenzi A, Marseglia C, Malcovati L et al. (2000) Haematological modifications after acute exposure to high altitude: possible applications for detection of recombinant erythropoietin misuse. *Br J Haematol*, **109**, 895–896.
21 Bowen AL, Hudson JG, Navia P, Rios-Dalenz J, Pollard AJ, Williams D and Heath D (1977) The effect of altitude on blood platelet count. *Br J Haematol*, **97**, Suppl 1, 83.
22 Carballo C, Foucar K, Swanson P, Papile LA and Watterberg KL (1992) Effect of high altitude on neutrophil counts in newborn infants. *J Pediatr*, **119**, 464–466.
23 Kristal-Bonch E, Froom P, Harari G, Shapiro Y and Green MS (1993) Seasonal changes in red blood cell parameters. *Br J Haematol*, **85**, 603–607.
24 Kristal-Bonch E, Froom P, Harari G and Ribak J (1997) Seasonal differences in blood cell parameters and the association with cigarette smoking. *Clin Lab Haematol*, **19**, 177–181.
25 Bertouch JV, Roberts-Thomson PJ and Bradley J (1983) Diurnal variation of lymphocyte subsets identified by monoclonal antibodies. *BMJ*, **286**, 1171–1172.
26 Philips D, Rezvani K and Bain BJ (2000) Exercise induced mobilisation of the marginated granulocyte pool in the investigation of ethnic neutropenia. *J Clin Pathol*, **53**, 481–483.
27 Bain BJ, Phillips D, Thomson K, Richardson D and Gabriel I (2000) Investigation of the effect of marathon running on leucocyte counts of subjects of different ethnic origins: relevance to the aetiology of ethnic neutropenia. *Br J Haematol*, **108**, 483–487.
28 Bain BJ (1992) Haematological effects of smoking. *J Smoking Rel Dis*, **3**, 99–108.
29 Milman N, Byg K-E, Mulvad G, Pedersen HS and Bjerregaard P (2001) Haemoglobin concentrations appear to be lower in indigenous Greenlanders than in Danes: assessment of haemoglobin in 234 Greenlanders and in 2804 Danes. *Eur J Haematol*, **67**, 23–29.
30 Wilson CA, Bekele G, Nicolson M, Ravussin E and Pratley RE (1997) Relationship of the white blood cell count to body fat: role of leptin. *Br J Haematol*, **99**, 447–451.
31 Nanji AA and Freeman JB (1985) Relationship between body weight and total leukocyte count in morbid obesity. *Am J Clin Pathol*, **84**, 346–347.

32 Cembrowski G, Qiu Y, Szkotak S, Clarke G and La M (2013) Variation in reference intervals of many complete blood count (CBC) constituents dependent on waist circumference (WC). *Int J Lab Hematol*, **35**, Suppl. 1, 15.

33 Waalen J, Felitti V and Beutler E (2002) Haemoglobin and ferritin concentrations in men and women: cross sectional study. *BMJ*, **325**, 137.

34 Nilsson-Ehle A, Jagenburg R, Landahl S and Svanborg A (2000) Blood hemoglobin declines in the elderly: implications for reference intervals for 70–88. *Eur J Haematol*, **65**, 297–305.

35 Troussard X, Vol S, Cornet E, Bardet V, Couaillac JP, Fossat C *et al.* for the French-Speaking Cellular Hematology Group (Groupe Francophone d'Hématologie Cellulaire, GFHC) (2014) Full blood count normal reference values for adults in France. *J Clin Pathol*, **67**, 341–344.

36 Nilsson-Ehle A, Jagenburg R, Landahl S, Svanborg A and Westin J (1988) Haematological abnormalities in a 75-year-old population. Consequences for health-related reference intervals. *Eur J Haematol*, **41**, 136–146.

37 Yamada M, Wong FL and Suzuki G (2003) Longitudinal trends of hemoglobin levels in a Japanese population – RERF's Adult Health Study subjects. *Eur J Haematol*, **70**, 129–135.

38 Beutler E and Waalen J (2006) Hemoglobin levels, altitude, and smoking. *Blood*, **108**, 2131–2132.

39 Wakeman L, Al-Ismail S, Benton A, Beddall A, Gibbs A, Hartnell S *et al.* (2007) Robust, routine haematology reference ranges for healthy adults, *Int J Lab Hematol*, **29**, 279–283.

40 Beutler E and Waalen J (2006) The definition of anemia: what *is* the lower limit of normal of the blood hemoglobin concentration? *Blood*, **107**, 1747–1750.

41 Fairbanks VF and Tefferi A (2001) Letter to the Editor. *Eur J Haematol*, **67**, 203–204.

42 Shaper AG and Lewis P (1971) Genetic neutropenia in people of African origin. *Lancet*, **ii**, 1021–1023.

43 Lugada ES, Mermin J, Haharuza F, Ulvestad E, Were W, Langeland N *et al.* (2004) Population-based hematologic and immunologic reference values for a healthy Ugandan population. *Clin Diagn Lab Immunol*, **11**, 29–34.

44 Eller LA, Eller MA, Ouma B, Kataaha P, Kyabaggu D, Tumusiime R *et al.* (2008) Reference intervals in healthy adult Ugandan blood donors and their impact on conducting international vaccine trials. *PLoS One*, **3**, e3919.

45 Saathoff E, Schneider P, Kleinfeldt V, Geis S, Haule D, Maboko L *et al.* (2008) Laboratory reference values for healthy adults from southern Tanzania. *Trop Med Int Health*, **13**, 612–625.

46 Tsegaye A, Messele T, Tilahun T, Hailu E, Sahlu T, Doorly R *et al.* (1999) Immunohematological reference ranges for adult Ethiopians. *Clin Diagn Lab Immunol*, **6**, 410–414.

47 Adetifa IMO, Hill PC, Jeffries DJ, Jackson-Sillah D, Ibanga HB, Bah G *et al.* (2009) Haematological values from a Gambian cohort – possible reference range for a West African population. *Int J Lab Hematol*, **31**, 615–622.

48 Karita E, Ketter N, Price MA, Kayitenkore K, Kaleebu P, Nanvubya A (2009) CLSI-derived hematology and biochemistry reference intervals for healthy adults in eastern and southern Africa. *PLoS One*, **4**, e4401.

49 Zeh C, Amornkul PN, Inzaule S, Ondoa P, Oyaro B, Mwaengo DM *et al.* (2011) Population-based biochemistry, immunologic and hematological reference values for adolescents and young adults in a rural population in Western Kenya. *PLoS One*, **6**, e21040.

50 Buseri FI, Siaminabo IJ and Jeremiah ZA (2010) Reference values of hematological indices of infants, children, and adolescents in Port Harcourt, Nigeria. *Path Lab Med Int*, **2**, 65–70.

51 Orfanakis NJ, Ostlund RE, Bishop CR and Athens JW (1970) Normal blood leukocyte concentration values. *Am J Clin Pathol*, **53**, 647–651.

52 Saxena S and Wong ET (1990) Heterogeneity of common hematologic parameters among racial, ethnic, and gender subgroups. *Arch Pathol Lab Med*, **114**, 715–719.

53 Freedman DS, Gates L, Flanders WD, Van Assendelft OW, Barboriack JJ, Joesoef MR and Byers T (1997) Black/White differences in leukocyte subpopulations in men. *Int J Epidemiol*, **26**, 757–764.

54 Lim E-M, Cembrowski G, Cembrowski M and Clarke G (2010) Race-specific WBC and neutrophil count reference intervals. *Int J Lab Hematol*, **32**, 590–597.

55 Rezvani K, Flanagan AM, Sarma U, Constantinovici N and Bain BJ (2000) Investigation of ethnic neutropenia by assessment of bone marrow colony-forming cells. *Acta Haematol*, **105**, 32–37.

56 Reich D, Nalls MA, Kao WH, Akylbekova EL, Tandon A, Patterson N *et al.* (2009) Reduced neutrophil count in people of African descent is due to a regulatory variant in the Duffy antigen receptor for chemokines gene. *PLoS Genet*, **5**, e1000360.

57 Hsieh M, Chin K, Link B, Stroncek D, Wang E, Everhart J *et al.* (2005) Benign ethnic neutropenia in individuals of African descent: incidence, granulocyte mobilization, and gene expression profiling. *Blood*, **106**, 858a–858b.

58 Hsieh MM, Everhart JE, Byrd-Holt DD, Tisdale JF and Rodgers GP (2007) Prevalence of neutropenia in the U.S. population: age, sex, smoking status, and ethnic differences. *Ann Intern Med*, **146**, 486–492.

59 Marks J, Gairdner D and Roscoe JD (1955) Blood formation in infancy. Part III. Cord blood. *Arch Dis Child*, **30**, 117–120.

60 Pranke P, Failace RR, Allebrandt WF, Steibel G, Schmidt F and Nardi NB (2001) Hematologic and immunophenotypic characterization of human umbilical cord blood. *Acta Haematol*, **105**, 71–76.

61 Matoth Y, Zaizov R and Varsano I (1971) Postnatal changes in some red cell parameters. *Acta Paediatr Scand*, **60**, 317–323.

62 Lanzkowsky P (1960). Effects of early and late clamping of umbilical cord on infant's haemoglobin level. *BMJ*, **ii**, 1777–1782.

63 www.beckman.com (accessed 2005).

64 Saarinem UM and Siimes MD (1978) Developmental changes in red blood cell counts and indices of infants after exclusion of iron deficiency by laboratory criteria and continuous iron supplementation. *J Pediatr*, **92**, 412–416.

65 Serjeant GR, Grandison Y, Mason K, Serjeant B, Sewell A and Vaidya V (1980) Hematological indices in normal Negro children: a Jamaican cohort from birth to five years. *Clin Lab Haematol*, **2**, 169–178.

66 Scott-Emuakpor AB, Okolo AA, Omene JA and Ukpe SI (1985) The limits of physiological anaemia in the African neonate. *Acta Haematol*, **74**, 99–103.

67 Gregory J and Hey E (1972) Blood neutrophil response to bacterial infection in the first month of life. *Arch Dis Child*, **47**, 747–753.

68 Weinberg AG, Rosenfeld CR, Manroe BL and Browne R (1985) Neonatal blood cell count in health and disease. II Values for lymphocytes, monocytes, and eosinophils. *J Pediatr*, **106**, 462–466.

69 Manroe BL, Weinberg AG, Rosenfeld CR and Brown R (1979) The neonatal blood count in health and disease. I. Reference values for neutrophilic cells. *J Pediatr*, **95**, 89–98.

70 Schmutz N, Henry E, Jopling J and Christensen RD (2008) Expected ranges for blood neutrophil concentrations of neonates: the Manroe and Mouzinho charts revisited. *J Perinatol*, **28**, 275–281.

71 Chan PCY, Hayes L and Bain BJ (1985) A comparison of the white cell counts of cord bloods from babies of different ethnic origins. *Ann Trop Paediatr*, **5**, 153–155.

72 Xanthou M (1970) Leucocyte blood picture in full-term and premature babies during neonatal period. *Arch Dis Child*, **45**, 242–249.

73 Cranendonk E, van Gennip AH, Abeling NGGM, Behrendt H and Hart AA (1985) Reference values for automated cytochemical differential count of leukocytes in children 0–16 years old: a comparison with manually obtained counts from Wright-stained smears. *J Clin Chem Clin Biochem*, **23**, 663–667.

74 Dallman PR and Siimes MA (1979) Percentile curves for hemoglobin and red cell volume in infancy and childhood. *J Pediatr*, **94**, 26–31.

75 Katsares V, Pararidis Z, Nikolaidou E, Karvounidou I, Ardean K-A, Drossas N et al. (2008) References ranges for umbilical cord blood hematological values. *Lab Med*, **40**, 437–439.

76 Aneja S, Manchanda R, Patwari A, Sagreiya K and Bhargava SK (1979) Normal hematological values in newborns. *Indian Pediatr*, **16**, 781–786.

77 Ezeilo GC (1978) A comparison of the haematological values of cord bloods of African, European and Asian neonates. *Afr J Med Sci*, **7**, 163–169.

78 Green DW and Mimouni F (1990) Nucleated erythrocytes in healthy infants and in infants of diabetic mothers. *J Pediatr*, **116**, 129–131.

79 Frazier JP, Cleary TG, Pickering LK, Kohl S and Ross PJ (1982) Leukocyte function in healthy neonates following vaginal and cesarean section deliveries. *J Pediatr*, **101**, 269–272.

80 Harrison KL (1979) The effect of maternal smoking on neonatal leucocytes. *Aust NZ J Obstet Gynaecol*, **19**, 166–168.

81 McIntosh N, Kempson C and Tyler RM (1988) Blood counts in extremely low birth weight infants. *Arch Dis Child*, **63**, 74–76.

82 Özyürek E, Çetintaş S, Ceylan T, Öğüş E, Haberal A, Gürakan B and Özbek N (2006) Complete blood count parameters for healthy, small-for-gestational-age, full-term newborns. *Clin Lab Haematol*, **28**, 97–104.

83 Green DW, Hendon B and Mimouni FB (1995) Nucleated erythrocytes and intraventricular haemorrhage in preterm neonates. *Pediatrics*, **96**, 475–478.

84 Playfair JHL, Wolfendale MR and Kay HEM (1963) The leucocytes of peripheral blood in the human foetus. *Br J Haematol*, **9**, 336–344.

85 Millar DS, Davis LR, Rodeck CH, Nicolaides KH and Mibashan RS (1985) Normal blood cell values in the early mid-trimester fetus. *Prenat Diagn*, **5**, 367–373.

86 Forestier F, Daffos F, Galactéros F, Bardakjian J, Rainaut M and Beuzard Y (1986) Haematological values of 163 normal fetuses between 18 and 30 weeks of gestation. *Paediatr Res*, **20**, 342–346.

87 Mari G, Zimmerman R and Oz U (2000) Non-invasive diagnosis of fetal anemia by Doppler ultrasonography. *N Engl J Med*, **343**, 67–68.

88 Srisupundit K, Piyamongkol W and Tongsong T (2008) Comparison of red blood cell hematology among normal, α-thalassemia-1 trait, and haemoglobin Bart's fetuses at mid-pregnancy. *Am J Hematol*, **83**, 908–910.

89 Hohlfeld P, Forestier F, Kaplan C, Tissot JD and Daffos F (1994) Fetal thrombocytopenia: a retrospective survey of 5,194 fetal blood samplings. *Blood*, **84**, 1851–1856.

90 Forestier F, Hohlfeld P, Vial Y, Olin V, Andreux J-P and Tissot J-D (1996) Blood smears and prenatal diagnosis. *Br J Haematol*, **95**, 278–280.

91 Coulombel L, Dehan M, Tchernia G, Hill C and Vial M (1979) The number of polymorphonuclear leucocytes in relation to gestational age in the newborn. *Acta Paediatr Scand*, **68**, 709–711.

92 Zaizov R and Matoth Y (1976) Red cell values on the first postnatal day during the last sixteen weeks of gestation. *Am J Hematol*, **1**, 275–278.

93 Castriota-Scanderberg A, Fedrazzi G, Mercadanti M, Stapane I, Butturini A and Izzi G (1992) Normal values of total reticulocytes and reticulocyte subsets in children and young adults. *Haematologica*, **77**, 363–364.

94 Dallman PR, Looker AC, Johnson CL and Carroll M (1996) Influence of age on laboratory criteria for the diagnosis of iron deficiency in infants and children. In: Hallberg L and Asp NG (eds) *Iron Nutrition in Health and Disease*. John Libbey, London, quoted by Wharton BA (1999) Iron deficiency in children: detection and prevention. *Br J Haematol*, **106**, 270–280.

95 Hinchliffe RF, Bellamy GJ, Bell F, Finn A, Vora AJ and Lennard L (2013) Reference intervals for red cell variables and platelet counts in infants at 2, 5 and 13 months of age: a cohort study. *J Clin Pathol*, **66**, 962–966.

96 Hunter RE and Smith NJ (1972) Hemoglobin and hematocrit values in iron deficiency in infancy. *J Pediatr*, **81**, 710–713.

97 Burman D (1972) Haemoglobin levels in normal infants aged 3 to 24 months, and the effect of iron. *Arch Dis Child*, **47**, 261–271.

98 Emond AM, Hawkins N, Pennock C, Golding J and the ALSPAC Children in Focus Study Team (1996) Haemoglobin and ferritin concentrations in infants at 8 months of age. *Arch Dis Child*, **74**, 36–69.

99 Sherriff A, Emond A, Hawkins N, Golding J and the ALSPAC Children in Focus Study Team (1999) Haemoglobin and ferritin concentrations in children aged 12 and 18 months. *Arch Dis Child*, **80**, 153–157.

100 Morley R, Abbott R, Fairweather-Tait S, MacFadyen U, Stephenson T and Lucas A (1999) Iron fortified follow on formula from 9 to 18 months improves iron status but not development or growth: a randomised trial. *Arch Dis Child*, **81**, 247–252.

101 Viteri FE, de Tuna V and Guzmán MA (1972) Normal haematological values in the Central American population. *Br J Haematol*, **23**, 189–204.

102 Natvig H and Vellar OD and Andersen J (1967) Studies on hemoglobin value in Norway. VII. Hemoglobin, hematocrit and MCHC values among boys and girls aged 7–20 years in elementary and grammar school. *Acta Med Scand*, **182**, 183–191.

103 Taylor MRH, Holland CV, Spencer R, Jackson JF, O'Connor GI and O'Donnell JR (1997) Haematological references ranges for schoolchildren. *Clin Lab Haematol*, **19**, 1–15.

104 Flegar-Mĕštrić Z, Nazor A and Jagarinic N (1999) Reference intervals for haematological parameters in urban school children. *Clin Lab Haematol*, **21**, 72–74.

105 Bellamy GJ, Hinchliffe RF, Crawshaw KJ, Finn AH and Bell F (2000) Total and differential leucocyte counts in infants at 2, 5 and 13 months of age. *Clin Lab Haematol*, **22**, 81–87.

106 Dallman PR (1991) Blood and blood forming tissues. In Rudolph AM and Hoffman JIE (eds), *Rudolph's Pediatrics*, 19th edn. Appleton & Lange, New York.

107 Osgood EE, Brownlee IE, Osgood MW, Ellis DM and Cohen W (1939) Total, differential and absolute leukocyte counts and sedimentation rates of healthy children four to seven years of age. *Am J Dis Child*, **58**, 61–70.

108 Osgood EE, Brownlee IE, Osgood MW, Ellis DM and Cohen W (1939) Total, differential and absolute leukocyte counts and sedimentation rates of healthy children. Standards for children eight to fourteen years of age. *Am J Dis Child*, **58**, 282–294.

109 Lundstrom U, Siimes MA and Dallman PR (1977) At what age does iron supplementation become necessary in low-birth-weight infants. *J Pediatr*, **91**, 878–883.

110 Andersson O, Hellström-Westas L, Andersson D and Domellöf M (2011) Effect of delayed versus early umbilical cord clamping on neonatal outcomes and iron status at 4 months: a randomised controlled trial. *BMJ*, **343**, 1244.

111 Caramihai E, Karayalcin G, Aballi AJ and Lanzkowsky P (1975) Leukocyte count differences in healthy white and black children 1 to 5 years of age. *J Pediatr*, **86**, 252–254.

112 Sadowitz PD and Oski FA (1983) Differences in polymorphonuclear cell counts between healthy white and black infants: response to meningitis. *Pediatrics*, **72**, 405–407.

113 Williams TN, Maitland K, Ganczakowski M, Peto TEA, Clegg JB, Weatherall DJ and Bowden DK (1996) Red blood cells phenotypes in the α⁺ thalassaemias from early childhood to maturity. *Br J Haematol*, **95**, 266–272.

114 Osta V, Caldirola MS, Fernandez M, Marcone MI, Tissera G, Pennesi S and Ayuso C (2013) Utility of new mature erythrocyte and reticulocyte indices in screening for iron-deficiency anemia in a pediatric population. *Int J Lab Hematol*, **35**, 400–405.

115 Milman N, Bergholt T, Byg K, Eriksen L and Hvas AM (2007) Reference intervals for haematological variables during normal pregnancy and postpartum in 434 healthy Danish women. *Eur J Haematol*, **79**, 39–46.

116 Cruikshank JM (1970) Some variations in the normal haemoglobin concentration. *Br J Haematol*, **18**, 523–529.

117 England JM and Bain BJ (1976) Annotation: total and differential leucocyte count. *Br J Haematol*, **33**, 1–7.

118 Brecher G and Cronkite EP (1950) Morphology and enumeration of human blood platelets. *J Appl Physiol*, **3**, 365–377.

119 Sloan AW (1951) The normal platelet count in man. *J Clin Pathol*, **4**, 37–46.

120 Miale JB (1982) *Laboratory Medicine Hematology*, 6th edn. CV Mosby, St Louis.

121 Bain BJ and Forster T (1980) A sex difference in the bleeding time. *Thromb Haemostas*, **43**, 131–132.

122 Giles C (1981) The platelet count and mean platelet volume. *Br J Haematol*, **48**, 31–37.

123 Bain BJ and Seed M (1986) Platelet count and platelet size in Africans and West Indians. *Clin Lab Haematol*, **8**, 43–48.

124 Payne BA and Pierre RV (1986) Using the three-part differential. Part 1. Investigating the possibilities. *Lab Med*, **17**, 459–462.

125 Gladwin AM, Trowbridge EA, Slater DN, Reardon D and Martin JF (1990) The size and number of bone marrow megakaryocytes in malignant lymphoma and their relationship to the platelet count. *Am J Hematol*, **35**, 225–231.

126 Brummitt DR and Barker HF (2000) The determination of a reference range for new platelet parameters produced by the Bayer ADVIA™ 120 full blood count analyser. *Clin Lab Haematol*, **22**, 103–107.

127 Giacomini A, Legovini P, Gessoni G, Antico F, Valverde S, Salvadego MM and Manoni F (2001) Platelet count and parameters determined by the Bayer ADVIA™ 120 in reference subjects and patients. *Clin Lab Haematol*, **23**, 181–186.

128 Adibi P, Faghih Imani E, Talaei M and Ghanei M (2007) Population-based platelet reference values for an Iranian population. *Int J Lab Hematol*, **29**, 195–199.

129 Takamatsu N, Yamamoto H, Onomura Y and Ichikawa N (1992) A study of the hematological reference ranges and changes with age using the automated hematology analyzer K-1000™. *Sysmex J Int*, **2**, 136–145.

130 Essien EM, Usanga EA and Ayeni O (1973) The normal platelet count and platelet factor 3 availability in some Nigerian population groups. *Scand J Haematol*, **10**, 378–383.

131 Gill GV, England A and Marshal C (1979) Low platelet counts in Zambians. *Trans R Soc Trop Med Hyg*, **73**, 111–112.

132 Bain BJ (1985) Platelet count and platelet size in men and women. *Scand J Haematol*, **35**, 77–79.

133 Biino G, Gasparini P, D'Adamo P, Ciullo M, Nutile T, Toniolo D et al. (2012) Influence of age, sex and ethnicity on platelet count in five Italian geographic isolates: mild thrombocytopenia may be physiological. *Br J Haematol*, **157**, 384–387.

134 Kim MJ, Park P-W, Seo Y-H, Kim K-H, Seo JY, Jeong JH et al. (2013) Reference intervals for platelet parameters in Korean adults using Advia 2120. *Ann Lab Med*, **33**, 364–366.

135 Wilson CA, Bekele G, Nicolson M, Ravussin E and Pralley RE (1997) Relationship of the white blood cell count to role of leptin. *Br J Haematol*, **99**, 447–451.

136 Sell EJ and Corrigan JJ (1973) Platelet counts, fibrinogen concentrations, and factor V and factor VII levels in healthy infants according to gestational age. *J Pediatr*, **82**, 1028–1032.

137 Soranzo N, Spector TD, Mangino M, Kühnel B, Rendon A, Teumer A et al. (2009) A genome-wide meta-analysis identified 22 loci associated with eight hematological parameters in the HaemGen consortium. *Nat Genet*, **41**, 1182–1190.

138 Latger-Cannard V, Hoarau M, Salignac S, Baumgart D, Nurden P and Lecompte T (2012) Mean platelet volume: comparison of three analysers towards standardization of morphological phenotype. *Int J Lab Hematol*, **34**, 300–310.

139 Pathepchotiwong K, Dhareruchta P and Adirojananon W (2001) Platelet parameter in healthy subjects analyzed by automation analyzer. *Thai J Hematol Transfus Med*, **11**, 93–100, cited by Latger-Cannard et al. [138].

140 Noris P, Klersy C, Zecca M, Arcaini L, Pecci A, Melazzini F et al. (2009) Platelet size distinguishes between inherited macrothrombocytopenias and immune thrombocytopenia. *J Thromb Haemost*, **7**, 2131–2136.

141 Hoffmann JJML, van den Broek NMA and Curvers J (2013) Reference intervals of reticulated platelets and other platelet parameters and their associations. *Arch Pathol Lab Med*, **137**, 1635–1640.

142 Doretto P, Biasioli B, Casolari B, Pasini L, Bulian P, Buttarello M et al. (2011) Conteggio reticulocitario automizzato: valutazione NCCLS H-44 ed ICSH su 5 strumenti. In: Cenci A and Cappelletti P (eds) *Appunti di Ematologia di Laboratorio*. MAF Servizi Editore, Turin.

143 Machin SJ and Briggs C (2010) Commentary: mean platelet volume: a quick, easy determinant of thrombotic risk? *J Thromb Haemostas*, **8**, 146–147.

144 Ko YJ, Kim H, Hur M, Choi SG, Moon H-W, Yun Y-M and Hong SN (2013) Establishment of reference interval for immature platelet fraction. *Int J Lab Hematol*, **35**, 528–533.

145 Crouch JY and Kaplow LS (1985) Relationship of reticulocyte age to polychromasia, shift cells and shift reticulocytes. *Arch Pathol Lab Med*, **109**, 325–329.

146 Deiss A and Kurth D (1970) Circulating reticulocytes in normal adults as determined by the new methylene blue method. *Am J Clin Pathol*, **53**, 481–484.

147 Lee GR (1981) Normal blood and bone marrow values in men. In: Wintrobe MM, Lee GR, Boggs DR, Bithell TC, Foerster J, Athens JW and Lukens IN (eds) *Clinical Hematology*, 8th edn. Lea & Febiger, Philadelphia.

148 Nobes PR and Carter AB (1990) Reticulocyte counting using flow cytometry. *J Clin Pathol*, **43**, 675–678.

149 Chin-Yee I, Keeney M and Lehmann C (1991) Flow cytometric reticulocyte analysis using thiazole orange: clinical experience and technical limitations. *Clin Lab Haematol*, **13**, 177–188.

150 Buttarello M, Bulian P, Farina G, Temporin V, Toffolo L, Trabuio E and Rizzotti P (2000) Flow cytometric reticulocyte counting: parallel evaluation of five fully automated analyzers: an NCCLS-ICSH approach. *Am J Clin Pathol*, **115**, 100–111.

151 Van den Bossche J, Devreese K, Malfait R, van de Vyvere M and Schouwer P (2001) Comparison of the reticulocyte mode of the Abx Pentra 120Retic, Coulter General-S, Sysmex SE 9500, Abbott CD 4000 and Bayer Advia 120 haematology analysers in a simultaneous evaluation. *Clin Lab Haematol*, **23**, 355–360.

152 Cappelletti P, Biasioli B, Buttarello M, Bulian P, Casolari B, Cenci A et al. (2011) Mean reticulocyte volume (MCVr): intervalli di riferimento e necessità di standardizzazione. In: Cenci A and Cappelletti P (eds) *Appunti di Ematologia di Laboratorio*. MAF Servizi Editore, Turin.

CHAPTER 6

Quantitative changes in blood cells

This chapter deals with quantitative changes in blood cells, first the causes of increased cell counts for each lineage, then the causes of decreased counts. An increase of a cell type usually results either from redistribution of cells or from increased bone marrow output; occasionally an increased count, most noticeably of red cells, can result from a decrease of plasma volume. A decreased count of any cell type can result from diminished bone marrow output, redistribution or shortened survival in the circulation.

Polycythaemia

The term polycythaemia, strictly speaking, should indicate an increase in the number of red cells in the circulation but, in practice, the term is used for an increase of the haemoglobin concentration (Hb) and haematocrit/packed cell volume (Hct/PCV) above that which is normal for the age and sex of the subject. Usually, the red blood cell count (RBC), Hb and Hct rise in parallel. Conventionally, the term polycythaemia does not refer to an increased RBC if the Hb is normal, as may be seen, for example, in thalassaemia trait. A raised Hb can be due to a decreased plasma volume occurring either acutely or chronically. An acute decrease in plasma volume can be caused by shock, when there is a loss of fluid from the intravascular compartment, or by dehydration. An intermittent apparent polycythaemia, which can be very striking, occurs in the idiopathic capillary leak syndrome [1]. It can also occur acutely in the toxic shock syndrome, resulting from a bacterial toxin, and in capillary leak syndromes associated with viral haemorrhagic fevers. Drinking a litre of water in a short period of time causes a transient increase in Hb due to increased sympathetic activity (which is followed by a gradual reduction) [2]; this is unlikely to be noted other than in an experimental situation. A chronic decrease in plasma volume is sometimes due to cigarette smoking,

but in many cases the cause is unknown. The phenomenon has been referred to as 'stress polycythaemia' but 'pseudopolycythaemia' or 'relative polycythaemia' is a better designation since there is no clear relationship to 'stress'.

Alternatively, a raised Hb can be due to true polycythaemia, i.e. to an increase in the total volume of circulating red cells usually referred to, inaccurately, as the 'red cell mass'. True polycythaemia can be primary or secondary. In primary polycythaemia there is an intrinsic bone marrow disorder, either inherited or acquired. Erythropoietin concentration is decreased. In contrast, secondary polycythaemia is generally mediated by increased erythropoietin production, usually occurring either as a physiological response to hypoxia or as a result of inappropriate secretion by a diseased kidney or by a tumour. Causes of polycythaemia are summarised in Table 6.1. The differential diagnosis of polycythaemia vera (PV) is discussed in Chapter 8. Neonates have higher Hbs than adults, but the Hb may rise even higher in pathological conditions. Some causes of polycythaemia that are peculiar to the neonatal period are summarised in Table 6.2.

Reticulocytosis

Either the percentage or absolute reticulocyte count or both may be increased. With rare exceptions, an increased reticulocyte percentage indicates an increased proportion of young erythrocytes. Again with rare exceptions, an increased absolute reticulocyte count indicates an increased marrow output of erythrocytes. Often both the percentage and absolute count are increased, but a patient with significant anaemia may have an increased percentage of reticulocytes without an increase in the absolute count.

Causes of an increased reticulocyte count are shown in Table 6.3.

Blood Cells A Practical Guide, Fifth Edition. By Barbara J. Bain © 2015 John Wiley & Sons, Ltd. Published 2015 by John Wiley & Sons, Ltd.
Companion Website: www.wiley.com/go/bain/bloodcells

Table 6.1 Some causes of polycythaemia.

Primary

Inherited

Erythroid progenitor cells with enhanced sensitivity to erythropoietin [3], sometimes caused by mutation of the erythropoietin receptor gene (*EPOR*) [4]; homozygosity for a R200W mutation in the *VHL* gene in mid-Volga (Chuvash) familial polycythaemia (which also occurs in occasional families in western Europe, Pakistan and Bangladesh and is endemic on the Italian island of Ischia) [4–6, 7] and for the H191D *VHL* mutation in Croatia [8] resulting in protection of HIP1α (hypoxia-inducible protein 1α) from degradation and consequent increased synthesis of erythropoietin; mutation in the *EGLN1* (*PHD2*) gene encoding HIF-prolyl hydroxylase, resulting in impaired hydroxylation of HIFα [9], gain-of-function mutation in *EPAS1* (*HIF2A*) [10]; familial inappropriate increase of erythropoietin synthesis [11,12], sometimes with preceding multiple paragangliomas [13]

Acquired

Polycythaemia vera (polycythaemia rubra vera)

Essential or idiopathic erythrocytosis

Secondary

Caused by tissue hypoxia

Inherited

Inadequate oxygen-carrying capacity

Caused by congenital deficiency of NAD-linked or NADH-linked methaemoglobin reductase with resultant methaemoglobinaemia

Haemoglobin M (structurally abnormal haemoglobins with tendency to form methaemoglobin)

Impaired release of oxygen from haemoglobin

High affinity haemoglobins including some methaemoglobins and hereditary persistence of fetal haemoglobin

Oxygen affinity of haemoglobin increased by very low levels of 2,3 DPG (2,3 diphosphoglycerate) resulting from *BPGM* mutation and deficiency of bisphosphoglycerate mutase or, occasionally, from deficiency of phosphofructokinase [14]

Acquired

Hypoxia

Residence at high altitude

Use of simulated high altitude in athletic training (hypoxic tent or 'high altitude bed')

Cyanotic heart disease

Chronic hypoxic lung disease

Sleep apnoea [15]* and other hypoventilation syndromes including morbid obesity (Pickwickian syndrome)

Hepatic cirrhosis (consequent on pulmonary arteriovenous shunting) [16]

Pulmonary arteriovenous malformations in hereditary haemorrhagic telangiectasia [17]

Inadequate oxygen-carrying capacity

Chronic carbon monoxide poisoning [18] or heavy cigarette smoking including water-pipe (Shisha) smoking [19]

Chronic methaemoglobinaemia or sulphaemoglobinaemia caused by drugs or chemicals

Consequent on inappropriate synthesis or administration of erythropoietin (proven or presumptive) or androgens [20,21]

Renal lesions including carcinoma (hypernephroma), Wilms tumour, renal adenoma, renal haemangioma, renal sarcoma, renal cysts including polycystic disease of the kidney, renal artery stenosis, renal vein thrombosis, post-transplant polycythaemia, hydronephrosis, horseshoe kidney, nephrocalcinosis (including that caused by hyperparathyroidism), Bartter syndrome, renal lymphangiectasis [22], perinephric lymphangioma [23]

Hyperparathyroidism [24]

Cerebellar haemangioblastoma

Meningioma

Hepatic lesions including hepatoma, hepatic hamartoma, hepatic angiosarcoma, hepatic haemangioma and early in infectious hepatitis [25]

Uterine leiomyoma (uterine fibroid)

Tumours of the adrenal gland, ovary, lung, thymus, parathyroid (carcinoma/adenoma)

Phaeochromocytoma [26]

Atrial myxoma [27]

Cushing syndrome and primary aldosteronism

Erythropoietin administration (e.g. illicit use in athletes)

Androgen administration or androgen-secreting tumours in women

Gestational hyperandrogenism [28]

Androgen abuse in males (e.g. in athletes) [29]

TEMPI syndrome (**T**elangiectasia, **E**levated erythropoietin, **M**onoclonal gammopathy, **P**erinephric fluid collection, **I**ntrapulmonary shunting) [30]

'Blood doping'

Illicit homologous transfusion or re-transfusion of autologous blood by athletes

Other mechanisms or unknown

Inherited

Some familial cases [31]

Acquired

Cobalt toxicity [32]

Monge disease (excessive erythrocytosis at altitude – possibly related to cobalt toxicity [33])

Associated with POEMS [34]

Administration of anti-vascular endothelial growth factor receptor (semaxanib) therapy in von Hippel-Lindau syndrome [35]

Romiplostim therapy [36]

Sorafenib and sunitinib therapy [37]

*Obstructive sleep apnoea causes only a minor increase in the haematocrit, which may represent relative polycythaemia [15]

NAD, nicotinamide adenine dinucleotide; NADH, reduced nicotinamide adenine dinucleotide; POEMS, **P**olyendocrinopathy, **O**rganomegaly, **E**ndocrinopathy, **M**-protein, **S**kin changes syndrome

Table 6.2 Some causes of polycythaemia of particular importance in or peculiar to the neonatal period.

Intra-uterine twin-to-twin transfusion
Intra-uterine maternal-to-fetal transfusion
Placental insufficiency and intrauterine hypoxia
Small-for-dates babies
Post-mature babies
Maternal pregnancy-associated hypertension
Maternal smoking
Maternal diabetes mellitus
Chromosomal abnormalities
Down syndrome
Trisomy 13 syndrome
Trisomy 18 syndrome
Neonatal thyrotoxicosis
Neonatal hypothyroidism
Congenital adrenal hyperplasia
Delayed cord clamping
Underwater labour with late cord clamping [38]

Table 6.3 Causes of reticulocytosis.

Common causes
Shortened red cell life span (i.e. haemolytic anaemia)
Recent blood loss
Response to therapy in a patient with deficiency of vitamin B_{12}, folic acid or iron
Recovery from bone marrow (or erythroid) suppression or failure
Administration of erythropoietin
Hypoxia
Diabetes mellitus (possibly representing compensated haemolysis) [39]
Rare causes
Delayed maturation of reticulocytes (in myelodysplastic syndrome)
Genetic haemochromatosis [40]

Leucocytosis

Leucocytosis is an increase in the total white blood cell count (WBC). It most often results from an increase in neutrophils, but sometimes from an increase in lymphocytes and occasionally from an increase in eosinophils or from the presence of abnormal myeloid or lymphoid cells in the blood. Leucocytosis cannot be interpreted without knowledge of the differential count, although it is sometimes used as a surrogate indicator of the neutrophil count when a differential count is not available. Leucocytosis is predictive of a worse prognosis in sickle cell disease [41]. It is an adverse prognostic indicator in acute coronary syndrome, stroke and pulmonary embolism [42]. The WBC is incorporated into the Alvarado score for the presumptive diagnosis of acute appendicitis [43].

Neutrophil leucocytosis – neutrophilia

Neutrophil leucocytosis or neutrophilia is the elevation of the absolute neutrophil count above that expected in a healthy subject of the same age, gender, ethnic origin and physiological status. Healthy neonates have both a higher neutrophil count than is normal at other stages of life and also a left shift. Similarly, women in the reproductive age range have somewhat higher neutrophil counts than men, the count varying with the menstrual cycle. During pregnancy, a marked rise in the neutrophil count occurs and this is further accentuated during labour and the postpartum period. In addition, pregnancy is associated with a left shift (with myelocytes and even a few promyelocytes appearing in the blood), with 'toxic' granulation and with Döhle bodies.

Neutrophil leucocytosis is usually due to redistribution of white cells or increased bone marrow output. Rarely, there is a prolongation of the period a neutrophil spends in the circulation. Exercise can alter the distribution of white cells within the circulation, with cells that were previously marginated (against the endothelium) being mobilised into the circulating blood. Vigorous exercise can double the neutrophil count. The absolute number of lymphocytes, monocytes, eosinophils and basophils also increases, but because of the more striking increase in neutrophil numbers the increase of other cell types may go unnoticed. If exercise is both severe and prolonged a left shift can occur, indicating that there is then increased bone marrow output in addition to redistribution. Patients do not usually undergo severe exercise before having a blood sample taken, but epinephrine (adrenaline) administration and epileptiform convulsions can mobilise neutrophils similarly and even severe pain can have an effect on the neutrophil count. Corticosteroids also alter neutrophil kinetics. The output from the bone marrow is increased and there is a concomitant decrease in egress to the tissues. Experiments in rabbits suggest there is also mobilisation of neutrophils from the marginated granulocyte pool [44]. A rise in the WBC starts within a few hours of intravenous administration or within 1 day of oral administration. WBCs as high as $20 \times 10^9/l$ occur, the elevation being predominantly due to neutrophilia but with some increase also in the absolute monocyte count, and with a fall in the absolute eosinophil and lymphocyte counts. Epinephrine and corticosteroids do not cause toxic granulation, Döhle bodies, left shift or neutrophil vacuolation.

Neutrophilia in pathological conditions usually results from increased output from the bone marrow, which more than compensates for any increased egress to the tissues. The major causes (and some minor causes) of neutrophilia are shown in Table 6.4 and

Table 6.4 Some causes of neutrophil leucocytosis.

Inherited

As a direct effect of the condition

Hereditary neutrophilia [45], some cases due to mutation of *CSF3R* encoding the receptor for granulocyte colony-stimulating factor [46]

Inherited deficiency of CR3 complement receptors [47]

Deficient surface expression of leucocyte adhesion molecules, CD11b or CD15 (leucocyte adhesion deficiencies types I and II) [48,49,50]

Defective integrin rearrangement in response to chemokines and chemo-attractants, kindlin 3 deficiency [51,52]

Associated with autosomal dominant thrombocytopenia due to mutation of *ANKRD26* [53]

As an indirect effect of the condition

Familial cold urticaria with leucocytosis [54]

Hyperimmunoglobulin D syndrome [55]

Familial periodic fever syndromes including familial Mediterranean fever, tumour necrosis factor receptor-associated periodic syndrome (TRAPS) [55] and hyperimmunoglobulin D with periodic fever

Autoinflammatory disease due to deficiency of interleukin 1 receptor antagonist [56]

Inherited metabolic disorders, e.g. ornithine transcarbamylase deficiency [57]

Acquired

Infections

Many acute and chronic bacterial infections, including miliary tuberculosis and some rickettsial infections, e.g. Rocky Mountain Spotted fever (*Rickettsia rickettsii* infection), *Rickettsia parkeri* infection and some cases of typhus and murine typhus

Toxic shock syndrome

Some viral infections, e.g. chicken pox, herpes simplex infection, rabies, poliomyelitis, St Louis encephalitis virus infection, Eastern equine encephalitis virus infection, hantavirus infection including hantavirus pulmonary syndrome (Sin Nombre virus infection) [58,59], Japanese encephalitis [60], cytomegalovirus infection [61]

Some fungal infections, e.g. actinomycosis, coccidioidomycosis, North American blastomycosis, nocardiosis [62], cepacia syndrome (colonization of the lungs by *Burkholderia cepacia* in cystic fibrosis) [63], cryptococcosis [64]

Some parasitic infections, e.g. liver fluke, hepatic amoebiasis, filariasis, malaria [65], some *Pneumocystis jirovecii* infections, *Cystoisospora belli* enteritis [66]

Tissue damage, e.g. trauma, surgery (particularly splenectomy), burns, acute hepatic necrosis, acute pancreatitis, haemolytic–uraemic syndrome, potassium cyanide poisoning [67]

Tissue infarction, e.g. myocardial infarction, pulmonary embolism causing pulmonary infarction, sickle cell crisis, atheroembolic disease

Acute inflammation and severe chronic inflammation, e.g. gout, pseudogout (calcium pyrophosphate crystal deposition disease), rheumatic fever, rheumatoid arthritis, Still disease, ulcerative colitis, enteritis necroticans ('pigbel'), polyarteritis nodosa, scleroderma, acute generalised exanthematous pustulosis [68]

Acute haemorrhage

Acute hypoxia

Heat stress [69]

Drowning and near drowning

Metabolic and endocrine disorders, e.g. diabetic ketoacidosis, acute renal failure, Cushing syndrome, thyrotoxic crisis

Malignant disease, e.g. carcinoma, sarcoma, melanoma, Hodgkin lymphoma (particularly but not only when there is extensive disease or tumour necrosis) – sometimes related to secretion of G-CSF by the tumour, e.g. in multiple myeloma [70] and spindle cell carcinoma of the kidney [71]

Myeloproliferative and leukaemic disorders, e.g. chronic myelogenous leukaemia, chronic myelomonocytic leukaemia, neutrophilic leukaemia, acute myeloid leukaemia (not commonly), other rare leukaemias, polycythaemia vera, essential thrombocythaemia, primary myelofibrosis (early in the disease process), systemic mastocytosis

Post-neutropenia rebound, e.g. following dialysis-induced neutropenia, recovery from agranulocytosis and cytotoxic chemotherapy, treatment of megaloblastic anaemia

Administration of cytokines such as G-CSF, GM-CSF, IL1, IL2 [72], IL3 [73], IL6 [74], IL10 [75]

Administration of drugs, e.g. epinephrine (adrenaline), corticosteroids, lithium, clozapine [76], desmopressin [77], initiation of rituximab therapy [78], plerixafor (CXCR4 antagonist) [79]

Poisoning by various chemicals and drugs, e.g. ethylene glycol [80], iron

Hypersensitivity reactions including those due to drugs

Envenomation, e.g. scorpion bite [81], 'killer bee' attack [82], snake bite [83]

Cigarette smoking [84]

Vigorous exercise

Acute pain, epileptic convulsions, electric shock, paroxysmal tachycardia

Eclampsia and pre-eclampsia (pregnancy-associated hypertension)

Kawasaki disease

Sweet syndrome [85]

Neuroleptic malignant syndrome [86]

Blood transfusion in critically ill patients [87]

Infusion of cryoprecipitate [88]

Chronic idiopathic neutrophilia [89]

G-CSF, granulocyte colony-stimulating factor; GM-CSF, granulocyte-macrophage colony-stimulating factor; IL, interleukin some causes of particular importance in the neonatal period in Table 6.5.

An increased neutrophil count can be of adverse prognostic significance. This is so for long-term prognosis in sickle cell anaemia and for short-term prognosis in unstable angina and following myocardial infarction.

Table 6.5 Significant causes of neutrophilia in the neonate.

Maternal factors
Maternal smoking
Maternal fever
Prolonged intrapartum oxytocin administration
Administration of dexamethasone
Fetal factors
Stressful delivery
Birth asphyxia or other hypoxia
Crying
Physiotherapy
Pain, e.g. lumbar puncture
Hypoglycaemia
Seizures
Infection
Haemolysis
Intraventricular haemorrhage
Meconium aspiration syndrome
Hyaline membrane disease with pneumothorax
Thrombocytopenia with absent radii

Eosinophil leucocytosis – eosinophilia

Eosinophil leucocytosis or eosinophilia is the elevation of the eosinophil count above levels observed in healthy subjects of the same age with no history of allergy. Eosinophil counts are higher in neonates than in adults. A slow decline in the eosinophil count occurs in elderly people. Eosinophil counts are the same in men and women. Contrary to earlier reports, counts do not differ between different ethnic groups. High eosinophil counts previously reported in Indians and Africans are attributable to environmental influences.

The absolute eosinophil count is increased with vigorous exercise, but not out of proportion to the increase in other leucocytes.

Some of the causes of eosinophilia are shown in Tables 6.6, 6.7 and 6.8, the commonest being allergic diseases (particularly asthma, hay fever and eczema)

and, in some parts of the world, parasitic infection. When the eosinophil count is greatly elevated (greater than $10 \times 10^9/1$) the likely causes are far fewer (Table 6.9). Allergic conditions causing eosinophilia are usually readily apparent from the patient's medical history but, in the case of parasitic infections, the laboratory detection of eosinophilia may be the finding that leads to the correct diagnosis. Migrants from the tropics and returning travellers should be investigated by examination of faeces for ova, cysts and parasites and should have strongyloides serology performed. Those who have been in areas of Africa where *Schistosoma haematobium* occurs should have serology plus microscopy of a terminal urine specimen.

In hospital patients, eosinophilia can be a useful sign of drug allergy. Following bone marrow transplantation, eosinophilia may be a feature of graft-versus-host disease and has been found to be predictive of extensive scleroderma-like changes [166].

The laboratory detection of eosinophilia in patients with lung disease (Table 6.10) is important in indicating relevant diagnostic possibilities and in excluding conditions, such as Wegener granulomatosis, which are not associated with eosinophilia. In patients with symptoms suggestive of obstructive pulmonary disease, the presence of eosinophilia usually indicates a reversible or asthmatic component, although it does not necessarily indicate allergic rather than other triggering factors [173]. In uncomplicated asthma the eosinophil count is rarely in excess of $2 \times 10^9/l$. Higher counts, often in association with deteriorating pulmonary function, may indicate either allergic aspergillosis

Table 6.6 Some of the more common causes of eosinophilia.

Allergic diseases, e.g. atopic eczema, asthma, allergic rhinitis (hay fever), acute urticaria, allergic bronchopulmonary aspergillosis and other bronchoallergic fungal infections, milk precipitin disease [90]
Drug hypersensitivity (particularly to gold, sulphonamides, penicillin, nitrofurantoin) including drug-induced Churg–Strauss syndrome or eosinophilia–myalgia syndrome [91,92]
Parasitic infection (particularly when tissue invasion has occurred) – see Table 6.7
Skin diseases, e.g. pemphigus vulgaris, bullous pemphigoid, dermatitis herpetiformis, herpes gestationalis, eosinophilic pustular folliculitis [93], familial peeling skin syndrome [94], acute generalised exanthematous pustulosis (some cases) [68]

Table 6.7 Parasitic infections known to cause eosinophilia.

Disease	Parasite	Usual degree of eosinophilia*
Protozoan		
Dientamoeba fragilis infection [95]	*Dientamoeba fragilis*	Absent or mild [96]
Isospora belli infection [95]	*Isospora belli*	Absent, in immunosuppressed patients, or mild [96]
Blastocystis hominis infection [97]	*Blastocystis hominis*	
Eosinophilic myositis	*Sarcocystis hominis*	Rarely causes marked eosinophilia [98]
Giardiasis	*Giardia lamblia*	Rarely causes marked eosinophilia [99]
Nematode (roundworm) infections		
Hookworm infection	*Ancylostoma duodenale* (Old World hookworm) *Necator americanus* (New World hookworm) *Ancylostoma ceylanicum* [100] *Ancylostoma caninum*	Absent in chronic infection, mild or moderate during stage of larval migration through the lung (Löffler syndrome) [96]
Cutaneous larva migrans	*Ancylostoma braziliense* (dog and cat hookworm) [101] *Ancylostoma caninum* (dog hookworm) [101] *Gnathostoma doloresi* [102]	Rarely associated with eosinophilia
Epidemic eosinophilic enteritis [103]	*Ancylostoma caninum* (dog hookworm)	
Ascariasis	*Ascaris lumbricoides* (large intestinal roundworm)	Absent during adult stage, moderate during stage of larval migration through the lungs (Löffler syndrome) [96]
Strongyloidiasis	*Strongyloides stercoralis* (threadworm)[†]	Absent, mild or moderate; moderate during stage of larval migration through the lungs (Löffler syndrome) [96]; usually present in strongyloides hyperinfection in immunosuppressed subjects
Trichuriasis [101]	*Trichuris trichiuria* (whipworm)	Absent or mild [96]
Trichinellosis, trichinosis [101]	*Trichinella spiralis* (trichina worm)	Moderate or marked during the acute phase [96]
Capillariasis [101,104,105]	Hepatic infection by *Capillaria hepatica* (*Calodium hepaticum*), a roundworm of rodents, or intestinal infection by *Capillaria philippinensis*	
Trichostrongyliasis [101,106]	*Trichostrongylus colubriformis* (a roundworm of sheep)	
Anisakidosis [107]	*Anisakis simplex* and *Anisakis pegreffi* (anasakiasis) *Contracaecum osculatum Pseudoterranova decipiens* (pseudoterranovosis)	Parasitic worms of fish
Enterobiasis	*Enterobius vermicularis* (pinworm or threadworm†)	Rarely causes eosinophilia but may do so when there is enteritis [108]
Filariasis (lymphatic filariasis including tropical pulmonary eosinophilia resulting from occult lymphatic filariasis)	*Wuchereria bancrofti* (Bancroft's filaria) *Brugia malayi* (Malayan filaria) *Brugia timori* (Timorian filariasis)	Mild, moderate or marked, marked in tropical pulmonary eosinophilia [96]
Loiasis [101]	*Loa loa* (eyeworm)	Moderate or marked [96]
Onchocerciasis (river blindness) [101]	*Onchocerca volvulus* (blinding filaria)	Mild, moderate or marked [96]
Mansonellosis [101]	*Mansonella perstans*	
Dirofilariasis (tropical eosinophilia, eosinophilic pneumonia)	*Dirofilaria immitis* (dog heartworm), *Dirofilaria repens* (roundworm of dogs, cats and foxes) [109]	
Dracunculiasis [101]	Subcutaneous infection by *Dracunculus medinensis* (Guinea worm) *Spirurina* type X infection [110]	

(continued)

Table 6.7 *(continued)*

Disease	Parasite	Usual degree of eosinophilia*
Angiostrongyloidiasis, eosinophilic meningitis [111,112]	*Angiostrongylus cantonensis* (rat lungworm)	Mild or moderate [96]
Eosinophilic enteritis [101]	*Angiostrongylus costaricensis* (rat roundworm)	
Gnathostomiasis [101] (including eosinophilic meningitis and visceral larva migrans)	*Gnathostoma spinigerum*	Mild, moderate or marked [96]
Visceral larva migrans (including toxocariasis, gnathostomiasis, capillariasis)	*Toxocara canis* or *Toxocara cati* (toxocariasis) *Baylisascaris procyonis* [113] *Gnathostoma* spp [113], e.g *Gnathostoma doloresi, Gnathostoma spinigerum* ? *Ascaris suum* [113,114] *Capillaria hepatica*	Moderate or marked
Eosinophilic myositis (Tasmania and Queensland)	*Haycocknema perplexum* [115]	Mild eosinophilia
Trematode (fluke) infection		
Clonorchiasis	*Clonorchis sinensis* (Oriental or Chinese liver fluke)	Absent or mild in chronic infection, may be moderate or marked in acute infection
Fascioliasis (liver fluke infection)	*Fasciola hepatica* (sheep liver fluke) [116] *Fasciola gigantica* [101] *Metorchis conjunctus* (North American liver fluke) [117]	Mild, moderate or marked during stage of larval migration [96]
Fasciolopsiasis (intestinal fluke infection)	*Fasciolopsis buski* (large intestinal fluke) [101,106]	Marked eosinophilia
Heterophyiasis or echinostomiasis [101]	*Heterophyes heterophyes* or Echinostoma spp (intestinal flukes)	
Opisthorchiasis [101]	*Opisthorchis viverrini* (a South-East Asian liver fluke) or *Opisthorchis felineus* (a Russian liver fluke, also found in Italy)	Usually absent or mild, may be moderate or marked in early infection
Paragonimiasis, distomiasis [101]	*Paragonimus westermani* (Oriental lung fluke) [118]	Marked eosinophilia
Schistosomiasis	*Schistosoma mansoni* *Schistosoma haematobium* *Schistosoma intercalatum* *Schistosoma mekongi*	Usually absent or mild but may be moderate to high in acute schistosomiasis (Katayama fever) [96]
Cestode (tapeworm) infection		
Cysticercosis	Larval stage of *Taenia solium* (pig tapeworm)	Absent or mild, may be moderate if encysted larvae die and release antigen [96]
Echinococcosis (hydatid cyst)	Larval stage of *Echinococcus granulosus* (dog tapeworm)	Absent or mild, may increase if cysts rupture or leak [96]
Coenurosis [101	*Coenurus cerebralis* (larval stage of a dog tapeworm, *Taenia multiceps*, which rarely occurs in man)	
Hymenolepsiasis [101]	*Hymenolepis nana* (dwarf tapeworm)	
Sparganosis [101]	Spirometra ssp, e.g. *Sparganum mansoni*	Absent or mild
Arthropods		
Scabies (ectoparasite) [119]	*Sarcoptes scabiei*	
Pentastomiasis (endoparasite) [120]	*Armillifer moniliformis, Porocephalus taiwana, Armillifer agkistrodontis* (tongue worms)	
Myiasis [121]	Cutaneous larvae of flies	

*Mild = 0.4–1.0 × 10^9/l, moderate = 1.0–3.0 × 10^9/l, marked = greater than 3.0 × 10^9/l
†The term 'threadworm' is used for two different parasites

Table 6.8 Some of the less common and rare causes of eosinophilia.

Hereditary eosinophilia [122]

Myeloid leukaemias, e.g. chronic myelogenous leukaemia and some other chronic myeloid leukaemias, systemic mastocytosis and less often other chronic myeloproliferative neoplasms, acute myeloid leukaemia (particularly FAB categories M2 and M4), chronic eosinophilic leukaemia (including that associated with a *FIP1L1-PDGFRA* [123], with rearrangement of *PDGFRB* or *FGFR1* [124] or with *PCM1-JAK1* or *ETV6-FLT3* fusion)

Lymphoproliferative disorders, e.g. acute lymphoblastic leukaemia (B-lineage, T-lineage and mixed T-B lineages [125]), non-Hodgkin lymphoma (particularly T-cell and including angioimmunoblastic T-cell lymphoma [126], mycosis fungoides and Sézary syndrome, enteropathy-associated T-cell lymphoma [127]), multiple myeloma [128], Hodgkin lymphoma

Presence of an occult T-cell clone secreting cytokines (such as IL3 and IL5) capable of increasing eosinophil production [129]

Autoimmune lymphoproliferative syndrome [130] (uncommonly)

Non-haematological malignant disease, e.g. carcinoma, sarcoma, glioma, mesothelioma, malignant melanoma, hepatoma, metastatic pituitary tumour [131]

Autoimmune and connective tissue disorders, e.g. Churg-Strauss variant of polyarteritis nodosa (eosinophilic granulomatosis with polyangiitis), systemic necrotising vasculitis (variant of polyarteritis nodosa), Crohn disease, ulcerative colitis, rheumatoid arthritis (uncommonly) [98], dermatomyositis (uncommonly) [98], Sjögren syndrome (uncommonly) [98], eosinophilic fasciitis (some cases caused by L-tryptophan) [132], eosinophilic cellulitis (Wells syndrome) [133], progressive systemic sclerosis [134], systemic lupus erythematosus, chronic active hepatitis [135], sclerosing cholangitis (uncommonly) [136], primary biliary cirrhosis (uncommonly) [98], autoimmune hepatitis [137], eosinophilic cholangitis [98], eosinophilic cholecystitis [98], eosinophilic cystitis [138], acute eosinophilic pneumonia (late in disease course) [139], chronic eosinophilic pneumonia, idiopathic pulmonary haemosiderosis [140], eosinophilic oesophagitis [98], eosinophilic enteritis [98] (including as a manifestation of graft-versus-host disease), IgG4-related disease [141]

Administration of cytokines (e.g. G-CSF [142], GM-CSF, IL2, IL3, IL5) that are capable of increasing eosinophil production or administration of cytokines (e.g. IL2 or IL15) that stimulate T-cell proliferation [143]

Immune deficiency states and other conditions with recurring infections, e.g. Wiskott–Aldrich syndrome, Job syndrome (hyperimmunoglobulin E syndrome), immunoglobulin A deficiency, hyperimmunoglobulin M syndrome, severe congenital neutropenia, HIV infection [144] (particularly if complicated by HTLV-2 infection [129])

Cyclical neutropenia

Cyclical eosinophilia with angio-oedema [145]

Miscellaneous, e.g. recovery from some bacterial and viral infections, premature neonates during the first few weeks of life, cytomegalovirus pneumonia of infancy [90], scarlet fever, tuberculosis (6–10% of patients), coccidioidomycosis, *Pneumocystis jirovecii* infection, disseminated histoplasmosis [146], cat-scratch disease [90], infectious lymphocytosis [90], *Borrelia burdorferi* infection [147], propanolol administration, drug abuse including cocaine inhalation [148,149], toxic oil syndrome [150], L-tryptophan toxicity (see above) [151], haemodialysis and occasionally peritoneal dialysis [90], atheroembolic disease [152,153], acute and chronic graft-versus-host disease, thrombocytopenia with absent radii syndrome, chronic pancreatitis, Omenn syndrome [154], hepatitis B vaccination [155], treatment of lymphoid malignancies with nucleoside analogues (fludarabine or cladribine) [156], angiolymphoid hyperplasia with eosinophilia, Kimura disease [157], adrenal insufficiency (Addison disease) [158] or hypopituitarism, arsenic toxicity [159], Whipple disease [160], mitochondrial cytopathy [161], organising subdural haematoma [98], sarcoidosis, hard metal pneumoconiosis [162], chronic active Epstein-Barr virus infection [163], Castleman disease [164], basidiobolomycosis (*Basiliobolus rananus* infection) [165]

Unknown – idiopathic hypereosinophilic syndrome [95]

FAB, French–American–British; G-CSF, granulocyte colony-stimulating factor; GM-CSF, granulocyte macrophage colony-stimulating factor; HIV, human immunodeficiency virus; HTLV-2, human T-cell lymphotropic virus 2; Ig, immunoglobin; IL, interleukin

Table 6.9 Some causes of marked eosinophilia.

Parasitic infections, e.g. toxocariasis, trichinosis, tissue migration by larvae of ascaris, ankylostoma or strongyloides

Drug hypersensitivity

Churg–Strauss variant of polyarteritis nodosa

Hodgkin lymphoma

Acute lymphoblastic leukaemia

Chronic eosinophilic leukaemia

Idiopathic hypereosinophilic syndrome

or the Churg–Strauss syndrome. The Churg–Strauss syndrome is a variant of polyarteritis nodosa characterised by pulmonary infiltrates and eosinophilia, neither of which is typical of classical polyarteritis nodosa [174]. Patients are also seen with some features of classical polyarteritis nodosa and some of the Churg–Strauss syndrome: this has been referred to as 'chronic necrotising vasculitis' or 'the overlap syndrome'. Eosinophilia of $1.5 \times 10^9/l$ or more is an important

Table 6.10 Some causes of eosinophilia with pulmonary infiltration.

Parasitic infections, e.g. toxocariasis, filariasis, schistosomiasis, larval migration stage of strongyloidiasis, ascariasis, ankylostomiasis
Asthma
Allergic bronchopulmonary aspergillosis
Hypersensitivity reactions to drugs (such as sulindac, fenoprofen, ibuprofen, diclofenac, tenidap [167], amoxicillin, clarithromycin [168]) and chemicals (such as zinc, chromium or beryllium)
Cocaine pneumonitis
Churg–Strauss variant of polyarteritis nodosa and systemic necrotising vasculitis
Infections
Tuberculosis (rarely), brucellosis [169], coccidioidomycosis (rarely), histoplasmosis [169], *Pneumocystis jirovecii* pneumonia (rarely)
Sarcoidosis [169]
Hodgkin lymphoma [169]
Carcinoma [170]
Cytokine (GM-CSF) administration [171]
Bronchocentric granulomatosis [172]
Chronic idiopathic eosinophilic pneumonia
Idiopathic hypereosinophilic syndrome

GM-CSF, granulocyte macrophage colony-stimulating factor

criterion in making the diagnosis of the Churg–Strauss syndrome or the overlap syndrome.

In some patients with eosinophilia and pulmonary infiltration no underlying condition can be found. Many such patients have a condition known as eosinophilic pneumonia; its cause is unknown, but chest radiology shows distinctive peripheral infiltration and there is a predictable response to corticosteroid therapy. The combination of the characteristic X-ray appearance with eosinophilia has been considered sufficient to make the diagnosis [175], whereas in the minority of patients lacking eosinophilia a lung biopsy is needed to establish the diagnosis.

Eosinophilia is a rare manifestation of non-haemopoietic malignancy. It is usually associated with widespread malignant disease, but rarely may provide a clue to a localised tumour. Eosinophilia may be mediated by interleukin (IL) 3, IL5, granulocyte colony-stimulating factor (G-CSF) or granulocyte-macrophage colony-stimulating factor (GM-CSF), sometimes demonstrated to be secreted by tumour cells [176,177]. Eosinophilia may also occur as a reaction

to lymphoid malignancy, particularly Hodgkin lymphoma, T-lineage non-Hodgkin lymphoma and T-lineage or B-lineage acute lymphoblastic leukaemia (ALL). Eosinophilia can precede other clinical evidence of non-Hodgkin lymphoma or ALL by 6–12 months [178], and can recur some weeks before relapse can be detected. In Hodgkin lymphoma, isolated eosinophilia has been associated with a better prognosis [179]. In some patients with an initially unexplained eosinophilia, an occult T-cell clone can be demonstrated [180].

In a minority of cases, eosinophilia is neoplastic rather than reactive. Eosinophilia is present in more than 90% of cases of chronic myelogenous leukaemia (CML) and in a lower percentage of other myeloid leukaemias and myeloproliferative neoplasms. It occurs occasionally in acute myeloid leukaemia (AML) and rarely in the myelodysplastic syndromes (MDS). In some patients with leukaemia, differentiation is predominantly to eosinophils and the term 'chronic eosinophilic leukaemia' is then applicable (see Chapter 9).

An absolute, or even a relative, eosinophilia can be useful in the intensive care ward setting, in alerting clinicians to the possibility of adrenal insufficiency. The presence of more than 3% eosinophils has been suggested as a criterion for further investigation [158,181,182].

Incidental eosinophilia in a blood count has been found to be sometimes predictive of Hodgkin lymphoma (if eosinophils are at least 1×10^9/l) or of a myeloproliferative neoplasm (if eosinophils are at least 0.5×10^9/l) and was also observed in patients with previously undiagnosed early chronic lymphocytic leukaemia (CLL); the presence of an eosinophil count above 0.5×10^9/l was associated with higher all-cause mortality [183].

There remains a group of patients with persistent, moderate or marked eosinophilia for which no cause can be found despite detailed investigation. This condition is designated the 'idiopathic hypereosinophilic syndrome (HES)' (see Chapter 9). This diagnosis should only be made when a patient has been fully investigated to exclude identifiable causes.

Basophil leucocytosis – basophilia

Some of the causes of basophilia are shown in Table 6.11. The detection of basophil leucocytosis is useful in making the distinction between a myeloproliferative neoplasm and a reactive condition, since only in

Table 6.11 Some causes of basophil leucocytosis.

Myeloproliferative and leukaemic disorders
  Chronic myelogenous leukaemia (almost invariably)
  Other chronic myeloid leukaemias
  Acute myeloid leukaemia (very rarely)
  Polycythaemia vera
  Essential thrombocythaemia
  Primary myelofibrosis
  Systemic mastocytosis
  Some cases of Ph-positive acute lymphoblastic leukaemia
  Basophilic leukaemia
Reactive basophilia
  Myxoedema (hypothyroidism)
  Ulcerative colitis
  Juvenile rheumatoid arthritis [90]
  Immediate hypersensitivity reactions
  Oestrogen administration
  Hyperlipidaemia
  Administration of interleukin 3 [73]
  Lymphoma [184]
Unknown nature
  Idiopathic hypereosinophilic syndrome

myeloproliferative neoplasms and certain leukaemias is a marked increase in the basophil count at all common. A rising basophil count in CML is of prognostic significance since it often indicates an accelerated phase of the disease and impending blast transformation. The occurrence of basophilia in association with ALL may indicate that the patient is Philadelphia-positive and in AML may indicate Philadelphia-positivity or the presence of t(6;9)(p23;q34.3), both karyotypic abnormalities being of adverse prognostic significance. Chronic basophilic leukaemia is often Philadelphia-positive and in this case should be regarded as a variant of CML.

Lymphocytosis

Lymphocytosis is an increase in the absolute lymphocyte count above that expected in a healthy subject of the same age. Since the lymphocyte counts of infants and children are considerably higher than those of adults, it is particularly important to use age-adjusted reference ranges. There are no gender or ethnic differences in the lymphocyte count. In an adult, a count greater than $3.5 \times 10^9/l$ may be considered abnormal. Some of the causes of lymphocytosis are shown in Table 6.12. The increase in the lymphocyte count that

occurs with exercise is due to an increase in all lymphocyte populations, B cells, CD4-positive and CD8-positive T cells, and NK cells [215]; this exercise-induced increase is enhanced by caffeine [216]. Studies of splenectomised subjects suggest that about two-thirds of the exercise-induced increase in T cells and NK cells is due to mobilisation from the spleen [217]. Using multivariate analysis, lymphocytosis has been found predictive of mortality in hospitalised patients with general trauma or central nervous system injury [218].

In assessing a lymphocytosis it is important to consider cytology as well as the lymphocyte count and both should be assessed in relation to the age and clinical features of the patient. Children are more prone than adults to both lymphocytosis and reactive changes in lymphocytes, and even apparently healthy children may have some lymphocytes showing atypical features.

Lymphocytosis can occur without there being any cytological abnormality. This is usual when lymphocytosis is due to redistribution of lymphocytes (e.g. following exercise or epinephrine injection or as an acute response to severe stress), in endocrine abnormalities and in 'acute infectious lymphocytosis' (see Table 6.12). Cytological abnormalities are also uncommon in whooping cough, but sometimes there are cleft cells resembling those of follicular lymphoma [219]. In other viral and bacterial infections there are often minor changes in lymphocytes, such as a visible nucleolus or increased cytoplasmic basophilia, which are often referred to as 'reactive changes'. Infectious mononucleosis and to a lesser extent other conditions are associated with much more striking reactive changes, the abnormal cells being referred to as 'atypical lymphocytes' or 'atypical mononuclear cells' (see Table 9.1). Post-splenectomy lymphocytosis is usually mild, with only minor atypical features. However, it is important to realise that post-splenectomy counts can be in excess of $10 \times 10^9/l$ and misdiagnosis as a lymphoproliferative disorder has occurred. Large granular lymphocytes are often prominent in post-splenectomy lymphocytosis. Many heavy cigarette smokers have a mild lymphocytosis without cytological abnormalities. A minority of smokers, mainly women, have a persistent polyclonal B-cell lymphocytosis. An increase of large granular lymphocytes can occur as a reactive change, e.g. in human immunodeficiency virus (HIV) infection [220] and chronic hepatitis B or Epstein–Barr virus (EBV) infection, sometimes without an increase in the total lymphocyte count. An increase of large granular lymphocytes

Table 6.12 Some causes of lymphocytosis.

Constitutional	Transient stress-related lymphocytosis, e.g. associated with myocardial infarction, cardiac arrest, trauma, obstetric complications, sickle cell crisis [202,203]
Defective integrin rearrangement in response to chemokines and chemo-attractants, kindlin 3 deficiency [51,52]	Epinephrine (adrenaline) administration
DiGeorge syndrome (polyclonal B lymphocytosis can occur) [185]	Plerixafor (CXCR4 antagonist) administration [79]
Autosomal dominant polyclonal B lymphocytosis due to *CARD11* mutation [186]	Vigorous muscular contraction, e.g. vigorous exercise, status epilepticus
	Cigarette smoking [85] causing either T-lymphocytosis (common) or persistent polyclonal B-lymphocytosis (uncommon) [204]
Acquired	Administration of cytokines, e.g. IL3 [73] or G-CSF [205]
Viral infections including measles (rubeola), German measles (rubella), mumps, chickenpox (varicella), influenza, infectious hepatitis (hepatitis A), infectious mononucleosis (EBV infection), CMV infection, infectious lymphocytosis (caused by infection by certain Coxsackie viruses, adenovirus types 1, 2 and 5, and echovirus 7) [187–191], HIV infection, infection by the human lymphotropic viruses (HTLV-1 and HTLV-2) [192]	Allergic reactions to drugs
	Serum sickness
	Splenectomy
	Endocrine disorders, e.g. Addison disease, hypopituitarism, hyperthyroidism [206]
	β thalassaemia intermedia [207]
	Gaucher disease [208]
	Thymoma [209]
Certain bacterial infections including whooping cough (pertussis, infection by *Bordetella pertussis*), brucellosis, tuberculosis, syphilis, plague (*Yersinia pestis* infection) [193], Lyme disease [194], human monocytic ehrlichiosis (recovery phase) [195], human granulocytic anaplasmosis (previously known as human granulocytic ehrlichiosis; recovery phase) [196], rickettsial infections including scrub typhus (*Rickettsia tsutsugamushi* – now known as *Orientia tsutsugamushi*) and murine typhus (*Rickettsia typhi*) [197,198], toxic shock syndrome [199] and bacterial infections in infants and young children	Autoimmune lymphoproliferative syndrome [210]
	Associated with rituximab-induced autoimmune neutropenia [211]
	Lymphoid leukaemias and other lymphoproliferative disorders, e.g. chronic lymphocytic leukaemia, non-Hodgkin lymphoma, Hodgkin lymphoma (rarely) [212], adult T-cell leukaemia/lymphoma, hairy cell leukaemia and hairy cell variant leukaemia, Waldenström macroglobulinaemia, heavy chain disease, mycosis fungoides and Sézary syndrome, large granular lymphocyte leukaemia
	Natalizumab (anti CD49b) therapy [213]
Malaria [65], hyper-reactive malarial splenomegaly [200] and the acute phase of Chagas disease [201]	Ibrutinib therapy in chronic lymphocytic leukaemia and mantle cell lymphoma [214]

CMV, cytomegalovirus; EBV, Epstein–Barr virus; G-CSF, granulocyte colony-stimulating factor; HIV, human immunodeficiency virus; HTLV-1 and HTLV-2, human T-cell lymphotropic viruses 1 and 2; IL3, interleukin 3

causing an absolute lymphocytosis has also been noted following dasatinib therapy for CML or Ph-positive ALL [221] and has been shown to be an expansion of a pre-existing monoclonal or oligoclonal population [222]; the lymphocytes may be CD3+CD8+ T cells or CD3-CD16/CD56+ NK cells.

In lymphoproliferative disorders, lymphocytosis is usually caused by the presence of considerable numbers of lymphoma cells in the peripheral blood. However, occasionally, e.g. in Hodgkin lymphoma, there is a lymphoma-associated polyclonal reactive lymphocytosis [212]. Neoplastic lymphocytes almost always show cytological abnormalities. The exception is large granular lymphocyte leukaemia, in which the neoplastic cells are usually cytologically indistinguishable from normal cells. It is often said that in CLL there is an increase in apparently normal, mature lymphocytes, but in fact subtle abnormalities are

present. The specific cytological features of this and other lymphoproliferative disorders are described in Chapter 9. In general, lymphoproliferative disorders have distinctive cytological features and can thus be readily distinguished from reactive changes in lymphocytes. An exception may occur in some low-grade non-Hodgkin lymphomas, particularly mantle cell lymphoma, some cases of which have neoplastic cells that can be confused with reactive lymphocytes. For this reason the term 'reactive changes' should be used with circumspection.

Monocytosis

Monocytosis is an increase of the monocyte count above that expected in a healthy subject of the same age. The absolute monocyte count is higher in neonates than at other stages of life. A rise occurs in pregnancy in parallel with the rise in the neutrophil count. Some of the common causes of monocytosis are shown in Table 6.13. In diffuse large B-cell lymphoma a monocyte count of above $0.8 \times 10^9/l$ [238] or of $0.63 \times 10^9/l$ or above [239] is associated with a worse prognosis. A monocyte count of above $0.9 \times 10^9/l$ in classical Hodgkin lymphoma [240] and above $0.6 \times 10^9/l$ in nodular lymphocyte predominant Hodgkin lymphoma [241] is of adverse prognostic significance. A monocyte count above $0.5 \times 10^9/l$ is of adverse significance in mantle cell lymphoma [242].

Table 6.13 Some causes of monocytosis [223].

Exercise
Caffeine [216]
Chronic infection including miliary tuberculosis [224], congenital syphilis [225], typhoid fever [226] and leishmaniasis [227]
Rocky Mountain spotted fever [90]
Malaria [65] and babesiosis [228]
Chronic inflammatory conditions including Crohn disease, ulcerative colitis, rheumatoid arthritis and systemic lupus erythematosus
Autoinflammatory disease due to deficiency of interleukin 1 receptor antagonist [229]
Carcinoma [230]
Administration of cytokines including G-CSF, GM-CSF, M-CSF, IL3, IL10 and FLT ligand [73,231–233]
Recovery from bone marrow suppression
Administration of desmopressin [77]
Myocardial infarction [234]
Neutropenia and immune deficiency syndromes of various causes, e.g. cyclical neutropenia, severe congenital neutropenia, chronic idiopathic neutropenia, autoimmune neutropenia
Noonan syndrome in infants
Long-term haemodialysis [235]
Plerixafor (CXCR4 antagonist) administration [79]
Lymphomatoid granulomatosis [236]
Autoimmune lymphoproliferative syndrome [237]
RAS-associated autoimmune leucoproliferative disorder [237]
Myeloproliferative and leukaemic conditions including CMML, atypical CML, JMML, CML,*MDS, systemic mastocytosis, AML
Diffuse large B-cell lymphoma [238]
Cigarette smoking [84]

*absolute but not relative monocytosis
AML, acute myeloid leukaemia; CML, chronic myelogenous leukaemia; CMML, chronic myelomonocytic leukaemia; G-CSF, granulocyte colony-stimulating factor; GM-CSF, granulocyte macrophage colony-stimulating factor; IL, interleukin; JMML, juvenile myelomonocytic leukaemia; M-CSF, macrophage colony-stimulating factor; MDS, myelodysplastic syndrome

In examining a film of a patient with an unexplained monocytosis, evidence of chronic infection or myelodysplasia should be sought. The presence of promonocytes and blasts suggests AML with monocytic differentiation.

Plasmacytosis

Plasmacytosis is the appearance in the blood of appreciable numbers of plasma cells. These may be reactive or neoplastic. Some of the causes of plasmacytosis are shown in Table 6.14.

In reactive plasmacytosis, the number of circulating plasma cells is usually low, but occasionally quite considerable numbers are present. A case of serum sickness due to tetanus antitoxin, for example, was found to have $3.2 \times 10^9/l$ plasma cells [243]. In reactive plasmacytosis the plasma cells are usually mature, but occasionally plasmablasts are present. Plasma cells can contain vacuoles or, occasionally, crystals. Atypical lymphocytes and plasmacytoid lymphocytes can also be present and cells of other lineages can show reactive changes.

Neoplastic plasma cells usually show more cytological abnormality than those produced in reactive states. The haematological features of plasma cell leukaemia and multiple myeloma and their differential diagnosis are discussed in Chapter 9.

Table 6.14 Some causes of peripheral blood plasmacytosis.

Reactive
Bacterial and viral infections and immunisation
Hypersensitivity reactions to drugs
Streptokinase administration
Serum sickness
Systemic lupus erythematosus
Neoplastic
Multiple myeloma and plasma cell leukaemia
Gamma heavy chain disease
Waldenström macroglobulinaemia (rarely)
Angioimmunoblastic T-cell lymphoma

Thrombocytosis

Thrombocytosis is an increase of the platelet count above that expected in a healthy subject of the same age and sex. Use of the term 'thrombocythaemia' is usually restricted to a thrombocytosis that represents a myeloproliferative neoplasm; the term 'essential thrombocytosis' is synonymous but is little used. Thrombocytosis is usually the result of increased marrow production of platelets, either autonomous or reactive. Following splenectomy and in hyposplenism, thrombocytosis is due to redistribution of platelets. Some of the causes of thrombocytosis are shown in Table 6.15 and the causes of a marked increase in the platelet count in Table 6.16. It should be noted that as more and more routine platelet counts are performed on very sick patients, the percentage of even very high platelet counts that are reactive is increasing and myeloproliferative neoplasms are now responsible for only 10–15% of counts greater than $1000 \times 10^9/l$.

Blood film and count

Increased platelet size, platelet anisocytosis, the presence of poorly granulated platelets, circulating megakaryocyte nuclei or micromegakaryocytes and an increased basophil count are all suggestive of a primary bone marrow disease rather than a reactive thrombocytosis. Large platelets are also seen in hyposplenism, whereas in reactive thrombocytosis platelets are generally small and normally granulated. The blood film may also show abnormalities of other lineages, which indicate the correct diagnosis. The features of hyposplenism should be specifically sought.

Table 6.15 Some causes of thrombocytosis.

Primary	Inflammation
Inherited	Haemorrhage
Familial thrombocytosis (sometimes caused by a mutation in the thrombopoietin gene (*TPHO*) with autosomal dominant inheritance [244], sometimes unlinked to thrombopoietin and showing either dominant [245] or recessive, possibly X-linked recessive, inheritance [246], sometimes resulting from a mutation in the *MPL* gene [247]); polymorphism of *MPL* (MPL-Baltimore) found in 7% of African-Americans, causing variable but sometimes marked thrombocytosis in heterozygotes and marked thrombocytosis in homozygotes [248]; in one family autosomal dominant due to *JAK2* V617I mutation [249] and in another resulting from *JAK2* R564Q [250]; infantile cortical hyperostosis (*COL1A1* mutation) [251]; Diamond–Blackfan syndrome [252]; some severely anaemic patients with cartilage-hair hypoplasia syndrome [253]	Surgery and trauma
	Malignant disease
	Kawasaki disease (peaking in second or third week) [256]
	Iron deficiency
	Lead poisoning (one case) [257]
	Rebound after cytotoxic chemotherapy
	Rebound after alcohol withdrawal
	Following treatment of severe megaloblastic anaemia
	Severe haemolytic anaemia, particularly after unsuccessful splenectomy
	Multicentric angiofollicular hyperplasia [258], Castleman disease [259] and POEMS [259]
	Chronic eosinophilic pneumonia [260]
	Epinephrine (adrenaline) administration
	Vinca alkaloid (e.g. vincristine) administration
Acquired	Administration of recombinant thrombopoietin or PEG-rHuMGDF [261]
Essential thrombocythaemia (all cases)	Administration of IL3 [73], IL6 [262], IL11 [263]
Chronic myelogenous leukaemia (most cases)	Administration of erythropoietin [264] or vitamin E to premature infants [265]
Primary myelofibrosis (early in the disease course)	In infants of drug-abusing mothers [266]
Polycythaemia vera (many cases)	Erdheim–Chester disease [267]
Myelodysplastic syndromes (a minority of cases of the 5q– syndrome)	Type Ib glycogen storage disease [268]
Myelodysplastic/myeloproliferative neoplasms (some cases), e.g. refractory anaemia with ring sideroblasts and thrombocytosis	Severe congenital neutropenia [269]
	Enzyme replacement in Gaucher disease [270]
Acute myeloid leukaemia (a minority of cases, particularly acute megakaryoblastic leukaemia including transient abnormal myelopoiesis in neonates with Down syndrome, some cases with inv(3)(q21q26) and acute hypergranular promyelocytic leukaemia during all-*trans*-retinoic acid therapy [254])	Anorexia nervosa, particularly but not only during refeeding [271]
	Redistributional
Secondary	Splenectomy and hyposplenism
Exercise	
Caffeine [216]	**Unknown mechanism**
Infection (including some patients with miliary tuberculosis) [255]	Premature infants at 4–6 weeks of age [272]
	Tidal platelet dysgenesis

IL, interleukin; PEG-rHuMGDF, pegylated recombinant human megakaryocyte growth and development factor; POEMS, **P**olyendocrinopathy, **O**rganomegaly, **E**ndocrinopathy, **M**-protein, **S**kin changes syndrome

Table 6.16 Some causes of markedly elevated platelet counts.

Platelet count	>1000 × 10⁹/l [273]	>900 × 10⁹/l [274]	>1000 × 10⁹/l [275]	>500 × 10⁹/l [276]
Patients (n)	102	526	280	**777**
Cause	Cases attributable (%)			
Malignant disease	45	27	11.5	5.9
Splenectomy or hyposplenism	40	20	16	1.9
Myeloproliferative neoplasm	28	26	14	3.4
Infection or inflammation	30	19	26	35
Connective tissue disorder	2	9		
Iron deficiency	4			
Trauma or other tissue damage			11.5	17.9
Blood loss			5	
Rebound			2.5	19.4

The degree of elevation of the platelet count is of some use in the differential diagnosis. Counts of greater than 1500×10^9/l are usually indicative of a myeloproliferative neoplasm, but reactive thrombocytosis with counts as high as 2000×10^9/l [275] and even 6000×10^9/l [277] have been reported. In primary thrombocytosis the automated blood count may show an increased mean platelet volume (MPV) and platelet distribution width (PDW), indicative of increased platelet size and platelet anisocytosis, respectively. In secondary or reactive thrombocytosis the MPV and PDW are more often normal.

Further tests

The cause of reactive thrombocytosis is usually readily apparent from the clinical history. When the cause is not apparent a bone marrow aspirate, trephine biopsy, cytogenetic analysis and analysis for *JAK2* V617F and a *CALR* mutation are indicated. Indirect evidence favouring a reactive thrombocytosis includes an increased erythrocyte sedimentation rate (ESR) and an increased concentration of C-reactive protein, fibrinogen, factor VIII and von Willebrand factor. It can sometimes be difficult to distinguish iron deficiency with a marked reactive thrombocytosis from polycythaemia vera with complicating iron deficiency and in these circumstances a judicious trial of iron therapy may be needed.

Anaemia

Anaemia is a reduction in the haemoglobin concentration in the peripheral blood below that expected for a healthy person of the same age, gender and physiological status (pregnant or not). It can be due to: (i) defective production of red cells; (ii) reduced red cell survival in the circulation due to haemolysis or blood loss; (iii) increased pooling of essentially normal red cells in a large spleen; or (iv) sequestration of abnormal red cells such as those in sickle cell anaemia or sickle cell/haemoglobin C disease, in the spleen or, less often, in the liver. Anaemia may be an isolated abnormality or there may be pancytopenia (see below).

Blood film and count

The blood film and count commonly give a clue to the cause of the anaemia by showing microcytosis, macrocytosis or a specific type of poikilocyte. Red cell disorders associated with these features are discussed in Chapter 8. The presence of polychromasia suggests an adequate bone marrow response to anaemia and indicates that anaemia may have been caused by haemolysis or haemorrhage. The differential diagnosis of a normocytic, normochromic anaemia and the peripheral blood features that may be helpful in suggesting the diagnosis are summarised in Table 6.17. Various other rare and curious causes of anaemia exist, e.g. that due to therapy with leeches, which sometimes necessitates blood transfusion [291]. Causes of pure red cell aplasia are detailed in Table 6.18. In some anaemic patients the blood film is leucoerythroblastic, i.e. granulocyte precursors and nucleated red blood cells (NRBC) are present. In these cases the differential diagnosis is more limited, as summarised in Table 6.19. A leucoerythroblastic blood film is normal in the neonatal period and pregnant women occasionally have NRBC in addition to the more usual granulocyte precursors. Otherwise a leucoerythroblastic

Table 6.17 Some causes of normocytic normochromic anaemia (other than conditions that usually cause pancytopenia, these being listed in Table 6.30).

Causative conditions	Peripheral blood features that may be useful in diagnosis
Early iron deficiency*	A few hypochromic cells may be present, RDW increased
Anaemia of chronic disease*	Increased rouleaux and ESR, occasionally increased platelet count or WBC, RDW often normal
Lead poisoning*†	Basophilic stippling, some cases have polychromasia
Double deficiency of iron and vitamin B_{12} or folic acid*	Hypersegmented neutrophils, increased RDW
Blood loss	If blood loss is severe and acute, anaemia is leucoerythroblastic; polychromasia, reticulocytosis and increased RDW develop within a few days
Non-spherocytic haemolytic anaemia*	Occasional poikilocytes, polychromasia, increased reticulocyte count, RDW increased
Malaria and babesiosis	Parasites present, sometimes also thrombocytopenia
Some congenital dyserythropoietic anaemias†	Striking anisocytosis and poikilocytosis
Paroxysmal nocturnal haemoglobinuria	Sometimes other cytopenias – particularly a low WBC, low neutrophil alkaline phosphatase score, polychromasia in some cases
Myelodysplastic syndromes†	Other features of myelodysplastic syndromes
Renal failure	Sometimes keratocytes or schistocytes
Liver failure†	Target cells, stomatocytes, acanthocytes, other cytopenias
Congestive cardiac failure	Nil
Hypothyroidism†	Sometimes acanthocytes
Addison disease and hypopituitarism	Lymphocytosis, eosinophilia, neutropenia, monocytopenia
Androgen ablation therapy, e.g. for carcinoma of the prostate	Nil
Hyperparathyroidism	Nil
Anorexia nervosa	Other cytopenia, acanthocytes, poikilocytosis, basophilic stippling
Pure red cell aplasia†	Normal RDW, reticulocyte count very low or reticulocytes absent
Pearson syndrome and other mitochondrial cytopathies)*† [161,278]	Nil
Cystinosis	Nil
Administration of IL2 , IL6 [279], IL11 [280] or IL12 [281]	Other features of cytokine administration
Bortezomib therapy	Nil
Autonomic failure [282] including dopamine-β-hydroxylase deficiency [283]	Nil
Vitamin D intoxication [284]	Nil
Hypervitaminosis A [285]	Platelet count also reduced
Arsenic poisoning	There may be basophilic stippling, neutropenia and thrombocytopenia [286]
Graft-versus-host disease [287]	Clinical features of graft-versus-host disease
Alemtuzumab (anti-CD52) therapy	Nil
Therapy with enalapril (an angiotensin-converting enzyme (ACE) inhibitor) [288]	Nil
Therapy with sartanes (e.g. losartan or irbesartan) in patient with renal insufficiency or on dialysis [289]	Nil
Colchicine toxicity [290]	Vacuolation and dysplastic nuclear changes
Copper deficiency*†	Neutropenia may coexist
Cartilage-hair hypoplasia syndrome†	Thrombocytosis can occur [253]

* can also be microcytic
† can also be macrocytic
ESR, erythrocyte sedimentation rate; IL, interleukin; RDW, red cell distribution width; WBC, white blood cell count

Table 6.18 Some causes of pure red cell aplasia.

Transient

Parvovirus B19-induced

Drug-induced [292], e.g. antibiotics, antithyroid drugs, anticonvulsants, azathioprine, tacrolimus [293], allopurinol [294], phenytoin, isoniazid, ribavirin [295]

Transient erythroblastopenia of childhood

Chronic

Constitutional

Diamond–Blackfan syndrome

Cases of cartilage-hair hypoplasia with severe anaemia [253]

Hereditary transcobalamin deficiency [296]

Acquired

Associated with chronic lymphocytic leukaemia, large granular lymphocyte leukaemia (T or NK cell), Hodgkin lymphoma, thymoma or autoimmune disease such as systemic lupus erythematosus, rheumatoid arthritis or autoimmune polyglandular syndrome

Tumour-associated [297]

Pregnancy-associated [298]

Chronic parvovirus B19 infection (in individuals with impaired immunity)

ABO-incompatible stem cell transplantation [299], particularly but not only with non-myelo-ablative conditioning [300]

Development of antibodies to erythropoietin after recombinant erythropoietin therapy [301]

Myelodysplastic syndrome and other myeloid neoplasm (e.g. refractory anaemia)

Table 6.19 Some causes of leucoerythroblastic anaemia.

Bone marrow infiltration in carcinoma, lymphoma (Hodgkin lymphoma, non-Hodgkin lymphoma), chronic lymphocytic leukaemia, multiple myeloma, acute lymphoblastic leukaemia or other malignant disease

Myeloproliferative neoplasms, particularly primary myelofibrosis and chronic myelogenous leukaemia

Acute myeloid leukaemia and the myelodysplastic syndromes

Bone marrow granulomas, e.g. in miliary tuberculosis

Storage diseases, e.g. Gaucher disease

Acute haemolysis (including erythroblastosis fetalis)

Shock, e.g. due to severe haemorrhage

Severe infection

Rebound following bone marrow failure or suppression

Crises of sickle cell anaemia

Bone marrow infarction

Thalassaemia major

Severe megaloblastic anaemia

Systemic lupus erythematosus [302]

Severe nutritional rickets [303]

Marble bone disease (osteopetrosis)

blood film, other than during an acute illness, is likely to indicate serious underlying disease.

In the perinatal period, the conditions responsible for anaemia differ somewhat from those operating later in life (Table 6.20). Other rare causes include anaemia

Table 6.20 Some causes of anaemia of importance in the fetus and neonate.

Severe inherited haemolytic anaemias (G6PD deficiency, sometimes following maternal ingestion of oxidants), triose phosphate isomerase deficiency, glucose phosphate isomerase deficiency, pyruvate kinase deficiency [304], hexokinase deficiency [305], hereditary xerocytosis [306], homozygosity for hereditary spherocytosis caused by band 3 Coimbra [307], homozygosity for haemoglobin Taybe [308]), South-East Asian ovalocytosis* [309]

Haemoglobin F-Poole [310]

Haemoglobin Bart's hydrops fetalis

εγδβ thalassaemia [311]

Congenital dyserythropoietic anaemia [312]

Diamond–Blackfan syndrome [313]

Congenital hypotransferrinaemia [314]

Haemolysis due to transplacental passage of alloantibodies, e.g. Rh or Kell antibodies, rarely ABO [315]

Pure red cell aplasia caused by transplacental passage of maternal anti-Kell or anti-M antibodies [316]

Parvovirus B19 infection

Cytomegalovirus infection

Malaria

Congenital leukaemia [317]

Transient abnormal myelopoiesis of Down syndrome

Feto-maternal haemorrhage (including following external cephalic version, amniocentesis, antepartum haemorrhage and abdominal trauma)

Twin-to-twin haemorrhage

Haemorrhage resulting from amniocentesis or cordocentesis

Neonate

Haemorrhage from the cord or the placenta or internal haemorrhage (e.g. cephalohaematoma, intracranial haemorrhage, ruptured liver or spleen), during or as a result of difficult birth

Twin–twin transfusion during birth

Haemolytic disease of the newborn (e.g. ABO haemolytic disease of the newborn)

Transient severe haemolysis in hereditary elliptocytosis

Haemolysis associated with disseminated intravascular coagulation caused by sepsis

Congenital infections, e.g. rubella, adenovirus infection [310]

Prematurity

Vitamin E deficiency [318]

Removal of inappropriately large amounts of blood for laboratory testing

*Causes haemolytic anaemia only in the neonate and infant

associated with cystic hygroma or chorioangioma and anaemia resulting from fetal haematuria caused by congenital mesoblastic nephroma [310]. Occasional neonates are anaemic as a result of haemoglobin H disease, Blackfan–Diamond syndrome, Pearson syndrome, cartilage-hair hypoplasia, congenital sideroblastic anaemia or osteopetrosis [310]. In the fetus and neonate, haemolytic anaemia may be the result of transplacental passage of antibodies (alloantibodies or, less often, maternal autoantibodies) or on intrauterine infections by micro-organisms that in later life do not usually cause anaemia (e.g. cytomegalovirus infection, toxoplasmosis, syphilis and rubella) [319]. The consequences of anaemia also differ from those at other periods of life. Severe anaemia in the fetus can lead to hydrops fetalis, a condition characterised by gross oedema of the fetus and placenta, often leading to intra-uterine death. In the neonate, because of the immaturity of the liver, severe haemolysis can lead to marked hyperbilirubinaemia with resultant brain damage. The identification of anaemia, particularly haemolytic anaemia, in the fetus and neonate is therefore of considerable importance.

Further tests

When the cause of anaemia is not apparent from the clinical history or the blood film and count, other tests are needed. Those most likely to be useful are: (i) a reticulocyte count; (ii) assay of serum ferritin or of serum iron and transferrin concentrations; (iii) serum B_{12} and red cell folate assays; and (iv) tests of renal, thyroid and hepatic function. If these investigations do not reveal the cause of the anaemia, a bone marrow aspirate is usually indicated. When there is an unexplained leucoerythroblastic anaemia, other than during an acute illness, a bone marrow aspirate and trephine biopsy are indicated without delay.

In the neonate, serological tests on mother and baby, a Kleihauer test to detect fetomaternal haemorrhage, haematological assessment of both parents and glucose-6-phosphate dehydrogenase (G6PD) assay may be useful.

Reticulocytopenia

Reticulocytopenia means that there is a reduction in the absolute reticulocyte count below that expected in a healthy subject of the same age. Usually the reticulocyte

Table 6.21 Some causes of reticulocytopenia.

Deficiency of vitamin B_{12}, iron or folic acid
Anaemia of chronic disease
Bone marrow suppression by cytotoxic chemotherapy or other bone marrow-damaging drugs
Aplastic anaemia
Pure red cell aplasia
Acute leukaemia
Myelodysplastic syndromes (most cases)

percentage is also reduced. In assessing the reticulocyte count it is important not only to consider whether the value falls within the reference range, but also whether it is appropriate to the degree of anaemia and to any shortening of red cell life span. Thus a patient with a haemolytic anaemia should have a reticulocyte count above the normal range; lack of reticulocytosis in such a patient may indicate pure red cell aplasia or folic acid deficiency.

Causes of reticulocytopenia are shown in Table 6.21.

Leucopenia

Leucopenia is a reduction of the total white cell count below that expected in a healthy subject of the same age, gender, physiological status and ethnic origin. It can result from a decrease in the neutrophil count, the lymphocyte count or both and cannot be interpreted without knowledge of the differential count. There are, however, certain infections that are associated with leucopenia rather than leucocytosis and the presence of leucopenia in a febrile patient can therefore be of some diagnostic use. They include dengue fever, rickettsial infections, typhoid fever and leishmaniasis.

Neutropenia

Neutropenia is a reduction of the absolute neutrophil count below that expected in a subject of the same age, gender, physiological status and ethnic origin. It is particularly important to use an appropriate reference range in individuals with African ancestry, to avoid a misdiagnosis of neutropenia, since Africans and, to a lesser extent Afro-Americans and Afro-Caribbeans, have neutrophil counts much lower than those of Caucasians. Neutropenia may be an isolated phenomenon or part of a pancytopenia. Mechanisms of neutropenia include: (i) inadequate production by the bone marrow because of reduced stem cell numbers, bone marrow replacement or ineffective granulopoiesis; (ii) destruction by bone marrow macrophages and other reticuloendothelial cells in haemophagocytic syndromes; (iii) defective release from the bone marrow as in myelokathexis; (iv) redistribution within the vasculature as occurs early during haemodialysis and can occur due to pulmonary sequestration following transfusion of blood containing an anti-neutrophil antibody, e.g. in transfusion-related acute lung injury [320]; (v) pooling in the spleen; (vi) shortened intravascular lifespan as in immune neutropenias; and (vii) rapid egress to the tissues when the bone marrow output cannot increase adequately, as in neonates with sepsis.

An unexpected apparent neutropenia on an automated counter should always be confirmed on a blood film since it may be factitious (see Chapter 4). The detection of unexpected neutropenia by the laboratory can be of vital importance, since drug-induced agranulocytosis can be rapidly fatal. In many clinical circumstances the likely cause of neutropenia will be readily apparent from the patient's medical history, including the history of drug intake. When the history and examination of the blood film do not reveal the cause, bone marrow investigation is usually necessary. The causes of neutropenia are summarised in Tables 6.22 and 6.23.

Table 6.22 Some inherited disorders causing neutropenia.

Reticular agenesis or dysgenesis (severe granulocytopenia, monocytopenia and lymphocytopenia with hypoplasia of thymus and lymph nodes and impaired cellular and humoral immunity; bi-allelic mutation in the *AK2* gene)

Neutropenia with pancreatic exocrine deficiency and dyschondroplasia – neutropenia may be intermittent (Shwachman or Shwachman–Diamond syndrome, resulting from mutations in the *SBDS* gene)

Mitochondrial disorders: neutropenia with pancreatic exocrine deficiency and sideroblastic erythropoiesis (Pearson syndrome) [278], Barth syndrome (cardiomyopathy, growth retardation and, variably, congenital neutropenia, which may be cyclical, resulting from mutation of the *TAZ* (G4.5) gene at Xq28) [321], Kearns–Sayre syndrome [161], fumarase deficiency [161]

Familial benign neutropenia

Familial severe neutropenia, previously known as infantile genetic agranulocytosis (autosomal recessive, autosomal dominant or X-linked – autosomal recessive cases known as Kostmann syndrome), some cases due to mutations in *ELANE* (elastase) gene or the *HAX1* gene; less often results from mutation in the gene encoding the G-CSF receptor [322], activating mutations of the *WAS* gene [323,324] or *GFI1* gene [325]; mutation in the *LAMTOR 2* (*MAPBPIP*) gene (autosomal recessive) [326]; one of two reported cases of mutation in *BLOC1S6* encoding pallidin, Hermansky–Pudlak syndrome type 9 (autosomal recessive) [327]

Familial cyclical neutropenia† (autosomal dominant) [328]; may result from mutation of the *ELANE* gene

Congenital dysgranulopoietic neutropenia [329]

Myelokathexis, also known as the WHIM (warts, hypogammaglobulinaemia, infections and myelokathexis) syndrome [330]

Lazy leucocyte syndrome (may actually represent childhood autoimmune neutropenia rather than being inherited) [90]

Chédiak–Higashi syndrome

Dyskeratosis congenita

Associated with X-linked agammaglobulinaemia (occurring in a third of cases)

Associated with hyper-immunoglobulin M syndrome [331]

Associated with cartilage-hair hypoplasia

Associated with severe combined immunodeficiency [332]

Cohen syndrome [333]

Bloom syndrome [334]

Diamond–Blackfan syndrome, during the course of the disease [335]

Griscelli syndrome, type 2 [336]

Hermansky–Pudlak syndrome due to mutation of *AP3B1* gene (Hermansky-Pudlak syndrome type 2) [337]

Associated with familial fragile site at 16q22 leading to mosaic del(16)(q22) [338]

Glutathione synthase deficiency [90]

Rothmund–Thomson syndrome [339]

Associated with certain inborn errors of metabolism: idiopathic hyperglycinaemia, isovaleric acidaemia, methylmalonic acidaemia, type Ib glycogen storage disease due to bi-allelic *SLC37A4* mutation, bi-allelic *G6PC3* mutation [340], carnitine deficiency [341], methylglutaconic aciduria [342], propionic acidaemia [343], hyperzincaemia with hypercalprotectinaemia [344], tyrosinaemia [90], mevalonate kinase deficiency (hyperimmunoglobulin D syndrome) [345]

G-CSF, granulocyte colony-stimulating factor

Table 6.23 Some acquired disorders causing neutropenia.

Infections
  Viral infections, e.g. measles, mumps, rubella including intrauterine rubella infection [346], MMR (measles, mumps and rubella) vaccination, influenza, avian influenza A [347], influenza vaccination [348], infectious hepatitis, infectious mononucleosis, cytomegalovirus infection including intra-uterine cytomegalovirus infection [346], human herpesvirus 6 infection [349,350], parvovirus B19 infection (occasionally) [351], yellow fever, dengue fever, Colorado tick fever, Venezuelan haemorrhagic fever [352], Crimean–Congo haemorrhagic fever [353], lymphocytic choriomeningitis virus infection [354], corona virus-associated severe acute respiratory distress syndrome (SARS; occasionally) [355], advanced HIV infection (AIDS), severe fever with thrombocytopenia syndrome virus (SFTSV, a Bunya virus) infection [356], Heartland virus (a phlebovirus) infection [357], chronic hepatitis C infection [358]
  Bacterial infections, e.g. typhoid [226], paratyphoid, brucellosis, tularaemia [359], some cases of miliary tuberculosis [223], some Gram-negative infections (early in the disease process), overwhelming bacterial infection – particularly but not only Gram-negative infection, bacterial infection in neonates, rickettsial infections including scrub typhus [360], rickettsial pox [361], *Rickettsia africae* infection [362] and some cases of typhus, human granulocytic anaplasmosis (previously known as human granulocytic ehrlichiosis) and human monocytic ehrlichiosis [363]
  Protozoal infection, e.g. malaria, visceral leishmaniasis (kala azar), trypanosomiasis, babesiosis [364]
  Fungal infections, e.g. histoplasmosis [365]
Drugs,* e.g. alkylating agents and other anticancer and related drugs (including methotrexate used for rheumatological and skin conditions, azathioprine, zidovudine and, rarely, neutropenia in infancy following perinatal exposure to zidovudine [367]), idiosyncratic reaction to drugs (most often with anti-thyroid drugs, sulphonamides, chlorpromazine, gold), interferon, alemtuzumab, rituximab (probably autoimmune) [368], bortezomib [369], sirolimus, imatinib [370], fostamatinib (R788) [371], thalidomide, lenalidomide, pomalidomide, levamisole, etanercept, clopidogrel, brodalumab [372], ixekizumab [373], granulocyte colony-stimulating factor (transient, about 30 minutes after administration) [374], ibrutinib [375]
Mustard gas exposure [376]
Administration of IL12 [281]
Irradiation
Bone marrow replacement, e.g. in ALL, multiple myeloma, or carcinoma
Primary and secondary myelofibrosis
Ineffective granulopoiesis, e.g. in most cases of AML and most MDS
Megaloblastic anaemia
Aplastic anaemia
Paroxysmal nocturnal haemoglobinuria
Acute anaphylaxis
Hypersplenism
Haemophagocytic syndromes
Immune neutropenia

Alloimmune neutropenia, following blood transfusion [377] or in neonates, as a result of transplacental passage of maternal alloantibody to human neutrophil antigens, HLA antigens or CD16 (FcγRIIIb; one case) [378]
Immune neutropenia in neonates, as a result of transplacental passage of maternal autoantibody [379]
Autoimmune neutropenia [380], including isolated autoimmune neutropenia and autoimmune neutropenia associated with autoimmune haemolytic anaemia, autoimmune thrombocytopenia, autoimmune lymphoproliferative syndrome, systemic lupus erythematosus, rheumatoid arthritis (Felty syndrome), scleroderma, hyperthyroidism, chronic active hepatitis, polyarteritis nodosa, primary biliary cirrhosis, thymoma, Hodgkin lymphoma, non-Hodgkin lymphoma, angioimmunoblastic T-cell lymphoma, large granular lymphocyte leukaemia (both T cell and NK cell) and increased activated T lymphocytes [381], viral infection (e.g. chronic parvovirus infection [382], HIV infection, infectious mononucleosis), Castleman disease, Sjögren syndrome, mannosidosis and hypogammaglobulinaemia
Autoimmune panleucopenia [383]
Autoimmune pure white cell aplasia [384] (may be associated with thymoma)
Graft-versus-host disease [287]
Administration of anti-Rh D for the treatment of autoimmune thrombocytopenic purpura [385]
Severe combined immunodeficiency, possibly due to graft-versus-host disease induced by maternal T lymphocytes [386]
Cyclical neutropenia, including adult onset cyclical neutropenia associated with large granular lymphocyte leukaemia (see above)
Haemodialysis and filtration leukapheresis (early during the procedures)
Transfusion-associated acute lung injury ('TRALI') [320,387]
Peripheral blood stem cell apheresis [388]
Endocrine disorders, e.g. hypopituitarism, Addison disease, hyperthyroidism [206]
Alcoholism [389]
Anorexia nervosa [271]
Kawasaki disease
Kikuchi disease (necrotising lymphadenitis) [390]
Copper deficiency [391,392]
Arsenic poisoning [286]
Hypercarotenaemia [393]
Placental insufficiency – babies with intrauterine growth retardation and babies born to hypertensive and diabetic mothers [394,395]
Babies with asphyxia neonatorum [395]
Rh haemolytic disease of the newborn [394]
Extracorporeal membrane oxygenation in neonates [396]
Administration of erythropoietin to premature babies [264]
Associated with transient erythroblastopenia of childhood [397]
Intravenous immunoglobulin infusion in infants [394]
Therapy with alemtuzumab [398]
Splenic sarcoidosis [399]
Intermittent severe neutropenia of uncertain mechanism in some patients with immune deficiency due to *STK4* mutation [400]

* Can result from inadvertent intake of drugs, e.g. levamisole used as a 'filler' in cocaine [366]
AIDS, acquired immune deficiency syndrome; ALL, acute lymphoblastic leukaemia; AML, acute myeloid leukaemia; HIV, human immunodeficiency virus; IL, interleukin; MDS, myelodysplastic syndrome

Eosinopenia

Eosinopenia is a reduction of the eosinophil count below that expected in a healthy subject of the same age. Eosinopenia is rarely noted on a routine blood film and cannot be detected on a routine 100-cell differential cell count, since the eosinophil is a relatively infrequent cell and the reference limits include zero. Since the introduction of automated differential counts, eosinopenia is far more often noted. However, it is a common non-specific abnormality, so its detection is not of much clinical significance.

A physiological fall in the eosinophil count occurs during pregnancy and there is a further fall during labour. Common causes of a low eosinophil count are shown in Table 6.24. The eosinophil count has been reported to be reduced in Down syndrome [401]. Rare causes that have been reported include thymoma, pure eosinophil aplasia [402] and apparent autoimmune destruction of eosinophils and basophils [403]. The eosinophil count is reduced in human T-cell lymphotropic virus 1 (HTLV-1) carriers [404].

Table 6.24 Some causes of eosinopenia

Acute stress including trauma, surgery, burns, epileptiform convulsions, acute infections, acute inflammation, myocardial infarction, anoxia and exposure to cold
Cushing syndrome
Administration of various drugs including corticosteroids and ACTH, epinephrine (adrenaline) and other β agonists, histamine and aminophylline
Haemodialysis (during procedure)

ACTH, adrenocorticotropic hormone

Basopenia

Basopenia is a reduction in the basophil count below that which would be expected in a healthy subject. Some of the causes are shown in Table 6.25. Basophils are so infrequent in normal blood that their reduction is not likely to be noticed on inspection of the film or on a routine 100-cell or even 500-cell differential count. In theory, basopenia can be detected on automated differential counters, since they have reference ranges for basophils that do not include zero. However, in practice, automated basophil counts are not very accurate and the observation of basopenia has not yet been found to be of any great importance in diagnosis.

Table 6.25 Some causes of basopenia.

Acute stress including infection and haemorrhage
Cushing syndrome and administration of ACTH
Administration of prednisone in healthy subjects [405]
Anaphylaxis, acute urticaria and other acute allergic reactions
Chronic urticaria (increased by prednisolone therapy) [405]
Hyperthyroidism
Progesterone administration

ACTH, adrenocorticotropic hormone

Monocytopenia

Monocytopenia is the reduction of the monocyte count below that expected in a healthy subject of the same age. It may accompany other cytopenias, e.g. in reticular agenesis and aplastic anaemia. Sporadic and autosomal dominant monocytopenia associated with a loss-of-function *GATA2* mutation may have an associated reduction of B lymphocytes, natural killer cells and dendritic cells and predisposes to MDS and AML (Mono-MAC syndrome) [406,407]. Monocytopenia is also associated with mild congenital neutropenia due to a *GATA2* mutation [408]. Circulating monocytes are absent in homozygosity for a rare mutation in the gene encoding interferon regulatory factor 8 [409]. The monocyte count is reduced in the WHIM (Warts, Hypogammaglobulinaemia, Infections, Myelokathexis) syndrome [79]. The monocyte counts falls after administration of corticosteroids and in acute infections associated with endotoxaemia [90]. Monocyte numbers are conspicuously reduced in hairy cell leukaemia. The monocyte count falls, together with the neutrophil count, in transfusion-associated acute lung injury ('TRALI') [387]. Alemtuzumab therapy causes monocytopenia.

Lymphocytopenia (lymphopenia)

Lymphopenia or, more correctly, lymphocytopenia is a reduction of the lymphocyte count below what would be expected in a healthy subject of the same age. It is important in assessing babies with suspected immunodeficiency to use an appropriate reference range; counts below $2.8 \times 10^9/l$ in a baby with infection raise the possibility of severe combined immunodeficiency [410].

Lymphocytopenia is extremely common as part of the acute response to stress, although it is often

Table 6.26 Some causes of lymphocytopenia.

Inherited Certain rare congenital immune deficiency syndromes including reticular dysgenesis, severe combined immunodeficiency, Swiss type agammaglobulinaemia, some case of thymic hypoplasia (diGeorge syndrome), ataxia telangiectasia, mutation in the CD2 gene [415], WHIM syndrome [79] Congenital dyserythropoietic anaemia, type I [416] **Acquired** Acute stress including trauma, surgery, burns, acute infection, fulminant hepatic failure (may be preceded by lymphocytosis) Acute and chronic renal failure (including patients on dialysis) Cushing syndrome and the administration of corticosteroids or ACTH Carcinoma (particularly with advanced disease) Hodgkin lymphoma (particularly with advanced disease) Some non-Hodgkin lymphomas Angioimmunoblastic T-cell lymphoma Acute HIV infection Acquired immune deficiency syndrome (AIDS) Cytotoxic and immunosuppressive therapy, particularly nucleoside analogue therapy, and also use of antilymphocyte and antithymocyte globulin and monoclonal antibody therapy directed at lymphocytes (e.g. alemtuzumab – anti-CD52); dimethyl fumarate (for psoriasis) [417]	Stem cell transplantation* Clozapine therapy [86] Quinine hypersensitivity [418] Erythropoietin therapy [419] IL12 administration [281] Influenza vaccination [420] Irradiation Alcoholism [389] Rheumatoid arthritis [421] and systemic lupus erythematosus [422] Sarcoidosis [423] Aplastic anaemia and agranulocytosis Megaloblastic anaemia The myelodysplastic syndromes [424,425][†] Anorexia nervosa [426] Intestinal lymphangiectasia and Whipple disease Peripheral blood stem cell apheresis [388] Iron deficiency anaemia [427] Chronic platelet apheresis [428] Graft-versus-host disease Administration of 'Lorenzo's oil' [429] Thymoma [430]

*A lymphocyte count of less than 0.75×10^9/l at day 100 is predictive of extensive and severe graft-versus-host disease after allogeneic transplantation

†A lymphocyte count of less than 1.2×10^9/l is of adverse prognostic significance in the myelodysplastic syndromes [425]

ACTH, adrenocorticotropic hormone; HIV, human immunodeficiency virus; IL12, interleukin 12; WHIM, Warts, Hypogammaglobulinaemia, Infections, Myelokathexis

overshadowed by the coexisting changes in neutrophils. It is more likely to be noticed when an automated differential count is performed and counts are expressed in absolute numbers. With the increasing importance of the diagnosis of the acquired immune deficiency syndrome (AIDS), characterised by increasingly severe lymphopenia with disease progression, it is important to realise how common this abnormality is in acutely ill patients, regardless of the nature of the underlying illness. In one study of patients with bacteraemia, lymphopenia was observed more consistently than neutrophilia [411]. In Hodgkin lymphoma, a lymphocyte count of less than 0.6×10^9/l is of adverse prognostic significance [412]. Lymphopenia is also of adverse significance in peripheral T-cell lymphoma, not otherwise specified [413]. Similarly, a lymphocyte count of 1×10^9/l or less at presentation of diffuse large B-cell lymphoma

is associated with a worse prognosis [414]. In diffuse large B-cell lymphoma, lymphopenia at the completion of first-line treatment is predictive of early relapse [414]. Causes of lymphocytopenia are summarised in Table 6.26.

Lymphocyte counts 3–6 days after irradiation exposure correlate with the severity of acute radiation sickness, ranging from $0.8–1.5 \times 10^9$/l during this period after exposure for those with mild disease to $0–0.1 \times 10^9$/l with no latent phase in those with lethal exposure [431].

Thrombocytopenia

Thrombocytopenia is a reduction of the platelet count below the level expected in a healthy subject of the same age and gender. Ethnic origin may also be relevant, since lower platelet counts have been observed in Africans and Afro-Caribbeans. Thrombocytopenia may be congenital or acquired and due to reduced production or to increased destruction, consumption or extravascular loss. The causes are summarised in Table 6.27. Information on drugs recognised as causing thrombocytopenia is available on a website, which is updated annually [534].

Table 6.27 Some causes of thrombocytopenia (excluding conditions that usually cause pancytopenia).

Failure of platelet production

Congenital (inherited or resulting from intra-uterine events)

May–Hegglin anomaly, Sebastian syndrome, Epstein syndrome, Fechtner syndrome (all resulting from a *MYH9* mutation)

Bernard–Soulier syndrome

Other inherited thrombocytopenias (see Tables 8.11–13)

Megakaryocytic hypoplasia, inherited or due to intrauterine events (including some mutations of the *MPL* gene encoding the thrombopoietin receptor), some cases of trisomy 13, trisomy 18 and trisomy 21 syndromes, thrombocytopenia with absent radii, thrombocytopenia with radio-ulnar synostosis (*HOXA11* mutation), thrombocytopenia with normal radii but with other physical abnormalities in 40% of cases and having an autosomal recessive or X-linked recessive inheritance [432], amegakaryocytic thrombocytopenia with Noonan syndrome [433], X-linked thrombocytopenia due to *GATA1* mutation

Reticular agenesis (variable thrombocytopenia)

Placental insufficiency – associated with fetal hypoxia/intrauterine growth retardation/babies of hypertensive or diabetic mothers [394,434]

Haemolytic disease of the newborn (Rh and, particularly, Kell) [435,436]

Transplacental passage of maternal anti-platelet antibodies inhibiting megakaryocytopoiesis, e.g. anti HPA-2b [437]

Inherited but not present at birth

Fanconi anaemia

Acquired

Following bone marrow damage by some of the drugs that can cause aplastic anaemia or as the first manifestation of aplastic anaemia or as a feature of mustard gas exposure [438]

Anticancer drugs – alkylating agents, nitrosoureas, anthracyclines, mitoxantrone, imatinib (rarely) [196], dasatinib [439], thalidomide, lenalidomide, bortezomib

Thiazide administration

Myelodysplastic syndromes

Severe iron deficiency (rarely)

Parvovirus infection (rarely) [440]

HHV6 infection [350] including delayed platelet engraftment following allogeneic transplantation associated with early HHV6 variant B infection [441]

Chronic hepatitis C virus infection (probably) [442]

Interferon therapy

Paroxysmal nocturnal haemoglobinuria

Alcohol abuse [443]

Anorexia nervosa [271]

Autoimmune acquired amegakaryocytic thrombocytopenia [443] including amegakaryocytic thrombocytopenia associated with large granular lymphocyte leukaemia and sometimes causing cyclical thrombocytopenia [444]

Graft-versus-host disease [287]

Chronic renal failure on haemodialysis and, to a lesser extent, on peritoneal dialysis [445]

Development of antibodies to thrombopoietin after administration of pegylated recombinant thrombopoietin [446]

Hypervitaminosis A [285]

Copper deficiency [392]

Arsenic poisoning [286]

Increased platelet consumption, destruction or removal (demonstrated or presumptive)

Immune mechanisms

Congenital

Alloimmune thrombocytopenia

Transplacental transfer of maternal autoantibody

Transplacental transfer of maternal anti GpIIb/IIIa (in the case of a mother with Glanzmann thrombasthenia) [447]

Transplacental transfer of maternal anti-CD36 isoantibodies from CD36-deficient mothers [448]

Transplacental transfer of maternal HLA antibodies (uncommon) [437]

Transplacental transfer of maternal ABO antibodies (rare) [437]

Maternal drug hypersensitivity

Acquired

Autoimmune thrombocytopenic purpura as an isolated abnormality or associated with other autoimmune disease (systemic lupus erythematosus, primary antiphospholipid syndrome, rheumatoid arthritis, autoimmune haemolytic anaemia (Evans syndrome), autoimmune lymphoproliferative syndrome), with a lymphoproliferative disease (chronic lymphocytic leukaemia, non-Hodgkin lymphoma, Hodgkin lymphoma, large granular lymphocyte leukaemia), sarcoidosis [448], common variable immune deficiency [449] or angioimmunoblastic lymphadenopathy

Alloimmune, e.g. caused by transfer of donor lymphocytes during stem cell transplantation [450], infusion of plasma containing platelet alloantibodies [451]

Drug-induced immune thrombocytopenia including heparin-induced thrombocytopenia, protamine-heparin induced thrombocytopenia [452], thrombocytopenia induced by quinine (including in Indian tonic water, bitter lemon and

(continued)

Table 6.27 *(continued)*

Dubonnet [453]), vancomycin and carbimazole [454] and thrombocytopenia induced by anti-platelet monoclonal antibodies such as abciximab* (anti-platelet glycoprotein IIb/IIIa) [455] and other drugs interfering with binding of fibrinogen to platelet glycoprotein IIb/IIIa – eptifibatide, orbofiban, roxifiban, tirofiban and xemilofiban [456], alemtuzumab (thrombocytopenia is transient)

Drug-induced autoimmune thrombocytopenia due to gold salts and possibly procainamide, sulphonamides and interferon alpha and beta [457]

Food-associated immune thrombocytopenia – tahina [458], *Lupinus termis* beans [459], cow's milk [453], cranberry juice [453]

Immune thrombocytopenia associated with Jui herbal tea (a traditional Chinese remedy) [460]

Immune thrombocytopenia associated with HIV infection

Immune thrombocytopenia associated with cytomegalovirus infection [461], HHV6 infection [462], hepatitis C infection [463], hepatitis E infection [464], *Mycoplasma pneumoniae* infection [465], scarlet fever (β haemolytic streptococcal infection) [466], tuberculosis [467,468], brucellosis [469], toxoplasmosis [469], *Helicobacter pylori* infection [470], Q-fever [471], H7N9 (avian origin) influenza virus infection [472], malaria, babesiosis

Post-infection thrombocytopenia, particularly after rubella but also after chicken pox (varicella), infectious mononucleosis, other viral infections and vaccinations, e.g. MMR vaccine

Post-transfusion purpura

Cocaine abuse [473]

Anaphylaxis

Onyalai [474]

Use of dialysers sterilised with electron beam radiation [475]

Non-immune mechanisms
Congenital

The Schulman–Upshaw syndrome [476,477]

Hereditary phytosterolaemia [478]

Kaposiform haemangioendothelioma [479] or tufted haemangioma (Kasabach–Merritt syndrome)

Intrahepatic infantile haemangioma [479]

Type IIB von Willebrand disease, particularly after DDAVP therapy, and platelet-type (pseudo) von Willebrand disease (inherited defect of platelet GpIb)

Mutation in *ITGB3* gene encoding GpIIb/IIa [480]

Acquired

Disseminated intravascular coagulation (including that associated with heat stroke, IL2 administration [481,482], trypanosomiasis [483] and angiosarcoma [484])

Thrombotic microangiopathy (thrombotic thrombocytopenic purpura and related conditions, see Table 8.8)

Post-transplant hepatic veno-occlusive disease [485]

Venous thrombo-embolism [486]

Viral haemorrhagic fevers – arenavirus infection (Lassa fever and Argentinian, Bolivian, Venezuelan and Brazilian haemorrhagic fevers), Bunyaviridae infections (Rift Valley fever, Crimean–Congo haemorrhagic fever, haemorrhagic fever with renal syndrome due to Hantaan, Seoul, Puumala and other viruses and hantavirus pulmonary syndrome due to Sin Nombre virus) [59], Black Creek Canal and other viruses infection, severe fever with thrombocytopenia syndrome virus (SFTSV) infection [356], Filoviridae infections (Marburg and Ebola haemorrhagic fevers), Flaviviridae infections (yellow fever [487], dengue, Kyasanur Forest disease and Omsk haemorrhagic fever) and certain other viral infections, e.g. Colorado tick fever (coltivirus infection), acute HIV infection, Cache valley virus infection [488], lymphocytic choriomeningitis virus infection [354], Nipah virus encephalitis [489], corona-virus associated severe acute respiratory distress syndrome (SARS) [354], avian influenza A infection [347], chikungunya fever [490], Heartland virus (a phlebovirus) infection [357], West Nile virus infection [491], Alkhumra virus infection [492]

Rickettsial infections, e.g. Rocky Mountain spotted fever, malignant Mediterranean spotted fever, Queensland tick typhus [493], scrub typhus [494], murine typhus [495]

Certain bacterial infections, e.g. Brazilian haemorrhagic fever (*Haemophilus aegypticus* infection), relapsing fever (*Borrelia recurrentis* infection), human monocytic ehrlichiosis (*Ehrlichia chaffeensis* infection), human granulocytic anaplasmosis (previously known as human granulocytic ehrlichiosis; *Anaplasma phagocytophilum* infection) and infection by *Ehrlichia ewingii* and ehrlichia species Wisconsin [496], *Bartonella quintana* infection (trench fever) [497], inhalational anthrax [498], brucellosis [499], typhoid fever [500], leptospirosis [501]

Certain protozoal infections, e.g. malaria and babesiosis

Extracorporeal circulation

Use of intra-aortic balloon pump [502]

Peripheral blood stem cell apheresis [388]

Massive transfusion

Kaposi sarcoma [503]

'Histiocytic sarcoma' of the spleen [504]

Administration of M-CSF [505]

Snake bite [83]

Envenomation by bees [506]

Acquired phytosterolaemia associated with soy-based parenteral nutrition [507]

Redistribution of platelets
Congenital

Hypersplenism

Acquired

Hypersplenism (including acute sequestration in sickle cell disease)

Administration of Lorenzo's oil [429,508]

Hypothermia [509]

Uncertain or complex mechanisms	Acquired
Congenital	Phototherapy in the neonate [518]
Extreme prematurity	Respiratory distress syndrome and mechanical ventilation in the
Wiskott–Aldrich syndrome	neonate [519,520]
The grey platelet syndrome	Neonatal herpes simplex infection
Chédiak–Higashi anomaly	Associated with cyanotic congenital heart disease
Griscelli syndrome, type 2 [469]	Neonatal hyperthyroidism [521]
Hermansky–Pudlak syndrome type II [510]	Miliary tuberculosis [255]
Cyclical thrombocytopenia and tidal platelet dysgenesis	Graves disease [522]
Mediterranean macrothrombocytosis	Hypothyroidism [523]
Jacobsen syndrome (Paris-Trousseau thrombocytopenia, terminal	Pregnancy-associated thrombocytopenia
deletion of 11q with q21-q24 breakpoint)	Monge disease (inappropriate altitude-related polycythaemia) [524]
Congenital infections (toxoplasmosis, cytomegalovirus infection,	Thrombocytopenia with exanthem in Japanese neonates [525]
rubella, syphilis, listeriosis, coxsackie B infection, herpes simplex	Wilson disease [526]
virus infection, relapsing fever (*Borrelia hermsii* infection) [511])	Paracetamol (acetaminophen) overdose [527]
Associated with certain inborn errors of metabolism (idiopathic	Drug-induced, non-immune (valproate, amrinone, linezolid
hyperglycinaemia [512], methylmalonic acidaemia [512], isovaleric	[457,528])
acidaemia [512], propionic acidaemia [343], hyperzincaemia	Drug-induced, unknown mechanism (infliximab, efalizumab,
with hypercalprotectinaemia [344], holocarboxylase synthetase	rituximab [457,529,530]), alemtuzumab, omalizumab (anti-
deficiency, mevalonic aciduria [513])	immunoglobulin E) therapy [531], trastuzumab [532], bortezomib
Mitochondrial cytopathies including Pearson syndrome, fumarase	[369], IL12 [281], sirolimus, ibrutinib [375]
deficiency and mitochondrial depletion syndrome [161,514]	Iodinated radiological contrast media [457]
Associated with factor V Quebec [515]	Use of Jui (traditional Chinese herbal medicine) (probably immune)
Congenital dyserythropoietic anaemia, type I (thrombocytopenia is	[533]
transient) [516]	Oroya fever [191]
Severe congenital neutropenia, during treatment with G-CSF [517]	

*but note that abciximab can also cause factitious thrombocytopenia as a result of platelet aggregation

DDAVP, 1-deamino-8-D-arginine vasopressin; HHV6, human herpesvirus 6; HIV, human immunodeficiency virus; HLA, human histocompatibility antigen; IL, interleukin; M-CSF, macrophage colony-stimulating factor

The platelet count is significantly lower and the mean platelet volume significantly higher in individuals with acute coronary syndromes in comparison with those with stable angina or non-cardiac pain [535].

Some causes of thrombocytopenia of particular importance in the fetus and the neonate are summarised in Tables 6.28 and 6.29. In fetuses with intra-uterine growth retardation, thrombocytopenia is indicative of a worse prognosis [537]. The most common cause of severe thrombocytopenia in neonates is alloimmune thrombocytopenia.

Blood film and count

In unexplained congenital thrombocytopenia both platelet size and granularity and white cell morphology should be assessed. A number of inherited conditions have thrombocytopenia associated with morphological abnormalities of platelets or neutrophils (see Chapter 9). In acquired thrombocytopenia, platelet size is also relevant since increased platelet consumption or destruction with increased bone marrow output is associated with increased platelet size, whereas bone marrow failure is associated with small or normal sized platelets. Red cells should be assessed for any evidence of a microangiopathic haemolytic anaemia, which may be associated with thrombocytopenia caused by a thrombotic microangiopathy. The blood film should also be examined for abnormal lymphocytes (indicative of viral infection or lymphoproliferative disorder), blast cells, immature granulocytes or NRBC (indicative of leukaemia or bone marrow infiltration) and dysplastic features (indicative of MDS or AML). Children with amegakaryocytic thrombocytopenia may have macrocytosis [433].

The automated blood count shows an increased MPV and PDW when there is increased platelet consumption or destruction and a low MPV when there is failure of bone marrow output. The count of 'reticulated

Table 6.28 Some causes of fetal thrombocytopenia (platelet count less than $150 \times 10^9/l$) [536,537]; the prevalence among fetuses with certain specified abnormalities is shown in brackets [536].

Category/mechanism	Frequency among instances of thrombocytopenia	Specific cause and % of cases of condition in which it is found
Intrauterine infection	28%	Toxoplasmosis (26%), cytomegalovirus infection (36%), rubella (20%), HIV infection
Immune	18%	Alloimmune thrombocytopenia, maternal autoimmune thrombocytopenia
Chromosomal abnormalities	17%	Trisomy 13 (54%), trisomy 18 (86%), trisomy 21 (6%), Turner syndrome (31%), triploidy (3/4)
Unknown and presumably heterogeneous mechanisms	12%	Associated with multiple congenital abnormalities without a chromosomal abnormality
Intrauterine growth retardation	6%	
Unknown mechanism	4%	Severe Rh haemolytic disease
Inherited	rare	Wiskott–Aldrich syndrome
		Congenital amegakaryocytic thrombocytopenia

Table 6.29 Some causes of thrombocytopenia of particular importance in the neonate (for mechanisms and other rare causes see Table 6.27).

Chronic fetal hypoxia (maternal hypertension, diabetes mellitus, idiopathic intrauterine growth retardation)*
Perinatal asphyxia (often associated with disseminated intravascular coagulation) [538]
Intrauterine infection
  Viral infection (cytomegalovirus infection, congenital rubella, HIV infection, herpes simplex infection, varicella-zoster infection, coxsackie B infection)
  Congenital syphilis
  Listeriosis
  Congenital toxoplasmosis
Perinatal infection (e.g. *Escherichia coli*, group B streptococcus) [538]
Maternal antiplatelet antibodies (autoantibodies, alloantibodies or drug-dependent antibodies)
Congenital leukaemia including transient abnormal myelopoiesis of Down syndrome
Disseminated intravascular coagulation (e.g. resulting from bacterial sepsis, acute asphyxia, respiratory distress syndrome, pulmonary hypertension, necrotising enterocolitis) [272]
Thrombosis (of aorta or renal vein) [537]
Kasabach–Merritt syndrome
Inherited (e.g. thrombocytopenia with absent radii, congenital amegakaryocytic thrombocytopenia, trisomy 13 [538], trisomy 18 [538], Noonan syndrome [539])
Metabolic disease (e.g. propionic and methylmalonicacidaemia, Gaucher disease) [536]
Exchange transfusion
Hyperbilirubinaemia and phototherapy [272]
Induced hypothermia [537]
Necrotising enterocolitis

*There may be associated polycythaemia, mild neutropenia and features of hyposplenism [537]

platelets' is increased when there is increased platelet turnover and decreased when there is failure of production.

Other tests

In congenital thrombocytopenia, the patient should be assessed for evidence of associated congenital defects and other family members should be assessed for platelet number and morphology and other evidence of inherited abnormalities. Children with amegakaryocytic thrombocytopenia may have an increased percentage of haemoglobin F and increased i antigen expression [433].

In acquired thrombocytopenia not readily explained by the clinical circumstances, a bone marrow aspiration, tests for autoantibodies (antinuclear factor, anti-DNA antibodies and the lupus anticoagulant) and coagulation tests to exclude disseminated intravascular coagulation can be useful. Testing for HIV antibodies should be considered.

Pancytopenia

Pancytopenia is a combination of anaemia (with reduction of the RBC), leucopenia and thrombocytopenia. Leucopenia is usually mainly due to a reduction in the neutrophil count, although the numbers of other granulocytes, monocytes and lymphocytes are often also reduced.

Pancytopenia is usually caused by bone marrow replacement or failure, but it sometimes results from splenic pooling or peripheral destruction of mature cells. Cyclical pancytopenia, probably cytokine-induced, is an unusual manifestation of Hodgkin lymphoma [540]. Some of the causes of pancytopenia are shown in Table 6.30. In hospital practice, pancytopenia is most often the result of cytotoxic or immunosuppressive drug therapy.

Blood film and count

When the aetiology is not readily apparent from the clinical history, the blood film should be carefully examined for blast cells, dysplastic features in any cell lineage, lymphoma cells, hairy cells, myeloma cells, increased rouleaux formation, macrocytes, hypersegmented neutrophils, NRBC and immature granulocytes. Blast cells should be

Table 6.30 Some causes of pancytopenia.

Inherited disorders	multiple myeloma, carcinoma, non-Hodgkin lymphoma, hairy cell leukaemia and hairy cell variant leukaemia
Inherited conditions causing aplastic anaemia: Fanconi anaemia, dyskeratosis congenita, WT syndrome of radioulnar hypoplasia, hypoplastic anaemia and susceptibility to leukaemia [541], xeroderma pigmentosa, late stages of Shwachman–Diamond syndrome, aplastic anaemia following congenital amegakaryocytic thrombocytopenia [432] including some patients with amegakaryocytic thrombocytopenia as a result of a defective thrombopoietin receptor (*MPL* mutation) [542], ataxia-pancytopenia syndrome [543], Jacobsen syndrome (terminal deletion of 11q with q21-q24 breakpoint), Dubowitz syndrome (microcephaly and other developmental defects with aplastic anaemia) [433], Seckel syndrome (microcephaly and dwarfism with aplastic anaemia) [433]	Hodgkin lymphoma (cytokine-induced) [540]
	Clonal disorders of haemopoiesis: the myelodysplastic syndromes, paroxysmal nocturnal haemoglobinuria, acute myelofibrosis, advanced primary myelofibrosis
	Ineffective haemopoiesis: acute or severe megaloblastic anaemia
	Arsenic poisoning [556]
	Acute infections: some cases of acute HIV infection [557], parvovirus infection [558], ehrlichiosis [559] and anaplasmosis [560], brucellosis [561], miliary tuberculosis, cytomegalovirus infection in bone marrow transplant recipients [562], human herpesvirus 6 infection [563], human herpesvirus 8 infection in immunosuppressed patients [564], toxoplasmosis in immunosuppressed patients [565], Legionnaires' disease [566], Mediterranean spotted fever [567], chronic active Epstein–Barr virus (EBV) infection [568] and following EBV infection in hosts subject to X-linked lymphoproliferative syndrome
Marble bone disease (osteopetrosis)	
Inherited metabolic disorders [544–548]: mannosidosis, Gaucher disease, adult Niemann–Pick disease, methylmalonic aciduria, oxalosis, isovaleric acidaemia, alpha methyl beta hydroxybutyric aciduria, propionic acidaemia, cystinosis	
Mitochondrial cytopathies including some cases of Pearson syndrome [278] and pancytopenia associated with necrotising encephalopathy [549]	Some chronic infections, especially visceral leishmaniasis (kala azar), when it is due to hypersplenism; rarely chronic parvovirus infection [569], miliary tuberculosis (a minority of patients) [255]
Other rare inherited conditions: cobalamin C deficiency [550], Griscelli syndrome, type 2 [551], thiamine-responsive anaemia [552], Wolfram syndrome (DIDMOAD—**D**iabetes **I**nsipidus **D**iabetes **M**ellitus **O**ptic **A**tropy **D**eafness syndrome), methylmalonicaciduria	Haemophagocytic syndromes (including familial and infection-related)
	Acquired immune deficiency syndrome (AIDS)
	Fusariosis [570]
	Systemic lupus erythematosus
Acquired disorders	Combined immunocytopenia [571]
Aplastic and hypoplastic anaemias including idiopathic, virus-induced, drug-induced and chemical-induced aplastic anaemia; hypopituitarism [553]; bone marrow aplasia preceding ALL; bone marrow aplasia associated with thymoma and large granular lymphocyte leukaemia; graft-versus-host disease including transfusion-associated graft-versus-host disease; donor lymphocyte infusion following haemopoietic stem cell transplantation; irradiation; use of alkylating agents and other anticancer and related drugs; imatinib therapy [554]; alemtuzumab; development of anti-thrombopoietin antibodies [555]	Autoimmune lymphoproliferative syndrome [572]
	Severe or chronic graft-versus-host disease [573]
	Drug-induced immune pancytopenia (e.g. caused by phenacetin, para-amino salicylic acid, sulphonamides, rifampicin and quinine)
	Hypersplenism (e.g. kala azar and *Schistosoma mansoni* infection)
	Acquired sea-blue histiocytosis during prolonged parenteral nutrition (the mechanism is probably hypersplenism) [574]
	Wilson disease [575]
	Hyperthyroidism (rarely) [576]
	Alcohol toxicity [389]
	Copper deficiency [576]
	Hypothermia [577]
Bone marrow infiltration, with or without associated fibrosis, including ALL, AML (ineffective haemopoiesis also contributes),	Paget disease [578]
	Hyperparathyroidism [579]

AIDS, acquired immune deficiency syndrome; ALL, acute lymphoblastic leukaemia; AML, acute myeloid leukaemia; HIV, human immunodeficiency virus specifically sought along the edges of the film. Blast cells and hairy cells may be very infrequent, but the presence of even small numbers is significant. In aplastic anaemia the red cells may be normocytic or macrocytic, polychromasia is absent and the platelets are usually small and uniform in size; occasionally poikilocytosis is quite marked.

Differential diagnosis

The presence of dysplastic features in the absence of administration of cytotoxic drugs and toxic chemicals suggests either HIV infection or MDS or AML. Macrocytosis may be present in liver disease and alcohol abuse, megaloblastic anaemia and hypoplastic and aplastic anaemias, MDS and following cytotoxic chemotherapy. Poikilocytic red cells and a leucoerythroblastic blood film (see Table 6.19) suggest bone marrow infiltration or primary myelofibrosis. A low reticulocyte count indicates failure of bone marrow output, whereas an elevated reticulocyte count suggests peripheral destruction, e.g. paroxysmal nocturnal haemoglobinuria or immune destruction of cells.

The full blood count (FBC) may show an elevated mean cell volume (MCV) and elevated red cell distribution width (RDW). An appropriately increased MPV and 'reticulated platelet' count suggest peripheral platelet destruction, whereas a reduced MPV and a low 'reticulated platelet' count despite thrombocytopenia suggest failure of bone marrow output.

Further tests

A reticulocyte count is indicated and a bone marrow aspirate is usually necessary. Unless a cellular aspirate is obtained, a trephine biopsy is also required. Bone marrow aspiration is needed urgently if the clinical history suggests the possibility of a haemophagocytic syndrome, acute infection or the rapid onset of megaloblastic anaemia. In the latter condition macrocytes and hypersegmented neutrophils may be infrequent or absent and only the bone marrow aspirate reveals the diagnosis. The other tests that are needed will be determined by the results of these initial investigations and by the specific diagnosis that is suspected.

TEST YOUR KNOWLEDGE

Visit the companion website for MCQs and EMQs
   on this topic:
www.wiley.com/go/bain/bloodcells

References

1 Doubek M, Brychtova Y, Tomiska M and Mayer J (2005) Idiopathic systemic capillary leak syndrome misdiagnosed and treated as polycythemia vera. *Acta Haematol*, **113**, 150–151.

2 Endo Y, Torii R, Yamazaki F, Sagawa S, Yamauchi K, Tsutsui Y *et al.* (2001) Water drinking causes a biphasic change in blood composition in humans. *Pflugers Arch*, **442**, 362–368.

3 Juvonen E, Ikkala E, Fyhrquist F and Ruutu T (1991) Autosomal dominant erythrocytosis caused by increased sensitivity to erythropoietin. *Blood*, **78**, 3066–3069.

4 Prchal JT and Sokol L (1996) "Benign erythrocytosis" and other familial and congenital polycythemias. *Eur J Haematol*, **57**, 263–268.

5 Ang SO, Chan H, Stockton DW, Sergueeva A, Gordeuk WF, Prchal JT (2001) Von Hippel-Lindau protein, Chuvash polycythemia and oxygen sensing. *Blood*, **98**, 748a.

6 Percy MJ, McMullin MF, Jowitt SN, Potter M, Treacy M, Watson WH and Lappin TRJ (2003) Chuvash-type congenital polycythaemia in 4 families of Asian and Western European ancestry. *Blood*, **102**, 1097–1099.

7 Perrotta S, Nobili B, Ferraro M, Migliaccio C, Borriello A, Cucciolla V *et al.* (2006) Von Hippel-Lindau-dependent polycythaemia is endemic on the island of Ischia: identification of a novel cluster. *Blood*, **107**, 514–519.

8 Tomasic NL, Piterkova L, Huff C, Bilic E, Yoon D, Miasnikova GY *et al.* (2013) The phenotype of polycythemia due to Croatian homozygous *VHL* (571C>G:H191D) mutation is different from that of Chuvash polycythemia (*VHL* 598C>T:R200W). *Haematologica*, **98**, 560–567.

9 Percy MJ, Zhao Q, Flores A, Harrison CN, Lappin TRJ, Maxwell PH *et al.* (2006) A family with erythrocytosis establishes a role for prolyl hydroxylase domain protein 2 in oxygen homeostasis. *Proc Natl Acad Sci USA*, **103**, 654–659.

10 Percy MJ, Furlow PW, Lucas GS, Li X, Lappin TR, McMullin MF and Lee FS (2008) A gain-of-function mutation in the *HIF2A* gene in familial erythrocytosis. *N Engl J Med*, **358**, 162–168.

11 Distelhorst CW, Wagner DS, Goldwasser E and Adamson JW (1981) Autosomal dominant familial erythrocytosis due to anomalous erythropoietin production. *Blood*, **58**, 1155–1158.

12 Manglani MV, DeGroff CG, Dukes PP and Ettinger LJ (1998) Congenital erythrocytosis with elevated erythropoietin level: an incorrectly set "erythrostat"? *J Pediatr Hematol Oncol*, **20**, 560–562.

13 Guan Y, Wu JK, Jastaniah W, Moss LG, Digman C, Mostacci S *et al.* (2004) A new polycythaemia syndrome: congenital polycythemia with high erythropoietin and propensity for malignant hypertension due to paraganglionoma. *Blood*, **104**, 171b.

14 Tanaka KR and Zerez CR (1990) Red cell enzymopathies of the glycolytic pathway. *Semin Hematol*, **27**, 165–185.

15 King AJ, Eyre T and Littlewood T (2013) Obstructive sleep apnoea and erythrocytosis. *Brit Med J*, **347**, 24–25.

16 Hutchinson DCS, Sapru RP, Sumerling MD, Donaldson GWK and Richmond J (1968) Cirrhosis, cyanosis and polycythemia: multiple pulmonary arteriovenous anastomoses. *Am J Med*, **45**, 139–151.

17 Gajra A and Grethlein SJ (1999) Hereditary haemorrhagic telangiectasia—an unusual cause of polycythemia in pregnancy. *Blood*, **94**, Suppl. 1, 14b.

18 di Marco AT (1989) Carbon monoxide poisoning presenting as polycythemia. *N Engl J Med*, **319**, 874.

19 Bonadies N, Tichelli A and Rovo A (2012) When water doesn't clear the smut from the smoke: secondary polyglobulia caused by accidental co-intoxication related to excessive water-pipe smoking. *Haematologica*, **97**, Suppl. 1, 703.

20 Hammond D and Winnick S (1974) Paraneoplastic erythrocytosis and ectopic erythropoietins. *Ann N Y Acad Sci*, **230**, 219–227.

21 Souid AK, Dubanshy AS, Richman P and Sadowitz PD (1993) Polycythemia: a review article and a case report of erythrocytosis secondary to Wilms' tumor. *Pediatr Hematol Oncol*, **10**, 215–221.

22 Bazari H, Attar EC, Dahl DM, Uppot RN and Colvin RB (2010) Case 23-2010: a 49-year-old man with erythrocytosis, perinephric fluid collections, and renal failure. *N Engl J Med*, **363**, 463–475.

23 Shaheen M, Hilgarth KA, Antony AC, Hawes D and Badve S (2003) A Mexican man with "too much blood'". *Lancet*, **362**, 806.

24 Eccersley LRC, Moule SP, Kargathra N, Abrahamson G, Philpott N, Baynes K and Brito-Babapulle F (2007) Hyperparathyroidism — associated polycythaemia: an analysis of 140 cases of hyperparathyroidism. *Br J Haematol*, **137**, Suppl. 1, 49.

25 Bank H and Passwell J (1974) Absolute erythrocytosis in early infectious hepatitis. *Med Chir Dig*, **3**, 321–323.

26 Jacobs P and Wood L (1994) Recurrent benign erythropoietin-secreting pheochromocytomas. *Am J Med*, **97**, 307–308.

27 Reynen K (1995) Cardiac myxomas. *N Engl J Med*, **333**, 1610–1617.

28 Nagajothi N and Sanmugarajah J (2006) Erythrocytosis and gestational hyperandrogenism. *Am J Hematol*, **81**, 984–985.

29 Dickerman RD, Pertusi R, Miller J and Zachariah NY (1999) Androgen-induced erythrocytosis: is it erythropoietin? *Am J Hematol*, **61**, 154–155.

30 Sykes DB, Schroyens W and O'Connell CO (2011) The TEMPI syndrome — a novel multisystem disease. *N Engl J Med*, **365**, 475–476.

31 Emanuel PD, Eaves CJ, Broody C, Papayannopoulo T, Moore MR, D'Andrea AD et al. (1992) Familial and congenital polycythemia in three unrelated families. *Blood*, **79**, 3019–3030.

32 Norberg G (1994) Assessment of risk in occupational cobalt exposures. *Sci Total Environ*, **150**, 201–207.

33 Jefferson JA, Escudero E, Hurtado M-E, Pando J, Tapia R, Swenson ER et al. (2002) Excessive erythrocytosis, chronic mountain sickness, and serum cobalt levels. *Lancet*, **359**, 407–408.

34 Nakanishi T, Sobue I, Tokokura Y, Nishitani H, Kuroiwa Y, Satayoshi L et al. (1984) The Crow-Fukase syndrome: a study of 102 cases in Japan. *Neurology*, **34**, 712–720.

35 Richard S, Croisille L, Yvart J, Casadeval N, Eschwège P, Aghakhani N et al. (2002) Paradoxical secondary polycythemia in von Hippel-Lindau patients treated with antivascular endothelial growth factor receptor therapy. *Blood*, **99**, 3851–3853.

36 Comont T, Delavigne K, Cougoul P, Challan-Belval T, Ollier S, Adoue D and Beyne-Rauzy O (2011) Secondary polycythemia during the course of immune thrombocytopenic purpura (ITP) treatment with romiplostim. *Haematologica*, **96**, Suppl. 2, 654.

37 Alexandrescu DT, McClure R, Farzanmehr H and Dasanu CA (2008) Secondary erythrocytosis produced by the tyrosine kinase inhibitors sunitinib and sorafenib. *J Clin Oncol*, **26**, 4947–4048.

38 Austin T, Bridges N, Markiewicz M and Abrahamson E (1997) Severe neonatal polycythaemia after third stage labour underwater. *Lancet*, **350**, 1445.

39 Hudson PR, Tandy SC, Child DF, Williams CP and Cavill I (2001) Compensated haemolysis: a consistent features of diabetes mellitus. *Br J Haematol*, **113**, Suppl. 1, 47.

40 Worwood M, Carter K, Jackson HA, Hutton RD and Cavill I (2001) Erythropoiesis and iron status in asymptomatic subjects homozygous for HFE C282Y. *Br J Haematol*, **113**, Suppl. 1, 63.

41 Platt OS, Brambilla DJ, Rosse WF, Milner PF, Castro O, Steinberg MH and Klug PP (1994) Mortality in sickle cell disease: life expectancy and risk factors for early death. *N Engl J Med*, **330**, 1639–1644.

42 Venetz C, Labarère J, Jiménez D and Aujesky D (2013) White blood cell count and mortality in patients with acute pulmonary embolism. *Am J Hematol*, **88**, 677–681.

43 Alvarado A (1986) A practical score for the early diagnosis of acute appendicitis. *Ann Emerg Med*, **15**, 557–564.

44 Nakagawa M, Terashima T, D'yachkova Y, Bondy GP, Hogg JC and van Eeden SF (1998) Glucocorticoid-induced granulocytosis: contribution of marrow release and demargination of intravascular granulocytes. *Circulation*, **98**, 2307–2313.

45 Herring WB, Smith LG, Walker RI and Herion JC (1974) Hereditary neutrophilia. *Am J Med*, **56**, 729–734.

46 Plo I, Zhang Y, Le Couedic J-P, Nakatake M, Boulet J-M, Itaya M et al. (2009) An activating mutation in the CSF3R gene induces a hereditary chronic neutrophilia. *J Exp Med*, **206**, 1701–1707.

47 Malech HL and Gallin JI (1987) Current concepts: immunology, neutrophils in human disease. *N Engl J Med*, **317**, 687–694.

48 Arnaout MA (1990) Structure and function of the leukocyte adhesion molecules CD11/CD18. *Blood*, **75**, 1037–1050.

49 Etzione A, Frydman M, Pollack S, Avidor I, Phillips ML, Paulson JC and Gershoni-Baruch R (1992) Recurrent severe infections caused by a novel leukocyte adhesion deficiency. *N Engl J Med*, **327**, 1789–1792.

50 Etzioni A, Doerschuk CM and Harlan JM (1999) Of man and mouse: leukocyte and endothelial adhesion molecule deficiencies. *Blood*, **94**, 3281–3288.

51 Alon R, Aker M, Feigelson S, Sokolovsky-Eisenberg M, Staunton DE, Cinamon G *et al.* (2003) A novel genetic leukocyte adhesion deficiency in subsecond triggering of integrin avidity by endothelial chemokines results in impaired leukocyte arrest on vascular endothelium under shear flow. *Blood*, **101**, 4437–4445.

52 Malinin NL, Plow EF and Byzova TV (2010) Kindlins in FERM adhesion. *Blood*, **115**, 4011–4017.

53 Noris P, Perrotta S, Seri M, Pecci A, Gnan C, Loffredo G *et al.* (2011) Mutations in ANKRD26 are responsible for a frequent form of inherited thrombocytopenia: analysis of 78 patients from 21 families. *Blood*, **117**, 6673–6680.

54 Tindall JP, Beeker SK and Rose WF (1969) Familial cold urticaria: a generalized reaction involving leucocytosis. *Arch Intern Med*, **124**, 129–134.

55 Drenth J and van der Meer JWM (2001) Hereditary periodic fever. *N Engl J Med*, **345**, 1748–1757.

56 Dinarello CA (2009) Interleukin-1β and the autoinflammatory diseases. *N Engl J Med*, **360**, 2467–2470.

57 Blans MJ, Vos PE, Faber HJ and Boers GH (2001) Coma in a young anorexic woman. *Lancet*, **357**, 1944.

58 Duchin JC, Koster FT, Peters CJ, Simpson GL, Tempest B, Zaki SR *et al.* (1994) Hantavirus pulmonary syndrome. *N Engl J Med*, **330**, 949–955.

59 Khan AS, Ksiazek TG and Peters CJ (1996) Hantavirus pulmonary syndrome. *Lancet*, **347**, 739–741.

60 Phoncharoensri D, Witoonpanich R, Tunlayadechanont S and Laothamatas J (2004) Confusion and paraparesis. *Lancet*, **363**, 1954.

61 Amory JK, Rosen H, Sukut C, Wallace F and Saint S (2006) A jaundiced eye. *N Eng J Med*, **354**, 1516–1520.

62 Case Records of the Massachusetts General Hospital (2000) Case 29-2000: A 69-year-old renal transplant recipient with low-grade fever and multiple pulmonary nodules. *N Engl J Med*, **343**, 870–877.

63 Dobbin CJ, Soni R, Jelihovsky T and Bye PTP (2000) Cepacia syndrome occurring following prolonged colonisation with *Burkholderia cepacia*. *Aust NZ J Med*, **30**, 288–289.

64 Case Records of the Massachusetts General Hospital (2002) A 46-year-old woman with extensive pulmonary infiltrates. *N Engl J Med*, **347**, 517–524.

65 Ladhani S, Lowe B, Cole AO, Kowuondo K and Newton CRJC (2003) Changes in white blood cells and platelets in children with falciparum malaria: relationship to disease outcome. *Br J Haematol*, **119**, 839–847.

66 Ryan ET, Cronin CG and Branda JA (2011) Case 38-2011: a 34-year-old man with diarrhoea and weakness. *N Engl J Med*, **365**, 2306–2316.

67 Matsuoka Y, Yasuda M and Hashizume M (2009) Lung injury and renal failure caused by potassium cyanide poisoning. *BMJ Case Reports*, doi: 10.1136/bcr.04.2009.1768.

68 Halevy S (2009) Acute generalized exanthematous pustulosis. *Curr Opin Allergy Clin Immunol*, **9**, 322–328.

69 Keatinge WR, Coleshaw SRK, Easton JC, Coller F, Mattock MB and Chelliah R (1986) Increased platelet and red cell counts, blood viscosity, and plasma cholesterol levels during heat stress, and mortality from coronary and cerebral thrombosis. *Am J Med*, **81**, 795–800.

70 Kohmura K, Miyakawa Y, Kameyama K, Kizaki M and Ikeda Y (2004) Granulocyte colony stimulating factor-producing multiple myeloma associated with neutrophilia. *Leuk Lymphoma*, **45**, 1475–1479.

71 Kanda S, Inoue T, Tsuruta H, Chiba S, Obara T, Saito M *et al.* (2011) [Granulocyte colony stimulating factor-producing spindle cell renal cell carcinoma successfully treated by chemotherapy consisting of gemcitabine and doxorubicin]. *Hinyokika Kiyo*, **57**, 385–359. (abstract only read)

72 Locker GJ, Kapiotis S, Veitl M, Mader RM, Stoiser B, Kofler J *et al.* (1999) Activation of endothelium by immunotherapy with interleukin-2 in patients with malignant disorders. *Br J Haematol*, **105**, 912–919.

73 Ganser A, Lindemann A, Siepelt G, Ottman OG, Herrmann F, Eder M *et al.* (1990) Effects of recombinant human interleukin-3 in patients with normal haematopoiesis and in patients with bone marrow failure. *Blood*, **76**, 666–676.

74 Asano S, Okano A, Ozawa K, Nakahata T, Ishibashi T, Koike K *et al.* (1990) *In vivo* effects of recombinant human interleukin-6 in primates: stimulated production of platelets. *Blood*, **75**, 1602–1605.

75 Huhn RD, Radwanski E, O'Connell SM, Sturgill MG, Clarke L, Cody RP *et al.* (1996) Pharmacokinetics and immunomodulatory properties of intravenously administered recombinant human interleukin-10 in healthy volunteers. *Blood*, **87**, 699–705.

76 Gershon SL (1993) Clozapine—deciphering the risks. *N Engl J Med*, **329**, 204–205.

77 Harrison P, Cardigan R, Harrison C, Addison I, Chavda N, Chitolie A and Machin SJ (1996) Delayed effect of desmopressin on circulating neutrophils and monocytes. *Br J Haematol*, **95**, 570–571.

78 Bienvenu J, Chvetzoff R, Salles G, Balter C, Tilly H, Herbrecht R *et al.* (2001) Tumour necrosis factor α release is a major biological event associated with rituximab treatment. *Hematol J*, **2**, 378–384.

79 Dale DC, Bolyard AA, Kelley ML, Westrup EC, Makaryan V, Aprikyan A *et al.* (2011) The CXCR4 antagonist plerixafor is a potential therapy for myelokathexis, WHIM syndrome. *Blood*, **118**, 4963–4966.

80 Sahoo S (2005) Pathologic quiz case: a 44-year-old man with acute renal failure. *Arch Pathol Lab Med*, **129**, e81–e83.

81 Berg RA and Tarantino MD (1991) Envenomation by scorpion *Centruroides exilicauda* (*C. sculpturatus*): severe and unusual manifestations. *Pediatrics*, **87**, 930–933.

82 Franca FOS, Benvenuti LA, Fan HW, Dos Santos DR, Hain SH, Picchi-Martins FR *et al.* (1994) Severe and fatal mass attack by 'killer' bees (Africanized honey bee—*Apis mellifera scutellata*) in Brazil: clinicopathological studies with measurement of serum venom concentrations. *Q J Med*, **87**, 269–282.

83 Warrell DA (1998) Antivenoms and treatment of snake-bite. *Prescribers J*, **38**, 10–18.

84 Mansoor MA, Stakkestad JA and Drabløs PA (2013) Higher leukocyte subpopulation counts in healthy smoker industrial workers than in nonsmoker industrial workers: possible health consequences. *Acta Haematol*, **129**, 218–222.

85 Cooper PH, Innes DJ and Greer KE (1983) Acute febrile neutrophilic dermatosis (Sweet's syndrome) and myeloproliferative disorders. *Cancer*, **51**, 1518–1526.

86 Rosenberg MR and Green M (1989) Neuroleptic malignant syndrome: review of response to therapy. *Arch Intern Med*, **149**, 1927–1931.

87 Fenwick JC, Cameron M, Naiman SC, Haley LP, Ronco JJ, Wiggs BR and Tweeddale MG (1994) Blood transfusion as a cause of leucocytosis in critically ill patients. *Lancet*, **344**, 855–856.

88 Mayne EE, Fitzpatrick J and Nelson SD (1970) Leucocytosis following administration of cryoprecipitate. *Acta Haematol*, **44**, 155–160.

89 Ward H and Reinhard D (1971) Chronic idiopathic leukocytosis. *Ann Intern Med*, **75**, 193–198.

90 Dinauer MC (2003) The phagocytic system and disorders of granulopoiesis and granulocyte function. In: Nathan DG, Orkin SH, Ginsburg D and Look AT, *Nathan and Oski's Hematology of Infancy and Childhood*, 6th edn, Saunders, Philadelphia.

91 Hübner C, Dietz A, Stremmel W, Stiehl A and Andrassy K (1997) Macrolide-induced Churg-Strauss syndrome in a patient with atopy. *Lancet*, **350**, 563.

92 Kränke B and Arberer W (1997) Macrolide-induced Churg–Strauss syndrome in patient with atopy. *Lancet*, **350**, 1551–1552.

93 Darmstadt GL, Tunnessen WW and Sweren RJ (1992) Eosinophilic pustular folliculitis. *Pediatrics*, **89**, 1095–1098.

94 Janin A, Copin MC, Dubos JP, Rouland V, Delaporte E and Blanchet-Bardon C (1996) Familial peeling skin syndrome with eosinophilia: clinical, histologic, and ultrastructural study of three cases. *Arch Pathol Lab Med*, **120**, 662–665.

95 Weller PF and Bubley GJ (1994) The idiopathic hypereosinophilic syndrome. *Blood*, **83**, 2759–2779.

96 Ryan ET, Wilson ME and Kain KC (2002) Illness after international travel. *N Engl J Med*, **347**, 505–516.

97 Sheehan DJ, Rancher BG and McKitrick JC (1986) Association of *Blastocystis hominis* with signs and symptoms of human disease. *J Clin Microbiol*, **24**, 548–550.

98 Nutman TB (2007) Evaluation and differential diagnosis of marked, persistent eosinophilia. *Immunol Aller Clin North Amer*, **27**, 529–549.

99 Ahmad RN, Sherjil A, Mahmood A and Rafi S (2011) Severe eosinophilia in a case of giardiasis. *Medit J Hemat Infect Dis*, **3**, e2011009.

100 Traub RJ (2013) *Ancylostoma ceylanicum*, a re-emerging but neglected parasitic zoonosis. *Int J Parasitol*, **43**, 1009–1015.

101 Leder K and Weller PF (2000) Eosinophilia and helminth infections. *Baillière's Clin Haematol*, **13**, 301–317.

102 Diaz Camacho SP, Zazueta Ramos M, Ponce Torrecillas E, Osuna Ramirez I, Castro Velazquez R, Flores Gaxiola A *et al.* (1998) Clinical manifestations and immunodiagnosis of gnathostomiasis in Culiacan, Mexico. *Am J Trop Med Hyg*, **59**, 908–915.

103 Prociv P and Croese J (1990) Epidemic eosinophilic enteritis in north Queensland caused by common dog hookworm, *Ancylostoma caninum*. *Aust NZ J Med*, **20**, 439.

104 Yfanti G, Andreadis E, Spiliadou C and Diamantopoulos EJ (1996) A woman with fever and a jejunal stricture. *Lancet*, **347**, 802.

105 Fan E, Soong C, Kain KC and Detsky AS (2008) A gut feeling. *N Engl J Med*, **359**, 75–80.

106 Petithory J-C (1998) Les éosinophilies familiales: apports de la parasitologie à leur diagnostic. *Bull Acad Natl Med*, **182**, 1823–1835.

107 Gomez B, Tabar AI, Tunon T, Larrinaga B, Alvarez MJ, Garcia BE and Olaguibel JM (1998) Eosinophilic gastroenteritis and anisakis. *Allergy*, **53**, 1148–1154.

108 Surmont I and Liu LX (1995) Enteritis, eosinophilia, and Enterobius vermicularis. *Lancet*, **346**, 1167.

109 Marty P (1997) Human dirofilariasis due to Dirofilaria repens in France. A review of reported cases. *Parassitologia*, **39**, 383–386.

110 Goto Y, Tamura A, Ishikawa O, Miyachi Y, Ishii T and Akao N (1998) Creeping eruption caused by a larva of the suborder Spirurina type X. *Br J Dermatol*, **139**, 315–318.

111 Paine M, Davis S and Brown G (1994) Severe forms of infection with Angiostrongylus cantonensis acquired in Australia and Fiji. *Aust NZ J Med*, **24**, 415–416.

112 Slom TJ, Cortese MM, Gerber SI, Jones RC, Holtz TH, Lopez AS *et al.* (2002) An outbreak of eosinophilic meningitis caused by *Angiostrongylus cantonensis* in travellers returning from the Caribbean. *N Engl J Med*, **346**, 668–675.

113 Petithory JC (1996) Can *Ascaris suum* cause visceral larva migrans? *Lancet*, **348**, 689.

114 Maruyama H, Nawa Y, Noda S, Mimori T and Choi WY (1996) An outbreak of visceral larva migrans due to *Ascaris suum* in Kyushu, Japan. *Lancet*, **347**, 1766–1767.

115 Dennett X, Andrews J, Siejka S, Beveridge I and Spratt D (1998). New muspiceoid nematode causes eosinophilic polymyositis: two case reports. *Aust Med J*, **168**, 226–227.

116 el-Karaksy H, Hassanein B, Okasha S, Behairy B and Gadallah I (1999) Human fascioliasis in Egyptian children: successful treatment with triclabendazole. *J Trop Pediatr*, **45**, 135–138.

117 MacLean JD, Arthur JR, Ward BJ, Gyorkos TW, Curtis MA and Kokoskin E (1996) Common-source outbreak of acute infection due to the North American liver fluke *Metorchis conjunctus*. *Lancet*, **347**, 154–158.

118 Burton K, Yogev R, London N, Boyer K and Shulman ST (1982) Pulmonary paragonimiasis in Laotian refugee children. *Pediatrics*, **70**, 246–248.

119 Seymour JF (1997) Splenomegaly, eosinophilia, and pruritis: Hodgkin's disease, or…? *Blood*, **90**, 1719–1720.

120 Wang HY, Zhu GH, Luo SS and Jiang KW (2013) Childhood pentastomiasis: a report of three cases with the following-up data. *Parasitol Int*, **62**, 289–292.

121 Navajas A, Cardenal I, Pinan MA, Ortiz A, Astigarraga I and Fdez-Teijeiro A (1998) Hypereosinophilia due to myiasis. *Acta Haematol*, **99**, 27–30.

122 Rioux JD, Stone VA, Daly MJ, Cargill M, Green T, Nguyen H *et al.* (1998) Familial eosinophilia maps to the cytokine gene cluster on human chromosomal region 5q31-q33. *Am J Hum Genet*, **63**, 1086–1094.

123 Cools J, DeAngelo DJ, Gotlib J, Stover EH, Legare RD, Cortes J *et al.* (2003) A tyrosine kinase created by the fusion of the PDGFRA and FIP1L1 genes as a therapeutic target of imatinib in idiopathic hypereosinophilic syndrome. *N Engl J Med*, **348**, 1201–1214.

124 Bain BJ, Gilliland DG, Horny H-P and Vardiman JW (2008) Myeloid and lymphoid neoplasms with eosinophilia and abnormalities of *PDGFRA*, *PDGFRB* and *FGFR1*. In: Swerdlow SH, Campo E, Harris NL, Jaffe ES, Pileri SA, Stein H *et al.* (eds), *World Health Organization Classification of Tumours of Haematopoietic and Lymphoid Tissues*, 4th edn, IARC Press, Lyon.

125 Bae SY, Yiin S-Y, Huh JH, Sung HJ and Choi IK (2007) Hypereosinophilia in biphenotypic (B-cell/T-cell) acute lymphoblastic leukemia. *Leuk Lymphoma*, **48**, 1417–1419.

126 Cullen MH, Stansfield AG, Oliver RTD, Lister TA and Malpas JS (1979) Angio-immunoblastic lymphadenopathy: report of ten cases and review of the literature. *Q J Med*, **48**, 151–177.

127 Jayakar V, Goldin RD and Bain BJ (2006) Teaching cases from the Royal Marsden and St Mary's Hospitals: eosinophilia and pruritis. *Leuk Lymphoma*, **47**, 2404–2405.

128 Glantz L, Rintels P, Samoszuk M and Medeiros LJ (1995) Plasma cell myeloma associated with eosinophilia. *Am J Clin Pathol*, **103**, 583–587.

129 Kaplan MH, Hall WW, Susin M, Pahwa S, Salahuddin SZ, Heilman C *et al.* (1991) Syndrome of severe skin disease, eosinophilia, and dermatopathic lymphadenopathy in patients with HTLV-II complicating human immunodeficiency virus infection. *Am J Med*, **91**, 300–309.

130 Aspinall AI, Pinto A, Auer IA, Bridges P, Luider J, Dimnik L *et al.* (2001) Identification of new fas mutations in a patient with autoimmune lymphoproliferative syndrome (ALPS) and eosinophilia. *Blood Cells Mos Diseas*, **25**, 227–238.

131 Lowe D, Jorizzo J and Hutt MSR (1981) Tumour-associated eosinophilia: a review. *J Clin Pathol*, **34**, 1343–1348.

132 Case records of the Massachusetts General Hospital (1992) Case 18–1992. *N Engl J Med*, **326**, 1204–1212.

133 Wells GC and Smith NP (1979) Eosinophilic cellulitis. *Br J Dermatol*, **100**, 101–109.

134 Don IJ, Khettry U and Canoso JJ (1978) Progressive systemic sclerosis with eosinophilia and a fulminant course. *Am J Med*, **65**, 346–348.

135 Panush RS, Wilkinson LS and Fagin RR (1973) Chronic active hepatitis associated with Coombs-positive hemolytic anemia. *Gastroenterology*, **64**, 1015–1019.

136 Neeman A and Kadish U (1987) Marked eosinophilia in a patient with primary sclerosing cholangitis. *Am J Med*, **83**, 378–379.

137 Chowdry S, Rubin E and Sass DA (2012) Acute autoimmune hepatitis presenting with peripheral blood eosinophilia. *Ann Hepatol*, **11**, 559–563.

138 Case Records of the Massachusetts General Hospital (1998) A 10-year-old girl with urinary retention and a filling defect in the bladder. *N Engl J Med*, **339**, 616–622.

139 Weschler ME (2007) Pulmonary eosinophilic syndromes. *Immunol Allergy Clin North Amer*, **27**, 477–492.

140 Ezekowitz RAB and Stockman JA (2003) Hematologic manifestations of systemic diseases. In: Nathan DG, Orkin SH, Ginsburg D and Look AT, *Nathan and Oski's Hematology of Infancy and Childhood*, 6th edn, Saunders, Philadelphia.

141 Stone JH, Zen Y and Deshpande V (2012) IgG4-related disease. *N Engl J Med*, **366**, 1646–1647.

142 Karawajczyk M, Höglund M, Ericsson J and Venge P (1997) Administration of G-CSF to healthy subjects: the effects on eosinophil counts and mobilization of eosinophil granule proteins. *Br J Haematol*, **96**, 259–265.

143 Means-Markwell M, Burgess T, de Keratry D, O'Neil K, Mascola J, Fleisher T and Lucey D (2000) Eosinophilia with aberrant T cells and elevated serum levels of interleukin-2 and interleukin-15. *N Engl J Med*, **342**, 1568–1571.

144 van der Graaf W and Borleffs JCC (1994) Eosinophilia in patients with HIV infection. *Eur J Haematol*, **52**, 246–247.

145 Gleich GJ, Schroeter AL, Marcoux P, Sachs MI, O'Connell EJ and Kohler PF (1984) Episodic angioedema associated with eosinophilia. *N Engl J Med*, **310**, 1621–1626.

146 Bullock WE, Artz RP, Bhathena D and Tung KSK (1979) Histoplasmosis: association with circulating immune complexes, eosinophilia, and mesangiocapillary glomerulonephritis. *Arch Intern Med*, **139**, 700–702.

147 Granter SR, Barnhill RL and Duray PH (1996) Borrelial fasciitis: diffuse fasciitis and peripheral eosinophilia associated with Borrelia infection. *Am J Dermatopathol*, **18**, 465–473.

148 Mayron LW, Alling S and Kaplan E (1972) Eosinophilia and drug abuse. *Ann Allergy*, **30**, 632–637.

149 Rubin RB and Neugarten J (1990) Cocaine-associated asthma. *Am J Med*, **88**, 438–439.

150 Gabriel LC, Escribano LM, Villa E, Leiva C and Valdes MD (1968) Ultrastructural studies of blood cells in toxic oil syndrome. *Acta Haematol*, **75**, 165–170.

151 Kilbourne EM, Swygert LA, Philen RM, Sun RK, Auerbach SB, Miller L *et al.* (1990) Interim guidance on the eosinophilia-myalgia syndrome. *Ann Intern Med*, **112**, 85–87.

152 Carvajal JA, Anderson R, Weiss L, Grismer J and Berman R (1967) Atheroembolism. An etiologic factor in renal insufficiency, gastrointestinal haemorrhages, and peripheral vascular diseases. *Arch Intern Med*, **119**, 593–599.

153 Cogan E, Schandene L, Papadopoulos T, Crusiaux A and Goldman M (1995) Interleukin-5 production by T lymphocytes in atheroembolic disease with hypereosinophilia. *Allergy Clin Immunol*, **96**, 427–429.

154 Omenn GS (1965) Familial reticuloendotheliosis with eosinophilia. *N Engl J Med*, **273**, 427–432.

155 Nagafuchi S, Tokiyama K, Kashiwagi S, Yayashi S, Imayama S and Niho Y (1993) Eosinophilia after intradermal hepatitis B vaccination. *Lancet*, **342**, 998.

156 Lärfars G, Uden-Blohmë AM and Samuelsson J (1996) Fludarabine, as well as 2-chlorodeoxyadenosine, can induce eosinophilia during treatment of lymphoid malignancies. *Br J Haematol*, **94**, 709–712.

157 Weiden PL, Bauermeister DE and Fatta EA (1998) An Asian man with enlarged glands. *Lancet*, **351**, 1098.

158 Angelis M, Yu M, Takanishi D, Hasaniya NWMA and Brown MR (1996) Eosinophilia as a marker of adrenal insufficiency in the surgical intensive care unit. *J Am Coll Surg*, **183**, 589–596.

159 Feussner JR, Shelburne JD, Bredhoeft S and Cohen HJ (1978) Arsenic-induced bone marrow toxicity: ultrastructural and electron-probe analysis. *Blood*, **53**, 820–827.

160 Fenollar F, Lepidi H and Raoult D (2001) Whipple's endocarditis: review of the literature and comparisons with Q fever, Bartonella infection, and blood culture-positive endocarditis. *Clin Infect Dis*, **33**, 1309–1316.

161 Finsterer J (2007) Hematological manifestations of primary mitochondrial disorders. *Acta Haematol*, **118**, 88–98.

162 Schwarz YA, Kivity S, Fischbein A, Ribak Y, Firemen E, Struhar D *et al.* (1994) Eosinophilic lung reaction to aluminium and hard metal. *Chest*, **105**, 1261–1263.

163 Klion AD, Mejia R, Cowen EW, Dowdell KC, Dunleavy K, Fahle GA *et al.* (2013) Chronic active Epstein-Barr virus infection: a novel cause of lymphocytic variant hypereosinophilic syndrome. *Blood*, **121**, 2364–2366.

164 Ishii T, Tatekawa T, Koseto M, Ishii M, Kobayashi H, Koike M *et al.* (2003) A case of multicentric Castleman's disease demonstrating severe eosinophilia and enhanced production of interleukin-5. *Eur J Haematol*, **70**, 115–118.

165 Hassan HA, Majid RA, Rashid NG, Nuradeen BE, Abdulkarim QH, Hawramy TA *et al.* (2013) Eosinophilic granulomatous gastrointestinal and hepatic abscesses attributable to basidiobolomycosis and fasciolias: a simultaneous emergence in Iraqi Kurdistan. *BMC Infect Dis*, **13**, 91.

166 Hildebrandt GC, Hahn J, Erdmann A, Grube M, Andreesen R and Holler E (2000) Eosinophilia after bone marrow transplantation as a predictor of extensive and sclerodermatous chronic graft versus host disease. *Blood*, **96**, 194a.

167 Martinez BM and Domingo P (1997) Acute eosinophilic pneumonia associated with tenidap. *BMJ*, **314**, 349.

168 Terzano C and Petroianni A (2003) Clarithromycin and pulmonary infiltration with eosinophilia. *BMJ*, **326**, 1377–1378.

169 Crofton JW, Livingstone IL, Oswald NC and Roberts ATM (1952) Pulmonary eosinophilia. *Thorax*, **7**, 1–35.

170 Horie S, Okubo Y, Suzuki J and Isobe M (1996) An emaciated man with eosinophilic pneumonia. *Lancet*, **348**, 166.

171 Donhuijsen K, Haedicke C, Hattenberger C and Freund M (1992) Granulocyte-macrophage colony-stimulating factor-related eosinophilia and Loeffler's endocarditis. *Blood*, **79**, 2798.

172 Allen JN and Davis WB (1994) Eosinophilic lung disease. *Am J Respir Crit Care Med*, **150**, 1423–1438.

173 Schatz M, Wasserman S and Patterson R (1982) The eosinophil and the lung. *Arch Intern Med*, **142**, 1515–1519.

174 Fauci AS, Harley JB, Roberts WC, Ferrans VJ, Gralnick HR and Bjornson BH (1982) NIH Conference. The idiopathic hypereosinophilic syndrome. *Ann Intern Med*, **97**, 78–92.

175 Dines DE (1978) Chronic eosinophilic pneumonia. *Mayo Clin Proc*, **53**, 129–130.

176 Pandit R, Scholnik A, Wulfekuhler L and Dimitrov N (2007) Non-small-cell lung cancer associated with excessive eosinophilia and secretion of interleukin-5 as a paraneoplastic syndrome. *Am J Hematol*, **82**, 234–237.

177 Todenhofer T, Wirths S, von Weyern CH, Heckl S, Horger M, Hennenlotter J *et al.* (2012) Severe paraneoplastic hypereosinophilia in metastatic renal cell carcinoma. *BMC Urology*, **12**, 7.

178 Rapanotti MC, Caruso R, Ammatuna E, Zaza S, Trotta L, Divona M *et al.* (2010) Molecular characterization of paediatric idiopathic hypereosinophilia. *Br J Haematol*, **151**, 440–446.

179 Vaughan Hudson B, Linch DC, Macintyre EA, Bennett MH, MacLennan KA, Vaughan Hudson G and Jelliffe AM (1987) Selective peripheral blood eosinophilia associated with survival advantage in Hodgkin's disease (BNLI Report No 31). British National Lymphoma Investigation. *J Clin Pathol*, **40**, 247–250.

180 Simon HU, Plötz SG, Dummer R and Blaser K (1999) Abnormal clones of interleukin-5-producing T cells in idiopathic eosinophilia. *N Engl J Med*, **341**, 1112–1120.

181 Beishuizen A, Vermes I, Hylkema BS and Haanen C (1999) Relative eosinophilia and functional adrenal insufficiency in critically ill patients. *Lancet*, **353**, 1675–1676.

182 Loughlin KR (2000) Hypereosinophilic syndrome. *N Engl J Med*, **342**, 442.

183 Andersen CL, Siersma VD, Hasselbalch HC, Lindegaard H, Vestergaard H, Felding P *et al.* (2013) Eosinophilia in routine blood samples and the subsequent risk of hematological malignancies and death. *Am J Hematol*, **88**, 843–847.

184 Tokuhira M, Watanabe R, Iizuka A, Sekiguchi Y, Nemote T, Hanzawa K *et al.* (2006) De novo CD5+ diffuse large B cell lymphoma with basophilia in the peripheral blood: successful treatment with autologous peripheral blood stem cell transplantation. *Am J Hematol*, **82**, 162–167.

185 Davies JK, Telfer P, Cavenagh JD, Foot N and Neat M (2003) Case Report. Autoimmune cytopenias in the 22q11.2 deletion syndrome. *Clin Lab Haematol*, **25**, 195–197.

186 Snow AL, Xiao W, Stinson JR, Lu W, Chaigne-Delalande B, Zheng L *et al.* (2012) Congenital B cell lymphocytosis explained by novel germline *CARD11* mutations. *J Exp Med*, **209**, 2247–2261.

187 Olson LC, Miller G and Hanshaw JB (1964) Acute infectious lymphocytosis presenting as a pertussis-like illness: its association with adenovirus type 12. *Lancet*, **i**, 200–201.

188 Anonymous (1968) Lymphocytopoietic viruses. *N Engl J Med*, **279**, 432–433.

189 Mandal BK and Stokes KJ (1973) Acute infectious lymphocytosis and enteroviruses. *Lancet*, **ii**, 1392–1393.

190 Nkrumah FK and Addy PAK (1973) Acute infectious lymphocytosis. *Lancet*, **i**: 1257–1258.

191 Horwitz CA, Henle W, Henle G, Polesky H, Balfour HH, Siem RA *et al.* (1977) Heterophile-negative infectious mononucleosis and mononucleosis-like illnesses. *Am J Med*, **63**, 947–957.

192 Rosenblatt JD, Plaeger-Marshall S, Giorgi JV, Swanson P, Chen ISY, Chin E *et al.* (1990) A clinical, hematologic, and immunologic analysis of 21 HTLV-I infected intravenous drug users. *Blood*, **76**, 409–417.

193 Rogers L (1905) The blood changes in plague. *J Pathol*, **10**, 291–295.

194 Kvasnicka HM, Thiele J and Ahmadi T (2003) Bone marrow manifestation of Lyme disease (Lyme borreliosis). *Br J Haematol*, **120**, 723.

195 Caldwell CW and Lacombe F (2000) *Evaluation of Peripheral Blood Lymphocytosis*. Academic Information Systems, Santa Cruz.

196 Heller HM, Telford SR and Branda JA (2005) Case records from the Massachusetts General Hospital: case 10-2005: a 73-year-old man with weakness and pain in the legs. *N Engl J Med*, **352**, 1358–1364.

197 McDonald JC, MacLean JD and McDade JE (1988) Imported rickettsial disease: clinical and epidemiologic features. *Am J Med*, **85**, 799–805.

198 Wilson ME, Brush AD and Meany MC (1989) Murine typhus acquired during short-term urban travel. *Am J Med*, **57**, 233–234.

199 Carulli G, Lagomarsini G, Azzarà A, Testi R, Riccioni R and Petrini M (2004) Expansion of TcRαβ+CD3+CD4-CD8- (CD4/CD8 double-negative) T lymphocytes in a case of staphylococcal toxic shock syndrome. *Acta Haematol*, **111**, 163–167.

200 Bates I, Bedu-Addo G, Bevan DH and Rutherford TR (1991) Use of immunoglobulin gene rearrangements to show clonal lymphoproliferation in hyper-reactive malarial splenomegaly. *Lancet*, **337**, 505–507.

201 Weatherall D and Kwiatkowski D (2003) Hematologic manifestations of systemic diseases in children in developing countries. In: Nathan DG, Orkin SH, Ginsburg D and Look AT, *Nathan and Oski's Hematology of Infancy and Childhood*, 6th edn. Saunders, Philadelphia.

202 Groom DA, Kunkel LA, Brynes RK, Parker JW, Johnson CS and Endres D (1990) Transient stress lymphocytosis during crisis of sickle cell anaemia and emergency trauma and medical conditions. *Arch Pathol Lab Med*, **114**, 570–576.

203 Wentworth P, Salonen V and Pomeroy J (1991) Transient stress lymphocytosis during crisis of sickle cell anaemia. *Arch Pathol Lab Med*, **115**, 211.

204 Chow K-C, Nacilla JQ, Witzig TE and Li C-Y (1992) Is persistent polyclonal B lymphocytosis caused by Epstein-Barr virus? A study with polymerase chain reaction and *in situ* hybridization. *Am J Hematol*, **41**, 270–275.

205 Kerrigan DP, Castillo A, Foucar K, Townsend K and Neidhart J (1989) Peripheral blood morphologic changes after high-dose antineoplastic chemotherapy and recombinant human granulocyte colony-stimulating factor administration. *Am J Clin Pathol*, **92**, 280–285.

206 Lascari AD (1984) *Hematologic Manifestations of Childhood Diseases*. Theme-Stratton, New York.

207 Kapadia A, de Sousa M, Markenson AL, Miller DR, Good RA and Gupta S (1980) Lymphoid cell sets and serum immunoglobulins in patients with thalassaemia intermedia: relationship to serum iron and splenectomy. *Br J Haematol*, **45**, 405–416.

208 Marti GE, Ryan ET, Papadopoulos NM, Filling-Katz M, Barton N, Fleischer TA *et al.* (1988) Polyclonal B-cell lymphocytosis and hypergammaglobulinaemia in patients with Gaucher's disease. *Am J Hematol*, **29**, 189–194.

209 Medeiros LJ, Bhagat SK, Naylor P, Fowler D, Jaffe E and Stetler-Stevenson M (1993) Malignant thymoma associated with T-cell lymphocytosis. *Arch Pathol Lab Med*, **117**, 279–283.

210 Sneller MC, Wang J, Dale JK, Strober W, Middelton LA, Choi Y *et al.* (1997) Clinical, immunologic, and genetic features of an autoimmune lymphoproliferative syndrome associated with abnormal lymphocyte apoptosis. *Blood*, **15**, 1341–1348.

211 Papadaki T, Stamatopoulos K, Stavroyianni N, Paterakis G, Phisphis M and Stefanoudaki-Sofianatou K (2002) Evidence for T-large granular lymphocyte-mediated neutropenia in Rituximab-treated lymphoma patients: report of two cases. *Leuk Research*, **26**, 597–600.

212 Mariette X, Tsapis A, Oksenhendlcr E, Daniel M-T, d'Agay M-F, Berger R and Brouet J-C (1993) Nodular lymphocyte predominance Hodgkin's disease featuring blood atypical polyclonal B-cell lymphocytosis. *Br J Haematol*, **85**, 813–815.

213 Lesesve J-F, Debouverie M, Decarvalho Bittencourt M and Béné M-C (2011) CD49d blockade by natalizumab therapy in patients with multiple sclerosis increases immature B-lymphocytes. *Bone Marrow Transplantation*, **46**, 1489–1491.

214 Chang BY, Francesco M, De Rooij MF, Magadala P, Steggerda SM, Huang MM *et al.* (2013) Egress of CD19(+) CD5(+) cells into peripheral blood following treatment with the Bruton tyrosine kinase inhibitor ibrutinib in mantle cell lymphoma patients. *Blood*, **122**, 2412–2424.

215 Fry RW, Morton AR, Crawford GP and Keast D (1992) Cell numbers and in vitro responses of leucocytes and lymphocyte subpopulations following maximal exercise and interval training sessions of different intensities. *Eur J Appl Physiol Occup Physiol*, **64**, 218–227.

216 Bassini-Cameron A, Sweet E, Bottino A, Bittar C, Veiga C and Cameron LC (2007) Effect of caffeine supplementation on haematological and biochemical variables in elite soccer players under physical stress conditions. *Br J Sports Med*, **41**, 523–530.

217 Nielsen HB, Secher NH, Kristensen JH, Christensen NJ, Espersen K and Pedersen BK (1997) Splenectomy impairs lymphocytosis during maximal exercise. *Am J Physiol*, **272**, R1847–R1852.

218 Kho AN, Hui S, Kesterson JG and McDonald CJ (2007) Which observations from the complete blood cell count predict mortality for hospitalized patients? *J Hosp Med*, **2**, 5–12.

219 Cook PD, Osborn CD, Helbert BJ and Rappaport ES (1991) Cleaved lymphocytes in pertussis. *Am J Clin Pathol*, **96**, 428.

220 Milne TM, Cavenagh JD, Macey MG, Dale C, Howes D, Wilkes S and Newland AC (1998) Large granular lymphocyte (LGL) expansion in 20 HIV infected patients: analysis of immunophenotype and clonality. *Br J Haematol*, **101**, Suppl. 1, 107.

221 Nagata Y, Ohashi K, Fukuda S, Kamata N, Akiyama H and Sakamaki H (2010) Clinical features of dasatinib-induced large granular lymphocytosis and pleural effusion. *Int J Hematol*, **91**, 799–807.

222 Kreutzman A, Juvonen V, Kairisto V, Ekblom M, Stenke L, Seggewiss R *et al.* (2010) Mono/oligoclonal T and NK cells are common in chronic myeloid leukemia patients at diagnosis and expand during dasatinib therapy. *Blood*, **116**, 772–782.

223 Maldonado J and Hanlon DG (1965) Monocytosis: a current appraisal. *Mayo Clin Proc*, **40**, 248–259.

224 Glaser RM, Walker RI and Herion JC (1970) The significance of hematologic abnormalities in patients with tuberculosis. *Arch Intern Med*, **125**, 691–695.

225 Dorfman DH and Glader JH (1990) Congenital syphilis presenting in infants after the newborn period. *N Engl J Med*, **323**, 1299–1302.

226 Piankijagum A, Visudhiphan S, Aswapokee P, Suwanagool S, Kruatrachue M and Na-Nakorn S (1977) Hematological changes in typhoid fever. *J Med Assoc Thai*, **60**, 828–838.

227 Bhatia P, Haldar D, Varma N, Marwaha RK and Varma S (2011) A case series highlighting the relative frequencies of the common, uncommon and atypical/unusual hematological findings on bone marrow examination in cases of visceral leishmaniasis. *Mediterr J Hematol Infect Dis*, **3**, e2011035.

228 Gutman JD, Kotton CN and Kratz A (2003) Case Records of the Massachusetts General Hospital, Case 29-2003: a 60-year-old man with fever, rigors, and sweats. *N Engl J Med*, **349**, 1168–1175.

229 Reddy S, Jia S, Geoffrey R, Lorier R, Suchi M, Broeckel U *et al.* (2009) An autoinflammatory disease due to homozygous deletion of the *IL1RN* locus. *N Engl J Med*, **360**, 2438–2444.

230 Barrett O'N (1970) Monocytosis in malignant disease. *Ann Intern Med*, **73**, 991–992.

231 Schmitz LL, McClure JS, Letz CE, Dayton V, Weisdorf DJ, Parkin IL and Brunning RD (1994) Morphologic and quantitative changes in blood and marrow cells following growth factor therapy. *Am J Clin Pathol*, **101**, 67–75.

232 Huhn RD, Radwanski E, O'Connell SM, Sturgill MG, Clarke L, Cody RP *et al.* (1996) Pharmacokinetics and immunomodulatory properties of intravenously administered recombinant human interleukin-10 in healthy volunteers. *Blood*, **87**, 699–705.

233 Lebsack ME, McKenna HJ, Hoek JA, Hanna R, Feng A, Marashovsky E and Hayes FA (1997) Safety of FLT3 ligand in healthy volunteers. *Blood*, **90**, Suppl. 1, 170a.

234 Meisel SR, Pauzner H, Shechter M, Zeidan Z and David D (1998) Peripheral monocytosis following acute myocardial infarction: incidence and its possible role as a bedside marker of the extent of cardiac injury. *Cardiology*, **90**, 52–57.

235 Raska K, Raskova J, Shea SM, Frankel RM, Wood RH, Lifter J *et al.* (1983) T cell subsets and cellular immunity in end-stage renal disease. *Am J Med*, **75**, 734–740.

236 Pisani RJ, Witzig TE, Li CY, Morris MA and Thibodeau SN (1990) Confirmation of lymphomatous pulmonary involvement by immunophenotypic and gene rearrangement analysis of bronchoalveolar lavage fluid. *Mayo Clin Proc*, **65**, 651–656.

237 Rao VK and Oliveira JB (2011) How I treat autoimmune lymphoproliferative syndrome. *Blood*, **118**, 5741–5751.

238 Tadmor T, Benyamini N, Avivi I, Attias D and Polliack A (2012) Absolute monocyte count is associated with adverse prognosis in diffuse large B-cell lymphoma: a validation study in a cohort of 219 patients from two centers. *Haematologica*, **97**, Suppl. 1, 127.

239 Aoki K, Tabata S, Yonetani N, Matsushita A and Ishikawa T (2013) The prognostic impact of absolute lymphocyte and monocyte counts at diagnosis of diffuse large B-cell lymphoma in the rituximab era. *Acta Haematol*, **130**, 242–246.

240 Porrata LF, Ristow K, Colgan JP, Habermann TM, Witzig TE, Inwards DJ *et al.* (2012) Peripheral blood lymphocyte/monocyte ratio at diagnosis and survival in classical Hodgkin's lymphoma. *Haematologica*, **97**, 262–269.

241 Porrata LF, Ristow K, Habermann TM, Witzig TE, Colgan JP, Inwards DJ *et al.* (2012) Peripheral blood lymphocyte/monocyte ratio at diagnosis and survival in nodular lymphocyte-predominant Hodgkin lymphoma. *Br J Haematol*, **157**, 321–330.

242 von Hohenstaufen KA, Conconi A, de Campos CP, Franceschetti S, Bertoni F, Casaluci G M *et al.* (2013) Prognostic impact of monocyte count at presentation in mantle cell lymphoma. *Br J Haematol*, **162**, 465–473.

243 Moake IL, Landry PR, Oren ME, Sayer BL and Heffner LT (1974) Transient peripheral plasmacytosis. *Am J Clin Pathol*, **62**, 8–15.

244 Ghilardi N, Wiestner A, Kikuchi M, Ohsaka A and Skoda RC (1999) Hereditary thrombocythaemia in a Japanese family is caused by a novel point mutation in the thrombopoietin gene. *Br J Haematol*, **107**, 310–316.

245 Fujiwara T, Hariqae H, Kameoka J, Yokoyama H, Takahashi S, Tomiya Y *et al.* (2004) A case of familial thrombocytosis: possible role of altered thrombopoietin production. *Am J Hematol*, **76**, 395–397.

246 Sturhmann M, Bashawri L, Ahmed MA, Al-Awamy BH, Kühnau W, Schmidtke J and El-Harith EA (2001) Familial thrombocytosis as a recessive, possibly X-linked trait in an Arab family. *Br J Haematol*, **112**, 616–620.

247 Ding J, Komatsu H, Wakita A, Kato-Uranishi M, Ito M, Satoh A *et al.* (2004) Familial essential thrombocythaemia associated with a dominant-positive activating mutation of the *c-MPL* gene, which encodes for the receptor for thrombopoietin. *Blood*, **103**, 4198–4200.

248 Moliterno AR, Williams DM, Gutierrez-Alamillo LI, Salvatori R, Ingersoll RG and Spivak JL (2004) Mpl Baltimore: a thrombopoietin receptor polymorphism associated with thrombocytosis. *Proc Natl Acad Sci USA*, **101**, 11444–11447.

249 Mead AJ, Rugless MJ, Jacobsen SE and Schuh A (2012) Germline *JAK2* mutation in a family with hereditary thrombocytosis. *N Engl J Med*, **366**, 967–969.

250 Etheridge L, Corbo LM, Kaushansky K, Chan E and Hitchcock IS (2011) A novel activating JAK2 mutation, JAK2R564Q, causes familial essential thrombocytosis (fET) via mechanism distinct from JAK2 V617F. *Blood*, **118**, 123. (ASH Annual Meeting Abstracts)

251 Pickering D and Cuddigan B (1969) Infantile cortical hyperostosis associated with thrombocythaemia. *Lancet*, **ii**, 464–465.

252 Gazda HT amd Sieff CA (2006) Recent insights into the pathogenesis of Diamond–Blackfan anaemia. *Br J Haematol*, **135**, 149–157.

253 Williams MS, Ettinger RS, Hermanns P, Lee B, Carlsson G, Taskinen M and Mäkitie O (2005) The natural history of severe anemia in cartilage-hair hypoplasia. *Am J Med Genet A*, **138**, 35–40.

254 Losada R, Espinosa E, Hernãndez C, Dorticos E and Hernãndez P (1996) Thrombocytosis in patients with acute promyelocytic leukaemia during all-*trans* retinoic acid treatment. *Br J Haematol*, **95**, 704–705.

255 Maartens G, Willcox PA and Benatar SR (1990) Miliary tuberculosis: rapid diagnosis, hematologic abnormalities, and outcome in 109 treated adults. *Am J Med*, **89**, 291–296.

256 Meade RH and Brandt L (1982) Manifestations of Kawasaki disease in New England outbreak of 1980. *J Pediatr*, **100**, 558–562.

257 Pol RJ and Howard MR (2014) Anemia and thrombocytopenia. *Blood*, **123**, 1783.

258 Feigert JM, Sweet DL, Coleman M, Variakojis D, Wisch N, Schulman J and Markowitz MH (1990) Multicentric angiofollicular lymph node hyperplasia with peripheral neuropathy, pseudotumor cerebri, IgA dysproteinaemia, and thrombocytosis in women: a distinct syndrome. *Ann Intern Med*, **113**, 362–367.

259 Gherardi RK, Maleport D and Degos J-D (1991) Castleman disease-POEMS syndrome overlap. *Ann Intern Med*, **114**, 520–521.

260 Brezis M and Lafair J (1979) Thrombocytosis in chronic eosinophilic pneumonia. *Chest*, **76**, 231–232.

261 Harker LA, Roskos LK, Marzec UM, Carter RA, Cherry JK, Sundell B *et al.* (2000) Effects of megakaryocyte growth development factor on platelet production, platelet life span, and platelet function in healthy volunteers. *Blood*, **95**, 2514–2533.

262 Weber J, Yang IC, Topalian SL, Parkinson DR, Schwartzentruber DS, Ettinghausen SE *et al.* (1993) Phase I trial of subcutaneous interIeukin-6 in patients with advanced malignancies. *J Clin Oncol*, **11**, 499–506.

263 Kaushansky K (1996) The thrombocytopenia of cancer. Prospects for effective cytokine therapy. *Hematol Oncol Clin North Am*, **10**, 431–455.

264 Halpérin DS, Wacker P, Lacourt G, Félix M, Babel J-F, Aapro M and Wyss M (1990) Effects of recombinant human erythropoietin in infants with anemia of prematurity: a pilot study. *J Pediatr*, **116**, 779.

265 Ritchie JH, Fish MB, McMasters V and Grossman M (1968) Edema and hemolytic anemia in premature infants. A vitamin E deficiency syndrome. *N Engl J Med*, **279**, 1185–1190.

266 Bornstein Y, Rausen AR and Peterson CM (1982) Duration of thrombocytosis in infants of polydrug (including methadone) users. *J Pediatr*, **100**, 506.

267 Case Records of the Massachusetts General Hospital (2000) A 41-year-old man with multiple bony lesions and adjacent soft tissue masses. *N Engl J Med*, **342**, 875–884.

268 Kuijpers TW, Maianaski NA, Tool ATJ, Smit PA, Rake JP, Roos D and Visser G (2003) Apoptotic neutrophils in the circulation of patients with glycogen storage disease type Ib (GSD1b). *Blood*, **101**, 5021–5024.

269 Dale DC, Person RE, Bolyard AA, Aprikyan AG, Bos C, Bonilla MA *et al.* (2000) Mutation in the gene encoding neutrophil elastase in congenital and cyclical neutropenia. *Blood*, **96**, 2317–2322.

270 Dweck A, Blickstein D, Elstein D and Zimran A (2002) Thrombocytosis associated with enzyme replacement therapy in Gaucher disease. *Acta Haematol*, **108**, 94–96.

271 Sabel AL, Gaudiani JL, Statland B and Mehler PS (2013) Hematological abnormalities in severe anorexia nervosa. *Ann Hematol*, **92**, 605–613.

272 Monagle P and Andrew M (2003) Developmental hemostasis: relevance to newborns and infants. In: Nathan DG, Orkin SH, Ginsburg D and Look AT, *Nathan and Oski's Hematology of Infancy and Childhood*, 6th edn, Saunders, Philadelphia.

273 Schilling RF (1980) Platelet millionaires. *Lancet*, **ii**, 372–373.

274 Jones MI and Pierre RV (1981) The causes of extreme thrombocytosis. *Am J Clin Pathol*, **76**, 349.

275 Buss DH, Cashell AW, O'Connor ML, Richards F and Case LD (1994) Occurrence, etiology, and clinical significance of extreme thrombocytosis: a study of 280 cases. *Am J Med*, **96**, 247–253.

276 Santhosh-Kumar CR, Yohannan MD, Higgy KE and al-Mashhadani SA (1991) Thrombocytosis in adults: analysis of 777 patients. *J Intern Med*, **229**, 493–495.

277 Spigel SC and Mooney LR (1977) Extreme thrombocytosis associated with malignancy. *Cancer*, **39**, 339–341.

278 Pearson HA, Lobel JS, Kocoshis SA, Naiman IL, Windmiller J, Lammi AT *et al.* (1979) A new syndrome of refractory sideroblastic anemia with vacuolation of marrow precursors and exocrine pancreatic dysfunction. *J Pediatr*, **95**, 976–984.

279 Nieken J, Mulder NH, Buter J, Vellenga E, Limburg PC, Piers DA and de Vries EG (1995) Recombinant human interleukin-6 induces a rapid and reversible anemia in cancer patients. *Blood*, **86**, 900–905.

280 Bussel JB, Mukherjee R and Stone AJ (2001) A pilot study of rhuIL-11 treatment of refractory ITP. *Am J Hematol*, **66**, 172–177.

281 Gołąb J, Zagożdżon R, Stoklosa T, Lasek W, Jakóbisiak M, Pojda Z and Machaj E (1998) Erythropoietin prevents the development of interleukin-12-induced anemia and thrombocytopenia but does not decrease its antitumor activity in mice. *Blood*, **91**, 4387–4388.

282 Biaggioni I, Robertson D, Krantz S, Jones M and Haile V (1994) The anemia of primary autonomic failure and its reversal with recombinant erythropoietin. *Ann Intern Med*, **121**, 181–186.

283 Gomes MER, Deinum J, Timmers HJLNM and Lenders JWM (2003) Occam's razor; anaemia and orthostatic hypotension. *Lancet*, **363**, 1282.

284 Puig J, Corcoy R and Rodriguez-Espinosa J (1998) Anemia secondary to vitamin D intoxication. *Ann Intern Med*, **128**, 602–603.

285 Perrotta S, Nobili B, Rossi F, Criscuolo M, Iolascon A, Di Pinto D *et al.* (2002) Infant hypervitaminosis A causes severe anemia and thrombocytopenia: evidence of a retinol-dependent bone marrow growth inhibition. *Blood*, **99**, 2017–2022.

286 Hammett-Stabler CA, Broussard LA, Winecker RE and Ropero-Miller JD (2002) New insights into an old poison, arsenic. *Lab Med*, **33**, 437–447.

287 Arai S and Vogelsang GB (2000) Management of graft-versus-host disease. *CME Bulletin Haematology*, **14**, 190–204.

288 Ishani A, Weinhandl E, Zhao Z, Gilbertson DT, Collins AJ, Yusuf S and Herzog CA (2005) Angiotensin-converting enzyme inhibitor as a risk factor for the development of anemia, and the impact of incident anemia on mortality in patients with left ventricular dysfunction. *J Am Coll Cardiol*, **45**, 391–399.

289 Schwarzbeck A, Wittenmeier KW and Hällfritzsch U (1998) Anaemia in dialysis patients as a side-effect of sartanes. *Lancet*, **352**, 286.

290 Dickinson M and Juneja S (2009) Haematological toxicity of colchicine. *Br J Haematol*, **146**, 465.

291 Steer A, Daley AJ and Curtis N (2005) Suppurative sequelae of symbiosis. *Lancet*, **365**, 188.

292 Fisch P, Handgretinger R and Schaefer H-E (2000) Pure red cell aplasia. *Br J Haematol*, **111**, 1010–1022.

293 Winkler M, Schulze F, Jost U, Ringe B and Pichlmayr R (1993) Anaemia associated with Fk-506 immunosuppression. *Lancet*, **341**, 1035–1036.

294 Lin Y-W, Okazaki S, Hamahata K, Watanabe K-i, Asami I, Yoshibayashi M *et al.* (1999) Acute pure red cell aplasia associated with allopurinol therapy. *Am J Hematol*, **61**, 209–211.

295 Tanaka N, Ishada F and Tanaka E (2004) Ribavirin-induced red-cell aplasia during treatment of hepatitis C. *N Engl J Med*, **350**, 1264–1265.

296 Niebrugge DJ, Benjamin DR, Christie D and Scott CR (1982) Hereditary transcobalamin II deficiency presenting as red cell hypoplasia. *J Pediatr*, **101**, 732–735.

297 Tauchi T, Iwama H, Kaku H, Kimura Y and Ohyashiki K (1999) Remission of pure-red-cell aplasia associated with operative cure of lung cancer. *Am J Hematol*, **61**, 157–158.

298 Baker RI, Manoharan A, de Luca E and Begley CG (1993) Pure red cell aplasia of pregnancy: a distinct clinical entity. *Br J Haematol*, **85**, 619–622.

299 Volin L and Ruutu T (1990) Pure red-cell aplasia of long duration after major ABO-incompatible bone marrow transplantation. *Acta Haematol*, **84**, 195–197.

300 Bolan CD, Leitman SF, Griffith LM, Wesley RA, Procter JL, Stroncek DF *et al.* (2001) Delayed donor red cell chimerism and pure red cell aplasia following major ABO-incompatible nonmyeloablative hematopoietic stem cell transplantation. *Blood*, **98**, 1687–1694.

301 Casadevall N, Nataf J, Viron B, Kolta A, Kiladjian J-J, Martin-Dupont P *et al.* (2002) Pure red cell aplasia and antierythropoietin antibodies in patients treated with recombinant erythropoietin. *N Engl J Med*, **346**, 469–475.

302 Lau KS and White JC (1969) Myelosclerosis associated with systemic lupus erythematosus in patients in West Malaysia. *J Clin Pathol*, **22**, 433–438.

303 Yetgin S and Ozsoylu S (1982) Myeloid metaplasia in vitamin D deficiency rickets. *Scand J Haematol*, **28**, 180–185.

304 Ravindranath Y, Paglia DE, Warrier I, Valentine W, Nakatani M and Brockway RA (1987) Glucose phosphate isomerase deficiency as a cause of hydrops fetalis. *N Engl J Med*, **316**, 258–261.

305 Kanno H, Ishikawa K, Fujii H and Miwa S (1997) Severe hexokinase deficiency as a cause of hemolytic anemia, periventricular leucomalacia and intrauterine death of the fetus. *Blood*, **90**, Suppl. 1, 8a.

306 Rodriguez V, Godwin JE, Ogburn PL, Smithson WEA and Fairbanks VF (1997) Severe anemia and hydrops fetalis in hereditary xerocytosis. *Blood*, **90**, Suppl. 1, 18b.

307 Ribeiro ML, Alloisio N, Almeida H, Gomez C, Texier P, Lemos C *et al.* (2000) Severe hereditary spherocytosis and distal renal tubular acidosis associated with total absence of band 3. *Blood*, **96**, 1602–1604.

308 Arnon S, Tamary H, Dgany O, Litmanovitz I, Regev R, Bauer R *et al.* (2004) Hydrops fetalis associated with homozygosity for hemoglobin Taybe (α 38/39 THR deletion) in newborn triplets. *Am J Hematol*, **76**, 263–266.

309 Laosombat V, Viprakasit V, Dissaneevate S, Leetanaporn R, Chotsampancharoen T, Wongchanchailert M *et al.* (2010) Natural history of Southeast Asian Ovalocytosis during the first 3 years of life. *Blood Cells Mol Dis*, **45**, 29–32.

310 Brugnara C and Platt OS (2003) The neonatal erythrocyte and its disorders. In: Nathan DG, Orkin SH, Ginsburg D and Look AT, *Nathan and Oski's Hematology of Infancy and Childhood*, 6th edn. Saunders, Philadelphia.

311 Game L, Bergounioux J, Close JP, Marzouka BE and Thein SL (2003) A novel deletion causing $(\varepsilon\gamma\delta\beta)^0$ thalassaemia in a Chilean family. *Br J Haematol*, **123**, 154–159.

312 Parez N, Dommergues M, Zupan V, Chambost H, Fieschi JB, Delaunay J *et al.* (2000) Severe congenital dyserythropoietic anaemia type I: prenatal management, transfusion support and alpha-interferon therapy. *Br J Haematol*, **110**, 420–421.

313 Van Hook JW, Gill P, Cyr D and Kapur RP (1995) Diamond–Blackfan anemia as an unusual cause of nonimmune hydrops fetalis: a case report. *J Reprod Med*, **40**, 850–854.

314 Goldwurm S, Casati C, Venturi N, Strada S, Santambrighio P, Indraccolo S *et al.* (2000) Biochemical and genetic defects underlying human congenital hypotransferrinemia. *Hematol J*, **1**, 390–398.

315 McDonnell M, Hannam S and Devane SP (1998) Hydrops fetalis due to ABO incompatibility. *Arch Dis Child Fetal Neonatal Ed*, **78**, F220–F221.

316 Nolan B, Hinchliffe R and Vora A (2000) Neonatal pure red cell aplasia due to maternal anti-M. *Blood*, **96**, 8a.

317 Gray ES, Balch NJ, Kohler H, Thompson WD and Simson JG (1986) Congenital leukaemia: an unusual cause of stillbirth. *Arch Dis Child*, **61**, 1001–1006.

318 Swann IL and Kendra JR (1998) Anaemia, vitamin E deficiency and failure to thrive in an infant. *Clin Lab Haematol*, **20**, 61–63.

319 Lasky EA (1991) Polycythaemia in the newborn infant. In: Hann IM, Gibson BES, Lasky EA (eds), *Fetal and Neonatal Haematology*. Baillière Tindall, London.

320 Benson AB, Moss M and Silliman CC (2009) Transfusion-related acute lung injury (TRALI): a clinical review with emphasis on the critically ill. *Br J Haematol*, **147**, 431–443.

321 Kuijpers TW, Maianski NA, Tool ATJ, Becker K, Plecko B, Valianpour F *et al.* (2004) Neutrophils in Barth syndrome (BTHS) avidly bind annexin-V in the absence of apoptosis. *Blood*, **103**, 3915–3923.

322 Sinha S, Watkins S and Corey SJ (2001) Genetic and biochemical characterization of a deletional mutation of the extra-cellular domain of the human G-CSF receptor in a child with severe congenital neutropenia unresponsive to Neupogen. *Blood*, **98**, 440a.

323 Ancliff PJ, Blundell MP, Gale RE, Liesner R, Hann IM, Thrasher AJ and Linch DC (2001) Activating mutations in the Wiskott Aldrich Syndrome protein may define a subgroup of severe congenital neutropenia (SCN) with specific and unusual laboratory features. *Blood*, **98**, 439a.

324 Ancliff PJ (2003) Congenital neutropenia. *Blood Rev*, **17**, 209–216.

325 Person RE, Li F-Q, Duan Z, Benson KF, Wechsler J, Papadaki HA *et al.* (2003) Mutations in proto-oncogene GFI1 cause human neutropenia and target ELA2. *Nature Genet*, **34**, 308–312.

326 Bohn G, Allroth A, Brandes G, Thiel J, Glocker E, Schäffer AA *et al.* (2007) A novel human primary immunodeficiency syndrome caused by deficiency of the endosomal adaptor protein p14. *Nat Med*, **13**, 38–45.

327 Badolato R, Prandini A, Caracciolo S, Colombo F, Tabellini G, Giacomelli M *et al.* (2012) Exome sequencing reveals a pallidin mutation in a Hermansky-Pudlak-like primary immunodeficiency syndrome. *Blood*, **119**, 3185–3187.

328 Sieff CA, Nisbet-Brown E and Nathan DG (2000) Congenital bone marrow failure syndromes. *Br J Haematol*, **111**, 30–42.

329 Parmley RT, Crist WM, Ragab AH, Boxer LA, Malluh A, Liu VK and Darby CP (1980) Congenital dysgranulopoietic neutropenia: clinical, serologic, ultrastructural and *in vitro* proliferative characteristics. *Blood*, **56**, 465–475.

330 Wetzler M, Talpaz M, Kleinerman ES, King A, Huh YO, Gutterman JU and Kurzrock R (1990) A new familial immunodeficiency disorder characterized by severe neutropenia, a defective marrow release mechanism, and hypogammaglobulinemia. *Am J Med*, **89**, 663–672.

331 Hadžić N, Pagliuca A, Rela M, Portmann B, Jones A, Veys P *et al.* (2000) Correction of the hyper-IgM syndrome after liver and bone marrow transplantation. *N Engl J Med*, **342**, 320–324.

332 Ziedler C (2005) Congenital cytopenias: congenital neutropenias. *Hematology*, **10**, Suppl. 1, 306–311.

333 Pitcher LA, Taylor KM, Bartold PM, Seow K, Tong YH and Fanning S (1996) Filgrastim used successfully for asymptomatic neutropenia in Cohen's syndrome. *Aust NZ J Med*, **26**, 258.

334 van den Tweel JG (1997) Preleukaemic disorders in children: hereditary disorders and myelodysplastic syndromes. *Current Diagnostic Pathol*, **4**, 45–50.

335 Casadevall N, Croisille L, Auffray I, Tchernia G and Coulombel L (1994) Age-related alterations in erythroid and granulopoietic progenitors in Diamond Blackfan anaemia. *Br J Haematol*, **87**, 369–375.

336 Aksu G, Kütükçüler N, Genel F, Vergin C and Omowaire B (2003) Griscelli syndrome without hemophagocytosis in an eleven-year-old girl: expanding the phenotypic spectrum of *Rab27A* mutations in humans. *Am J Med Genet*, **116A**, 329–333.

337 Corral J, Gonzalez-Conejero R, Pujol-Moix N, Domenech P and Vicente V (2004) Mutation analysis of HPS1, the gene mutated in Hermansky-Pudlak syndrome, in patients with isolated platelet dense-granule deficiency. *Haematologica*, **89**, 325–329.

338 Glasser L, Meloni-Ehrig A, Joseph P and Mendiola J (2006) Benign chronic neutropenia with abnormalities involving 16q22, affecting mother and daughter. *Am J Hematol*, **81**, 262–270.

339 Porter WM, Hardman CM, Abdalla SH and Powles AV (1999) Haematological disease in siblings with Rothmund-Thomson syndrome. *Clin Exp Dermatol*, **24**, 452–454.

340 Roe TF, Coates TD, Thomas DW, Miller JH and Gilsanz V (1992) Treatment of chronic inflammatory bowel disease in glycogen storage disease type Ib with colony-stimulating factors. *N Engl J Med*, **326**, 1666–1669.

341 Ino T, Sherwood G, Cutz E, Benson LN, Rose IV and Freedman RM (1988) Dilated cardiomyopathy with neutropenia, short stature and abnormal carnitine metabolism. *J Pediatr*, **113**, 511–514.

342 Ronghe M, Cantlay AM, Chasty RC, Allen JT, Pennock CA, Oakhill A and Steward CG (1998) Exclusion of organic acid disorders in children with chronic idiopathic neutropenia. *Br J Haematol*, **101**, Suppl. 1, 74.

343 Susa JS, Bennett MJ and Jones PM (2003) Lethargy, failure to thrive, and vomiting in a neonate. *Lab Med*, **34**, 775–778.

344 Sampson B, Fagerhol MK, Sunderkötter C, Golden BE, Richmond P, Klein N et al. (2003) Hyperzincaemia with hypercalprotectinaemia: a new disorder of zinc metabolism. *Lancet*, **360**, 1742–1745.

345 Parvaneh N, Ziaee V, Moradinejad MH, Touitou I (2014) Intermittent neutropenia as an early feature of mild mevalonate kinase deficiency. *J Clin Immunol*, **34**, 123–126.

346 Al Mulla ZS and Christensen RD (1995) Neutropenia in the neonate. *Clin Perinatol*, **22**, 711–739.

347 Hien TT, Liem NT, Dung NT, San LT, Mai PP, Chau N N van V et al. (2004) Avian influenza A (H5N1) in 10 patients in Vietnam. *N Engl J Med*, **350**, 1179–1188.

348 Griffin M and Makris M (2013) Vaccination induced neutropenia. *Int J Lab Hematol*, **35**, e33.

349 Penchansky L and Jordan JA (1997) Transient erythroblastopenia of childhood associated with human herpesvirus type 6, variant B. *Am J Clin Pathol*, **108**, 127–132.

350 Hashimoto H, Maruyama H, Fujimoto K, Sakakura T, Seishu S and Okuda N (2002) The hematologic findings associated with thrombocytopenia during the acute phase of exanthem subitum confirmed by primary human herpesvirus-6 infection. *J Pediatr Hematol Oncol*, **24**, 211–214.

351 Pont J, Puchhammer-Stockl E, Chott A, Popow-Kraupp T, Kienzer H, Postner G and Honetz N (1992) Recurrent granulocytic aplasia as clinical presentation of a persistent parvovirus B19 infection. *Br J Haematol*, **80**, 160–165.

352 Salas R, de Manzione N, Tesh RB, Rico-Hesse R, Shope RE, Betancourt A et al. (1991) Venezuelan haemorrhagic fever. *Lancet*, **338**, 1033–1036.

353 Fisher-Hoch SP, Khan JA, Rehman S, Mirza S, Khurshid M and McCormick JB (1995) Crimean Congo-haemorrhagic fever treated with oral ribavirin. *Lancet*, **346**, 472–475.

354 Schanen A, Gallou G, Hincky JM and Saron MF (1998) A rash, circulating anticoagulant, then meningitis. *Lancet*, **351**, 1856.

355 Lee N, Hui D, Wu A, Chan P, Cameron P, Joynt GM et al. (2003) A major outbreak of severe acute respiratory syndrome in Hong Kong. *N Engl J Med*, **348**, 1986–1994.

356 Yu XJ, Liang MF, Zhang SY, Liu Y, Li JD, Sun YL et al. (2011) Fever with thrombocytopenia associated with a novel bunyavirus in China. *N Engl J Med*, **364**, 1523–1532.

357 McMullan LK, Folk SM, Kelly AJ, MacNeil A, Goldsmith CS, Metcalfe MG et al. (2012) A new phlebovirus associated with severe febrile illness in Missouri. *N Engl J Med*, **367**, 834–841.

358 Sheehan V, Weir A and Waters B (2013) Severe neutropenia in patients with chronic hepatitis C: a benign condition. *Acta Haematol*, **129**, 96–100.

359 Pullen RL and Stuart BM (1945) Tularemia. *JAMA*, **129**, 495–500.

360 Sheehy TW, Hazlett D and Turk RE (1973) Scrub typhus: a comparison of chloramphenicol and tetracycline in its treatment. *Arch Intern Med*, **132**, 77–80.

361 Brettman LR, Lewin S, Holzman RS, Goldman WD, Marr JS, Kechijian P and Schinella R (1981) Rickettsial pox: report of an outbreak and a contemporary review. *Medicine*, **60**, 363–372.

362 Parola P, Jourdan J and Raoult D (1998) Tick-borne infection caused by *Rickettsia africae* in the West Indies. *N Engl J Med*, **338**, 1391.

363 Goodman JL, Nelson C, Vitale B, Madigan JE, Dumler JS, Kurtti TJ and Munderloh UG (1996) Direct cultivation of the causative agent of human granulocytic ehrlichiosis. *N Engl J Med*, **334**, 209–215.

364 Tencic S (2011) Babesiosis in a returned traveller – the first Australian case. AIMS/NZIMLS Congress, Gold Coast.

365 Goodwin RA, Shapiro JL, Thurman GH, Thurman SS and des Prez RM (1980) Disseminated histoplasmosis: clinical and pathological correlations. *Medicine*, **59**, 1–33.

366 Perkisas S, Vrelust I, Martin M, Gadisseur A and Schroyens W (2011) A warning about agranulocytosis with the use of cocaine adulterated with levamisole. *Acta Clin Belg*, **66**, 226–227.

367 Blanche S, Tardieu M, Rustin P, Slama A, Barret B, Firtion G et al. (1999) Persistent mitochondrial dysfunction and perinatal exposure to antiretroviral nucleoside analogues. *Lancet*, **354**, 1084–1089.

368 Voog E, Morschhauser F and Solal-Céligny P (2003) Neutropenia in patients treated with rituximab. *N Engl J Med*, **348**, 2691–2694.

369 Richardson PG, Barlogie B, Berenson J, Singhal S, Jagannath S, Irwin D et al. (2003) A phase 2 study of bortezomib in relapsed refractory myeloma. *N Engl J Med*, **348**, 2609–2617.

370 Demetri GD, von Mehren M, Blanke CD, Van den Abbeele AD, Eisenberg B, Roberts PJ et al. (2002) Efficacy and safety of imatinib mesylate in advanced gastrointestinal stromal tumours. *N Engl J Med*, **347**, 472–480.

371 Weinblatt ME, Kavanaugh A, Genovese MC, Musser TK, Grossbard EB and Magilavy DB (2010) An oral spleen tyrosine kinase (Syk) inhibitor for rheumatoid arthritis. *N Engl J Med*, **363**, 1303–1312.

372 Papp KA, Leonardi C, Menter A, Ortonne JP, Krueger JG, Kricorian G et al. (2012) Brodalumab, an anti-interleukin-17-receptor antibody for psoriasis. *N Engl J Med*, **366**, 1181–1189.

373 Leonardi C, Matheson R, Zachariae C, Cameron G, Li L, Edson-Heredia E *et al.* (2012) Anti-interleukin-17 monoclonal antibody ixekizumab in chronic plaque psoriasis. *N Engl J Med*, **366**, 1190–1199.

374 DeJesus CE, Egen J, Metzger M, Alvarez X, Combs CA, Malide D *et al.* (2011) Transient neutropenia after granulocyte-colony stimulating factor administration is associated with neutrophil accumulation in pulmonary vasculature. *Exp Hematol*, **39**, 142–150.

375 Wang ML, Rule S, Martin P, Goy A, Auer R, Kahl BS *et al.* (2013) Targeting BTK with ibrutinib in relapsed or refractory mantle-cell lymphoma. *N Engl J Med*, **369**, 507–516.

376 Eisenmenger W, Drasch G, von Clarmann M, Kretschmer E and Roider G (1991) Clinical and morphological findings on mustard gas [bis(2-chloroethyl)sulfide] poisoning. *J Forensic Sci*, **36**, 1688–1698.

377 Wallis JP, Haynes S, Stark G, Green FA, Lucas GF and Chapman CD (2002) Transfusion-related alloimmune neutropenia: an undescribed complication of blood transfusion. *Lancet*, **360**, 1073–1074.

378 Mariani M, Cattaneo A, Bottelli G, Pugni L, Mosca F, Comonbo F *et al.* (2011) Severe neonatal alloimmune neutropenia in a newborn delivered by a CD16 deficient Gypsy woman. *Haematologica*, **96**, Suppl. 2, 341.

379 Kameoka J, Funato T, Miura T, Harigae H, Saito J, Yokoyama H *et al.* (2001) Autoimmune neutropenia in pregnant women causing neonatal neutropenia. *Br J Haematol*, **114**, 198–200.

380 Bux J and Mueller-Eckhardt C (1992) Autoimmune neutropenia. *Semin Hematol*, **29**, 45–53.

381 Papadaki HA, Stamatopoulos K, Damianaki A, Anagnostopoulos A, Papadaki T, Eliopoulos AG and Eliopoulos GD (2005) Activated T-lymphocytes with myelosuppressive properties in patients with chronic idiopathic neutropenia. *Br J Haematol*, **128**, 863–876.

382 McClain K, Estrov Z, Chen H and Mahoney DH (1993) Chronic neutropenia of childhood: frequent association with parvovirus infection and correlations with bone marrow culture studies. *Br J Haematol*, **85**, 57–62.

383 Cline MI, Opelz G, Saxon A, Fahey JL and Golde DW (1976) Autoimmune panleukopenia. *N Engl J Med*, **295**, 1489–1493.

384 Levitt LJ, Ries CA and Greenberg PL (1983) Pure white cell aplasia: antibody-mediated autoimmune inhibition of granulopoiesis. *N Engl J Med*, **308**, 1141–1146.

385 Longhurst HJ, O'Grady C, Evans G, De Lord C, Hughes A, Cavenagh J and Helbert MR (2002) Anti-D immunoglobulin treatment for thrombocytopenia associated with primary antibody deficiency. *J Clin Pathol*, **55**, 64–66.

386 Niehues T, Schwarz K, Schneider M, Schroten H, Schroder E, Stephan V and Wahn V (1996) Severe combined immunodeficiency (SCID) associated neutropenia: a lesson from monozygotic twins. *Arch Dis Child*, **74**, 340–342.

387 Marques MB, Tuncer HH, Divers SG, Baker AC and Harrison DK (2005) Acute transient leucopenia as a sign of TRALI. *Am J Hematol*, **80**, 90–91.

388 Anderlini P, Przepiorka D, Champlin R and Körbling M (1996) Peripheral blood stem cell apheresis in normal donors: the neglected side. *Blood*, **88**, 3663–3664.

389 Liu YK (1973) Leukopenia in alcoholics. *Am J Med*, **54**, 605–610.

390 Kubota M, Tsukamoto R, Kurokawa K, Imai T and Furusho K (1996) Elevated serum interferon gamma and interleukin-6 in patients with necrotizing lymphadenitis (Kikuchi's disease). *Br J Haematol*, **95**, 613–615.

391 Cordano A, Placko RP and Graham GG (1966) Hypocupremia and neutropenia in copper deficiency. *Blood*, **28**, 280–283.

392 Miyoshi I, Saito T and Iwahara Y (2004) Copper deficiency anaemia. *Br J Haematol*, **125**, 106.

393 Shoenfeld Y, Shaklai M, Ben-Baruch N, Hirschorn M and Pinkhas J (1982) Neutropenia induced by hypercarotenaemia. *Lancet*, **i**, 1245.

394 Koenig IM and Christensen RD (1989) Incidence, neutrophil kinetics, and natural history of neonatal neutropenia associated with maternal hypertension. *N Engl J Med*, **321**, 557–562.

395 Engle WD and Rosenfeld CR (1984) Neutropenia in high-risk neonates. *J Pediatr*, **105**, 982–986.

396 Zach TL, Steinhorn RH, Georgieff MK, Mills MM and Green TP (1990) Leukopenia associated with extracorporeal membrane oxygenation in newborn infants. *J Pediatr*, **116**, 440–443.

397 Rogers ZR, Bergstrom SK, Amylon MD, Buchanan GR and Glader BE (1989) Reduced neutrophil counts in children with transient erythroblastopenia of childhood. *J Pediatr*, **115**, 746–748.

398 Lundin J, Kimby E, Björkholm M, Broliden P-A, Gelsing F, Hjalmar V *et al.* (2002) Phase II trial of subcutaneous anti-CD53 monoclonal antibody alemtuzumab (Campath 1H) in the first-line treatment of chronic lymphocytic leukemia (B-CLL). *Blood*, **100**, 768–773.

399 Cuilliere-Dartigues P, Meyohas MC, Balladur P, Gorin NC and Coppo P (2010) Splenic sarcoidosis: an unusual aetiology of agranulocytosis. *Am J Hematol*, **85**, 891.

400 Abdollahpour H, Appaswamy G, Kotlarz D, Diestelhorst J, Beier R, Schäffer AA *et al.* (2012) The phenotype of human STK4 deficiency. *Blood*, **119**, 3450–3457.

401 Archer RK, Engisch HJC, Gaha T and Ruxton J (1971) The eosinophil leucocytes in the blood and bone marrow of patients with Down's anomaly. *Br J Haematol*, **21**, 271–276.

402 Nakahata T, Spicer SS, Leary AG, Ogawa M, Franklin W and Goetzl EJ (1984) Circulating eosinophil colony-forming cells in pure eosinophil aplasia. *Ann Intern Med*, **101**, 321–324.

403 Juhlin LL and Michaelsson G (1977) A new syndrome characterized by absence of eosinophils and basophils. *Lancet*, **i**, 1233–1235.

404 Welles SL, Mueller N, Tachibana N, Shishime E, Okayama A, Murai K and Tsuda K (1991) Decreased eosinophil numbers in HTLV-I carriers. *Lancet*, **337**, 987.

405 Grattan CEH, Dawn G, Gibbs S and Francis DM (2003) Blood basophil numbers in chronic ordinary urticaria and healthy controls: diurnal variation, influence of loratadine and prednisolone and relationship to disease activity. *Clin Exp Immunol*, **33**, 337–341.

406 Vinh DC, Patel SY, Uzel G, Anderson VL, Freeman AF, Olivier KN et al. (2010) Autosomal dominant and sporadic monocytopenia with susceptibility to mycobacteria, fungi, papillomaviruses, and myelodysplasia. *Blood*, **115**, 1519–1529.

407 Hsu AP, Sampaio EP, Khan J, Calvo KR, Lemieux JE, Patel SY et al. (2011) Mutations in *GATA2* are associated with the autosomal dominant and sporadic monocytopenia and mycobacterial infection (MonoMAC) syndrome. *Blood*, **118**, 2653–2655.

408 Pasquet M, Bellanné-Chantelot C, Tavitian S, Prade N, Beaupain B and Larochelle O (2013) High frequency of GATA2 mutations in patients with mild chronic neutropenia evolving to MonoMac syndrome, myelodysplasia, and acute myeloid leukemia. *Blood*, **121**, 822–829.

409 Hambleton S, Salem S, Bustamante J, Bigley V, Boisson-Dupuis S, Azevedo J et al. (2011) IRF8 mutations and human dendritic-cell immunodeficiency. *N Engl J Med*, **365**, 127–138.

410 Gossage DL and Buckley RH (1990) Prevalence of lymphocytopenia in severe combined immunodeficiency. *N Engl J Med*, **323**, 1422–1423.

411 Wyllie DH, Bowler ICJW and Peto TEA (2004) Relation between lymphopenia and bacteraemia in UK adults with medical emergencies. *J Clin Pathol*, **57**, 950–955.

412 Hasenclever D and Diehl V (1998) A prognostic score for advanced Hodgkin's disease. International Prognostic Factors Project on Advanced Hodgkin's Disease. *N Engl J Med*, **339**, 1506–1514.

413 Kim YR, Kim JS, Kim SJ, Jung HA, Kim SJ, Kim WS et al. (2011) Lymphopenia is an important prognostic factor in peripheral T-cell lymphoma (NOS) treated with anthracycline-containing chemotherapy. *J Hematol Oncol*, **4**, 34.

414 Aoki T, Nishiyama T, Imahashi N and Kitamura K (2011) Lymphopenia following the completion of first-line therapy predicts early relapse in patients with diffuse large B cell lymphoma. *Ann Hematol*, **91**, 375–382.

415 Tashima M, Nishikikori M, Kitawaki T, Hishizawa M, Izumi T, Fujiwara Y et al. (2010) Idiopathic CD4 lymphocytopenia due to loss of heterozygosity of the mutant CD2 gene. *Blood*, **116**, 1143–1144.

416 Wickramasinghe SN (1998) Congenital dyserythropoietic anaemias: clinical features, haematological morphology and new biochemical data. *Blood Rev*, **12**, 178–200.

417 Mrowietz U and Reich K (2013) Case reports of PML in patients treated for psoriasis. *N Engl J Med*, **369**, 1080–1081.

418 Hou M, Horney E, Stockelberg D, Jacobsson S, Kutti J and Wadenvik H (1997) Multiple quinine-dependent antibodies in a patient with episodic thrombocytopenia, neutropenia, lymphocytopenia, and granulomatous hepatitis. *Blood*, **90**, 4806–4811.

419 Berglund B and Ekblom B (1991) Effect of recombinant human erythropoietin treatment on blood pressure and some haematological parameters in healthy men. *J Intern Med*, **229**, 125–130.

420 Cummins D, Wilson ME, Foulgar KJ, Dawson D and Hogarth AM (1995) Effects of influenza vaccination on the blood counts of people aged over 65: case report and prospective study. *Br J Haematol*, **101**, Suppl. 1, 54.

421 Symmons DPM, Farr M, Salmon M and Bacon PA (1989) Lymphopenia in rheumatoid arthritis. *J Roy Soc Med*, **82**, 462–463.

422 Budman DR and Steinberg AD (1977) Hematologic aspects of systemic lupus erythematosus. *Ann Intern Med*, **86**, 220–229.

423 Daniele RP and Rowlands DT (1976) Lymphocyte subpopulations in sarcoidosis: correlation with disease activity and duration. *Ann Intern Med*, **85**, 593–600.

424 Bynoe AG, Scott CS, Ford P and Roberts BE (1983) Decreased T helper cells in the myelodysplastic syndromes. *Br J Haematol*, **54**, 97–102.

425 Jacobs NL, Holtan SG, Porrata LF, Markovic SN, Tefferi A and Steensma DP (2010) Host immunity affects survival in myelodysplastic syndromes: independent prognostic value of the absolute lymphocyte count. *Am J Hematol*, **85**, 160–163.

426 Bowers TK and Eckert E (1978) Leukopenia in anorexia nervosa: lack of an increased risk of infection. *Arch Intern Med*, **138**, 1520–1523.

427 Santos PC and Falcao RP (1990) Decreased lymphocyte subsets and K-cell activity in iron deficiency anemia. *Acta Haematol*, **84**, 118–121.

428 Robbins G and Brozovic B (1985) Lymphocytopenia in regular platelet apheresis donors. *Br J Haematol*, **61**, 558–559.

429 Unkrig CJ, Schroder R and Scharf RE (1994) Lorenzo's oil and thrombocytopenia. *N Engl J Med*, **330**, 577.

430 Masci AM, Palmieri G, Vitiello L, Montella L, Perna F, Orlandi P et al. (2003) Clonal expansion of CD8 $^+$BV8 T lymphocytes in bone marrow characterizes thymoma-associated B lymphopenia. *Blood*, **101**, 3106–3108.

431 Christodouleas JP, Forrest RD, Ainsley CG, Tochner Z, Hahn SM and Glatstein E (2011) Short-term and long-term health risks of nuclear-power-plant accidents. *N Engl J Med*, **364**, 2334–2341.

432 Lackner A, Basu O, Bierings M, Lassay L, Schaefer UW, Révész T et al. (2000) Haematopoietic stem cell transplantation for amegakaryocytic thrombocytopenia. *Br J Haematol*, **109**, 773–775.

433 Alter B (2003) Inherited bone marrow failure syndromes. In: Nathan DG, Orkin SH, Ginsburg D and Look AT, *Nathan and Oski's Hematology of Infancy and Childhood*, 6th edn. Saunders, Philadelphia.

434 Roberts IA and Murray NA (1999) Management of thrombocytopenia in neonates. *Br J Haematol*, **105**, 864–870.

435 Koenig JM and Christensen RD (1989) Neutropenia and thrombocytopenia in infants with Rh hemolytic disease. *J Pediatr*, **114**, 625–631.

436 Wagner T, Bernaschek G and Geissler G (2000) Inhibition of megakaryopoiesis by Kell-related antibodies. *N Engl J Med*, **343**, 72.

437 Blanchette VS, Johnson J and Rand M (2000) The management of alloimmune neonatal thrombocytopenia. *Baillière's Clin Haematol*, **13**, 365–390.

438 AbelmanW and Virchis A (2005) An unusual cause of thrombocytopenia. *Clin Lab Haematol*, **27**, 215–216.

439 Mazharian A, Ghevaert C, Zhang L, Massberg S and Watson SP (2011) Dasatinib enhances megakaryocyte differentiation but inhibits platelet formation. *Blood*, **117**, 5198–5206.

440 Bhattacharyya J, Kumar R, Tyagi S, Kishore J, Mahapatra M and Choudhry VP (2005) Human parvovirus B19-induced acquired pure amegakaryocytic thrombocytopenia. *Br J Haematol*, **128**, 128–129.

441 Radonić A, Oswald O, Thulke S, Brockhaus N, Nitsche A, Siegert W and Schetelig J (2005) Infections with human herpesvirus 6 variant B delay platelet engraftment after allogeneic haematopoietic stem cell transplantation. *Br J Haematol*, **131**, 480–482.

442 Garcia-Suárez J, Burgaleta C, Hernanz N, Albarran F, Tobaruela P and Alvarez-Mon M (2000) HCV-associated thrombocytopenia: clinical characteristics and platelet response after recombinant α2b-interferon therapy. *Br J Haematol*, **110**, 98–103.

443 Hoffman R (1991) Acquired pure amegakaryocytic thrombocytopenic purpura. *Semin Hematol*, **28**, 303–312.

444 Fogarty PF, Stetler-Stevenson M, Pereira A and Dunbar CE (2005) Large granular lymphocytic proliferation-associated cyclic thrombocytopenia. *Am J Hematol*, **79**, 334–336.

445 Ando M, Iwamoto Y, Suda A, Tsuchiya K and Nihei H (2001) New insights into the thrombopoietic status of patient on dialysis through the evaluation of megakaryocytopoiesis in bone marrow and of endogenous thrombopoietin levels. *Blood*, **97**, 915–921.

446 Li J, Yang C, Xia Y, Bertino A, Glaspy J, Roberts M and Kuter DJ (2001) Thrombocytopenia caused by the development of antibodies to thrombopoietin. *Blood*, **98**, 3241–3248.

447 Curtis BR, Ali S, Aitman TJ, Ebert DD, Lenes BA and Aster RH (2001) Maternal isoimmunization against CD36 (GPIV) should be considered in unresolved cases of apparent immune neonatal thrombocytopenia. *Blood*, **98**, 710a.

448 Dickerman JD, Holbrook PR and Zinkham WH (1972) Etiology and therapy of thrombocytopenia associated with sarcoidosis. *J Pediatr*, **81**, 758–764.

449 Parameswaran R, Cavenagh JD, Davies JK and Newland AC (1999) Immune cytopenias as the presenting feature of common variable immune deficiency. *Br J Haematol*, **105**, Suppl. 1, 51.

450 West KA, Anderson DR, McAlister VC, Hewlett TJ, Belitsky P, Smith JW and Kelton JG (1999) Alloimmune thrombocytopenia after organ transplantation. *N Engl J Med*, **341**, 1504–1507.

451 Solenthaler M, Krauss JK, Boehlen F, Koller R, Hug M and Lammle B (1999) Fatal fresh frozen plasma infusion containing HPA-1a alloantibodies. *Br J Haematol*, **106**, 258–259.

452 Bakchoul T, Zöllner H, Amiral J, Panzer S, Selleng S, Kohlmann T *et al.* (2013) Anti-protamine-heparin antibodies: incidence, clinical relevance, and pathogenesis. *Blood*, **121**, 2821–2827.

453 Royer DJ, George JN and Terrell DR (2010) Thrombocytopenia as an adverse effect of complementary and alternative medicines, herbal remedies, nutritional supplements, foods, and beverages. *Eur J Haematol*, **84**, 421–429.

454 Warkentin TE (2007) Drug-induced immune-mediated thrombocytopenia — from purpura to thrombosis. *N Engl J Med*, **356**, 891–893.

455 Jubelirer SJ, Koenig BA and Bates MC (1999) Acute profound thrombocytopenia following C7E3 Fab (Abciximab) therapy: case reports, review of the literature and implications for therapy. *Am J Hematol*, **62**, 205–208.

456 Bougie DW, Wilker PR, Wuitschick ED, Curtis BR, Malik M, Levine S *et al.* (2002) Acute thrombocytopenia after treatment with tirofiban or eptifibatide is associated with antibodies specific for ligand-occupies GPIIb/IIIa. *Blood*, **100**, 2071–2076.

457 Aster RH and Bougie DW (2007) Drug-induced immune thrombocytopenia. *N Engl J Med*, **357**, 580–587.

458 Arnold J, Ouwehand WH, Smith GA and Cohen H (1998) A young woman with petechiae. *Lancet*, **351**, 618.

459 Lavy R (1964) Thrombocytopenic purpura due to lupinus termis bean. *J Allergy Clin Immunol*, **35**, 386–389.

460 Azuno Y, Taga K, Sasayama T and Kimoto K (1996) Thrombocytopenia induced by Jui, a traditional Chinese herbal medicine. *Lancet*, **354**, 394–305.

461 Wright JG (1992) Severe thrombocytopenia secondary to asymptomatic cytomegalovirus infection in an immunocompetent host. *J Clin Pathol*, **45**, 1037–1038.

462 Kitamura K, Ohta H, Ihara T, Kamiya H, Ochiai H, Yamanishi K and Tanaka K (1994) Idiopathic thrombocytopenic purpura after human herpesvirus 6 infection. *Lancet*, **344**, 830.

463 Bauduer F, Marty F, Larrouy M and Ducout L (1998) Immunologic thrombocytopenic purpura as presenting symptom of hepatitis C infection. *Am J Hematol*, **57**, 338–340.

464 Singh NM and Gangappa M (2007) Acute immune thrombocytopenia associated with hepatitis E in an adult. *Am J Hematol*, **82**, 942–943.

465 Beanie RM (1993) Mycoplasma and thrombocytopenia. *Arch Dis Child*, **68**, 250.

466 Castagnola E, Dufour C, Timitilli A and Giacchino R (1994) Idiopathic thrombocytopenic purpura associated with scarlet fever. *Arch Dis Child*, **70**, 164.

467 al-Majed SA, al-Momen AK, al-Kassimi FA, al-Zeer A, Kambal AM and Baaqil H (1995) Tuberculosis presenting as immune thrombocytopenic purpura. *Acta Haematol*, **94**, 135–138.

468 Spedini P (2002) Tuberculosis presenting as immune thrombocytopenic purpura. *Haematologica*, **87**, ELT09.

469 Gürkan E, Başlamişli F, Güvenç B, Bozkurt B and Ünsal Ç (2003) Immune thrombocytopenic purpura associated with *Brucella* and *Toxoplasma* infections. *Am J Hematol*, **74**, 52–54.

470 Franchini M and Veneri D (2003) *Helicobacter pylori* infection and immune thrombocytopenic purpura. *Haematologica*, **88**, 1087–1091.

471 Munckhof WJ, Runnegar N, Gray TJ, Taylor C, Palmer C and Holley A (2007) Two rare severe and fulminant presentations of Q fever in patients with minimal risk factors for this disease. *Intern Med J*, **37**, 775–778.

472 Gao H-N, Lu H-Z, Cao B, Du B, Shang H, Gan J-H *et al.* (2013) Clinical findings in 111 cases of influenza A (H7N9) virus infection. *N Engl J Med*, **368**, 2277–2285.

473 Leissinger CA (1990) Severe thrombocytopenia associated with cocaine abuse. *Ann Intern Med*, **112**, 708–710.

474 Hesseling PB (1992) Onyalai. *Bailliere's Clin Haematol*, **5**, 457–473.

475 Kiaii M, Djurdjev O, Farah M, Levin A, Jung B and MacRae J (2011) Use of electron-beam sterilized hemodialysis membranes and risk of thrombocytopenia. *JAMA*, **306**, 1679–1687.

476 Schulman I, Pierce M, Lukens A and Currimbhoy Z (1960) Studies on thrombopoiesis I. A factor in normal human plasma required for platelet production; chronic thrombocytopenia due to its deficiency. *Blood*, **16**, 943–957.

477 Upshaw JD (1978) Congenital deficiency of a factor in normal plasma that reverses microangiopathic hemolysis and thrombocytopenia. *N Engl J Med*, **298**, 1350–1352.

478 Rees DC, Iolascon A, Carella M, O'Marcaigh AS, Kendra JR, Jowitt SN *et al.* (2005) Stomatocytic haemolysis and macrothrombocytopenia (Mediterranean stomatocytosis/macrothrombocytopenia) is the haematological presentation of phytosterolaemia. *Br J Haematol*, **130**, 297–309.

479 Mulliken, JB, Anupindi S, Ezekowitz RAB and Mihm MC (2004) Case records of the Massachusetts General Hospital, Case 13-2004: a newborn girl with a large cutaneous lesion, thrombocytopenia, and anemia. *N Engl J Med*, **350**, 1764–1775.

480 Watkins NA, Rankin A, Smith GA, Schaffner-Reckinger E, Kieffer N, Laffan M and Ouwehand WH (2006) A novel inherited form of familial thrombocytopenia due to an autosomal dominant mutation in the cytoplasmic domain of the platelet beta3integrin that is associated with expression of activation dependent alphaIIb/beta3 epitopes. *Brit J Haematol*, **133**, Suppl. 1, 19.

481 Paciucci PA, Mandeli J, Oleksowicz L, Ameglio F and Holland JF (1990) Thrombocytopenia during immunotherapy with interleukin-2 by constant infusion. *Am J Med*, **89**, 308–312.

482 Locker GJ, Kapiotis S, Veitl M, Mader RM, Stoiser B, Kofler J *et al.* (1999) Activation of endothelium by immunotherapy with interleukin-2 in patients with malignant disorders. *Br J Haematol*, **105**, 912–919.

483 Maddocks S and O'Brien R (2000) African trypanosomiasis in Australia. *N Engl J Med*, **342**, 1254.

484 Lee JJ, Levitt L and Lin AY (2012) Case 2-2012: dyspnoea and rapidly progressive respiratory failure. *N Engl J Med*, **366**, 1647.

485 McDonald GB, Sharma P, Matthews DE, Shulman HM and Thomas ED (1984) Venocclusive disease of the liver after bone marrow transplantation: diagnosis, incidence, and predisposing factors. *Hepatology*, **4**, 116–122.

486 Kitchens CS (2004) Thrombocytopenia due to acute venous thromboembolism and its role in expanding the differential diagnosis of heparin-induced thrombocytopenia. *Am J Hematol*, **76**, 69–73.

487 Van der Stuyft P, Gianella A, Pirard M, Cespedes J, Lora J, Peredo C *et al.* (1999) Urbanisation of yellow fever in Santa Cruz, Bolivia. *Lancet*, **354**, 1559–1562.

488 Sexton DJ, Rollin PE, Breitschwerdt EB, Corey GR, Myers SA, Dumais MR *et al.* (1997) Life-threatening Cache Valley virus infection. *N Engl J Med*, **336**, 547–549.

489 Goh KJ, Tan CT, Chew NK, Tan PSK, Kamarulzaman A, Sarji SA *et al.* (2000) Clinical features of Nipah virus encephalitis among pig farmers in Malaysia. *N Engl J Med*, **342**, 1229–1235.

490 Charrel RN, de Lamballerie X and Raoult D (2007) Chikungunya outbreaks — the globalization of vectorborne diseases. *N Engl J Med*, **356**, 769–771.

491 Vyas JM, González RG and Pierce VM (2013) Case records of the Massachusetts General Hospital. Case 15-2013. A 76-year-old man with fever, worsening renal function, and altered mental status. *N Engl J Med*, **368**, 1919–1927.

492 Madani TA, Azhar EI, Abuelzein el-TM, Kao M, Al-Bar HM, Abu-Araki H *et al.* (2011) Alkhumra (Alkhurma) virus outbreak in Najran, Saudi Arabia: epidemiological, clinical, and laboratory characteristics. *J Infect*, **62**, 67–76.

493 Pinn TG and Sowden D (1998) Queensland tick typhus. *Aust NZ J Med*, **28**, 824–826.

494 Thiebaut MM, Bricaire F and Raoult D (1997) Scrub typhus after a trip to Vietnam. *N Engl J Med*, **336**, 1613–1614.

495 Roberts SA and Ellis-Pegler RB (1997) Murine typhus in the Kaukapakapa area again. *Aust NZ J Med*, **27**, 446–447.

496 Pritt BS, Sloan LM, Johnson DKH, Munderloh UG, Paskewitz SM, McElroy KM *et al.* (2011) Emergence of a new pathogenic Ehrlichia species, Wisconsin and Minnesota, 2009. *N Engl J Med*, **365**, 422–429.

497 Brouqui P, Lascola B, Roux V and Raoult D (1999) Chronic *Bartonella quintana* bacteremia in homeless patients. *N Engl J Med*, **340**, 184–189.

498 Bush LM, Abrams BH, Beall A and Johnson CC (2001) Index case of fatal inhalational anthrax due to bioterrorism in the United States. *N Engl J Med*, **345**, 1607–1610.

499 Sevinc A, Kutlu NO, Kuku I, Ozgen U, Aydogdu I and Soylu H (2000) Severe epistaxis in brucellosis-induced isolated thrombocytopenia: a report of two cases. *Clin Lab Haematol*, **22**, 373–375.

500 Serefhanoglu K, Kaya E, Sevinc A, Aydogdu I, Kuku I and Ersoy Y (2003) Isolated thrombocytopenia: the presenting feature of typhoid fever. *Clin Lab Haematol*, **25**, 63–65.

501 Tunbridge AJ, Dockrell DH, Channer KS and McKendrick MW (2002) A breathless triathlete. *Lancet*, **359**, 130.

502 Vonderheide RH, Thadhani R and Kuter DJ (1996) Association of thrombocytopenia and the use of intra-aortic balloon pump. *Blood*, **88**, Suppl. 1, 63b.

503 Turnbull A and Almeyda J (1970) Idiopathic thrombocytopenic purpura and Kaposi's sarcoma. *Proc R Soc Med*, **63**, 603–605.

504 Kimura H, Nasu K, Sakai C, Shiga Y, Miyamoto E, Shintaku M *et al.* (1998) Histiocytic sarcoma of the spleen associated with hypoalbuminemia, hypoγ-globulinemia and thrombocytopenia as a possibly unique clinical entity — report of three cases. *Leuk Lymphoma*, **31**, 217–224.

505 Baker GR and Levin J (1998) Transient thrombocytopenia produced by administration of macrophage colony-stimulating factor: investigations of the mechanism. *Blood*, **91**, 89–99.

506 Diaz-Sánchez CL, Lifshitz-Guinzberg A, Ignacio-Ibarra G, Halabe-Cherem J and Quinones-Galvan A (1998) Survival after massive (>2000) Africanized honeybee stings. *Arch Intern Med*, **158**, 925–927.

507 Clayton PT, Bowron A, Mills KA, Massoud A, Casteels M and Milla PJ (1993) Phytosterolaemia in children with parenteral nutrition-associated cholestatic liver disease. *Gastroenterology*, **105**, 1806–1813.

508 Auborg P (1994) Lorenzo's oil and thrombocytopenia. *N Engl J Med*, **330**, 577.

509 O'Brien H, Amess JAL and Mollin JD (1982) Recurrent thrombocytopenia, erythroid hypoplasia and sideroblastic anaemia associated with hypothermia. *Br J Haematol*, **51**, 451–456.

510 Jung J, Bohn G, Allroth A, Boztug K, Brandes G, Sandrock I *et al.* (2006) Identification of a homozygous deletion in the AP3B1 gene causing Hermansky-Pudlak syndrome, type 2. *Blood*, **108**, 362–369.

511 Dittman WA (2000) Congenital relapsing fever (*Borrelia hermsii* infection). *Blood*, **96**, 3333.

512 Willoughby MLN (1977) *Paediatric Haematology*. Churchill Livingstone, Edinburgh.

513 Neven B, Valayannopoulos V, Quartier P, Blanche S, Prieur AM, Debre M *et al.* (2007) Allogeneic bone marrow transplantation in mevalonic aciduria. *N Engl J Med*, **356**, 2700–2703.

514 Bader-Meunier B, Breton-Gorius B, Cramer E, Mielot F, Rötig A, Dommergues JP and Tchernia G (1997) Hematology: a clue to the diagnosis of mitochondrial cytopathies. *Blood*, **96**, Suppl. 1, 9b.

515 Hayward CP, Rivard GE, Kane WH, Drouin J, Zheng S, Moore JC and Kelton JG (1996) An autosomal dominant,

qualitative platelet disorder associated with multimerin deficiency, abnormalities in platelet factor V, thrombospondin, von Willebrand factor, and fibrinogen and an epinephrine aggregation defect. *Blood*, **87**, 4967–4978.

516 Shalev H, Kapelushnik J, Moser A, Dgany O, Krasnov T and Tamary H (2004) A comprehensive study of the neonatal manifestations of congenital dyserythropoietic anemia type I. *J Pediatr Hematol Oncol*, **26**, 746–748.

517 Zeidler C (2005) Congenital neutropenia. *Hematology*, **10**, Suppl. 1, 306–311.

518 Maurer HM, Fratkin M, McWilliams NB, Kirkpatrick D, Draper DW, Haggins JC and Hunter CR (1976) Effects of phototherapy on platelet counts in lowbirthweight infants and on platelet production and life span in rabbits. *Pediatrics*, **57**, 506–512.

519 Ballin A, Korea G, Kohelet D, Burger R, Greenwald M, Bryan AC and Zipursky A (1987) Reduction in platelet counts induced by mechanical ventilation in the newborn infants. *J Pediatr*, **111**, 445–449.

520 Yang J, Lee C-H, Yang M, Li K, Ng P-C, Yuen M-P and Fok T-F (2001) Association between thrombocytopenia and mechanical ventilation in infants with respiratory distress syndrome. *Blood*, **98**, 37a.

521 Carroll DN, Kamath P and Stewart L (2005) Congenital viral infection? *Lancet*, **365**, 1110.

522 Kurata Y, Nishioeda Y, Tsubakio T and Kitani T (1980) Thrombocytopenia in Graves' disease: effect of T_3 on platelet kinetics. *Acta Haematol*, **63**, 185–190.

523 Bowles KM, Turner GE and Wimperis JZ (2004) Resolution of chronic severe refractory thrombocytopenia after treatment of hypothyroidism. *J Clin Pathol*, **57**, 995–996.

524 Pei SX, Chen XJ, Si Ren BZ, Liu YH, Cheng XS, Harris EM *et al.* (1989) Chronic mountain sickness in Tibet. *Q J Med*, **71**, 555–574.

525 Takahashi N and Nishida H (1997) New exanthematous disease with thrombocytopenia in neonates. *Arch Dis Child Fetal Neonatal Ed*, **77**, F79.

526 Prella M, Baccalà R, Horisberger J-D, Belin D, di Raimondo F, Invernizzi R *et al.* (2001) Haemolytic onset of Wilson's disease in a patient with homozygous truncation of ATP7B at ARG1319. *Br J Haematol*, **114**, 230–232.

527 Fischereder M and Jaffe JP (1994) Thrombocytopenia following acute acetaminophen overdose. *Am J Hematol*, **45**, 258–259.

528 Acharya S and Bussel JB (2000) Hematologic toxicity of sodium valproate. *J Pediatr Hematol Oncol*, **22**, 62–65.

529 Pamuk GE, Donmez S, Turgut B, Demir M and Vural O (2005) Rituximab-induced acute thrombocytopenia in a patient with prolymphocytic leukemia. *Am J Hematol*, **78**, 81.

530 Shah C and Grethlein SJ (2004) Case report of rituximab-induced thrombocytopenia. *Am J Hematol*, **75**, 263.

531 Smith KA, Nelson PN, Warren P, Astley SJ, Murray PG and Greenman J (2004) Demystified… recombinant antibodies. *J Clin Pathol*, **57**, 912–917.

532 Cathomas R, Goldhirsch A and von Moos R (2007) Drug-induced immune thrombocytopenia. *N Engl J Med*, **358**, 1869–1870.

533 Azuno Y, Yaga K, Sasayama T and Kimoto K (1999) Thrombocytopenia induced by Jui, a traditional Chinese herbal medicine. *Lancet*, **354**, 304–305.

534 http://www.ouhsc.edu/platelets/index.html (accessed June 2014).

535 Ranjith MP, Divya R, Mehta VK, Krishnan MG, KamalRaj R and Kavishwar A (2009) Significance of platelet volume indices and platelet count in ischaemic heart disease. *J Clin Pathol*, **62**, 830–833.

536 Hohlfeld P, Forestier F, Kaplan C, Tissot JD and Daffos F (1994) Fetal thrombocytopenia: a retrospective survey of 5,194 fetal blood samplings. *Blood*, **84**, 1851–1856.

537 Roberts I, Stanworth S and Murray NA (2008) Thrombocytopenia in the neonate. *Blood Rev*, **22**, 173–186.

538 Chakravorty S and Roberts I (2012) How I manage neonatal thrombocytopenia. *Br J Haematol*, **156**, 155–162.

539 Nunes P, Palaré MJ, Aguilar S, Ferrao A, Medeira A and Morais A (2011) Serious thrombocytopenia as hematological manifestation of Noonan syndrome. *Haematologica*, **96**, Suppl. 2, 651.

540 Chng WJ and Howard MR (2001) Pel-Ebstein fever with cyclical pancytopenia. *J R Soc Med*, **94**, 84–85.

541 Gonzalez CH, Durkin-Stamm MV, Geimer NF, Shahidi NT, Schilling RF, Rubira F and Opitz JM (1977) The WT syndrome—a "'new" autosomal dominant pleiotropic trait of radial/ulnar hypoplasia with high risk of bone marrow failure and/or leukemia. *Birth Defects Orig Artic Ser*, **13**(3B), 31–38.

542 Ihara K, Ishii I, Eguchi M, Takada H, Suminoe A, Good RA and Hara T (1999) Identification of mutations in the c-mpl gene in congenital amegakaryocytic thrombocytopenia. *Proc Natl Acad Sci USA*, **96**, 3132–3136.

543 González-del Angel A, Cervera M, Gómez L, Pérez-Vera P, Orozco L, Carnevale A, Del Castillo V (2000) Ataxia-pancytopenia syndrome. *Am J Med Genet*, **90**, 252–254.

544 Press OW, Fingert H, Lott IT and Dickersin R (1983) Pancytopenia in mannosidosis. *Arch Intern Med*, **143**, 1266–1268.

545 Hricik DE and Hussain R (1984) Pancytopenia and hepatosplenomegaly in oxalosis. *Arch Intern Med*, **144**, 167–168.

546 Kelleher JF, Yudkoff M, Hutchinson R, August CS and Cohn RM (1980) The pancytopenia of isovaleric acidemia. *Pediatrics*, **65**, 1023–1027.

547 Walter MJ and Dang CV (1998) Pancytopenia secondary to oxalosis in a 23-year-old woman. *Blood*, **91**, 4394.

548 Emadi A, Burns KH, Confer B and Borowitz MJ (2008) Hematological manifestations of nephropathic cystinosis. *Acta Haematol*, **19**, 169–172.

549 Blatt J, Katerji A, Barmada M, Wenger SL and Penchansky L (1994) Pancytopenia and vacuolation of marrow precursors associated with necrotizing encephalopathy. *Br J Haematol*, **86**, 207–209.

550 Kind T, Levy J, Lee M, Kaicker S, Nicholson J and Kane SA (2002) Cobalamin C disease presenting as hemolytic-uremic syndrome in the neonatal period. *J Pediatr Hematol Oncol*, **24**, 327–329.

551 Çetin M, Hiçsönmez G and Gögüs S (1998) Myelodysplastic syndrome associated with Griscelli syndrome. *Leuk Res*, **22**, 859–862.

552 Bazarbachi A, Muakkit S, Ayas M, Taher A, Salem Z, Solh H and Haidar JH (1998) Thiamine-responsive myelodysplasia. *Br J Haematol*, **102**, 1098–1100.

553 Ferrari E, Ascari E, Bossolo PA and Barosi G (1976) Sheehan's syndrome with complete bone marrow aplasia: long-term results of substitution therapy with hormones. *Br J Haematol*, **33**, 575–582.

554 Srinivas U, Pillai LS, Kumar R, Pati HP and Saxena R (2007) Bone marrow aplasia—a rare complication of imatinib therapy in CML patients. *Am J Hematol*, **82**, 314–316.

555 Basser RL, O'Flaherty E, Green M, Edmonds M, Nichol J, Menchaca DM et al. (2002) Development of pancytopenia with neutralizing antibodies to thrombopoietin after multicycle chemotherapy supported by megakaryocyte growth and development factor. *Blood*, **99**, 2599–2602.

556 Resuke WH, Anderson C, Pastuszak WT, Conway SR and Firshein SI (1991) Arsenic intoxication presenting as a myelodysplastic syndrome: a case report. *Am J Hematol*, **36**, 291–293.

557 Case records of the Massachusetts General Hospital (1989) Case 33–1989. *N Engl J Med*, **321**, 454–463.

558 Millá F, Feliu E, Ribera JM, Junta J, Flores A, Vidal J et al. (1993) Electron microscopic identification of parvovirus virions in erythroid and granulocytic-line cells in a patient with human parvovirus B19 induced pancytopenia. *Leuk Lymphoma*, **10**, 483–487.

559 Harkess JR (1993) Ehrlichiosis: a cause of bone marrow hypoplasia in humans. *Am J Hematol*, **30**, 265–266.

560 Gaines P, Thomas V, Fikrig E and Berliner N (2005) Infection with *Anaplasma phagocytophilum* inhibits proliferation and differentiation of myeloid progenitors: new insights into infection-related pancytopenia. *Blood*, **106**, 858a.

561 Al-Eissa YA, Assuhaimi SA, Al-Fawaz IM, Higgy KE, AI-Nasser MN and Al-Mobaireck KF (1993) Pancytopenia in children with brucellosis: clinical manifestations and bone marrow findings. *Acta Haematol*, **89**, 132–136.

562 Bilgrami S, Almeida GD, Quinn JJ, Tuck D, Bergstrom S, Dainiak N et al. (1994) Pancytopenia in allogeneic marrow transplant recipients: role of cytomegalovirus. *Br J Haematol*, **87**, 357–362.

563 Gompels UA, Luxton J, Knox KK and Carrigan DR (1994) Chronic bone marrow suppression in immunocompetent adult by human herpesvirus 6. *Lancet*, **343**, 735–736.

564 Thaunat O, Mamzer-Bruneel MF, Agbalika F, Valensi F, Venditto M, Lebbe C et al. (2006) Severe human herpesvirus-8 primary infection in a renal transplant patient successfully treated with anti-CD20 monoclonal antibody. *Blood*, **107**, 3009–3010.

565 Silveira P, Esteves I, Assis R, Pires F, Alanna A, Colombini M *et al.* (2010) Toxoplasmosis as a cause of pancytopenia in immunosuppressed patients. *Haematologica,* **95**, Suppl. 2, 734.

566 Martinez E, Domingo P and Ruiz D (1991) Transient aplastic anaemia associated with legionnaires' disease. *Lancet,* **338**, 264.

567 Ozkan A, Ozkalemkas F, Ali R, Karadogan S, Ozkocaman V, Ozcelik T and Tunali A (2006) Mediterranean spotted fever: presentation with pancytopenia. *Am J Hematol,* **81**, 646–647.

568 Cohen JI, Jaffe ES, Dale JK, Pittaluga S, Heslop HE, Rooney CM *et al.* (2011) Characterization and treatment of chronic active Epstein-Barr virus disease: a 28-year experience in the United States. *Blood,* **117**, 5835–5849.

569 Hasle H, Kerndrup G, Jacobsen BB, Heegaard ED, Hornsleth A and Lillevang ST (1994) Chronic parvovirus infection mimicking myelodysplastic syndrome in a child with subclinical immunodeficiency. *Am J Pediatr Hematol Oncol,* **16**, 329–333.

570 Hoagland HC and Goldstein NP (1978) Hematologic (cytopenic) manifestations of Wilson's disease (hepatolenticular degeneration). *Mayo Clin Proc,* **53**, 498–500.

571 Wiesneth M, Pflieger H, Frickhofen N and Heimpel H (1985) Idiopathic combined immunocytopenia. *Br J Haematol,* **61**, 339–348.

572 van der Werff ten Bosch J, Delabie J, Böhler T, Verschuere J and Thielemans K (1999) Revision of the diagnosis of T-zone lymphoma in the father of a patient with autoimmune lymphoproliferative syndrome type II. *Br J Haematol,* **106**, 1045–1048.

573 Barrett AJ (1987) Graft-versus-host disease: a review. *J Roy Soc Med,* **80**, 368–373.

574 Bigorgne C, Le Tourneau A, Messing B, Rio B, Giraud V, Molina T *et al.* (1996) Sea-blue histiocyte syndrome in bone marrow secondary to total parenteral nutrition including fat-emulsion sources: a clinicopathologic study of seven cases. *Br J Haematol,* **95**, 258–262.

575 Talansky AL, Schulman P, Vinciguerra VP, Margouleff D, Budman DR and Degman TJ (1981) Pancytopenia complicating Graves' disease and drug-induced hypothyroidism (sic). *Arch Intern Med,* **141**, 544–545.

576 Ruocco L, Baldi N, Ceccone A, Marini A, Azzara A, Ambrogi F and Grassi B (1986) Severe pancytopenia due to copper deficiency. *Acta Haematol,* **76**, 224–226.

577 Lo L, Singer S and Vichinsky E (2002) Pancytopenia induced by hypothermia. *J Pediatr Hematol Oncol,* **24**, 681–684.

578 Murrin RJA and Harrison P (2004) Abnormal osteoclasts and bone marrow fibrosis in Paget's disease of bone. *Br J Haematol,* **124**, 3.

579 Lim D-J, Oh EJ, Park C-W, Kwon H-S, Hong E-J, Yoon K-H *et al.* (2007) Pancytopenia and secondary myelofibrosis could be induced by primary hyperparathyroidism. *Int J Lab Hematol,* **29**, 464–468.

CHAPTER 7
Important supplementary tests

Peripheral blood cells can be used for many other tests, which supplement the full blood count (FBC) and May–Grünwald–Giemsa (MGG)-stained blood film. These include cytochemical tests, immunophenotyping, cytogenetic analysis, molecular genetic analysis and ultrastructural examination. Only those techniques that involve counting or examining cells will be dealt with in any detail in this chapter.

Cytochemical techniques

Some recommended techniques for cytochemical stains are given in Table 7.1. Reticulocyte counting and staining are dealt with in Chapter 2. The application of other cytochemical stains will be discussed in this chapter.

Table 7.1 Some recommended methods for cytochemical stains.

Procedure	Recommended method
Heinz body preparation	Rhodanile blue with 2 minutes' incubation [1] or methyl violet
Haemoglobin H preparation	Brilliant cresyl blue with 2 hours' incubation [1]
Haemoglobin F-containing cells	Acid elution [1]
Perls reaction for iron	Potassium ferrocyanide [1]
Myeloperoxidase	p-phenylenediamine + catechol + H_2O_2 [2]
Sudan black B	Sudan black B [1]
Naphthol AS-D chloroacetate esterase (chloroacetate esterase)	Naphthol AS-D chloroacetate + hexazotised fuchsin [3] or fast blue BB [4] or Corinth V
α naphthyl acetate esterase	α naphthyl acetate + hexazotised pararosaniline [3] or fast blue RR
Neutrophil alkaline phosphatase	Naphthol AS-MX phosphate + fast blue RR
Periodic acid–Schiff (PAS)	Periodic acid + Schiff's reagent [1]
Acid phosphatase and tartrate-resistant acid phosphatase	Naphthol AS-BI phosphate + fast garnet GBC, with and without tartaric acid [5]

Reagents suitable for cytochemical stains can be purchased from Sigma–Aldrich

Heinz bodies

Heinz bodies are red cell inclusions composed of denatured haemoglobin. They can be seen as refractile bodies in dry unstained films viewed with the condenser lowered. Their presence can often be suspected from features seen on an MGG-stained film. They can be stained by a number of vital dyes, including methyl violet, cresyl violet, 'new methylene blue', brilliant cresyl blue, brilliant green and rhodanile blue. Their characteristic shape and size (Fig. 7.1; see also Table 2.3) aid in their identification. Heinz bodies are not seen in normal subjects since they are removed by the splenic macrophages in a process often known as 'pitting'. Small numbers are seen in the blood of splenectomised subjects. Larger numbers are found following exposure to oxidant drugs, particularly in subjects who are glucose-6-phosphate dehydrogenase (G6PD) deficient or who have been splenectomised. They may also be seen post-splenectomy in patients with an unstable haemoglobin. Patients with an unstable haemoglobin

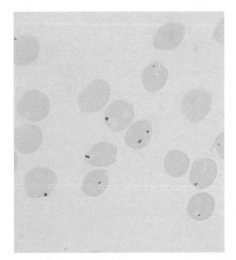

Fig. 7.1 A methyl violet preparation showing Heinz bodies in a patient exposed to the oxidant drug, dapsone. By courtesy of the late Dr David Swirsky and Mr David Roper, London.

Blood Cells A Practical Guide, Fifth Edition. By Barbara J. Bain © 2015 John Wiley & Sons, Ltd. Published 2015 by John Wiley & Sons, Ltd.
Companion Website: www.wiley.com/go/bain/bloodcells

who have not been splenectomised sometimes, but not always, show Heinz bodies; in some patients they form *in vitro* during prolonged incubation.

A stain for Heinz bodies is indicated when Heinz body-haemolytic anaemia is suspected. However, sometimes this diagnosis is readily evident from the clinical history and the MGG-stained film and the test is then redundant.

Haemoglobin H inclusions

Haemoglobin H (an abnormal haemoglobin with no α chains but with a β chain tetramer) is denatured and stained by the same vital dyes that stain reticulocytes. The characteristic regular 'golf-ball' inclusions (Fig. 7.2a) take longer to appear than the reticulum of

a reticulocyte. An incubation period of 2 hours is recommended. It is important that either new methylene blue or brilliant cresyl blue is used to demonstrate the characteristic inclusions. Methylene blue (which has been sold by manufacturers wrongly identified as new methylene blue) does not give the typical appearance [6]. Patients with haemoglobin H disease who have not been splenectomised show the characteristic golf-ball appearance, whereas post-splenectomy patients have, in addition, Heinz bodies that represent preformed inclusions of haemoglobin H (Fig. 7.2b). Cells containing haemoglobin H are readily detected in patients with haemoglobin H disease, in whom they may form the majority of cells. In patients with α thalassaemia trait,

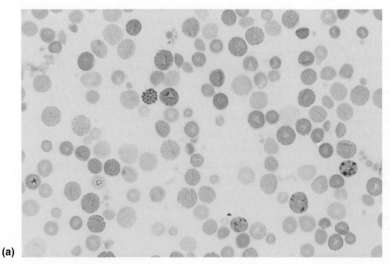

(a)

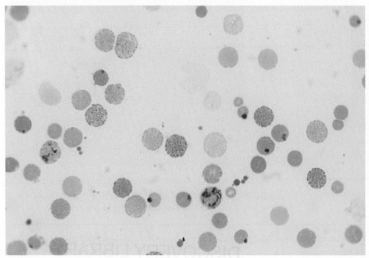

(b)

Fig. 7.2 Haemoglobin H preparations showing: (a) haemoglobin H-containing cells (containing multiple small pale blue inclusions) and reticulocytes (with a purple reticular network) in a patient with haemoglobin H disease; and (b) haemoglobin H-containing cells, a reticulocyte and Heinz bodies (large peripherally placed blue inclusions) in the blood of a patient with haemoglobin H disease who had been splenectomised.

their frequency is of the order of 1 in 1000 cells (when two of the four α genes are missing) or less (when one of the four α genes is missing); even when a prolonged search is made, they are not always detectable, particularly in individuals who lack only a single α gene. Haemoglobin H inclusions are not found in the red cells of haematologically normal subjects; apparently similar cells may be seen, however, in very occasional cells in normal subjects so that a control normal sample should be incubated in parallel with the patient's sample.

The identification of occasional haemoglobin H-containing cells may be useful in the diagnosis of α thalassaemia. However, the search for infrequent inclusion-containing cells is very time-consuming and, when the diagnosis is important, e.g. for genetic counselling, definitive confirmation by DNA analysis is required.

Haemoglobin F-containing cells

Haemoglobin F-containing cells are identified cytochemically by their resistance to haemoglobin elution in acid conditions (Fig. 7.3); the procedure is commonly referred to as a Kleihauer test from its originator, although Kleihauer's method is often modified. The test is useful for detecting fetal cells in the maternal circulation and thus for detecting and quantitating fetomaternal haemorrhage; it is indicated for the detection of fetomaternal haemorrhage in unexplained neonatal anaemia and for quantifying fetomaternal haemorrhage from an Rh D-positive fetus to an Rh D-negative mother. The Kleihauer test will also detect autologous cells containing appreciable quantities of haemoglobin F, such as may be seen in hereditary persistence of fetal haemoglobin and β thalassaemia, and in some patients with thalassaemia major, δβ thalassaemia trait, sickle cell disease, juvenile chronic myelomonocytic leukaemia, myelodysplastic syndromes (MDS) and various other conditions. The distribution of haemoglobin F in adult cells may be homogeneous (in some types of hereditary persistence of fetal haemoglobin) or heterogeneous (in other types of hereditary persistence of fetal haemoglobin and in other conditions). Both a positive and a negative control should be tested in parallel with the sample under investigation. A positive control can be prepared by mixing together adult and fetal cells.

It should be noted that a Kleihauer test cannot be used for detection of fetal cells in the maternal circulation if the mother already has a positive Kleihaeur test as a result of a high level of haemoglobin F.

Perls reaction for iron

Perls stain is based on a reaction between acid ferrocyanide and the ferric ion (Fe^{3+}) of haemosiderin to form ferric ferrocyanide, which has an intense blue colour (Prussian blue). Ferritin, which is soluble, does not give a positive reaction. Perls stain is most often performed on the bone marrow, but it can be used to stain peripheral blood cells in order to detect sideroblasts and siderocytes.

On a Romanowsky-stained blood film, haemosiderin appears as small blue granules, designated Pappenheimer bodies (see Chapter 3). On a Perls stain they are

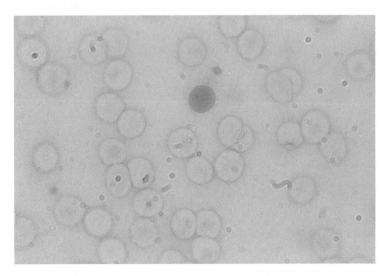

Fig. 7.3 Acid elution technique (Kleihauer test) for haemoglobin F-containing cells; the blood specimen was taken from a post-partum woman and shows that a fetomaternal haemorrhage had occurred. A single stained fetal cell is seen against a background of ghosts of maternal cells.

referred to as siderotic granules and the cells containing them are known as siderocytes (Fig. 7.4a). Siderocytes are rarely detected in the blood of normal subjects; siderotic granules are present in reticulocytes newly released from the bone marrow, but disappear during maturation of the reticulocyte in the spleen, probably because the haemosiderin is utilised for further haemoglobin synthesis. When haematologically normal subjects are splenectomised, small numbers of siderocytes are seen in the blood. When red cells containing abnormally large or numerous siderotic granules are released from the bone marrow, as in sideroblastic anaemia or in thalassaemia major, many of the abnormal inclusions are 'pitted' by the spleen. Some remain detectable in the

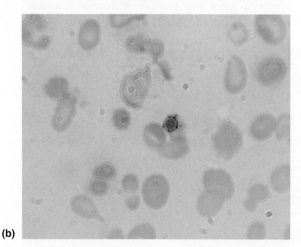

(a)

(b)

Fig. 7.4 Perls stain showing: (a) siderocytes (cells containing fine blue dots) in the blood of a patient with thalassaemia major; and (b) a ring sideroblast in the blood of a patient with sideroblastic anaemia.

peripheral blood, both in reticulocytes and in mature red cells. If a patient with a defect of iron incorporation has been splenectomised or is hyposplenic for any reason, very numerous siderocytes are seen.

A sideroblast is a nucleated red blood cell (NRBC) that contains siderotic granules. Sideroblasts are normally present in the bone marrow, but NRBCs do not normally circulate and it is therefore unusual to see sideroblasts in the peripheral blood. When they do appear, they may be morphologically normal, containing only one or a few fine granules, or abnormal, with the granules being increased in number, size or both. Abnormal sideroblasts include ring sideroblasts in which siderotic granules are present in a ring immediately adjacent to the nuclear membrane (Fig. 7.4b). When NRBCs are present in the peripheral blood, the film can be stained with a Perls stain to allow any siderotic granules present to be identified reliably. Abnormal sideroblasts may be detected in the peripheral blood in sideroblastic anaemia, megaloblastic anaemia and β thalassaemia major. They are seen in larger numbers when there is also an absent or hypofunctional spleen. Sideroblastic anaemia is usually diagnosed by bone marrow aspiration, but strong support for the diagnosis is obtained if ring sideroblasts are detected in the peripheral blood, if necessary in a buffy coat preparation in which any NRBCs are concentrated.

Glucose-6-phosphate dehydrogenase

A cytochemical stain for G6PD is useful in detecting females who are heterozygous for G6PD deficiency [7]. Although the G6PD assay may be normal, a cytochemical stain shows that there is a population of normal cells and a population of deficient cells.

Cytochemical stains used in the diagnosis and classification of leukaemias

Cytochemical stains used in the diagnosis and classification of leukaemias can be applied to both the bone marrow and peripheral blood. Studies of peripheral blood cells are needed when bone marrow aspiration is difficult or impossible. In other circumstances, studies of peripheral blood and bone marrow are complementary. Cytochemical stains for neutrophil alkaline phosphatase are performed on the peripheral blood. Cytochemical stains are much less needed for the investigation of leukaemia since flow cytometric immunophenotyping has become widely available, but remain important when there is no ready access to immunophenotyping. A myeloperoxidase or Sudan black B (SBB) stain remains useful for the identification of Auer rods.

Neutrophil alkaline phosphatase

This stain is redundant if there is access to molecular or cytogenetic analysis for the detection of *BCR-ABL1* or t(9;22)(q34;q11.2).

Mature neutrophils, but not eosinophils, have alkaline phosphatase in specific cytoplasmic organelles [8], which have been called secretory vesicles or phosphosomes. Neutrophil alkaline phosphatase (NAP) has sometimes been referred to as leucocyte alkaline phosphatase, but the former designation is more accurate since it is the neutrophils that are assessed. A number of cytochemical stains can be used for demonstrating NAP activity. One suitable stain is that recommended by Ackerman [9], which permits grading of alkaline phosphatase activity, as shown in Table 7.2 and Fig. 7.5, to give an NAP score that falls between 0 and 400. The normal range is dependent on the substrate used. With the above method it is of the order of 30–180. It is preferable for NAP scores to be determined on either native or heparinised blood. The cytochemical reaction should be carried out within 8 hours of obtaining the blood specimen but, if this is not possible, the films can be fixed and stored, in the dark, at room temperature. Ethylenediaminetetra-acetic acid (EDTA)-anticoagulated blood is not ideal as enzyme activity is inhibited; if it is used, the films should be made within 10–20 minutes of obtaining the blood, but even then there is some loss of activity. Low, normal and high controls should be stained in parallel with the patient's sample. A low control can be obtained from a patient

with chronic myelogenous leukaemia (CML), or can be prepared by immersing an appropriately fixed film of normal blood in boiling water for 1 minute. A high control can be obtained from a patient with infection or from a pregnant or postpartum woman or from a woman taking oral contraceptives. Positive and negative control films, which have been appropriately fixed and wrapped in Parafilm, can be stored at −70°C for at least 1 year.

Some of the causes of high and low NAP scores are shown in Table 7.3. Synthesis of NAP messenger ribonucleic acid (mRNA) is stimulated by granulocyte colony-stimulating factor (G-CSF) but inhibited by granulocyte-macrophage colony-stimulating factor (GM-CSF), interleukin 3 (IL3) and interferon. The low NAP score sometimes seen in viral infections may reflect the effect of interferon. Neonates have very high NAP scores, usually exceeding 200. A fall to levels more typical of childhood occurs between 5 and 10 months of age [15]. Premature and low birth-weight babies have lower scores than full-term babies. Children have higher NAP scores than adults, with a gradual fall to adult levels occurring before puberty [16]. Women in the reproductive age range have higher NAP scores than men, with the score varying with the menstrual cycle (Fig. 7.6). After the menopause, NAP scores of women approach those of men (Fig. 7.7) [16,17].

The NAP score is low in 95% of patients with CML. The test is useful in distinguishing between CML and other chronic myeloproliferative neoplasms, which usually have a normal or elevated NAP score, and between CML and reactive neutrophilia, since the latter almost invariably has a high score. Patients with CML may have a normal or elevated NAP during pregnancy, postoperatively (particularly following splenectomy), during bacterial infection, when the bone marrow is rendered hypoplastic by

Table 7.2 Scoring neutrophil alkaline phosphatase (NAP) activity (after Kaplow [10]); 100 neutrophils are scored as shown.

Score of cell	Percentage of cytoplasm occupied by precipitated dye	Size of granules	Intensity of staining	Cytoplasmic background
0	None	–	None	Colourless
1	50	Small	Faint to moderate	Colourless to very pale blue
2	50–80	Small	Moderate to strong	Colourless to pale blue
3	80–100	Medium to large	Strong	Colourless to blue
4	100	Medium and large	Very strong	Not visible

Following the scoring of individual neutrophils, the scores are summed to produce the final NAP score. This is most easily done by multiplying each score by the number of cells having that score and adding the results together.

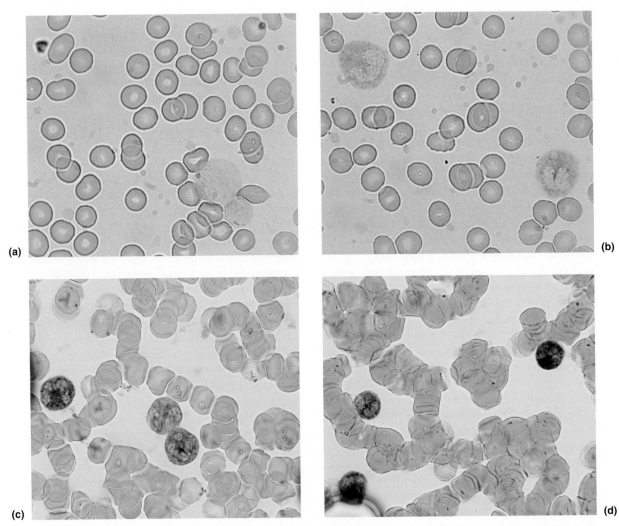

Fig. 7.5 Neutrophil alkaline phosphatase (NAP) reaction (method of Ackerman [9]) showing cells with reactions graded 0 to 4: (a) neutrophil with a score of 0 plus a lymphocyte, which is also negative; (b) two band cells with a score of 1; (c) two neutrophils with a score of 2 and one with a score of 3; and (d) two neutrophils with a score of 4 and one with a score of 2.

chemotherapy, and following the onset of transformation. However, it should be noted that, when cytogenetic and molecular genetic analysis are available, the NAP score is redundant even in the investigation of suspected CML.

The NAP score may be of use in distinguishing between polycythaemia vera, which usually has an elevated score, and secondary polycythaemia, in which the score is more likely to be normal. However, when molecular analysis for a *JAK2* mutation is available, the NAP is redundant. In multiple myeloma, the increased NAP score correlates with disease activity.

Myeloperoxidase

Peroxidases are enzymes that catalyse the oxidation of substrates by hydrogen peroxide. The granules of neutrophils and eosinophils contain peroxidases, which are designated leucocyte peroxidase or myeloperoxidase (MPO). The demonstration of MPO activity is useful in establishing and confirming the diagnosis of acute myeloid leukaemia (AML), since lymphoblasts are uniformly negative. Myeloperoxidase was initially demonstrated with benzidine or one of its derivatives as a substrate. A suitable non-carcinogenic substrate used in the method

Table 7.3 Some causes of high and low neutrophil alkaline phosphatase (NAP) scores [4,10].

High NAP	Low NAP
Inherited conditions	
Down syndrome	Inherited hypophosphatasia (NAP absent)
	Specific granule (lactoferrin) deficiency [11]
	Isolated primary NAP deficiency [12]
	Grey platelet syndrome (some families) [13]
Physiological effects	
Cord blood and neonate	
Mid-cycle in menstruating females	
Oral contraceptive intake	
Pregnancy and the postpartum period	
Reactive changes	
Bacterial infection	Some cases of infectious mononucleosis and other viral
Inflammation	infections
Surgery and trauma, tissue infarction, burns and other tissue damage	
Corticosteroids and ACTH administration and acute stress	
Leukaemoid reactions including those due to ectopic secretion of G-CSF, e.g. in multiple myeloma [14]	
Administration of G-CSF	
Carcinomatosis	
Acute lymphoblastic leukaemia	
Most cases of aplastic anaemia	Some cases of aplastic anaemia
Hairy cell leukaemia	
Some cases of chronic lymphocytic leukaemia	
Some cases of monoclonal gammopathy of undetermined significance	
Hodgkin lymphoma	
Hepatic cirrhosis (particularly when decompensated)	
Myeloid neoplasms	
Neutrophilic leukaemia	Chronic myelogenous leukaemia
Some cases of atypical chronic myeloid leukaemia	Most cases of atypical chronic myeloid leukaemia
Some cases of AML, particularly acute monoblastic leukaemia	Some cases of AML, particularly when there is differentiation
Most cases of primary myelofibrosis	Some cases of primary myelofibrosis
Some cases of MDS	Some cases of MDS
Some cases of JMML	Some cases of JMML
Some cases of essential thrombocythaemia	Paroxysmal nocturnal haemoglobinuria
Most cases of polycythaemia vera	

ACTH, adrenocorticotropic hormone; AML, acute myeloid leukaemia; G-CSF, granulocyte colony-stimulating factor; JMML, juvenile myelomonocytic leukaemia; MDS, myelodysplastic syndrome

of Hanker *et al.* [2] is p-phenylene diamine, which produces a brownish-black reaction product. Myeloperoxidase is demonstrated in neutrophils and their precursors (Fig. 7.8), eosinophils and their precursors and the precursors of basophils. In neutrophils and eosinophils the primary granules have peroxidase activity and in eosinophils this is also true of secondary granules. Neutrophil and eosinophil peroxidases differ from each other, e.g. in their pH optima and in their sensitivity to inhibition by cyanide. The peroxidase activity of eosinophils is stronger than that of neutrophils. Auer rods are peroxidase-positive. In the

monocyte lineage, peroxidase activity is detectable at the promonocyte stage. Monocytes and promonocytes have fewer peroxidase-positive granules than neutrophils and their precursors. Inherited deficiency of neutrophil peroxidase is quite common. Deficiencies of eosinophil peroxidase and monocyte peroxidase also occur.

An acquired peroxidase deficiency may be seen in AML and MDS. Although it cannot be excluded that a patient has acute lymphoblastic leukaemia (ALL) and a coincidental congenital peroxidase deficiency, the demonstration of peroxidase-deficient mature cells

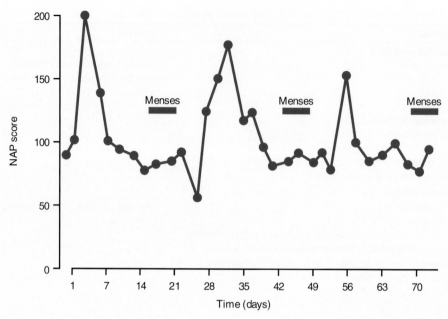

Fig. 7.6 Changes in NAP score during the menstrual cycle.

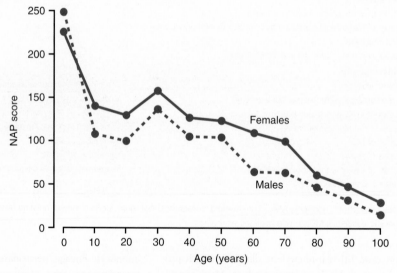

Fig. 7.7 Changes in NAP score with age in men and women. Data from Stavridis *et al.* [17].

nevertheless provides indirect evidence that an apparently undifferentiated leukaemia is actually AML of French–American–British (FAB) M0 category.

It should be noted that when a laboratory uses an automated haematology analyser employing peroxidase cytochemistry, such as Siemens H.1 and Advia series instruments, the instrument scatterplots can be useful for detecting both peroxidase activity in blast cells and peroxidase-deficient neutrophils.

Sudan black B

Sudan black B (SBB) (Fig. 7.9) has an affinity for poly-morphonuclear and monocyte granules. In general, the intensity of a positive staining reaction parallels

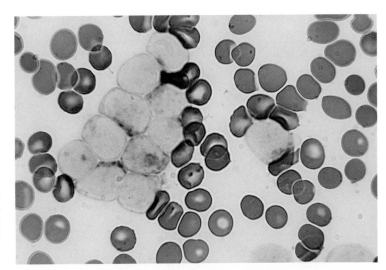

Fig. 7.8 Leukaemic blast cells stained by the Hanker technique [2] for myeloperoxidase showing a brownish-black deposit in the cytoplasm. This was a case of acute myeloid leukaemia (AML) of French–American–British (FAB) M2 category.

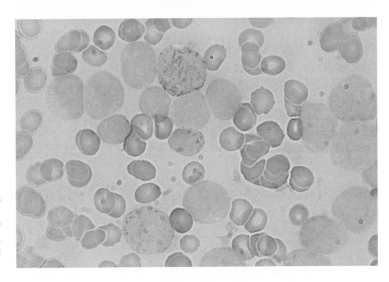

Fig. 7.9 Leukaemic blasts cells stained with Sudan black B (SBB). One large blast cell contains both granules and Auer rods. Several other blasts contain granules. The cells of this case, which was acute myeloid leukaemia of FAB M1 category, had very few granules and only rare Auer rods visible on a May–Grünwald–Giemsa (MGG)-stained film.

MPO activity. SBB staining is slightly more sensitive than MPO in the detection of myeloblasts. SBB stains the granules of neutrophils (both the primary and the specific granules) and the specific granules of eosinophils and, to a variable extent, the specific granules of basophils. The staining of eosinophil granules may be peripheral, with the central core remaining unstained. Auer rods are stained. Monoblasts are either negative or show a few small SBB-positive granules. Promonocytes and monocytes have a variable number of fine, positively staining granules. In hereditary neutrophil, eosinophil and monocyte peroxidase deficiencies, the granules of cells of the deficient lineages are SBB-negative. Lymphoblasts can have occasional fine positive dots, which may represent mitochondria [4]. Very rarely a stronger reaction is seen in the lymphoblasts of ALL [18] or in lymphoma cells of T or B lineage [19]. MPO and SBB staining can be used not only to demonstrate that an apparently undifferentiated leukaemia is myeloid, but also to provide evidence of granulocytic dysplasia, when mature neutrophil are shown to be negative [20] (Fig. 7.10). For practical purposes these two stains are equivalent and a laboratory needs only one or the other.

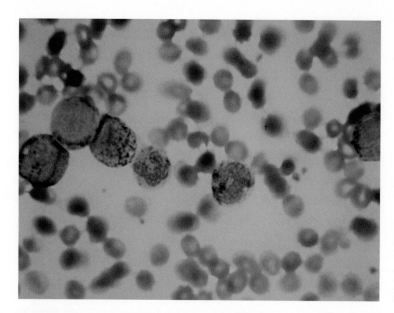

Fig. 7.10 Peripheral blood film from a patient with acute myeloid leukaemia stained with SBB, showing two blast cells that are positive. The presence of neutrophils that are largely or entirely SBB-negative demonstrates dysplastic neutrophil maturation.

Naphthol AS-D chloroacetate esterase

Naphthol AS-D chloroacetate esterase ('chloroacetate esterase', CAE) activity is found in neutrophils and their precursors (Fig. 7.11) and in mast cells. Auer rods are sometimes positive, but this stain is much less useful that the SBB and MPO reactions for the detection of

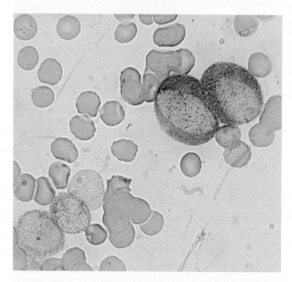

Fig. 7.11 Leukaemic blast cells stained for chloroacetate esterase (CAE) activity, using Corinth V as the dye. This was a case of AML of FAB M2 category.

Auer rods. Normal eosinophils and basophils are negative, but the eosinophils of certain types of eosinophil leukaemia may be positive. Monocytes are usually negative, but may show a weak reactivity. CAE is generally less sensitive than either MPO or SBB in the detection of myeloblasts, although occasional cases have been noted to be positive for CAE despite being MPO-negative [3,4].

Non-specific esterases

Esterase activity is common in haemopoietic cells. Nine isoenzymes have been demonstrated, of which four are found in neutrophils and are responsible for their CAE activity. Five are found in monocytes and a variety of other cells and the esterase activity of these cells has been designated 'non-specific' esterase [4,21]. Different isoenzymes are preferentially detected by different substrates and at different pHs. The most useful cytochemical reaction to detect the esterase activity of monocytes is α-naphthyl acetate esterase (ANAE) activity at acid pH (Fig. 7.12). α-naphthyl butyrate esterase (ANBE) activity is quite similar. With ANAE, strongly positive reactions are given by monocytes and their precursors and by megakaryocytes and platelets. Weaker reactions are given by plasma cells. ANBE is more often negative with megakaryocytes and platelets than is ANAE. Monocyte and megakaryocyte non-specific esterase activity can also be detected as naphthol AS-D acetate

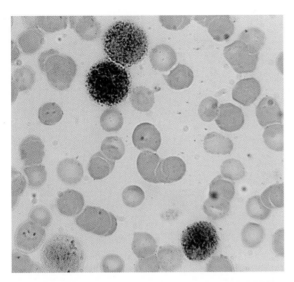

Fig. 7.12 Leukaemic blast cells stained for α-naphthyl acetate esterase (ANAE) activity using fast RR as the dye. This was a case of AML of FAB M5 category.

(NASDA) esterase activity or the very similar naphthol AS acetate (NASA) esterase. NASDA esterase is weakly positive in neutrophils and their precursors. It is therefore less suitable than ANAE for differentiating between the monocyte lineage and the neutrophil lineage; the specificity of the test can be improved by carrying out the reaction with and without fluoride, since the monocyte and megakaryocyte enzymes are inhibited by fluoride whereas the neutrophil enzyme is fluoride-resistant. The ANAE activity of monocytes and megakaryocytes is also fluoride-sensitive, but ANAE permits a clearer distinction between monocytes and neutrophils and the addition of fluoride is not necessary. Non-specific esterase activity is often demonstrable in normal T lymphocytes and also in acute and chronic leukaemias of T lineage. With ANAE, a characteristic dot positivity is often demonstrable in T-lineage ALL and T-prolymphocytic leukaemia; ANAE is superior to NASDA esterase in this regard [15], but this use of esterase cytochemistry is largely redundant since immunophenotyping is now widely available. The abnormal erythroblasts of erythroleukaemia or megaloblastic anaemia may also have non-specific esterase activity.

Combined esterase

A combined reaction for ANAE and CAE activities permits both reactions to be studied on the one blood film and is useful in characterising acute leukaemias. The monocytic and granulocytic differentiation of FAB M4 AML (acute myelomonocytic leukaemia) is clearly seen. The demonstration of an increased percentage (more than 3%) of cells staining for both chloroacetate esterase and non-specific esterase can provide evidence of MDS and in one reported patient provided evidence that an apparently undifferentiated leukaemia was actually myeloid, of FAB M0 category [22].

Periodic acid-Schiff reaction

The periodic acid-Schiff (PAS) reaction stains a variety of carbohydrates, including the glycogen that is often found in haemopoietic cells. The main clinical application of the stain is in the differential diagnosis of the acute leukaemias, but its role has diminished considerably with the increasing use of immunophenotyping. Lymphoblasts of ALL are PAS-positive in the great majority of cases, this positivity often being in the form of coarse granules or large blocks on a clear background (Fig. 7.13). A negative PAS reaction is more often seen in T-lineage than in B-lineage ALL. Myeloblasts and monoblasts may be PAS-negative or may have faint diffuse or granular positivity. Block positivity is rare in AML, but it has been observed in basophil precursors, monoblasts, megakaryoblasts and erythroblasts.

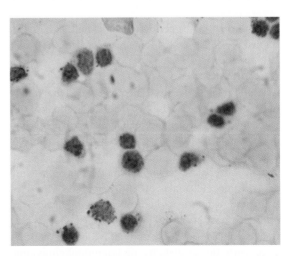

Fig. 7.13 Periodic acid–Schiff (PAS) reaction showing block positivity in the blast cells of a case of B-lineage acute lymphoblastic leukaemia (ALL) of FAB L1 category. By courtesy of Dr Ayed Eden, Southend-on-Sea.

Many other haemopoietic cells are PAS-positive, but the reaction is rarely of diagnostic importance. The reaction has a limited application in the diagnosis of erythroleukaemias, megakaryoblastic leukaemia and acute promyelocytic leukaemia. Platelets, mega-karyocytes and the more mature megakaryoblasts are positive. Megakaryoblasts may have PAS-positive granules within cytoplasmic blebs. Normal erythro-blasts are PAS-negative. Strong diffuse or block PAS positivity may be seen in erythroleukaemia. How-ever, quite strong reactions, either diffuse or granu-lar, may also be seen in β thalassaemia major and iron deficiency, and weaker reactions in sideroblastic anaemia, severe haemolytic anaemia and a number of other disorders of erythropoiesis. Acute promye-locytic leukaemia has moderately strong diffuse cytoplasmic positivity, appearing as a 'cytoplasmic blush'. Mature neutrophils have fine positive gran-ules, which appear to pack the cytoplasm, whereas eosinophils and basophils have a positive cytoplasmic reaction contrasting with the negative granules. Most normal lymphocytes are PAS-negative. Lympho-cytes containing PAS-positive granules become more numerous in reactive conditions, such as infectious mononucleosis and other viral infections, and in lym-phoproliferative disorders such as chronic lympho-cytic leukaemia (CLL) and non-Hodgkin lymphoma. A circlet of PAS-positive granules surrounding the nucleus, likened to rosary beads, may be found in Sézary cells.

A PAS stain can be performed on a film that has been stained previously with a Romanowsky stain.

Acid phosphatase

Acid phosphatase activity is demonstrated by a variety of haemopoietic cells. The two main applications of this reaction are in the diagnosis of hairy cell leukaemia and in the diagnosis of T-lineage leukaemias, particularly T-lineage ALL.

Acid phosphatase activity is usually stronger in acute and chronic leukaemias of T lineage than in those of B lineage, where it is often negative. T-lineage ALL often demonstrates focal positivity (Fig. 7.14), which is of some use in confirming this diagnosis. How-ever, with the availability of immunophenotyping, its importance has declined greatly. Acid phosphatase activity is also demonstrable in granulocytes and their precursors, in the monocyte lineage, and in platelets,

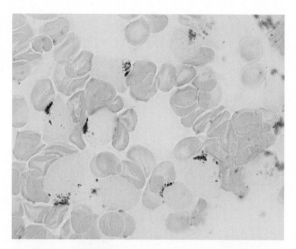

Fig. 7.14 Acid phosphatase stain by the method of Janckila *et al.* [5] showing focal positivity in the blast cells of a patient with T-lineage ALL.

megakaryocytes and the more mature megakaryo-blasts. Auer rods are positive.

A number of isoenzymes of acid phosphatase are found in haemopoietic cells. That of hairy cells is characteristically tartrate-resistant, whereas that of other cells is sensitive to inhibition by tartrate. The demonstration of tartrate-resistant acid phos-phatase (TRAP) activity remains useful in the diag-nosis of hairy cell leukaemia. It is present in the great majority of cases and is uncommon in other lym-phoproliferative disorders; however, TRAP positivity has also been reported in occasional cases of infec-tious mononucleosis, CLL, prolymphocytic leukae-mia (PLL), non-Hodgkin lymphoma and the Sézary syndrome. If immunophenotyping, for CD11c, CD25, CD103 and CD123, and molecular analysis, for a *BRAF1* mutation, are available, the TRAP reaction is redundant. The monocytes of patients with Gaucher disease are TRAP-positive but normal monocytes are not [23].

Flow cytometric immunophenotyping

Immunophenotyping is now usually performed by flow cytometry, using antibodies directly labelled with a fluorochrome (Fig. 7.15). This permits simultaneous analysis of the expression of two, three or four anti-gens together with an assessment of the strength of

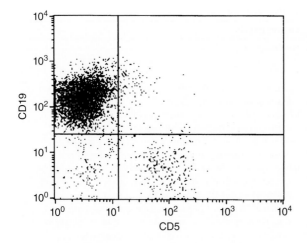

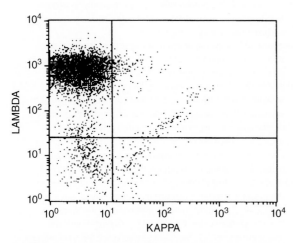

Fig. 7.15 Immunophenotyping by flow cytometry in a case of follicular lymphoma. The lower plot demonstrates clonality, cells being kappa-negative and lambda-positive, and shows that surface membrane immunoglobulin is strongly expressed. The upper plot demonstrates that the lymphoma cells are CD19 positive and CD5 negative, thus differing from both chronic lymphocytic leukaemia and mantle cell lymphoma. By courtesy of Mr Ricardo Morilla, London.

antigen expression. Flow cytometry immunophenotyping is used mainly for characterising neoplastic cells in leukaemia and lymphoma, but there are multiple other applications (Table 7.4). Flow cytometric immunophenotyping is of major importance in the diagnosis and further classification of leukaemia and lymphoma. It is essential for confirmation of the diagnoses of ALL and mixed phenotype acute leukaemia. When acute leukaemia is obviously myeloid,

immunophenotyping is unnecessary for diagnosis but, in the case of AML with no cytochemical evidence of myeloid differentiation (FAB M0 AML) and acute megakaryoblastic leukaemia (FAB M7 AML), it is essential. Even when not essential for diagnosis, immunophenotyping at diagnosis is required if it is to be used for monitoring of minimal residual disease.

Immunophenotyping is often very important to avoid diagnostic errors in the chronic lymphoproliferative disorders.

Immunophenotyping of the neoplastic cells in leukaemia and lymphoma is carried out with a panel of antibodies, mainly monoclonal antibodies, which detect antigens on the surface membrane or, if the cell is lightly fixed or 'permeabilised', cytoplasmic or nuclear antigens. With such panels, cells can be assigned to T-cell, B-cell or myeloid lineages. Certain specific antibodies can identify cells of erythroid, megakaryocyte and natural killer (NK) lineages. The use of secondary panels of antibodies permits the establishment of characteristic profiles that are very useful in the identification of specific types of lymphoproliferative disorder. Typical immunophenotypic findings in haematological neoplasms are shown in Tables 9.14–9.16. For a more detailed analysis of the role of immunophenotyping in haematological neoplasms, the reader is referred to reference 37.

An important but more specialised application of immunophenotyping is when expression of an antigen is used for the enumeration of cells of a specific type or for demonstrating antigenic abnormalities of cells, as summarised in Table 7.4.

Immunocytochemistry

Immunophenotyping can also be carried out on fixed cells in blood films or on cytospin preparations, using antibodies that are detected by either an immunoperoxidase (Fig. 7.16) or an alkaline phosphatase–anti-alkaline phosphatase (APAAP) technique (Fig. 7.17). Using these techniques, surface membrane, cytoplasmic and nuclear antigens are readily detected. These techniques have some advantages over flow cytometry since the cytological features of positive cells can be appreciated, but they are labour-intensive and thus are less suitable for routine use and are now rarely used.

Table 7.4 Applications of flow cytometric immunophenotyping of peripheral blood cells.*

Applications	Specific details
Immunophenotyping of abnormal cells in suspected leukaemia or lymphoma – for diagnosis, classification and minimal residual disease monitoring	See Chapter 9
Confirmation that stem cells are increased in peripheral blood, permitting harvesting for autologous transplantation	Counting of CD34-positive cells with weak expression of CD45 and low forward and side light scatter
Detection of circulating non-haemopoietic tumour cells for diagnosis or staging	Detection of circulating neuroblastoma cells by their CD81-positive, CD56-positive, CD45-negative immunophenotype
Exclusion of the presence of contaminating carcinoma cells, leukaemic cells or lymphoma cells in a peripheral blood stem cell harvest	Detection of cells expressing cytokeratin or aberrant antigen expression characteristic of cells of leukaemia or lymphoma
Diagnosis of paroxysmal nocturnal haemoglobinuria [24]	Detection of lack of expression of CD55 and CD59 by peripheral blood cells (erythrocytes, granulocytes, platelets) or lack of expression of FLAER (fluorescein-labelled proaerolysin) (granulocytes, monocytes, platelets); CD16 and CD66b are also reduced on neutrophils
Diagnosis of hereditary spherocytosis	Reduced binding of eosin-5-maleimide, which binds specifically to band 3 of the erythrocyte membrane† (see Chapter 8)
Detection and quantification of fetomaternal haemorrhage [25]	Enumeration of Rh D-positive cells in pregnant women in whom a high haemoglobin F invalidates a Kleihauer test; an alternative to a Kleihauer test in other women
	Detection of fetal cells by an anti-haemoglobin F antibody, the distinction from elevation of haemoglobin F in maternal cells being on the basis of the strength of the signal
	Detection of fetal cells by dual colour flow cytometry, using an antibody to haemoglobin F and an antibody to the i antigen; the expression of the i antigen on fetal cells permits the distinction of fetal cells from maternal cells; similarly a polyclonal antibody to carbonic anhydrase can be used together with an antibody to haemoglobin F, carbonic anhydrase being strongly expressed in maternal cells but quite weakly expressed in fetal cells [26]
Diagnosis of inherited platelet defects with reduction or absence of specific glycoproteins, e.g. Glanzmann thrombasthenia, Bernard–Soulier homozygotes and heterozygotes, Wiskott–Aldrich syndrome and X-linked thrombocytopenia	Lack of expression of platelet glycoproteins, e.g. lack of expression of glycoprotein IIb/IIIa in Glanzmann thrombasthenia, lack of expression of glycoprotein Ib/IX/V in Bernard–Soulier syndrome, lack of expression of the WAS protein in Wiskott–Aldrich and related syndromes [27], lack of expression of the thrombin receptor, PAR1, lack of expression of collagen receptors Ia/IIa and VI
Diagnosis of platelet δ-storage pool disease	Greatly reduced platelet serotonin content [28]
Diagnosis of leucocyte adhesion deficiency	Lack of expression of CD18 in type 1 disease and CD15 expression in type 2 disease
Detection of acquired platelet abnormalities, e.g. in MDS	Abnormal expression of platelet antigens or antigens do not show an appropriately increased or decreased expression in response to platelet agonists
Detection of activated platelets	Expression of CD61P and neo-epitopes on glycoprotein IIb/IIIa [29]
Tracking of transfused platelets	Two-colour immunofluorescence can be used to determine the survival of transfused platelets [30]
Diagnosis and monitoring of immunodeficiency (congenital or acquired)	Enumeration of T, B and NK lymphocytes and subset analysis, as appropriate, in suspected congenital or acquired immunodeficiency – detection of lack of expression of HLA-DR in 'bare lymphocyte syndrome'; detection of lack of expression of CD19 in some patients with congenital agammaglobulinaemia; detection of lymphocyte activation and increased expression of TCR-γδ in Omenn syndrome and severe combined immunodeficiency with maternofetal engraftment; lack of expression of Bruton tyrosine kinase (Btk) on some platelets in carrier females of X-linked agammaglobulinaemia; enumeration of CD4-positive cells in initial assessment and follow-up of the acquired immune deficiency syndrome (AIDS)

Applications	Specific details
Diagnosis of autoimmune lymphoproliferative syndrome	Distinctive immunophenotype with increased CD8-positive T cells, increased CD8-positive CD57-positive T cells, increased αβ-positive CD4-negative CD8-negative cells, increased γδ-positive CD4-negative CD8-negative cells, increased CD3-positive HLA-DR-positive T cells, decreased CD3-positive CD25-positive T cells and increased B cells including CD5-positive B cells [31]
Diagnosis of familial haemophagocytic lymphohistiocytosis type 2	Lack of expression of perforin by CD8-positive and CD56-positive lymphocytes [32]
Diagnosis of X-linked lymphoproliferative syndrome	Lack of expression of either SAP protein [33] or XIAP protein [34]
Detection of HLA-B27 histocompatibility antigens	Useful in supporting the diagnosis of ankylosing spondylitis, Reiter syndrome, psoriatic arthropathy and inflammatory bowel disease
T-cell monitoring and detection of T cells sensitised to an antigen	Monitoring of T-cell subsets following transplantation or immunosuppressive treatment; detection of antigen-specific T cells by their expression of the activation marker CD69 following exposure to the antigen
Quantification of CD46 on granulocytes	Diagnosis of one form of atypical haemolytic–uraemic syndrome [35]
Quantification of degree of parasitaemia in malaria	Quantification of the percentage of parasitised cells and of multiply infected cells in *Plasmodium falciparum* malaria [36]

*The role of immunophenotyping is greater when bone marrow cells are also available for study, e.g. for monitoring of minimal residual disease, for establishing clonality of plasma cells with anti-kappa and anti-lambda antibodies or for confirming a diagnosis of mastocytosis by demonstration of CD117-positive mast cells that express CD2 and CD25

†This test does not use an antibody but nevertheless permits recognition of a specific antigenic structure on the red cell membrane

MDS, myelodysplastic syndrome

Cytogenetic analysis

The peripheral blood can be used for cytogenetic analysis for the identification of constitutional disorders and for the investigation of leukaemia and lymphoma.

When investigating suspected constitutional abnormalities, e.g. Down syndrome, peripheral blood lymphocytes can be stimulated with phytohaemagglutinin (PHA) to induce mitosis and provide analysable metaphases. Cytogenetic techniques can also be applied to the diagnosis of Fanconi anaemia, susceptibility to clastogenic agents being shown.

In investigating leukaemias and lymphomas, the bone marrow is usually a more suitable tissue for analysis, but successful results are sometimes possible with peripheral blood cytogenetic analysis, in the case of

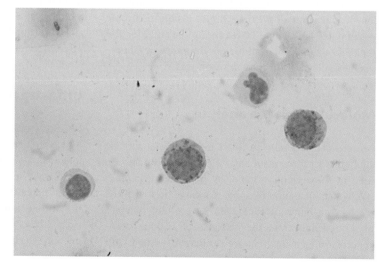

Fig. 7.16 Immunophenotyping using a monoclonal antibody to CD13 and the immunoperoxidase technique. The blast cells of this case gave negative reactions with myeloperoxidase (MPO), SBB and CAE, but were identified as myeloid (FAB M0 category) by the positivity with CD13 and negativity with monoclonal antibodies directed at lymphoid antigens. By courtesy of Professor Daniel Catovsky, London.

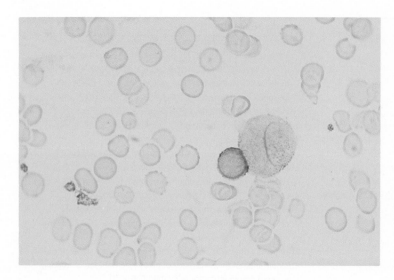

Fig. 7.17 Immunophenotyping using a monoclonal antibody to CD42 (antiplatelet glycoprotein Ib) and the alkaline phosphatase-anti-alkaline phosphatase (APAAP) technique. Positive reactions are given by two platelets, by a lymphocyte-sized micro-megakaryocyte and by a larger hypolobated megakaryocyte.

acute leukaemias, when there are a large number of circulating immature cells, or in the case of mature B-lineage and T-lineage lymphoproliferative disorders, when B-cell and T-cell mitogens respectively are employed.

For a detailed analysis of the role of cytogenetic analysis in haematological neoplasms, the reader is referred to reference 37.

Fluorescence *in situ* hybridisation

Fluorescence *in situ* hybridisation (FISH) can be performed on peripheral blood cells. Applications include the detection of abnormalities typical of haematological neoplasms, e.g. *PML-RARA* fusion in acute promyelocytic leukaemia or *FIP1L1-PDGFRA* fusion in chronic eosinophilic leukaemia. FISH can also be used for the rapid detection of constitutional chromosome abnormalities, such as trisomy 18 or trisomy 21.

Molecular genetic analysis

Peripheral blood cells are used for molecular genetic analysis with three main aims. Firstly, such studies are used to show clonality (and, by implication, neoplasia) by demonstration of clonal rearrangement of T-cell receptor or immunoglobulin genes. Secondly, they are used to demonstrate the presence of various oncogene rearrangements that are strongly associated with

specific haematological neoplasms; for example, *BCR-ABL1* can be used to monitor response to therapy in CML and *FIP1L1-PDGFRA* fusion can be used to identify one specific type of eosinophilic leukaemia. Thirdly, molecular techniques can be used to demonstrate inherited abnormalities of genes, e.g. α and β globin genes, that cause haematological abnormalities.

Molecular diagnostic techniques that may be employed include Southern blot analysis, the polymerase chain reaction (PCR) and comparative genomic hybridisation (CGH), for the analysis of deoxyribonucleic acid (DNA), and reverse-transcriptase-PCR (RT-PCR) for the investigation of ribonucleic acid (RNA). Real-time quantitative-PCR (RQ-PCR) can be used to quantitate the product of a specific fusion gene in a haematological neoplasm. For further details on the principles and applications of these techniques, the reader is referred to references 37–39.

Ultrastructural examination

Ultrastructural examination of peripheral blood cells by electron microscopy is labour-intensive and therefore is not often employed in routine diagnostic haematology. Scanning electron microscopy has been useful in increasing understanding of the actual shapes of the various abnormal erythrocytes seen in fixed and stained blood films (see Chapter 3). In the past, transmission electron microscopy has been used for the

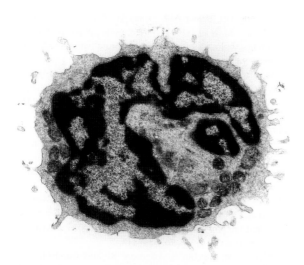

Fig. 7.18 Ultrastructural examination in Sézary syndrome showing a Sézary cell with a highly irregular nuclear outline. By courtesy of Dr Estella Matutes, Barcelona.

demonstration of the lineage of neoplastic cells (e.g. megakaryoblasts or myeloblasts) and for the detection of Sézary cells by demonstration of their characteristic nuclear form (Fig. 7.18), but these uses are now redundant. Transmission electron microscopy remains useful in distinguishing the various congenital thrombocytopenia syndromes resulting from mutation of the *MYH9* gene, and in identifying those that lack visible leucocyte inclusions by light microscopy.

TEST YOUR KNOWLEDGE

Visit the companion website for MCQs and EMQs on this topic:
www.wiley.com/go/bain/bloodcells

References

1 Bain BJ and Swirsky D (2012) Erythrocyte and leucocyte cytochemistry. In: Bain BJ, Bates I, Laffan MA and Lewis SM. *Dacie and Lewis Practical Haematology*, 11th edn. Churchill Livingstone, Edinburgh.

2 Hanker JS, Yates PE, Metz CB and Rustioni A (1977) A new, specific, sensitive and non-carcinogenic reagent for the demonstration of horseradish peroxidase. *Histochem J*, **9**, 789–792.

3 Yam LT, Li CY and Crosby WH (1971) Cytochemical identification of monocytes and granulocytes. *Am J Clin Pathol*, **55**, 283–290.

4 Hayhoe FGJ and Quaglino D (1980) *Haematological Cytochemistry*. Churchill Livingstone, Edinburgh.

5 Janckila A, Li C-Y, Lam K-W and Yam LT (1978) The cytochemistry of tartrate-resistant acid phosphatase technical considerations. *Am J Clin Pathol*, **70**, 45–55.

6 Gadson D, Hughes M, Dean A and Wickramasinghe SN (1986) Morphology of redox-dye-treated HbH-containing red cells: confusion caused by wrongly identified dyes. *Clin Lab Haematol*, **8**, 365–366.

7 Roper D and Layton M (2012) Investigation of the hereditary haemolytic anaemias: membrane and enzyme abnormalities. In: Bain BJ, Bates I, Laffan MA and Lewis SM. *Dacie and Lewis Practical Haematology*, 11th edn. Churchill Livingstone, Edinburgh.

8 Rustin GJS, Wilson PD and Peters TJ (1979) Studies on the subcellular localization of human neutrophil alkaline phosphatase. *J Cell Sci*, **36**, 401–412.

9 Ackerman GA (1962) Substituted naphthol AS phosphate derivatives for the localization of leukocyte alkaline phosphatase activity. *Lab Invest*, **11**, 563–567.

10 Kaplow LS (1968) Leukocyte alkaline phosphatase cytochemistry: applications and methods. *Ann NY Acad Sci*, **155**, 911–947.

11 Breton-Gorius J, Mason DY, Buriot D, Vilde J-L and Griscelli C (1980) Lactoferrin deficiency as a consequence of a lack of specific granules in neutrophils from patient with recurrent infections. *Am J Pathol*, **99**, 413–419.

12 Repine JE, Clawson CC and Brunning D (1976) Primary leucocyte alkaline phosphatase deficiency in an adult with repeated infections. *Br J Haematol*, **34**, 87–94.

13 Drouin A, Favier R, Massé J-M, Debili N, Schmitt A, Elbin C *et al.* (2001) Newly recognized cellular abnormalities in the gray platelet syndrome. *Blood*, **98**, 1382–1391.

14 Kohmura K, Miyakawa Y, Kameyama K, Kizaki M and Ikeda Y (2004) Granulocyte colony stimulating factor-producing multiple myeloma associated with neutrophilia. *Leuk Lymphoma*, **45**, 1475–1479.

15 O'Kell RT (1968) Leukocyte alkaline phosphatase activity in the infant. *Ann NY Acad Sci*, **155**, 980–982.

16 Rosner F, Lee SL, Schultz FS and Gorfien PC (1968) The regulation of leukocyte alkaline phosphatase. *Ann NY Acad Sci*, **155**, 902–910.

17 Stavridis J, Creatsas G, Lolis D, Traga G, Antonopoulos M and Kaskarelis D (1981) Relationships between leucocyte alkaline phosphatase and nitroblue tetrazolium reduction activities in the peripheral blood polymorphonuclear leucocytes in normal individuals. *Br J Haematol*, **47**, 157–159.

18 Stein P, Peiper S, Butler D, Melvin S, Williams D and Stass S (1983) Granular acute lymphoblastic leukaemia. *Am J Clin Pathol*, **79**, 426–430.

19 Savage RA, Fishleder J and Tubbs SRR (1983) Confirming myeloid differentiation. *Am J Clin Pathol*, **80**, 412.

20 Bain BJ (2010) Neutrophil dysplasia demonstrated on Sudan black B staining. *Am J Hematol*, **85**, 707.

21 Catovsky D (1980) Leucocyte enzymes in leukaemia. In: SRoath (ed.) *Topical Reviews in Haematology, Vol. 1.* John Wright, Bristol.

22 Elghetany MT (1999) Double esterase staining of the bone marrow contributes to lineage identification in a case of minimally differentiated acute myeloid leukaemia (AML M0). *Clin Lab Haematol*, **21**, 293–295.

23 Beutler E (1988) Gaucher disease. *Blood Rev*, **2**, 59–70.

24 Brodsky RA (2008) Advances in the diagnosis and therapy of paroxysmal nocturnal hemoglobinuria. *Blood Rev*, **22**, 65–74.

25 Gómez-Arbonés X, Pinacho A, Ortiz P, Maciá J, Gallart M, Araguás C *et al.* (2002) Quantification of foetomaternal haemorrhage. An analysis of two cytometric techniques and a semi-quantitative gel agglutination test. *Clin Lab Haematol*, **24**, 47–53.

26 Merz WM, Patzwaldt F, Fimmers R, Stoffel-Wagner B and Gembruch U (2012) Dual-colour flow cytometry for the analysis of fetomaternal haemorrhage during delivery. *J Clin Pathol*, **65**, 186–187.

27 Balduini CL, Cattaneo M, Fabris F, Gresele P, Iolascon A, Pulcinelli FM and Savoia A (2003) Inherited thrombocytopenias: a proposed diagnostic algorithm from the Italian Gruppo di Studio delle Piastrine. *Haematologica*, **89**, 325–329.

28 Maurer-Spurej E, Pittendreigh C and Wu JK (2007) Diagnosing platelet delta-storage pool disease in children by flow cytometry. *Am J Clin Pathol*, **127**, 626–632.

29 Roshan TM, Normah J, Rehman A and Naing L (2005) Effect of menopause on platelet activation markers determined by flow cytometry. *Am J Hematol*, **80**, 257–261.

30 Hughes DL, Evans G, Metcalfe P, Goodall AH and Williamson LM (2005) Tracking and characterisation of transfused platelets by two colour, whole blood flow cytometry. *Br J Haematol*, **130**, 791–794.

31 Bleesing JJH, Brown MR, Straus SE, Dale JK, Siegel RM, Johnson M *et al.* (2001) Immunophenotypic profiles in families with autoimmune lymphoproliferative syndrome. *Blood*, **98**, 2466–2473.

32 Suga N, Takada H, Nomura A, Ohga S, Ishii E, Ihara K *et al.* (2002) Perforin defects of primary haemophagocytic lymphohistiocytosis in Japan. *Br J Haematol*, **116**, 346–349.

33 Tabata Y, Villanueva J, Lee SM, Zhang K, Kanegane H, Miyawaki T *et al.* (2005) Rapid detection of intracellular SH2D1A protein in cytotoxic lymphocytes from patients with X-linked lymphoproliferative disease and their family members. *Blood*, **105**, 3066–3071.

34 Marsh RA, Villanueva J, Zhang K, Snow AL, Su HC, Madden L *et al.* (2009) A rapid flow cytometric screening test for X-linked lymphoproliferative disease due to XIAP deficiency. *Cytometry B Clin Cytom*, **76**, 334–344.

35 Taylor CM, Machin S, Wigmore SJ and Goodship TH; working party from the Renal Association, the British Committee for Standards in Haematology and the British Transplantation Society (2010) Clinical practice guidelines for the management of atypical haemolytic uraemic syndrome in the United Kingdom. *Br J Haematol*, **148**, 37–47.

36 Bei AK, Desimone TM, Badiane AS, Ahouidi AD, Dieye T, Ndiaye D *et al.* (2010) A flow cytometry-based assay for measuring invasion of red blood cells by Plasmodium falciparum. *Am J Hematol*, **85**, 234–237.

37 Bain BJ (2010) *Leukaemia Diagnosis*, 4th edn. Wiley–Blackwell, Oxford.

38 Bain BJ, Clarke DAC and Wilkins BS (2010) *Bone Marrow Pathology*, 4th edn. Wiley–Blackwell, Oxford.

39 Bain BJ (2005) *Haemoglobinopathy Diagnosis*, 2nd edn. Blackwell Publishing, Oxford.

CHAPTER 8
Disorders of red cells and platelets

Disorders of red cells

Disorders of red cells are most often divided into three broad categories, depending on whether the erythrocytes are: (i) microcytic and hypochromic; (ii) normocytic and normochromic; or (iii) macrocytic. Red cell disorders can also be classified as congenital or acquired. Anaemia can be further categorised according to the mechanism, whether due predominantly to a failure of production or to shortened red cell survival, and if the latter whether it is caused by an intrinsic defect of the red cell or by extrinsic factors. Anaemia can also be the result of pooling of red cells in an enlarged spleen and, in an acute situation, loss of blood from the body. In this chapter red cell disorders will be discussed in groups that relate mainly to the morphological features of the cells, including their size and degree of haemoglobinisation.

Hypochromic and microcytic anaemias and thalassaemias

Disorders resulting from a defect in haem synthesis
Iron deficiency anaemia
Iron deficiency develops when: (i) iron intake is inadequate for needs (e.g. during growth spurts or during pregnancy); (ii) there is malabsorption of iron; (iii) there is increased loss of iron, usually consequent on gastrointestinal or uterine blood loss; (iv) there is urinary loss of haemosiderin, as a result of chronic intravascular haemolysis; (v) there is a combination of these factors; or, rarely, (vi) there is sequestration of iron at an inaccessible site, as in idiopathic pulmonary haemosiderosis. In countries where *Schistosoma haematobium* infection occurs, urinary loss of blood can also be causative. Iron deficiency can be the presenting feature of autoimmune gastritis, presenting years in advance of megaloblastic anaemia due to vitamin B_{12} deficiency [1]. Anaemia occurs when a lack of reticuloendothelial storage iron and an inadequate rate of delivery of iron to

developing erythroid cells in the marrow leads to reduced synthesis of haem and therefore reduced production of haemoglobin and red blood cells. Clinical features include those attributable to anaemia, such as fatigue, pallor and exertional dyspnoea. More specific features of iron deficiency, apparent only when iron deficiency is severe, include koilonychia (spoon-shaped nails), angular cheilosis (cracks in the skin at the corners of the mouth) and glossitis (inflammation of the tongue).

Hereditary iron-refractory iron deficiency anaemia is the result of bi-allelic, or occasionally mono-allelic, mutation in the *TMPRSS6* gene [2]. Features of the blood film and count are the same as in other case of iron deficiency.

It is also necessary to recognise functional iron deficiency, defined as a state when there is insufficient iron available for erythropoiesis despite a normal serum ferritin and the presence of storage iron in the bone marrow [3]. This is one feature of the anaemia of chronic disease (see below), but is otherwise mainly recognised in renal patients given erythropoiesis-stimulating agents.

Blood film and count
In iron deficiency, a normocytic normochromic anaemia with anisocytosis precedes the development of anisochromasia, hypochromia and microcytosis. Morphological changes are not usually marked until haemoglobin concentration (Hb) falls below 100–110 g/l when characteristic features start to appear (Fig. 8.1). Poikilocytes include elliptocytes, particularly very narrow elliptocytes, which are often referred to as pencil cells. Poikilocytes designated 'pre-keratocytes', i.e. erythrocytes with preserved central pallor with a sharply defined submembranous vacuole, are often present and are more common than in β thalassaemia trait or anaemia of chronic disease [4]. Target cells are often present [4], although their numbers are generally lower than in β thalassaemia trait. Numerous target cells may be seen in iron deficient patients with haemoglobin C or S trait who sometimes develop target cells only when they become iron deficient. Teardrop poikilocytes may be

Blood Cells A Practical Guide, Fifth Edition. By Barbara J. Bain © 2015 John Wiley & Sons, Ltd. Published 2015 by John Wiley & Sons, Ltd.
Companion Website: www.wiley.com/go/bain/bloodcells

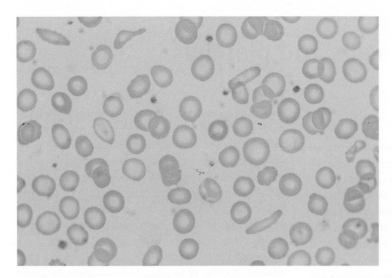

Fig. 8.1 The blood film of a patient with iron deficiency anaemia showing anisocytosis, poikilocytosis (including elliptocytes), hypochromia and microcytosis. The full blood count (FBC, Coulter S Plus IV) was: red blood cell count (RBC) $4.22 \times 10^{12}/l$, haemoglobin concentration (Hb) 70 g/l, haematocrit (Hct) 0.29 l/l, mean cell volume (MCV) 67 fl, mean cell haemoglobin (MCH) 16.6 pg, mean cell haemoglobin concentration (MCHC) 245 g/l.

present, particularly as anaemia becomes more severe. Basophilic stippling is infrequent. Polychromasia is sometimes present.

With most automated full blood counters, the earliest evidence of iron deficiency is an increase in the red cell distribution width (RDW). This is indicative of the anisocytosis that precedes anaemia. The next change observed is a fall in the Hb, red blood cell count (RBC) and haematocrit (Hct) followed by a fall in the mean cell haemoglobin (MCH) and the mean cell volume (MCV). In a study using one of two impedance counters (Sysmex K4500 or Coulter S890), an MCH of less than 26 pg was found to be a more sensitive indicator of iron deficiency than an MCV of less than 80 fl; sensitivity to a reduced serum ferritin was 97% and 85% respectively [5]. In early iron deficiency anaemia, the RBC is occasionally elevated rather than decreased, particularly in children. A low mean cell haemoglobin concentration (MCHC) is a sensitive indicator of iron deficiency when it is calculated from the Hb and a packed cell volume (microhaematocrit) and when it is measured by current Siemens instruments. When measured by impedance-based instruments (such as Coulter or Sysmex instruments) it is insensitive, but more specific for iron deficiency. With Siemens H.1 series and later automated counters the appearance of a population of hypochromic cells (%Hypo) and an increase in the haemoglobin distribution width (HDW) is the earliest change detected; a fall in the MCH and MCHC precedes any fall in the MCV [6]. The recent Sysmex instrument, the XE-5000, also measures the haemoglobin concentration in individual cells and produces a measurement that is analogous to that of Siemens instruments, designated %Hypo He, which is similarly low in iron deficiency. Other red cell variables that are reduced in iron deficiency include the RBC-Y on Sysmex instruments and the Low Haemoglobin Density (LHD) on the Coulter 750 (a mathematical transformation of the MCHC).

The reticulocyte percentage may be normal or elevated in iron deficiency anaemia, while the absolute reticulocyte count is normal or reduced. A low reticulocyte haemoglobin content (CHr) on Siemens instruments precedes any fall in Hb, MCH or MCV [7]. Similarly, the reticulocyte haemoglobin equivalent (Ret-He) on Sysmex instruments is an early sign of iron deficiency.

Patients with iron deficiency not infrequently have an increased platelet count, which may be resultant on the iron deficiency itself, on blood loss or on an underlying malignant disease. In severe iron deficiency the platelet count is sometimes low. Leucopenia and thrombocytopenia occur in up to 10% of patients. Hypersegmented neutrophils are sometimes present and are not necessarily indicative of coexisting vitamin B_{12} or folate deficiency. In geographical regions where hookworm (*Necator americanus* or *Ankylostoma duodenalis*) infection occurs, the observation of eosinophilia may suggest that this is the cause of the iron deficiency. The presence of hyposplenic features may suggest coeliac disease as the underlying cause.

Other automated instrument measurements that are useful in the recognition of functional iron deficiency include 6% or more hypochromic red cells (%HRC) or a reticulocyte haemoglobin content (CHr) < 29 pg measured on Siemens instruments, or a Ret-He value < 30.6 pg measured on Sysmex instruments [3]. The Sysmex %Hypo-He and the Beckman–Coulter LHD% are comparable to the Siemens %HRC (see Chapter 2).

Differential diagnosis

The important differential diagnoses of iron deficiency anaemia are thalassaemia trait and the anaemia of chronic disease. The blood film and count are of some use in distinguishing these disorders, but specific tests are needed for a precise diagnosis. Prominent target cells and basophilic stippling favour thalassaemia trait, whereas anisochromasia, pencil cells and prekeratocytes favour iron deficiency; increased rouleaux formation, background staining and other signs of inflammation suggest the anaemia of chronic disease. A high RBC and a low MCV despite a normal Hb are characteristic of thalassaemia trait, but very similar red cell indices occur in patients with polycythaemia vera who are iron deficient. The RDW is usually elevated in iron deficiency and most often normal in thalassaemia trait [8]. A low MCHC on the less sensitive impedance counters is strongly suggestive of iron deficiency since it is usually normal in thalassaemia trait and in the anaemia of chronic disease (although it is low in haemoglobin H disease). Copper deficiency, a rare cause of a microcytic anaemia, is associated with a low serum iron, normal transferrin concentration and normal ferritin [9]. The equally rare acaeruloplasminaemia is associated with a normochromic normocytic or hypochromic microcytic anaemia, low serum iron, normal transferrin concentration and moderately elevated serum ferritin. Other rare conditions that can cause a microcytic anaemia are listed in Table 3.1.

Further tests

In uncomplicated iron deficiency anaemia, the diagnosis can be confirmed by either (i) a low serum ferritin or (ii) a low serum iron coexisting with an increased transferrin concentration or serum iron binding capacity. It should be noted that a low serum iron by itself gives little useful information since it is found in both iron deficiency and anaemia of chronic disease. When iron deficiency and chronic inflammation coexist there may be no elevation in transferrin concentration and iron binding capacity, and serum ferritin may be in the lower part of the normal range rather than reduced. Whereas a serum ferritin of less than 20 µg/l is useful for the diagnosis of iron deficiency anaemia when there are no complicating factors, a cut-off

of 50 µg/l has been suggested in patients with liver disease [10] and of 70 µg/l in patients with chronic inflammation [11]. It should be noted that ferritin can be misleadingly normal in patients with iron deficiency anaemia as a result of idiopathic pulmonary haemosiderosis; iron deficiency anaemia can still be confirmed by a low serum iron, increased transferrin and absent bone marrow iron [12]. The hereditary hyperferritinaemia-cataract syndrome is not usually associated with any haematological abnormality. However, coincidental iron deficiency can occur and there is then a hypochromic microcytic anaemia with a high ferritin but low iron saturation [13]. In iron-refractory iron deficiency anaemia due to a *TMPRSS6* mutation, serum iron and transferrin saturation are low but serum ferritin is normal [2].

An elevated free erythrocyte protoporphyrin or zinc protoporphyrin concentration is found in iron deficiency anaemia, in the anaemia of chronic disease and in lead poisoning, but is less often found in thalassaemia trait. It is useful for supporting the diagnosis of iron deficiency in clinical situations where uncomplicated iron deficiency is common, e.g. in children or obstetric patients, and since it can be measured on a very small volume of blood can be useful in field surveys.

Soluble transferrin receptor in serum is increased in iron deficiency and not in the anaemia of chronic disease. However, the usefulness of this test is reduced by the fact that the concentration is also increased whenever erythropoiesis is expanded, e.g. in megaloblastic anaemia, haemolytic anaemias, thalassaemia trait and myelodysplastic syndromes (MDS). The soluble transferrin receptor/log serum ferritin gives improved discrimination between iron deficiency and other conditions; this ratio is increased in iron deficiency but not in anaemia of chronic disease [14] or β thalassaemia trait [15] or when erythropoiesis is expanded in MDS [15]. This ratio is particularly useful in the elderly in whom standard tests for iron deficiency are insensitive, probably because of the frequency of chronic inflammation [16]. Another ratio, the log[soluble transferrin receptor/serum ferritin] shows a linear relationship with body iron stores [17] and also gives improved separation of iron deficiency (with or without chronic inflammation) from other conditions. If measurement of soluble transferrin receptor is not available, it is possible to identify most iron deficient patients accurately by means of a graph of serum ferritin plotted against the erythrocyte sedimentation rate (ESR) [18]. The World Health Organization has recommended serum ferritin as the standard test for

Table 8.1 A comparison of laboratory tests in iron deficiency anaemia, the anaemia of chronic disease and thalassaemia trait.

	Iron deficiency anaemia	Anaemia of chronic disease	Anaemia of chronic disease plus iron deficiency	Thalassaemia trait
Serum iron	Reduced	Reduced	Reduced	Normal
Serum transferrin/serum iron binding capacity	Increased	Normal or Reduced	Variable	Normal
Transferrin saturation	Reduced, sometimes markedly	Reduced	Reduced	Normal
Serum ferritin	Reduced, less than 20 µg/l	Normal or increased	Normal or reduced, generally less than 70 µg/l	Normal
Red cell zinc protoporphyrin	Increased	Increased	Increased	Normal or somewhat increased
Soluble transferrin receptor	Increased	Normal or reduced	Normal or increased	Increased
Soluble transferrin receptor/ log serum ferritin	Increased	Normal	Probably increased	Normal
Log[soluble transferrin receptor/serum ferritin]	Increased	Normal	Increased	Normal
Bone marrow iron	Absent	Present, often increased	Absent	Present

iron deficiency, but with this test being supplemented by soluble transferrin receptor measurements in countries in which infection is common. In complicated cases the definitive test is the demonstration of absent bone marrow iron. Biochemical abnormalities of iron deficiency anaemia are summarised in Table 8.1.

Red cell survival is moderately reduced, e.g. to 46–85 days [19].

Iron deficiency should not be regarded as a satisfactory diagnosis until the underlying cause has been identified by clinical history, physical examination and supplementary tests. There is a very significant incidence of unsuspected coeliac disease (around 10%) in unselected UK adults presenting with iron deficiency anaemia. Screening for coeliac disease may therefore be justifiable, particularly if there is no obvious cause for iron deficiency [20]. Iron deficiency coexisting with autoimmune thyroid disease or diabetes mellitus suggests underlying autoimmune gastritis, possibly triggered by *Helicobacter pylori* infection [1]. The possibility of occult gastrointestinal cancer and, in areas of endemicity, of parasitic infections should also be considered and appropriately investigated. Relevant parasites include hookworm and *Blastocystis hominis*. In patients with iron deficiency anaemia that is found to be refractory to oral iron therapy, the diagnoses that particularly need to be considered are coeliac disease, autoimmune gastritis and *H. pylori* infection, the latter two conditions sometimes occurring together. The

rare cases of hereditary iron-refractory iron deficiency anaemia can be confirmed by gene sequencing in a reference laboratory.

Anaemia of chronic disease

'Anaemia of chronic disease' is a term used to describe anaemia that is the result of chronic infection or inflammation or, less often, of malignant disease and that is characterised by: (i) low serum iron concentration and defective incorporation of iron into haemoglobin despite adequate bone marrow stores of iron; (ii) a blunted erythropoietin response to anaemia; and (iii) some shortening of red cell survival [21]. Clinical features are attributable to the primary disease, the effects of anaemia or both.

Blood film and count

Anaemia of chronic disease, when mild, is normocytic and normochromic, but as it becomes more severe hypochromia and microcytosis develop (Fig. 8.2). In severe chronic inflammation, the degree of microcytosis may be just as marked as in iron deficiency. The RDW has been reported to be normal in anaemia of chronic disease [3], but this has not been a consistent observation [22]. The absolute reticulocyte count is reduced. Associated features indicative of chronic inflammation may be present, e.g. neutrophilia, thrombocytosis, increased rouleaux formation and increased background staining. Pencil cells and prekeratocytes are

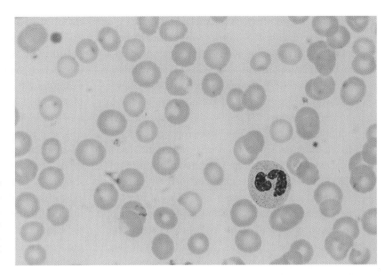

Fig. 8.2 The blood film of a patient with the anaemia of chronic disease consequent on a lymphoma, showing mild anisocytosis, poikilocytosis and hypochromia. The FBC (Coulter S Plus IV) was: RBC $3.10 \times 10^{12}/l$, Hb 74 g/l, Hct 0.23 l/l, MCV 75.6 fl, MCH 23.8 pg, MCHC 315 g/l.

less frequent than in iron deficiency and target cells are less frequent than in either iron deficiency anaemia or β thalassaemia trait [4]. Basophilic stippling is present in a minority of patients, fewer than in β thalassaemia trait [4].

Differential diagnosis

The differential diagnosis is iron deficiency anaemia (see above) and other causes of normochromic normocytic and hypochromic microcytic anaemia.

Further tests

Serum iron and serum transferrin (or iron binding capacity) are reduced. Serum ferritin is increased, consequent on synthesis of apoferritin by inflammatory or neoplastic cells. Associated features indicative of chronic inflammation are useful in making the diagnosis. In addition to blood film features, these commonly include elevated ESR and C-reactive protein, a reduced serum albumin concentration and an increased concentration of fibrinogen, α_2 macroglobulin and γ globulins. Red cell free protoporphyrin or zinc protoporphyrin is increased, so that this test is not useful in distinguishing between iron deficiency and the anaemia of chronic disease. Soluble serum transferrin receptor is generally reduced or normal.

It is not uncommon for a patient with anaemia of chronic disease due to malignancy or chronic inflammation to develop iron deficiency, usually as a result of gastrointestinal blood loss. The usual results of laboratory tests in anaemia of chronic disease, in iron deficiency anaemia and when both conditions are present are shown in Table 8.1. However, it may not always be possible to recognise the combination of iron deficiency and anaemia of chronic disease on the basis of the blood film and biochemical tests. A bone marrow aspiration will allow a correct appraisal.

Congenital sideroblastic anaemia

Congenital sideroblastic anaemia is a rare inherited condition. In most families it has an X-linked inheritance and is therefore largely confined to males. Rarely it occurs in women as a result of skewed X-chromosome inactivation and onset may then be delayed till old age [23]. Pyridoxine-responsive X-linked sideroblastic anaemia usually results from a defect in haem synthesis as a result of a mis-sense mutation in the erythroid-specific 5-amino laevulinic acid synthase gene, *ALAS2* [24]. Mutation in an erythroid-specific *ALAS* enhancer located in the first intron of the *ALAS* gene can also be responsible and in this case the condition is refractory to pyridoxine [25]. In addition, autosomal recessive pyridoxine-refractory sideroblastic anaemia can result from mutation in the *SLC25A38* gene [26] or the *GLRX5* gene [27]. Autosomal dominant inheritance with the genetic basis being unknown has also been described in one family. In non-syndromic cases of congenital sideroblastic anaemia, the clinical features are those of anaemia, sometimes complicated by iron overload. Only cases resulting from *ALAS2* mutation respond to pyridoxine [28].

Various syndromes of which sideroblastic anaemia is a part have been described. X-linked recessive sideroblastic anaemia due to a mutation in *ABCB7*, a gene encoding a mitochondrial transporter protein, is associated with spinocerebellar ataxia [29]. Autosomal recessive sideroblastic anaemia with myopathy and lactic acidosis can be due to mutation in either the *PUS1* gene or the *YARS2* gene [28]. A syndrome of severe congenital sideroblastic anaemia with B-cell immune deficiency, periodic fever and developmental delay (SIFD syndrome) has been described [30]; the molecular basis has not yet been defined. Erythropoietic porphyria, due to coinheritance of a loss-of-function mutation in the *FECH* gene and a low expression allele of the same gene, is associated with hypochromic microcytic anaemia in 20–60% of patients [31]. In a single family, transfusion-dependent congenital sideroblastic anaemia was the result of inheritance of a mutated *STEAP3* gene together with a low expression allele of the same gene [32]. In Pearson syndrome, resulting from mutation in a mitochondrial gene, there are ring sideroblasts associated with a normocytic or macrocytic anaemia rather than microcytic anaemia [33]. Similarly, in two other rare inherited syndromes there is macrocytosis associated with erythropoiesis that is both sideroblastic and megaloblastic; these syndromes are thiamine-responsive megaloblastic anaemia with diabetes mellitus and sensorineural deafness, due to a mutation in the *SLC19A2* gene, and the **D**iabetes **I**nsipidus, **D**iabetes **M**ellitus **O**ptic **A**trophy and **D**eafness (DIDMOAD) syndrome (also known as Wolfram syndrome), due to a mutation in the *WFS1* gene [34].

Blood film and count

The Hb ranges from 30–40 g/l to almost normal. Severity of anaemia differs according to the genetic defect; patients with an *SLC25A38* mutation, for example, are generally transfusion dependent. The blood film (Fig. 8.3) may be dimorphic or show uniform hypochromia and microcytosis. Occasionally, target cells and basophilic stippling are present. Poikilocytosis is sometimes marked and Pappenheimer bodies may be detectable. In older subjects, hypersplenism due to iron overload may cause mild leucopenia and thrombocytopenia. In the SIFD syndrome, dimorphism was not noted; the film features were hypochromia, microcytosis, schistocytes, basophilic stippling, frequent nucleated red blood cells and lymphopenia [30].

The MCV and MCH are reduced and the MCHC is sometimes reduced. Red cell histograms and cytograms may show two populations of red cells.

Rarely maternally inherited sideroblastic anaemia (with a low percentage of ring sideroblasts) is associated with macrocytosis [35] as is also seen in Pearson syndrome, thiamine-responsive megaloblastic anaemia and the DIDMOAD syndrome. In Pearson syndrome there is not only a normocytic or macrocytic anaemia but, in about a quarter of patients, neutropenia or thrombocytopenia [33].

Female carriers of X-linked sideroblastic anaemia resulting from an *ALAS2* mutation who are not themselves anaemic may have a minor population of hypochromic microcytic cells (Fig. 8.4). Rarely, females

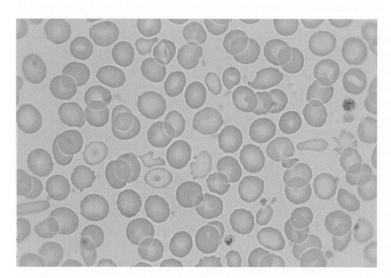

Fig. 8.3 A dimorphic blood film from a patient with congenital sideroblastic anaemia. There is a minor population of cells that are hypochromic and microcytic with a tendency to target cell formation; there is also poikilocytosis. The patient had previously responded to pyridoxine with a rise of Hb and was taking pyridoxine when this blood specimen was obtained.

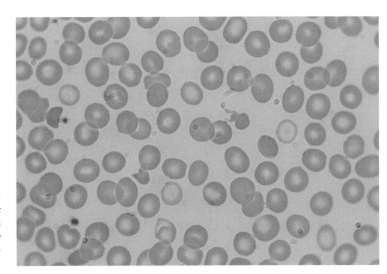

Fig. 8.4 Blood film obtained from a non-anaemic carrier of congenital sideroblastic anaemia, the daughter of a patient with moderately severe microcytic anaemia. The film is dimorphic, showing a minor population of hypochromic microcytes.

have a hypochromic microcytic anaemia similar to that observed in males, as a result of skewed X-chromosome inactivation. The dimorphism of the blood film and corresponding red cell cytograms and histograms may be more evident in heterozygous females than in hemizygous males [36]. Carriers of the *ABCB7* mutation may also have a population of hypochromic macrocytes [29].

Differential diagnosis

The differential diagnosis of X-linked sideroblastic anaemia includes iron deficiency anaemia and thalassaemia trait. Serum iron and ferritin are normal or elevated, high performance liquid chromatography (HPLC) and haemoglobin electrophoresis are normal and haemoglobin A_2 concentration is not increased. There is usually no difficulty distinguishing between congenital and acquired sideroblastic anaemia, since the latter is usually characterised by predominantly normocytic or macrocytic cells with only a small population of hypochromic microcytes.

The differential diagnosis of Pearson syndrome includes congenital bone marrow failure syndromes. The differential diagnosis of thiamine-responsive megaloblastic anaemia and the DIDMOAD syndrome includes other causes of megaloblastic anaemia.

Further tests

Diagnosis is by bone marrow aspiration; a Perls stain demonstrates ring sideroblasts. Pearson syndrome

shows, in addition to ring sideroblasts, erythroid hypoplasia with vacuolation of erythroid and granulocytic precursors. Biochemical assays of enzymes involved in haem synthesis will help to categorise cases further. Deoxyribonucleic acid (DNA) analysis of relevant genes is used for confirmation. Serum ferritin should also be monitored, to permit the early detection of iron overload.

Lead poisoning

Excess lead interferes with haem synthesis and also causes haemolysis. Patients with significant haematological effects often have other symptoms and signs of lead poisoning such as abdominal pain, constipation and a lead line on the gums. The clinical history and physical examination can thus be helpful in making the diagnosis. The source may be lead-glazed pottery, cosmetics or 'herbal' and other alternative remedies.

Blood film and count

Anaemia is usually mild or moderate in severity. The blood film may show hypochromia and microcytosis or normocytic normochromic red cells with some polychromasia. Basophilic stippling is often prominent (Fig. 8.5). Pappenheimer bodies may also be present since lead poisoning causes sideroblastic erythropoiesis. The reticulocyte percentage and absolute count may be elevated.

Red cell indices may be normal or there may be a reduction in the MCV, MCH and MCHC.

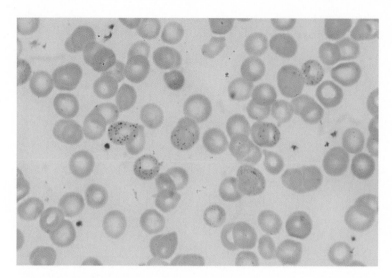

Fig. 8.5 The blood film of a patient with lead poisoning showing anisocytosis, hypochromia and prominent basophilic stippling. The FBC (Coulter S Plus IV) was: RBC $2.99 \times 10^{12}/1$, Hb 83 g/l, Hct 0.25 l/l, MCV 85 fl, MCH 27.8 pg, MCHC 327 g/l. The reticulocyte count was $281 \times 10^9/1$.

Differential diagnosis

The differential diagnosis includes other causes of hypochromic microcytic anaemia and also haemolytic anaemias, particularly that due to inherited pyrimidine 5′ nucleotidase deficiency in which basophilic stippling is also prominent. It should be noted that lead poisoning and iron deficiency often coexist.

Further tests

An appropriately elevated serum lead concentration is confirmatory. Erythrocyte free protoporphyrin or zinc protoporphyrin is increased, since ferrochelatase is inhibited by lead, but this test is not useful in making a distinction from iron deficiency. When there is a haemolytic element there is likely to be increased serum transferrin receptor, so this test is also not helpful in making a distinction from iron deficiency.

Disorders resulting from a defect in β globin chain synthesis

β thalassaemia trait

β thalassaemia trait refers to heterozygosity for β thalassaemia, an inherited condition in which a mutation in a β globin gene or, less often, the deletion of a β globin gene leads to a reduced rate of synthesis of β globin chains. There is consequently a reduced rate of synthesis of haemoglobin. Compensatory erythroid hyperplasia leads to the production of increased numbers of red cells of reduced size and haemoglobin content. The mutations giving rise to β thalassaemia are very numerous and very heterogeneous. In some cases the abnormal gene leads to no β chain

production ($β^0$ thalassaemia), whereas in others the abnormal gene permits β chain synthesis at a reduced rate ($β^+$ thalassaemia). Different mutations producing defects of varying severity are prevalent in different parts of the world.

β thalassaemia trait occurs in virtually all ethnic groups, although in northern European Caucasians it is very infrequent. It is common in Greece and Italy where the prevalence in some regions reaches 15–20%. There is a similar prevalence in Cyprus among both Greek and Turkish Cypriots. The prevalence in some parts of India, Thailand and other parts of South-East Asia reaches 5–10%. In Black Americans the prevalence is about 0.5% and in Afro-Caribbeans it is about 1%.

Heterozygosity for β thalassaemia is usually clinically inapparent and for this reason the term 'thalassaemia minor' is sometimes used to describe it. Occasional patients have mild splenomegaly or signs or symptoms of anaemia.

An acquired deficiency of pyrimidine 5′ nucleotidase has been found to be common in β thalassaemia heterozygosity, possibly resulting from oxidant damage to the enzyme [37].

Blood film and count

The majority of subjects with β thalassaemia trait have a normal Hb; a minority are mildly anaemic, particularly during pregnancy or intercurrent infections. Anaemia is more common among Greeks and Italians than among those with African ancestry. Despite the lack of anaemia, microcytosis is usually marked. The blood film (Figs 8.6 & 8.7) may or may not show hypochromia in

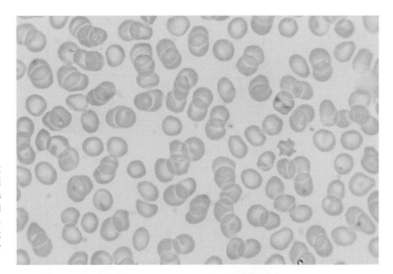

Fig. 8.6 The blood film of a healthy subject with β thalassaemia trait showing minimal morphological abnormalities – microcytosis and mild poikilocytosis. The diagnosis could easily be missed without the red cell indices. The FBC (Coulter S Plus IV) was RBC $7.3 \times 10^{12}/1$, Hb 143 g/l, Hct 0.43 l/l, MCV 59 fl, MCH 19.7 pg, MCHC 328 g/l.

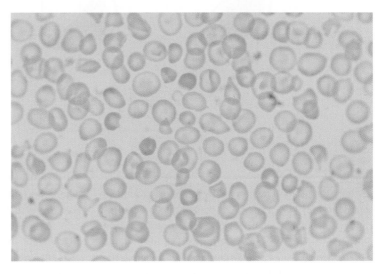

Fig. 8.7 The blood film of a healthy subject with β thalassaemia trait showing more marked morphological abnormalities – anisocytosis, poikilocytosis, hypochromia, microcytosis, occasional target cells and several irregularly contracted cells. The FBC (Coulter S Plus IV) was: RBC $5.78 \times 10^{12}/l$, Hb 105 g/l, Hct 0.32 l/l, MCV 56 fl, MCH 18.2 pg, MCHC 323 g/l.

addition to microcytosis. The haemoglobin concentration of cells may appear very uniform, in contrast to the anisochromasia that is usual in iron deficiency. Poikilocytosis varies from trivial to marked. Target cells may be prominent, but in some patients they are infrequent or absent. A few irregularly contracted cells are seen in some patients. Occasional patients have marked elliptocytosis but, in general, elliptocytes are not a feature. Basophilic stippling is quite common in Mediterranean subjects with β thalassaemia trait, but is less often seen in those of African or Chinese/South-East Asian ancestry. Acquired deficiency of pyrimidine 5′ nucleotidase (see above) provides a possible explanation of the frequency of basophilic stippling. The reticulocyte percentage and

absolute count are often somewhat elevated [38]. In uncomplicated cases the white cell and platelet counts are normal.

The red cell indices of β thalassaemia trait are very characteristic and it is often easier to make a correct provisional diagnosis from the red cell indices than from the blood film. The Hb and Hct are normal or close to normal while the MCV and MCH are usually markedly reduced. The MCHC is usually normal when measured by impedance counters such as Sysmex and Coulter instruments, but is often somewhat reduced when measured by Siemens H.1 and Advia series instruments. When the numbers of hypochromic cells and microcytic cells are measured independently, the percentage of microcytes

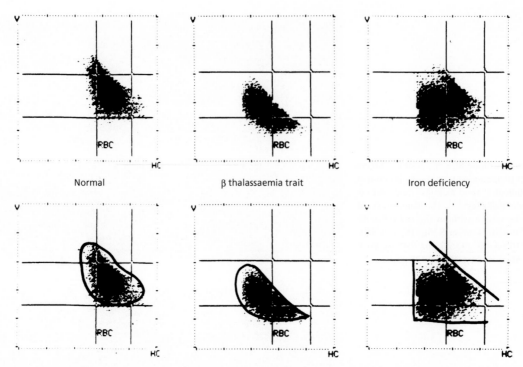

Fig. 8.8 Red cell cytograms from a Bayer H.2 counter showing the relationship between haemoglobinisation (*x*-axis) and volume (*y*-axis) of individual red cells in a normal subject (left) and patients with β thalassaemia trait (centre) and iron deficiency (right). The 'comma' shape of β thalassaemia trait is apparent and has been emphasised by the sketched outlines of the cytograms in the lower series of scatter plots.

usually exceeds the percentage of hypochromic cells in thalassaemia trait, whereas the reverse is found in iron deficiency [39]. The red cell cytogram characteristically has a 'comma' shape (Fig. 8.8). In contrast to iron deficiency, the RDW is usually normal [8], but when a patient with β thalassaemia trait becomes anaemic the RDW tends to rise [8], so that this measurement is least useful when most needed. Other observers have often found the RDW to be elevated even in non-anaemic patients [22].

The diagnosis of thalassaemia trait is more difficult in pregnant patients for two reasons. Firstly, the red cell indices are less characteristic since haemodilution, which is a physiological effect of pregnancy, lowers the Hb, RBC and Hct; the Hb may fall as low as 50–60 g/l [40]. The rise in MCV that occurs in pregnancy also contributes to the red cell indices being less characteristic than in a non-pregnant subject. Secondly, iron deficiency anaemia has an increased prevalence during pregnancy and when the two conditions coexist diagnosis is more complicated.

Differential diagnosis

The important differential diagnoses of β thalassaemia trait are α thalassaemia trait and iron deficiency anaemia. Various formulae have been devised in an attempt to separate iron deficiency from β thalassaemia trait [41–48]. Although such formulae may be useful in separating uncomplicated cases into the two diagnostic groups, they are not generally applicable to pregnant women [49] or children and are not useful in patients who have both iron deficiency *and* thalassaemia trait, a not uncommon situation with patients from the Indian subcontinent. Although these formulae are useful in suggesting the most likely diagnosis, there is little choice but to carry out specific diagnostic tests in circumstances where the diagnosis of thalassaemia trait is important, e.g. for antenatal, pre-conceptual or pre-marital genetic counselling. In this situation either the MCV (< 79 fl) or the MCH (< 27 pg) can be used as a screening test with all patients whose test results fall below an arbitrary limit having HPLC or an equivalent test performed. Occasional patients with mild variants of β thalassaemia trait have only a very trivial reduction of the MCV and MCH and if such cases are to be identified, it is necessary to test all patients whose results fall below the lower limit of the reference range. Even this will not detect all cases, since in some mild thalassaemic variants there is no apparent haematological defect in heterozygotes; such cases cannot be diagnosed on the basis of the blood film and indices. However, except when genetic counselling is being carried out in high incidence areas, it is generally necessary to have a cut-off point for further investigation that is at or below the lower limit of the reference range in order to avoid having a very high percentage of negative tests with a very low yield of positive diagnoses.

It is not possible on the basis of the blood film and count to distinguish β thalassaemia trait from δβ or εγδβ thalassaemia trait or from cases of α thalassaemia trait in which two of the four α genes are deleted. Cases of α thalassaemia trait in which only one of the four α genes is deleted have only minor haematological abnormalities and are less likely to be confused with β thalassaemia trait. Occasional patients with a blood film and red cell indices suggestive of thalassaemia trait have either a highly unstable globin chain or an abnormal haemoglobin that is synthesised at a reduced rate. The commonest of the latter group is haemoglobin E; red cell indices suggestive of β thalassaemia trait can result from heterozygosity for this variant haemoglobin and such indices are typical of homozygotes. The much less common haemoglobin Lepore, resulting from a δβ fusion gene, is synthesised at a greatly reduced rate and the blood count resembles that of β thalassaemia trait. Sickle cell trait and haemoglobin C trait are also not infrequently associated with microcytosis, although this may be only because of associated α thalassaemia trait.

The red cell indices in iron deficient polycythaemia may be indistinguishable from those of thalassaemia trait, but the RDW is more likely to be elevated and there may be associated features that are useful in the differential diagnosis, such as neutrophilia, basophilia, thrombocytosis and the presence of giant platelets. The characteristic indices of thalassaemia can also be simulated by iron deficiency anaemia undergoing treatment. A marked elevation of the RDW (and HDW) or the detection of two cell populations on a blood film or on the graphical output of an automated counter suggests that the correct diagnosis is iron deficiency.

Anaemia of chronic disease can usually be readily distinguished from β thalassaemia because of the greater degree of anaemia and retention of a normal MCV until significant anaemia has developed.

Further tests

Definitive diagnosis of β thalassaemia trait is usually by HPLC (which quantitates haemoglobin A_2 as well as detecting variant haemoglobins); alternative techniques are capillary electrophoresis and cellulose acetate electrophoresis, the latter supplemented by quantification of haemoglobin A_2 by microcolumn chromatography. Haemoglobin F is elevated in one third to one half of patients but is less specific than an increased percentage of haemoglobin A_2 and quantification is not necessary for diagnosis. δβ or $^A\gamma\delta\beta^0$ thalassaemia trait is diagnosed when there are thalassaemic indices with a normal or low haemoglobin A_2 and an elevated haemoglobin F. Diagnosis of the rare cases of εγδβ thalassaemia (also known as γδβ thalassaemia) trait requires DNA analysis. Haemoglobin Lepore trait is diagnosed when there are thalassaemic indices with a normal or reduced haemoglobin A_2 and with a minor abnormal haemoglobin having the same mobility as haemoglobin S at alkaline pH, the same mobility as haemoglobin A at acid pH and a retention time on HPLC that is similar to that of haemoglobin A_2. Haemoglobins E, C and S will also be detected on HPLC or electrophoresis.

Because iron deficiency causes a reduction of the haemoglobin A_2 percentage, some cases of mild β thalassaemia trait may be missed if tests are done when the patient has a coexisting iron deficiency. Except in pregnant patients when immediate diagnosis is needed, it is better **not** to carry out electrophoresis in patients who appear to have uncomplicated iron deficiency, but rather to check that the full blood count (FBC) returns to normal after treatment.

Most of the tests used to confirm a diagnosis of iron deficiency are normal in β thalassaemia trait (Table 8.1). However, zinc protoporphyrin is somewhat increased and soluble transferrin receptor is increased to similar levels to those seen in iron deficiency [15].

β thalassaemia major

β thalassaemia major is an inherited disease resulting from homozygosity or compound heterozygosity for β thalassaemia that leads to a severe reduction or total lack of synthesis of β globin chains. Consequently, there is a marked reduction or total failure to synthesise haemoglobin A. There is marked erythroid hyperplasia and ineffective haemopoiesis resulting from damage to developing erythroblasts by excess free α chains. Clinical features are severe anaemia, hepatomegaly, splenomegaly and expansion of marrow-containing bones leading to frontal bossing of the skull and deformity of the jaw bones. There is significant growth retardation. Treatment of β thalassaemia major by blood transfusion ameliorates many of the clinicopathological features seen in the untreated patient but, in the absence of effective chelation therapy, leads to iron overload, resultant organ damage and premature death.

Blood film and count

Anaemia is severe, with the Hb sometimes being as low as 20–30 g/l. The blood film (Fig. 8.9) shows very marked anisocytosis and poikilocytosis, with the poikilocytes including target cells, teardrop cells, elliptocytes, fragments and many cells of bizarre shape. Hypochromia is very striking, but microcytosis is not always so obvious on the blood film since the cells are very flat and red cell diameter is thus greater than would be expected from the red cell size. Basophilic stippling and Pappenheimer bodies are present. Sometimes a minority of cells have inclusions with the same staining characteristics as haemoglobin; these represent precipitates of excess α chains and are much more readily identified on a Heinz body preparation. Nucleated red blood cells (NRBC) are frequent. The circulating erythroblasts are micronormoblastic and show dyserythropoietic features, defective haemoglobinisation and the presence of Pappenheimer bodies. There is often leucocytosis, resulting from neutrophilia and, in younger children,

lymphocytosis. The platelet count may be normal or increased. In advanced disease with marked splenomegaly, the platelet count falls.

Following splenectomy (which may be performed because of discomfort from splenomegaly or to reduce transfusion requirement), the total nucleated cell count (TNCC), white blood cell count (WBC) and platelet count rise; the blood film is even more strikingly abnormal, with many abnormal NRBC and numerous target cells, Pappenheimer bodies and Howell–Jolly bodies. Post-splenectomy, Heinz body preparations show ragged inclusions in 10–20% of cells; these represent α chain precipitates and differ from the Heinz bodies consequent on oxidant stress in that they are not attached to the red cell membrane and are present in NRBC as well as mature erythrocytes [50]. Following splenectomy, there is often an exaggerated lymphocytosis or neutrophilia in response to intercurrent infections.

When patients are adequately transfused, the blood film is dimorphic with the percentage of the patient's own abnormal cells being low.

The blood count shows a severe microcytic anaemia, with the MCV, MCH and MCHC being greatly reduced and the RDW and HDW being increased. The TNCC, when measured on automated counters that do not correct for the presence of NRBC, is greatly increased; a true leucocytosis is also often present. The TNCC may be erroneous since, with some automated instruments, some but not all NRBC are included in the count. More recent instruments do not have this problem since NRBC are enumerated separately from WBC.

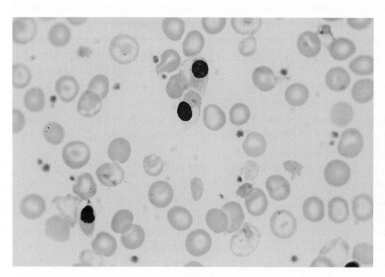

Fig. 8.9 The blood film of a patient with β thalassaemia major who has been splenectomised and is receiving intermittent blood transfusions. The blood film is dimorphic with about two-thirds of the erythrocytes being donor cells. The patient's own red cells show marked anisocytosis, poikilocytosis and hypochromia. There are several target cells and three nucleated red blood cells (NRBC). Some cells contain Pappenheimer bodies and in two cells (a very hypochromic cell and an NRBC) there are inclusions that represent precipitated α chains.

Differential diagnosis

Thalassaemia intermedia is distinguished from thalassaemia major on clinical rather than haematological grounds. It is a genetically heterogeneous condition but most often results from homozygosity or compound heterozygosity for mild β^+ thalassaemia. The Hb is usually above 70–80 g/l and other peripheral blood features are also intermediate between those of thalassaemia major and of thalassaemia minor. The compound heterozygous state for β thalassaemia and haemoglobin E can also have haematological features that resemble those of thalassaemia major.

Further tests

Diagnosis requires HPLC or haemoglobin electrophoresis, which show only haemoglobins F and A_2 when the genotype is β^0/β^0 and haemoglobins F and A_2 with a variable amount of haemoglobin A when the genotype is β^0/β^+ or β^+/β^+. Some cases of thalassaemia intermedia have a relatively high percentage of haemoglobin A, while others have almost exclusively haemoglobin F. Patients with severe disease as a result of compound heterozygosity for haemoglobin E and β thalassaemia are distinguished from thalassaemia major by HPLC or haemoglobin electrophoresis.

β thalassaemia intermedia

β thalassaemia intermedia refers to a clinical phenotype with diverse genetic explanations [48]. The genetic defect may be the presence of two alleles for mild β^+ thalassaemia, coinheritance of β thalassaemia and haemoglobin E or the presence of a single β thalassaemia allele with an aggravating factor such as coinheritance of triple α ($\alpha\alpha/\alpha\alpha\alpha$ or $\alpha\alpha\alpha/\alpha\alpha\alpha$). The patient is symptomatic from anaemia, often has splenomegaly and sometimes has bony deformities. However, in contrast to β thalassaemia major, the patient is not transfusion-dependent. β thalassaemia intermedia varies in severity, from a disabling condition in which survival without transfusion is barely possible to a condition only slightly more severe than β thalassaemia minor.

Blood film and count

There is a moderately severe microcytic anaemia. The blood film shows features similar to those of typical β thalassaemia trait, but the abnormalities are more severe (Figs 8.10 & 8.11). Polychromasia and circulating NRBC may be present.

Differential diagnosis

The differential diagnosis is β thalassaemia minor and β thalassaemia major. Diagnosis depends on clinical as well as laboratory features.

Other tests

HPLC or haemoglobin electrophoresis shows the presence of considerable amounts of haemoglobin F. The proportion of haemoglobin A_2 is increased. In some patients there is also some haemoglobin A. In cases dues to compound heterozygosity for β thalassaemia and haemoglobin E, haemoglobins F, E and A_2 will be present with or without some haemoglobin A.

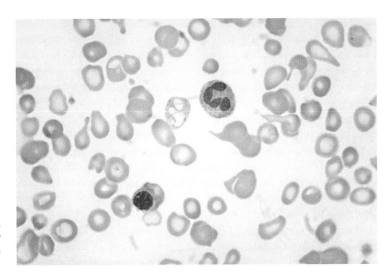

Fig. 8.10 The blood film of a patient with β thalassaemia intermedia caused by homozygosity for a mild β thalassaemia variant.

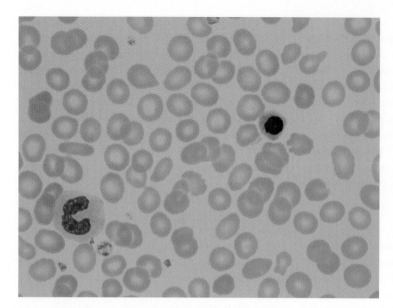

Fig. 8.11 The blood film of a patient with β thalassaemia intermedia caused by heterozygosity for β thalassaemia coinherited with duplication of alpha genes (αα/ααα) showing microcytosis, mild anisocytosis and poikilocytosis and the presence of a micronormoblast. Red cell indices were: RBC 4.94 × 10^{12}/l, Hb 94 g/l, Hct 0.30 l/l, MCV 61 fl, MCH 19 pg and MCHC 313 g/l with haemoglobin A_2 of 5.8% and haemoglobin F 3.1%.

Disorders resulting from a defect in α globin chain synthesis

α thalassaemia trait

Haematologically normal subjects have four α genes. α thalassaemia trait is an imprecise term used to indicate deletion of either one or two of the four α genes. The genotype –α/αα is designated α^+ thalassaemia. The genotype – –/αα is designated α^0 thalassaemia. Homozygosity for α^+ thalassaemia, i.e. –α/–α, or heterozygosity for the much less common non-deletional α thalassaemia trait, $\alpha^T\alpha/\alpha\alpha$ or $\alpha\alpha^T/\alpha\alpha$, produces a phenotype similar to that of α^0 thalassaemia heterozygosity. α thalassaemia is common among many ethnic groups. A high incidence is found among various South-East Asian populations, particularly among Thais and Chinese, who have both the –α/αα and the – –/αα genotypes. The – –/αα genotype also occurs in Greeks, Cypriots, Turks and Sardinians. Among Black Americans 25–30% have –α/αα and 1–2% have –α/–α [51]. In Jamaicans the prevalence is approximately 30% and 3%, respectively [52]. In Nigerians the prevalence is even higher, with 35% having –α/αα and 8% –α/–α [53]. –α/αα occurs in about 7% of Greeks [54] and is common in Cyprus and in some regions of Italy. On some Pacific islands the prevalence of –α/αα is as high as 85%.

A similar haematological phenotype is also produced by several α chain variant haemoglobins that are synthesised at a greatly reduced rate and thus represent non-deletional α thalassaemia; the commonest of these is haemoglobin Constant Spring, which is not uncommon in South-East Asia and is also found in the Caribbean area, around the Mediterranean, in the Middle East and in the Indian subcontinent. An α thalassaemia phenotype can also result from certain rare, highly unstable α chains variants that are largely degraded before haemoglobin can be formed.

α thalassaemia trait produces no clinically evident effects but can be of genetic significance.

Blood film and count

α^0 thalassaemia heterozygosity and α^+ thalassaemia homozygosity produce haematological features similar to those of β thalassaemia trait, although basophilic stippling and target cells are often not prominent (Fig. 8.12). An exception is non-deletional α thalassaemia due to the presence of haemoglobin Constant Spring, $\alpha^{CS}\alpha$, when basophilic stippling is prominent. α^+ thalassaemia heterozygosity produces a lesser abnormality and often there is no discernible abnormality in the blood film.

The red cell indices of individuals with only two α genes are similar to those of β thalassaemia trait. The indices in individuals with three rather than four α genes may be either normal or abnormal, in the latter case overlapping the values seen in those with only two α genes.

Differential diagnosis

The differential diagnosis of α thalassaemia trait is β thalassaemia trait and iron deficiency.

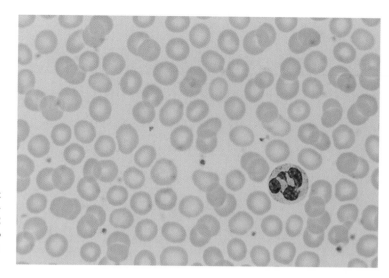

Fig. 8.12 The blood film of a healthy subject with α thalassaemia trait showing microcytosis and mild hypochromia. The FBC (Coulter S) was: RBC $6.24 \times 10^{12}/l$, Hb 141 g/l, Hct 0.45 l/l, MCV 72 fl, MCH 23 pg, MCHC 313 g/l.

Further tests

HPLC and haemoglobin electrophoresis are normal in α thalassaemia trait, except during the neonatal period when a low percentage of haemoglobin Bart's (γ_4) and haemoglobin H (β_4) may be detected. Haemoglobin Constant Spring can be detected electrophoretically and by HPLC, although sometimes with difficulty since the percentage of the abnormal haemoglobin is usually low. In adults the diagnosis of α thalassaemia trait should be suspected when a subject of an appropriate ethnic group who is not iron deficient has indices suggestive of thalassaemia trait with normal HPLC or haemoglobin electrophoresis and a normal or low haemoglobin A_2 percentage. The demonstration of haemoglobin H inclusions in a very small percentage of red cells supports the diagnosis, but this test is quite time-consuming and it may be negative, particularly in heterozygotes, and to a lesser extent homozygotes, for α^+ thalassaemia. When diagnosis is important, as when genetic counselling is required in a patient of South-East Asian, Greek, Turkish, Cypriot or Sardinian ethnic origin, DNA analysis is necessary.

Haemoglobin H disease

The lack of three of the four α genes (genotype – –/–α) or a functionally similar disorder [40] causes haemoglobin H disease. This most often occurs in subjects of South-East Asian origin including Thais, Chinese and Indonesians, but it is also seen in Greeks and Cypriots and less often in a variety of other ethnic groups. Clinical features are of a chronic haemolytic anaemia

with splenomegaly and sometimes hepatomegaly. In patients with more severe disease there is sometimes bony deformity similar to that seen in β thalassaemia major. Rarely there is transfusion dependency.

Blood film and count

The diagnosis of haemoglobin H disease can usually be suspected from the blood film and red cell indices. There is anaemia of moderate degree; the Hb is typically 60–100 g/l but it is lower during pregnancy, during intercurrent infections and following exposure to oxidant drugs. The blood film (Fig. 8.13) shows marked hypochromia, microcytosis and poikilocytosis, often including target cells, teardrop cells and fragments. Basophilic stippling and polychromasia are present. The reticulocyte percentage and absolute count are elevated. The coinheritance of haemoglobin H disease and hereditary elliptocytosis (see Fig. 3.25) causes striking poikilocytosis in addition to microcytosis.

The red cell indices show marked reduction of the MCV and MCH and reduction of the MCHC, which are demonstrated by the red cell cytogram (Fig. 8.14). The RDW and HDW are elevated.

Differential diagnosis

The differential diagnosis of haemoglobin H disease is β thalassaemia and other dyserythropoietic and haemolytic anaemias, particularly hereditary pyropoikilocytosis. The blood film and red cell indices are much more abnormal than in most β thalassaemia heterozygotes, but may be similar to those in β thalassaemia intermedia; the

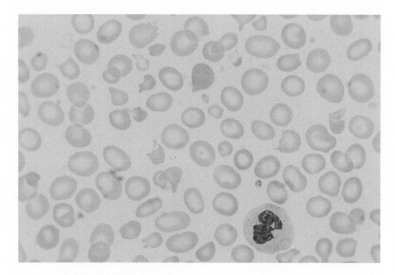

Fig. 8.13 The blood film of a patient with haemoglobin H disease showing anisocytosis, marked poikilocytosis, microcytosis and hypochromia. The FBC (Coulter S Plus IV) was: RBC $4.95 \times 10^{12}/l$, Hb 96 g/l, Hct 0.30 l/l, MCV 60.5fl, MCH 19.4 pg, MCHC 321 g/l, red cell distribution width (RDW) 25.7%. The corresponding haemoglobin H preparation is shown in Fig. 7.2a.

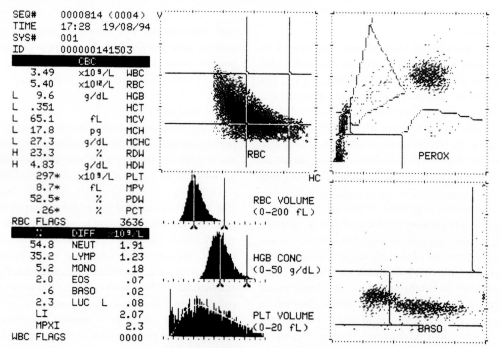

Fig. 8.14 Bayer H.2 scatter plots and histograms of a patient with haemoglobin H disease. The red cell cytogram and histograms show severe hypochromia and microcytosis. The white cell scatter plots are normal.

elevated reticulocyte count and the usual lack of NRBC in haemoglobin H disease are useful in making the distinction from β thalassaemia intermedia. The MCHC is reduced, irrespective of the method of measurement, whereas in β thalassaemia trait it is not reduced when measured by impedance counters, but is reduced when measured by Siemens H.1 and Advia series instruments.

Congenital dyserythropoietic anaemias and hereditary pyropoikilocytosis can show a similar degree of poikilocytosis to haemoglobin H disease, but the former group of disorders have normocytic or macrocytic red cells and no reticulocytosis, while the blood film in the latter condition shows specific types of poikilocyte such as microspherocytes, elliptocytes and red cells with bud-like

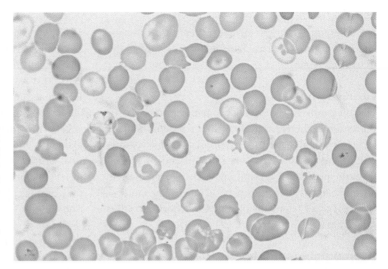

Fig. 8.15 The blood film of a patient with acquired haemoglobin H disease as part of a myelodysplastic syndrome showing anisocytosis, poikilocytosis, microcytosis and some hypochromic cells and target cells. One of the hypochromic cells contains Pappenheimer bodies. The FBC was: white blood cell count (WBC) 9.2×10^9/l, Hb 102 g/l, MCV 66 fl and platelet count 53×10^9/l. By courtesy of Dr A. Hendrick, South Shields.

projections. Acquired haemoglobin H disease, which can be a manifestation of MDS, should also be mentioned in the differential diagnosis of the inherited condition; it is differentiated by the age of onset, the lack of a relevant family history and the demonstration of other features of MDS (Fig. 8.15).

Further tests

The diagnosis is confirmed by the demonstration of haemoglobin H inclusions in red cells (see Fig. 7.2) and by HPLC or haemoglobin electrophoresis, which shows 2–40% of haemoglobin H. These procedures will also identify cases with both haemoglobin Constant Spring and haemoglobin H; such cases have the genotype $\alpha^{CS}\alpha/--$ or $\alpha^{CS}\alpha/\alpha^{CS}\alpha$, which produces clinical and haematological features similar to deletional haemoglobin H disease, although often somewhat more severe.

Haemoglobin Bart's hydrops fetalis

Haemoglobin Bart's hydrops fetalis is a syndrome resulting from an absence of all four α genes (α genotype $--/--$) and a resultant total lack of α globin chain synthesis. This results in severe anaemia, extramedullary haemopoiesis and hypoalbuminaemia, causing stillbirth or early neonatal death of a hydropic fetus.

Blood film and count

There is severe anaemia and the blood film (Fig. 8.16) shows striking hypochromia, microcytosis, poikilocytosis and the presence of NRBC.

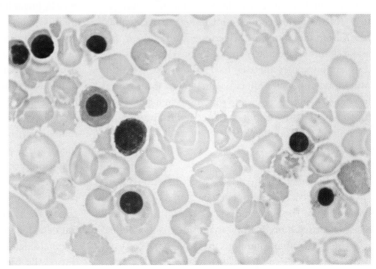

Fig. 8.16 The blood film of neonate with haemoglobin Bart's hydrops fetalis showing anisocytosis, poikilocytosis and NRBC. By courtesy of Dr Mary Frances McMullin, Belfast.

Differential diagnosis

The differential diagnosis includes other causes of severe anaemia in the fetus (see Table 6.20) and other causes of hydrops fetalis.

Further tests

The diagnosis is confirmed by demonstration of α^0 thalassaemia heterozygosity in both parents and by HPLC or haemoglobin electrophoresis, which shows only haemoglobins Bart's, H and Portland. Diagnosis in early pregnancy, permitting early termination of an affected pregnancy, can be achieved by molecular analysis of fetal cells obtained by chorionic villus sampling.

Haemoglobinopathies

Haemoglobinopathies are inherited abnormalities of globin chain synthesis. Some haematologists use this term broadly to cover all such abnormalities, including the thalassaemias. Others classify disorders of globin chain synthesis as 'haemoglobinopathies' when there is a structural abnormality and as 'thalassaemias' when the principal abnormality is a reduced rate of synthesis of one of the globin chains. There is necessarily some overlap between 'haemoglobinopathies' and 'thalassaemias' since some abnormal haemoglobins (e.g. haemoglobin E) are synthesised at a reduced rate. Abnormal haemoglobins may also be formed in thalassaemias as a result of unbalanced chain synthesis (e.g. haemoglobin Bart's and haemoglobin H in various α thalassaemia syndromes). The most convenient approach is therefore to regard thalassaemia as a subtype of haemoglobinopathy. Haemoglobinopathies (including thalassaemias) result from mutations in the genes encoding the α, β, γ and δ chains of haemoglobin. Mutations of α genes produce abnormalities affecting haemoglobins A, A_2 and F. Mutations in β genes affect haemoglobin A, mutations in γ genes haemoglobin F and mutations in δ genes haemoglobin A_2. Only mutations affecting α and β genes are important in adult life.

Sickle cell anaemia

Sickle cell anaemia is the disease caused by homozygosity for the β chain variant, haemoglobin S or sickle cell haemoglobin. The genotype is $\beta^S\beta^S$. The term 'sickle cell disease' is used more broadly than 'sickle cell anaemia' to include also other conditions that lead to red cell sickling, such as sickle cell/β thalassaemia.

Haemoglobin S is prone to polymerise in conditions of low oxygen tension, causing the red cell to become sickle shaped and less deformable. There are associated changes in the red cell membrane and in endothelial cells. The resulting obstruction of small blood vessels leads to tissue infarction, which underlies the dominant clinical feature of the disease, the recurrent painful crises affecting fingers and toes (in young children), limbs, abdomen and chest. Other clinical features are anaemia, which results largely from the low oxygen affinity of haemoglobin S, and splenomegaly, which is present only during childhood and is followed by splenic infarction and fibrosis leading to hyposplenism.

The β^S gene and therefore sickle cell anaemia have their greatest frequency in individuals with African ancestry, but the gene also occurs in Indian, Greek, Italian, Turkish, Cypriot, Spanish, Arab, North African, Central and South American and some Indian subcontinent populations.

Blood film and count

In sickle cell anaemia [55] the Hb is usually of the order of 70–80 g/l, but with a range of 40–110 g/l or even wider. Higher Hbs are characteristic of Arabs with sickle cell anaemia. A typical blood film (Fig. 8.17) shows anisocytosis, anisochromasia, sickle cells, boat-shaped cells (pointed at both ends but not crescent shaped), target cells, polychromasia, basophilic stippling, NRBC and sometimes occasional irregularly contracted cells or spherocytes. Scanning electron micrography shows the characteristic form of the sickle cell (see Fig. 3.56). There may be linear fragments of sickle cells (see Fig. 3.50). Once infancy is past, the features of hyposplenism – Howell–Jolly bodies, Pappenheimer bodies and more numerous target cells – are also present. Acanthocytes, which are usually present in hyposplenic states, are not a feature of hyposplenism caused by sickle cell disease. The reticulocyte count is usually 10–20%. The WBC, neutrophil, lymphocyte, monocyte and platelet counts are higher than in control subjects of the same ethnic group; counts tend to rise with age [56]. Occasional monocytes and neutrophils contain phagocytosed red cells.

At birth, when only a small amount of haemoglobin S is present, the Hb, red cell indices and blood count are normal. The blood film is usually normal, but occasionally sickle cells are seen, even in neonates. Haematological abnormalities usually become apparent during the first year of life [57,58]. The Hb falls below

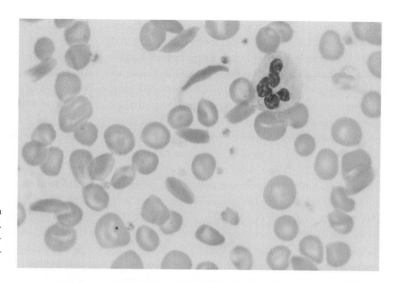

Fig. 8.17 The blood film of a patient with sickle cell anaemia showing anisocytosis, poikilocytosis, one sickle cell, several boat-shaped cells and a cell containing a Howell–Jolly body.

the normal range at 1–6 months of age. A few sickle cells and other features of sickle cell anaemia appear at 4–6 months of age; features of hyposplenism usually appear at 9–12 months of age, but sometimes as early as 6 months. The features of hyposplenism appear at about the time that splenomegaly is detected. In early infancy hyposplenism can be reversed by blood transfusion, but later it cannot. Circulating NRBC only become common after 12 months of age.

Some subjects, although homozygous for β^S, have a normal or near normal Hb and very few signs or symptoms of sickle cell anaemia; they are mainly Arabs with an unusually high percentage of haemoglobin F, which ameliorates the condition. In such subjects the morphological abnormalities may also be slight. When α thalassaemia trait coexists with sickle cell anaemia there are subtle differences in the red cell indices, but only when groups of patients are considered. Individuals cannot be distinguished on haematological grounds. In a group with coexisting α thalassaemia trait, the mean Hb and RBC are higher, whereas the mean MCV, MCH, MCHC, reticulocyte count and degree of polychromasia and number of sickle cells are less. Treatment with hydroxycarbamide causes a rise in the MCV and MCH and reduces the degree of blood film abnormality.

During painful crises there is leucocytosis (with the WBC sometimes as high as 40–50 × 10^9/l), neutrophilia, a minor fall in the Hb, increasing polychromasia and a rise in the number of NRBC and the reticulocyte count. There is an increase in the number of sickle cells

in the blood film, but recognition of this requires careful counting and a knowledge of the baseline values for an individual patient. Irregularly contracted cells become much more numerous during pulmonary infarction with hypoxia.

Because of the shortened red cell survival, patients with sickle cell anaemia are prone to acute worsening of the anaemia when complicating conditions develop. The blood film and count may give some clues as to the cause of this. In acute splenic sequestration, which is largely confined to infants, there is a very acute fall of the Hb and the platelet count also falls. Subsequently, there are increased numbers of NRBC, increasing polychromasia and an elevation of the reticulocyte count. In older subjects, acute sequestration may involve the liver rather than the spleen. In bone marrow infarction the WBC and platelet count may fall, there are prominent leucoerythroblastic features and some circulating megakaryocytes may be seen. In parvovirus B19 infection, white cells and platelets are rarely affected; there is a disappearance of both NRBC and polychromasia and the reticulocyte count is very low. During the recovery phase there is an outpouring of NRBC and a rise in the WBC, neutrophil count and reticulocyte count. The suppression of reticulocyte production is usually less when other infections lead to worsening of anaemia, which acquires the characteristics of the anaemia of chronic disease. In megaloblastic anaemia due to folate deficiency, some circulating megaloblasts, macrocytes and hypersegmented neutrophils may be seen. The reticulocyte count falls. In acute chest crisis, the Hb and platelet count fall, with a platelet count of less than 200 × 10⁹/l being an indicator of likely further complications [59]. Erythrophagocytosis may be observed in patients with hyperhaemolysis following blood transfusion [60]. The presence of red cell ghosts may alert the haematologist to haemolysis due to a coexisting glucose-6-phosphate dehydrogenase deficiency [61].

The blood count in sickle cell anaemia shows the Hb, RBC and Hct to be reduced. The MCV is normal or elevated, but is not increased to a degree commensurate with the increase in the reticulocyte count [62]; this may be regarded as a relative microcytosis. The RDW and HDW are increased. Red cell cytograms of Siemens H.1 (Fig. 8.18) and Advia (Fig. 8.19) series instruments show a population of dense cells representing irreversibly sickled cells and may show a population of hypodense cells representing reticulocytes. Although hyperdense cells are detected, their percentage may be underestimated because irreversibly sickled cells are incapable of undergoing the sphering that should occur

prior to measurement of red cell variables by these instruments [51,63]. Impedance counters fail to detect the increased MCHC of the most dense cells [63]. Further changes in red cell indices occur during, and sometimes 1–3 days before, painful crises [64]. The slight fall in the Hb and rise in the reticulocyte count are accompanied by further increases in the RDW and HDW. There is an increase in the MCHC and the percentage of abnormally dense cells.

Differential diagnosis

The differential diagnosis of sickle cell anaemia is mainly sickle cell/haemoglobin C disease (see below) and sickle cell/β thalassaemia. Sickle cell/β° thalassaemia cannot be distinguished from sickle cell anaemia on HPLC or haemoglobin electrophoresis since there is no haemoglobin A in either condition. The distinction is made on the basis of family studies and the lower MCV and MCH in the compound heterozygous state. Sickle cell/β⁺ thalassaemia may show a less abnormal blood count and blood film than sickle cell anaemia, depending on

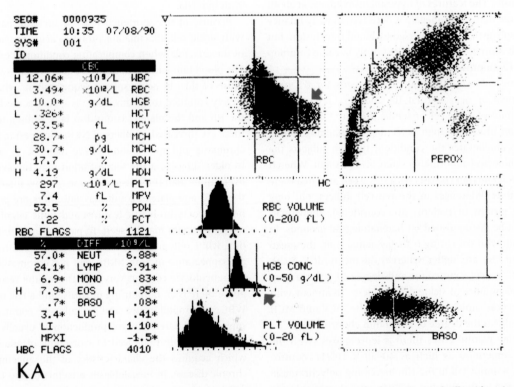

Fig. 8.18 Bayer H.1 red cell scatter plots and histograms of a patient with sickle cell anaemia; the presence of cells with an increased haemoglobin content is apparent on both the red cell cytogram and on the histogram of haemoglobin concentration (green arrows).

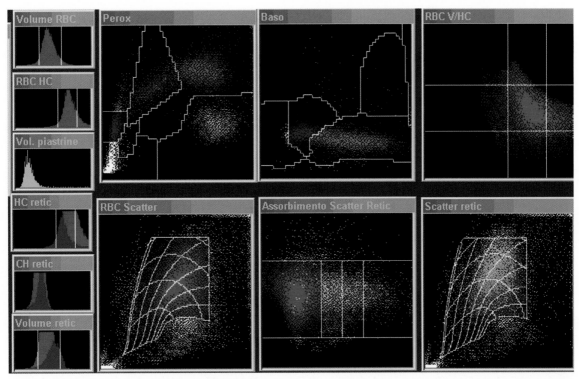

Fig. 8.19 Siemens Advia series cytogram and histograms from a patient with sickle cell anaemia. The FBC was: WBC 9.3×10^9/l, RBC 3.07×10^{12}/l, Hb 94 g/l, Hct 0.27 l/l, MCH 30.6 pg, MCHC 349 g/l, cellular haemoglobin concentration mean (CHCM) 365 g/l, RDW 19.7%, platelets 575×10^9/l, reticulocyte count 18.5%, 568×10^9/l. The red cell cytogram and haemoglobin concentration histogram (RBC HC) show an increase in cells with an increased haemoglobin concentration (to the right of the right-hand vertical threshold) and there was a +++ hyperchromia flag. There was also a flag indicating the presence of NRBC. The reticulocyte scatter plot shows increased mature, intermediate and immature reticulocytes (turquoise dots). Note that there is an incidental hypereosinophilia: 18.9%, 1.76×10^9/l. By courtesy of Professor Gina Zini, Rome.

the amount of haemoglobin A that is present; haemoglobin electrophoresis or HPLC is diagnostic. The blood film of compound heterozygotes for haemoglobin S and either haemoglobin D-Punjab or haemoglobin O-Arab cannot be distinguished from that of sickle cell anaemia. Compound heterozygosity for haemoglobin S and hereditary persistence of fetal haemoglobin can be distinguished by the milder clinical and haematological phenotype, family studies and haemoglobin electrophoresis or HPLC. Sickle cell trait should not be confused with sickle cell anaemia, since the Hb is normal and there are no sickle cells in the blood film, but heterozygotes for several rare variants, e.g. Hb S-Antilles, may have sickle cells on routine blood films [65] and heterozygotes for haemoglobin S-Oman have characteristic Napoleon hat cells – fat in the middle but pointed at both ends.

Further tests

Diagnosis is based on a sickle solubility test and either HPLC or haemoglobin electrophoresis, although it should be noted that if there are obvious sickle cells in a blood film the sickle solubility test could be considered redundant. Haemoglobin S predominates, with smaller amounts of haemoglobins F and A_2 and no haemoglobin A. Haemoglobin F varies from 2% to around 15% and haemoglobin A_2 may be minimally elevated. If haemoglobin electrophoresis is the primary analytical method, it is necessary for this to be performed at acid as well as alkaline pH to distinguish compound heterozygous states such as S/D-Punjab (S/D-Los Angeles) and S/Lepore from sickle cell anaemia; D-Punjab/Los Angeles and Lepore both move with S at alkaline pH, but at acid pH move with haemoglobin A. If the primary analytical method is HPLC, then these two variant haemoglobins are not confused with haemoglobin S. In infants, the percentage of haemoglobin S may be too low for the sickle solubility test to be positive and diagnosis then rests on HPLC, with confirmation by electrophoresis or isoelectric focusing, or by electrophoresis at acid and alkaline pH.

Diagnostic tests for sickle cell anaemia and other forms of sickle cell disease are recommended in all neonates of appropriate ethnic origin, since early parenteral education, appropriate vaccinations and prophylactic penicillin therapy significantly reduce mortality. In the UK routine testing is done in the early neonatal period using Guthrie spots (spots of dried blood from a heelprick specimen on filter paper).

Sickle cell trait

Sickle cell trait indicates heterozygosity for β^S so that both haemoglobin S and haemoglobin A are present. The genotype is $\beta\beta^S$. Sickle cell trait is usually asymptomatic, but is of genetic significance and is relevant if a patient is likely to become hypoxic. Occasional patients have clinical manifestations such as haematuria, loss of renal concentrating ability or splenic infarction at altitude.

Blood film and count

The blood film may be normal or show microcytosis or target cell formation. Although classical sickle cells are not seen, there may be small numbers of plump cells that are pointed at both ends [66]; such cells are observed in about 96% of individuals with sickle cell trait in comparison with 4% of normal subjects. Very rarely true sickle cells are seen. This has been reported in a patient with acute lymphoblastic leukaemia with a very high WBC and was attributed to *in vitro* consumption of oxygen by the leukaemic cells [67]. The blood count is either normal or shows reduction of the MCV and MCH. Reduction of the MCV is commoner in those with sickle cell trait than in other individuals of African ancestry [68]. This appears to be due to the slightly higher incidence of α thalassaemia trait in subjects with sickle cell trait [69], since no difference in red cell indices is observed between those with and without sickle cell trait when individuals with iron deficiency or α thalassaemia trait are excluded from the analysis [70].

Differential diagnosis

The main differential diagnosis is other conditions that cause microcytosis (see Table 3.1) and other causes of target cell formation (see Table 3.7).

Further tests

The blood film and count must not be relied on for diagnosis. Diagnosis requires both HPLC or haemoglobin electrophoresis (which shows A and S but with the percentage of A being greater than the percentage of S) and a sickle solubility test (which shows that the abnormal haemoglobin is haemoglobin S rather than another abnormal haemoglobin with the same mobility or retention time). Haemoglobin S is usually 25–45% of total haemoglobin. The diagnosis of sickle cell trait should not be excluded on the basis of a negative sickle solubility test alone; if this is done in an emergency, e.g. before anaesthesia, it must be followed by HPLC or haemoglobin electrophoresis to confirm the negative test. Diagnosis in the first 6 months of life, when the haemoglobin S percentage may be too low for a positive sickle solubility test, requires the use of two independent methods to confirm the nature of the variant haemoglobin, e.g. (i) HPLC, supplemented by isoelectric focusing or electrophoresis, or (ii) electrophoresis at both acid and alkaline pH.

Sickle cell/β thalassaemia

Patients who are heterozygous for haemoglobin S and either β^0 or β^+ thalassaemia cannot be distinguished reliably from sickle cell anaemia on the basis of clinical features, although those with $\beta^S\beta^+$ thalassaemia tend to have milder disease and splenomegaly is more likely to persist beyond early childhood.

Blood film and count

The blood films and counts of compound heterozygotes for haemoglobin S and β thalassaemia cannot be reliably distinguished from sickle cell anaemia, particularly sickle cell anaemia with coexisting α thalassaemia trait, but as a group some differences are apparent. Those with $\beta^S\beta^0$ thalassaemia show more microcytosis and hypochromia than is usual in sickle cell anaemia and Pappenheimer bodies may be more prominent (Fig. 8.20). Otherwise blood films are similar. The blood films of compound heterozygotes with $\beta^S\beta^+$ thalassaemia generally show less marked abnormalities, depending on the percentages of haemoglobins A and F; target cells are numerous but sickle cells are less frequent. When there is persistent

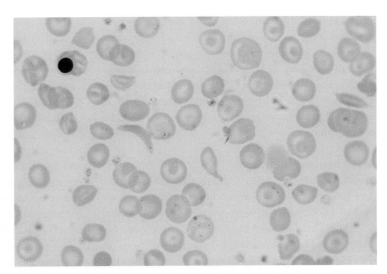

Fig. 8.20 The blood film of a patient with sickle cell/β⁰ thalassaemia compound heterozygosity showing anisocytosis, poikilocytosis, one sickle cell, one boat-shaped cell and one NRBC. Many of the red cells contain Pappenheimer bodies.

splenomegaly, leucopenia and thrombocytopenia can occur as a consequence of hypersplenism.

The blood counts in compound heterozygotes, particularly those with $\beta^S\beta^+$ thalassaemia, as a group show a higher Hb, RBC and Hct than patients with sickle cell anaemia and a lower MCV, MCH, MCHC, reticulocyte percentage and reticulocyte absolute count [71,72].

Differential diagnosis

The differential diagnosis is sickle cell anaemia and sickle cell/haemoglobin C disease.

Further tests

The diagnosis of $\beta^S\beta^+$ thalassaemia can be confirmed by HPLC or haemoglobin electrophoresis, which demonstrates haemoglobins S and A but, in contrast to sickle cell trait, the S percentage is higher than the A percentage. Haemoglobin F may also be increased, but does not usually exceed 10–15%. $\beta^S\beta^0$ thalassaemia cannot be distinguished readily from sickle cell anaemia by HPLC or haemoglobin electrophoresis, since in neither condition is there any haemoglobin A. Diagnosis of cases with microcytosis and haemoglobins S and F requires family studies and, if necessary, DNA analysis.

Haemoglobin S/hereditary persistence of fetal haemoglobin (HPFH) compound heterozygosity

Patients with compound heterozygosity for haemoglobin S and deletional HPFH, β^SHPFH genotype, have a mild clinical condition in which painful crises are infrequent or absent.

Blood film and count

The Hb is normal. Cells are normocytic and normochromic and features of hyposplenism are usually absent. There is anisocytosis, target cells are present and there are infrequent sickle cells.

The blood count is normal or shows very minor abnormalities.

Differential diagnosis

The differential diagnosis is sickle cell anaemia and sickle cell/β thalassaemia. The blood film shows much less abnormality than in either of the other conditions.

Further tests

HPLC or haemoglobin electrophoresis shows haemoglobin S and haemoglobin F. F constitutes 20–30% of total haemoglobin. The F percentage is generally higher than in S/β thalassaemia compound heterozygotes, who usually have a haemoglobin F of less than 15%. The F percentage is also generally higher than in sickle cell anaemia in which levels of 0.5–15% are usual; however, it should be noted that some Arab patients with sickle cell anaemia have higher levels of haemoglobin F, as do patients under treatment with hydroxycarbamide.

Sickle cell/haemoglobin C disease

Haemoglobin C is a β chain variant that originated in West Africa, west of the Niger River, and is also present in some Afro-Caribbeans and African Americans and, less commonly, in other ethnic groups such as North Africans, Sicilians, Italians and Spaniards. Compound heterozygotes for haemoglobin S and haemoglobin C, genotype $\beta^S\beta^C$, have a sickling disorder of very variable severity, ranging from virtually asymptomatic to a severity comparable with that of sickle cell anaemia. Splenomegaly is present in childhood and may persist into adult life. Retinal abnormalities and ischaemic necrosis of major bones are more common than in sickle cell anaemia.

Blood film and count

In sickle cell/haemoglobin C disease the Hb is higher than in sickle cell anaemia with little overlap, levels of 80–140 g/l being seen in women and 80–170 g/l in men [71]. Sickle cell/haemoglobin C disease can usually be distinguished from sickle cell anaemia on the basis of the blood film (Fig. 8.21), although it may not always be possible to distinguish it from haemoglobin C disease [73]. There are few sickle cells and, in comparison with sickle cell anaemia, fewer NRBC, less polychromasia and less evidence of hyposplenism, which tends to develop later in life. Target cells and boat-shaped cells are numerous. Irregularly contracted cells are more prominent and many patients have unusual poikilocytes that are specific to sickle cell/haemoglobin C disease; these resemble sickle cells in being dense and having some degree of curvature, but they differ in that they have some straight edges or are angulated or branched [73,74]. Specific SC poikilocytes are sometimes present in large numbers, but more often they are infrequent. Rare cells containing haemoglobin C crystals can also be found in a significant minority of patients.

In patients who are heterozygous for $\alpha^{G\ Philadelphia}$ as well as for β^S and β^C, morphological features differ [75]. Haemoglobin C crystals are longer and once the cell membrane has ruptured the crystal acquires a scalloped appearance, which has been likened to sugar cane.

A sudden fall in Hb may be due to superimposed megaloblastic anaemia, bone marrow necrosis or parvovirus B19-induced pure red cell aplasia. Megaloblastic anaemia and bone marrow necrosis are particularly likely during pregnancy. When these conditions are suspected as a complication of sickle cell/haemoglobin C disease, the same features should be sought as were described under sickle cell anaemia.

The Hb, RBC and Hct are higher than in sickle cell anaemia. The MCV is generally lower and may be below the normal range, even in those who do not have coexisting α thalassaemia trait [76]. The MCHC is higher than in sickle cell disease, often above the normal range, and red cell cytograms identify a population of hyperdense cells. The RDW and HDW are increased. The reticulocyte count is lower, averaging 3% in contrast to 10% in sickle cell anaemia [55].

The WBC and neutrophil and monocyte counts are higher than in Black controls [56].

Haemoglobin C disease

Homozygotes for haemoglobin C, genotype $\beta^C\beta^C$, have chronic haemolysis and usually haemolytic anaemia. The spleen is enlarged and the incidence of gallstones is increased.

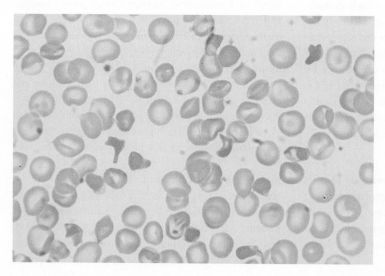

Fig. 8.21 The blood film of a patient with sickle cell/haemoglobin C compound heterozygosity showing numerous specific SC poikilocytes.

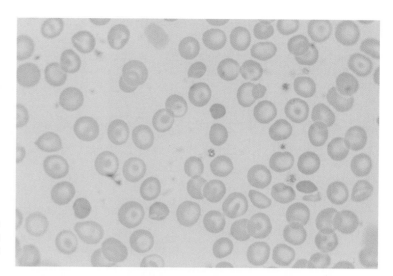

Fig. 8.22 The blood film of a patient with haemoglobin C disease showing a mixture of irregularly contracted cells and target cells.

Blood film and count

There is usually a mild to moderate anaemia. The blood film generally shows large numbers of both target cells and irregularly contracted cells (Fig. 8.22). The latter cells resemble spherocytes, but closer inspection shows that the majority are irregular in shape. Polychromasia and some NRBC may be noted. Some patients have hypochromia and microcytosis. Haemoglobin C crystals are uncommon, but when present are sufficiently distinctive to confirm the presence of this haemoglobin. They are rhomboidal with parallel sides and triangular or obliquely sloping ends (see below). They are usually contained in a cell that appears to be otherwise empty of haemoglobin. A minority of patients have a lesser degree of blood film abnormality with smaller numbers of target cells and irregularly contracted cells.

The Hb, RBC and Hct are normal or mildly to moderately reduced. A marked reduction of MCV and MCH is common, with the MCHC being increased [76]. The low MCV and MCH occur even in the absence of coexisting α thalassaemia trait. The RDW and HDW are increased and red cell cytograms show a population of hyperdense cells. The reticulocyte count is increased.

Differential diagnosis

The differential diagnosis is sickle cell/haemoglobin C disease and haemoglobin C/β thalassaemia compound heterozygosity. The blood film of haemoglobin C trait is also occasionally sufficiently abnormal to resemble that of milder cases of haemoglobin C disease.

Further tests

The diagnosis can usually be strongly suspected from the blood film, but confirmation requires a sickle solubility test and HPLC or haemoglobin electrophoresis. The haemoglobins present are C, A_2 (which cannot be easily distinguished from C on cellulose acetate electrophoresis, but separates on capillary electrophoresis) and small amounts of haemoglobin F. In microcytic cases, family studies or molecular genetic analysis are needed to make the distinction from compound heterozygosity for haemoglobin C and β° thalassaemia. If haemoglobin electrophoresis is the primary diagnostic method, a secondary method is needed to distinguish SC from S-O-Arab, since haemoglobin O-Arab moves with haemoglobin C at alkaline pH.

Haemoglobin C trait

Haemoglobin C trait, genotype $ββ^C$, is an asymptomatic abnormality of no significance apart from the possibility of more severe disease in offspring.

Blood film and count

The Hb is normal. The blood film (Fig. 8.23) may be normal or may show target cells, varying from occasional to frequent, or occasional irregularly contracted cells. Red cells are often hypochromic and microcytic, even in

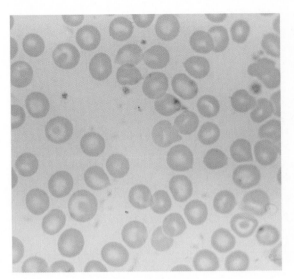

Fig. 8.23 The blood film of a patient with haemoglobin C trait showing several target cells and an irregularly contracted cell.

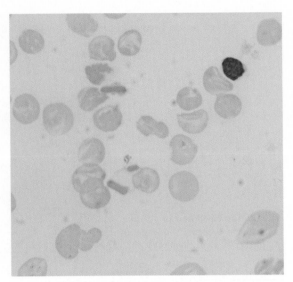

Fig. 8.24 The blood film of a patient with haemoglobin C/β^0 compound heterozygosity showing crystals of haemoglobin C within cells that otherwise appear empty of haemoglobin.

the absence of coexisting α thalassaemia trait [76]. The reticulocyte count is normal. The blood count is either normal or shows a reduced MCV and MCH.

Differential diagnosis
The differential diagnosis includes other causes of target cells (see Table 3.7) and sometimes other causes of irregularly contracted cells (see Table 3.4).

Further tests
Since the blood film and blood count may be normal, HPLC or haemoglobin electrophoresis is required to confirm or exclude haemoglobin C trait. One of these tests is therefore indicated if genetic counselling is required in West Africans, Afro-Caribbeans or Black Americans, even when a negative sickle solubility test has excluded the presence of haemoglobin S.

Haemoglobin C/β thalassaemia
The compound heterozygous state for haemoglobin C and β^0 or β^+ thalassaemia may cause symptomatic anaemia and splenomegaly.

Blood film and count
There is a moderate anaemia. The blood film (Fig. 8.24) shows microcytosis, hypochromia, target cells and irregularly contracted cells. Haemoglobin C crystals may be present. The blood count shows reduction of the Hb, RBC, Hct, MCV and MCH.

Differential diagnosis
The differential diagnosis is haemoglobin C disease and various thalassaemic conditions.

Further tests
The diagnosis is dependent on HPLC or haemoglobin electrophoresis, if necessary supplemented by family studies or molecular genetic analysis to distinguish haemoglobin C disease from haemoglobin C/β^0 thalassaemia.

Haemoglobin E disease
Haemoglobin E is a β chain variant that is common in Thailand, Burma, Laos, Cambodia, Vietnam and Malaysia and to a lesser extent in other countries in South-East Asia stretching from Indonesia to Nepal and including Sri Lanka. It has a very low frequency in Northern European Caucasians and individuals of African origin, although occasional cases are observed in Afro-Caribbeans. Haemoglobin E disease, genotype $\beta^E\beta^E$, is usually asymptomatic [77].

Blood film and count
There is a mild anaemia or a normal haemoglobin concentration. The blood film (Fig. 8.25) shows hypochromia and microcytosis, a variable number of target cells and sometimes irregularly contracted cells. The

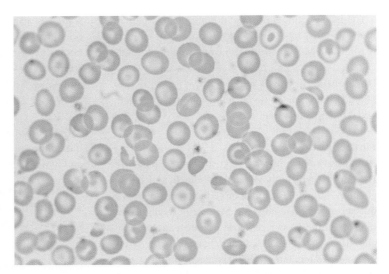

Fig. 8.25 The blood film of a patient with haemoglobin E homozygosity showing hypochromia, microcytosis, target cells and occasional irregularly contracted cells and other poikilocytes. The FBC (Coulter S) was: RBC $6.84 \times 10^{12}/1$, Hb 119 g/l, Hct 0.37 l/l, MCV 54 fl, MCH 17.4 pg, MCHC 267g/l.

reticulocyte count is usually normal. The blood count is often similar to that of β thalassaemia trait, with a mild anaemia or a normal Hb, elevated RBC and reduced MCV and MCH.

Differential diagnosis

The differential diagnosis is haemoglobin E/β thalassaemia compound heterozygosity, β thalassaemia trait and iron deficiency. Haemoglobin C disease would also be included in the differential diagnosis were it not for the fact that there is very little overlap between the ethnic groups in which these two haemoglobinopathies occur. Haemoglobin Eβ^0 thalassaemia is clinically more severe and often has a greater degree of anaemia and microcytosis than does haemoglobin E disease and also more NRBC. Haemoglobin Eβ^+ thalassaemia and the other conditions included in the differential diagnosis are excluded by haemoglobin electrophoresis or HPLC.

Further tests

Diagnosis requires HPLC or haemoglobin electrophoresis, which shows mainly haemoglobin E with up to 5–10% haemoglobin F. In haemoglobin E/β^0 thalassaemia the percentage of haemoglobin F is higher. Haemoglobin E has the same mobility as haemoglobin C at alkaline pH and the same mobility as haemoglobin A at acid pH. Haemoglobin E can be distinguished from haemoglobins A and C by HPLC, although it may have the same retention time as haemoglobin A$_2$. On capillary electrophoresis, haemoglobins E and A$_2$ separate.

Haemoglobin E trait

Haemoglobin E trait, genotype $\beta\beta^E$, is a completely asymptomatic condition that is only of importance because of its potential genetic significance.

Blood film and count

The blood film (Fig. 8.26) may be normal, but more often shows microcytosis or a few target cells or irregularly contracted cells.

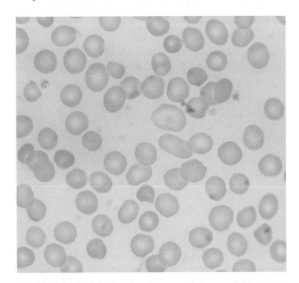

Fig. 8.26 The blood film of a patient with haemoglobin E trait showing hypochromia, microcytosis and occasional irregularly contracted cells. The FBC (Coulter S Plus IV) was: RBC $4.39 \times 10^{12}/1$, Hb 110 g/l, Hct 0.32 l/l, MCV 74 fl, MCH 25.1 pg, MCHC 332 g/l.

The blood count is normal in a minority of patients. In the majority (about 90%) it shows a minor reduction of MCV and MCH, with the Hb usually being normal.

Differential diagnosis
The differential diagnosis includes mild iron deficiency and β thalassaemia trait.

Further tests
Diagnosis is dependent on HPLC or haemoglobin electrophoresis, which show haemoglobin E and haemoglobin A, but with haemoglobin E being only about one quarter of total haemoglobin because of its diminished rate of synthesis. On cellulose acetate electrophoresis and HPLC, haemoglobin E and haemoglobin A_2 cannot be separated, but on capillary electrophoresis, when they separate, haemoglobin A_2 is found to be increased.

Haemoglobin E/β thalassaemia
Haemoglobin E/β thalassaemia compound heterozygosity, genotype $β^Eβ^0$ or $β^Eβ^+$ thalassaemia, is in general considerably more severe than haemoglobin E disease. It occurs in South-East Asia and in India and, following migration, in Europe and North America. Severity varies from a mild anaemia to a condition resembling thalassaemia intermedia or thalassaemia major, with hepatomegaly, splenomegaly, anaemia and often transfusion-dependence.

Blood film and count
Anaemia is usually moderate with an Hb of 70–90 g/l, though it varies from 20 to 130 g/l [78]. Marked hypochromia and microcytosis are usual (Fig. 8.27). Red cells of some cases show basophilic stippling, anisocytosis and poikilocytosis. Poikilocytes may include target cells, keratocytes, teardrop cells, fragments and irregularly contracted cells. The reticulocyte percentage is increased and some NRBC may be present. The Hb, RBC, Hct, MCV and MCH are all reduced and often also the MCHC.

Complicating conditions that may affect the blood film and count are aplastic crisis, megaloblastic anaemia and hypersplenism.

Differential diagnosis
The differential diagnosis includes haemoglobin E disease and various thalassaemic conditions.

Further tests
Diagnosis is dependent on HPLC or haemoglobin electrophoresis, which may need to be supplemented by family studies or molecular genetic analysis. In haemoglobin $Eβ^0$ thalassaemia, haemoglobins E and F are present, with haemoglobin F levels ranging from around 10% to well over 50%. In haemoglobin E/$β^+$ thalassaemia there is also haemoglobin A, usually constituting around 30% of total haemoglobin.

Unstable haemoglobins
Heterozygosity for an unstable haemoglobin produces mild, moderate or severe haemolytic anaemia, depending on the severity of the molecular defect. Haemolysis may be chronic or precipitated or aggravated by infection or exposure to oxidant drugs. The spleen is sometimes enlarged and patients may pass dark urine after episodes of haemolysis. Some unstable haemoglobins

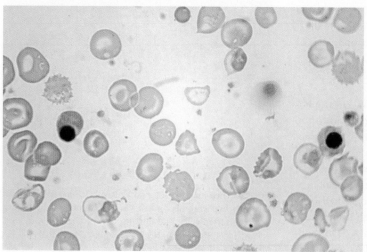

Fig. 8.27 The blood film of a patient with haemoglobin E/β thalassaemia compound heterozygosity.

also have a high oxygen affinity and can therefore cause polycythaemia. If the dominant clinical effect is usually polycythaemia rather than haemolysis, the variant haemoglobin is conventionally designated a high affinity haemoglobin rather than an unstable haemoglobin.

Blood film and count

The Hb varies from normal to markedly reduced, in cases with normal oxygen affinity, whereas the less common cases with a high affinity unstable haemoglobin may have a normal Hb. In some patients the blood film is normal or shows only macrocytosis associated with an elevated reticulocyte count. In others there is anisocytosis, poikilocytosis, hypochromia, variable numbers of irregularly contracted cells (Fig. 8.28), 'bite cells', basophilic stippling or polychromasia. During haemolytic crises, features of hyposplenism may appear. Non-splenectomised subjects may be thrombocytopenic, sometimes to a degree that seems out of proportion to the expected degree of hypersplenism.

The FBC shows a reduced Hb, elevated MCV and RDW, and often reduced MCH and MCHC, the latter abnormalities as a result of removal of Heinz bodies by the spleen. In some cases a discrepancy has been noted between lowered MCH and MCHC and a lack of hypochromia in the blood film. This has been attributed to the fact that an unstable haemoglobin may lose some of its haem groups; the staining of red cells is attributable to their globin content, whereas the biochemical measurement of Hb requires the presence of haem [79]. The reticulocyte count is elevated, sometimes out of proportion to the degree of anaemia. This occurs if an unstable haemoglobin also has an increased oxygen affinity, since this will aggravate the tissue hypoxia and stimulate erythropoiesis.

Differential diagnosis

The differential diagnosis includes other causes of irregularly contracted cells and other causes of haemolytic anaemia.

Further tests

Heinz bodies are detected following splenectomy and during haemolytic crises in some non-splenectomised patients. Definitive diagnosis requires a test for an unstable haemoglobin such as a heat or isopropanol instability test. HPLC or haemoglobin electrophoresis should also be performed. On HPLC, the undenatured haemoglobin often has the same retention time as haemoglobin A, but there may be a small peak with a longer retention time representing denatured haemoglobin. Cellulose acetate electrophoresis often shows normal mobility, but the band in the position of haemoglobin A may be blurred because of the presence of some denatured variant haemoglobin.

Macrocytic anaemias

Macrocytic anaemias result from abnormal erythropoiesis, which may be either megaloblastic or macronormoblastic. Megaloblastic erythropoiesis is characterised by dyserythropoiesis, increased size of erythroid precursors and asynchronous maturation of nucleus and cytoplasm,

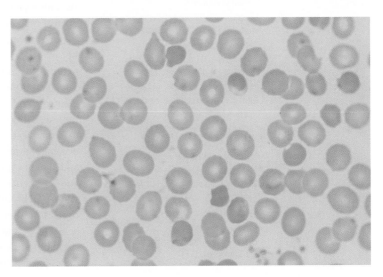

Fig. 8.28 The blood film of a patient who was heterozygous for haemoglobin Köln showing several irregularly contracted cells including one in which the haemoglobin appears to be retracted from the red cell margin. The FBC (Coulter S Plus IV) was: RBC $4.04 \times 10^{12}/1$, Hb 119 g/l, Hct 0.40 l/l, MCV 100 fl, MCH 29.5 pg, MCHC 294 g/l.

so that cytoplasmic maturation is in advance of nuclear maturation. Macronormoblastic anaemia is characterised by increased size of erythroid precursors with or without other features of dyserythropoiesis. The commonest causes of macrocytic anaemia are excess alcohol intake, liver disease, megaloblastic anaemia and MDS.

Megaloblastic anaemia

Megaloblastic anaemia usually results from deficiency of vitamin B_{12} or folic acid or the administration of drugs that interfere with DNA synthesis (see Table 3.2). Some causes are particularly important in infancy and childhood [80] (Table 8.2). The most frequent

Table 8.2 Some causes of megaloblastic anaemia of particular importance in infants and young children.

Nature of defect	Causes
Vitamin B_{12} deficiency	Maternal vitamin B_{12} deficiency (vegan mother or occult pernicious anaemia), particularly if baby is breast-fed
	Absent or non-functional intrinsic factor (*GIF* mutation)
	Imerslund-Gräsbeck syndrome (*CUBN* or *AMN* mutation)
	Absent or non-functional transcobalamin (*TCN2* mutation)
	Ileal resection for necrotising enterocolitis
Inborn errors in vitamin B_{12} metabolism	Methylmalonicaciduria due to combined deficiency of adenosylcobalamin and methylcobalamin
	Methionine synthase deficiency
Folate deficiency	Premature babies, particularly with coexisting haemolytic anaemia
	Babies weaned onto goat's milk
Inborn errors of folate metabolism	Hereditary folate malabsorption (some cases due to *SLC46A1* mutation)
	Glutamate formiminotransferase deficiency (*FTCD* mutation)
	Methylene tetrahydrofolate reductase deficiency (*MTHFR* mutation)
Other inborn errors of metabolism	Thiamine-responsive megaloblastic anaemia
	Diabetes **I**nsipidus, **D**iabetes **M**ellitus **O**ptic **A**trophy and **D**eafness (DIDMOAD) syndrome (Wolfram syndrome)
	Lesch-Nyhan syndrome (*HPRT1* mutation) [81]

causes of vitamin B_{12} deficiency in the adult are pernicious anaemia and food-B_{12} malabsorption [82]. The most frequent causes of folic acid deficiency are dietary deficiency and malabsorption, but the former is becoming infrequent as folic acid fortification of food is becoming increasingly prevalent worldwide. Excess alcohol intake may be complicated by dietary folic acid deficiency, but alcohol can produce macrocytosis even in the absence of folate deficiency; in these cases erythropoiesis may be macronormoblastic or mildly megaloblastic. Megaloblastic erythropoiesis can also occur in MDS and erythroleukaemia, but in these conditions macronormoblastic erythropoiesis is more usual.

The clinical features observed in patients with deficiency of vitamin B_{12} or folic acid include the usual features of anaemia but, in addition, there may be glossitis, mild splenomegaly and jaundice, the latter being the result of ineffective haemopoiesis. Patients with vitamin B_{12} deficiency may suffer, in addition, from optic atrophy, dementia, peripheral neuropathy and subacute combined degeneration of the spinal cord (causing spastic paraparesis and reduced proprioception). In some patients with megaloblastic anaemia as a result of vitamin deficiency there are no symptoms and the diagnosis is made incidentally when a blood count is performed for another reason.

Blood film and count

The haematological features of vitamin B_{12} and folate deficiency are indistinguishable. Characteristic blood film features (Figs 8.29 & 8.30) are anaemia, macrocytosis, anisocytosis, poikilocytosis (including the presence of oval macrocytes and teardrop cells) and neutrophil hypersegmentation. Neutrophil hypersegmentation is not invariably present but, in its absence, a chromatin pattern that is more open than normal may be noted. The macrocytes have increased thickness as well as diameter and central pallor is therefore lacking. There may also be occasional hypersegmented eosinophils, macropolycytes and basophilic stippling. As anaemia becomes more severe, there is increasing anisocytosis and poikilocytosis with the appearance of microcytes and fragments. There may be hypochromic microcytes and hypochromic fragments – as a feature of dyserythropoiesis rather than being indicative of coexisting iron deficiency. Small numbers of Howell–Jolly bodies and circulating megaloblasts and granulocyte precursors may appear. The WBC and platelet count fall with the

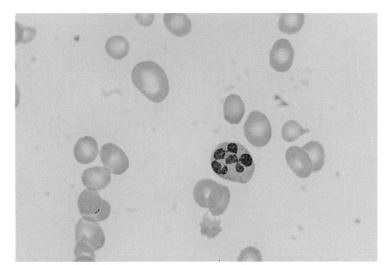

Fig. 8.29 The blood film of an elderly woman with both malabsorption of vitamin B_{12} and dietary deficiency of folic acid showing marked anisocytosis, macrocytosis, several oval macrocytes, a teardrop poikilocyte and a hypersegmented neutrophil. The FBC (Coulter S Plus IV) was: WBC 4.2×10^9/l, RBC 0.76×10^{12}/l, Hb 36 g/l, Hct 0.10 l/l, MCV 133 fl, MCH 47.4 pg, MCHC 356 g/dl, platelet count 50×10^9/l.

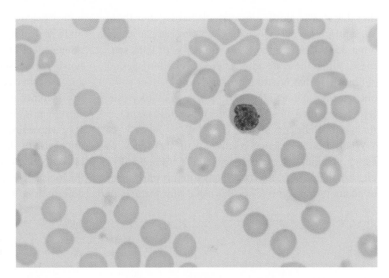

Fig. 8.30 The blood film of a patient with pernicious anaemia showing macrocytosis and a circulating megaloblast.

development of moderate neutropenia and mild lymphopenia. There is usually no polychromasia despite severe anaemia and the reticulocyte count is low. When megaloblastic anaemia develops acutely there may be a sudden failure of bone marrow output of cells. There is pancytopenia with a normal MCV and with few or no macrocytes or hypersegmented neutrophils. Polychromasia is absent and the reticulocyte count is very low. Such 'megaloblastic arrest' is seen in acutely ill patients, often in association with pregnancy, surgery or sepsis. Rarely, in other patients with severe megaloblastic anaemia, the MCV is normal [83]. In patients with minimal haematological features of vitamin B_{12} or folic acid

deficiency, e.g. some patients presenting with the neurological complications of vitamin B_{12} deficiency, the only haematological features may be occasional round or oval macrocytes and occasional hypersegmented neutrophils. Sometimes macrocytosis is associated with prominent features of hyposplenism, particularly with the presence of Pappenheimer bodies and with large and numerous Howell–Jolly bodies (Fig. 8.31); in a patient who has not had a splenectomy this suggests underlying coeliac disease with splenic atrophy as the cause of vitamin B_{12} or, more often, folate deficiency.

Megaloblastic anaemia resulting from folic acid antagonists such as methotrexate is indistinguishable from

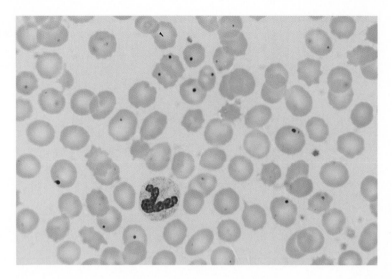

Fig. 8.31 The blood film of a splenectomised post-renal transplant patient with megaloblastic anaemia caused by azathioprine therapy showing macrocytosis, acanthocytes and prominent Howell–Jolly bodies.

that due to vitamin B_{12} or folate deficiency, but there are subtle differences when megaloblastosis is caused by other drugs that interfere more directly with DNA synthesis. When these are administered over a long period of time there may be striking macrocytosis with or without anaemia. Sometimes there is also stomatocytosis. Hypersegmented neutrophils are much less common than in the deficiency states.

When iron deficiency coexists with deficiency of either vitamin B_{12} or folic acid, blood film features are variable. There may be hypochromic microcytes in addition to macrocytes or the blood film features of iron deficiency may dominate, with only the presence of hypersegmented neutrophils suggesting a possible double deficiency. Hypersegmented neutrophils may, however, be seen in uncomplicated iron deficiency and for other reasons (see Chapter 3). Iron deficiency is sometimes unmasked when vitamin B_{12} or folic acid treatment is given to a patient with megaloblastic anaemia whose iron stores are inadequate. Following an initial rise of Hb and the production of well haemoglobinised cells, iron stores are exhausted, hypochromic microcytes are produced and the blood film becomes dimorphic (Fig. 8.32). Thalassaemia trait, like iron

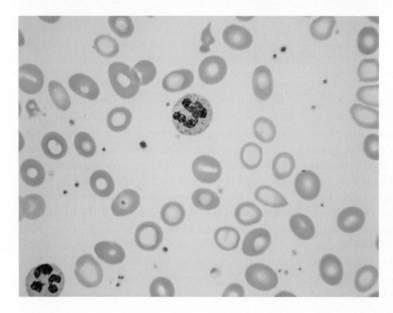

Fig. 8.32 A dimorphic peripheral blood film during treatment of megaloblastic anaemia. Iron stores have been exhausted and there is a population of hypochromic microcytes in addition to the original population of well-haemoglobinised macrocytes. By courtesy of Dr James Uprichard, London.

deficiency, can prevent the development of macrocytosis in megaloblastic anaemia. The MCV may rise into the normal range rather than above it.

When effective treatment is given to a patient with megaloblastic anaemia there is a lag phase of a few days and then a rise in the WBC and platelet count, followed by the production of polychromatic macrocytes and then a rise in Hb. If the patient has been pancytopenic there may be a rebound thrombocytosis, often associated with a left shift or a leucoerythroblastic blood film. Hypersegmented neutrophils persist in the peripheral blood for 5–7 days or even longer and in those who were cytopenic they may actually increase.

The blood count in megaloblastic anaemia shows reduction in the Hb, Hct and RBC. There is a parallel increase in the MCV and MCH. The MCHC is normal and the RDW increased. The increase in RDW precedes a rise in the MCV. As anaemia becomes more severe, the presence of severe poikilocytosis with red cell fragmentation may lead to a paradoxical decrease of the MCV; the RDW is then very high. On Siemens H.1 and Advia series instruments, megaloblastic anaemia is associated with an increased HDW, an increased mean peroxidase index (MPXI) (indicating an increased mean peroxidase activity of neutrophils) and a reduction of the lobularity index (indicating an immature structure of nuclear chromatin) [84] (Fig. 8.33). The red cell cytogram shows an increase in normochromic macrocytes and, when anaemia is severe, also increased microcytes (Fig. 8.34). On impedance counters the mean platelet volume (MPV) remains relatively low when thrombocytopenia is caused by megaloblastic anaemia, whereas it is increased when thrombocytopenia results from decreased platelet lifespan [85].

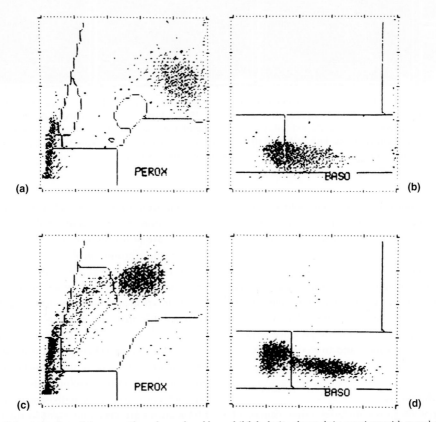

Fig. 8.33 Bayer H.1 scatter plots of the peroxidase channel and basophil/lobularity channels in a patient with megaloblastic anaemia (a, b) and a normal subject (c, d). In the peroxidase channel the neutrophil cluster is displaced to the right indicating a high peroxidase activity, which is reflected in a high mean peroxidase index (MPXI). In the basophil lobularity channel the abnormal chromatin structure of the neutrophils has led to a loss of the normal valley between the mononuclear cluster (left) and the granulocyte cluster (right), which is reflected in a low 'lobularity index'.

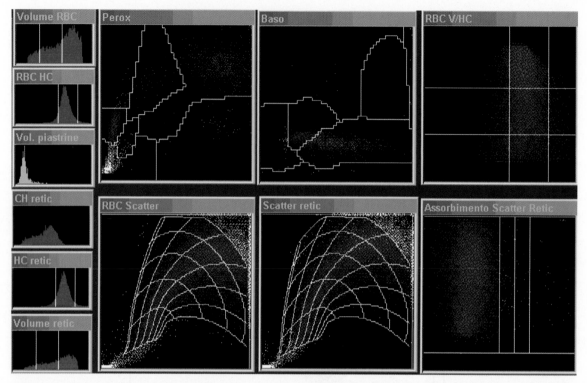

Fig. 8.34 Siemens Advia scatter plots and histograms in severe megaloblastic anaemia. The FBC was: WBC 2.1×10^9/l, RBC 0.86×10^{12}/l, Hb 36 g/l, Hct 0.10 l/l, MCV 118 fl, MCH 41.6 pg, MCHC 353 g/l, RDW 32.5%, haemoglobin distribution width (HDW) 3.7 g/l (increased), platelets 106×10^9/l. The red cell cytogram (top right) and histogram (top left) show an increase of macrocytes and a lesser increase in microcytes. The high RDW and HDW and the increased number of microcytes are the result of dyserythropoiesis. The reticulocyte count was very low at 13×10^9/l, consistent with the low number of hypochromic macrocytes present. By courtesy of Professor Gina Zini.

The various methods of assessing neutrophil hypersegmentation are discussed on p. 96. In a study comparing B_{12} or folate deficient patients who had megaloblastic erythropoiesis with patients who were not vitamin deficient, the index proposed by Edwin was found to be the most sensitive indicator of megaloblastosis [84]. Next most sensitive was the percentage of neutrophils with at least five lobes. In equal third place were the mean lobe count (Arneth score), the presence of neutrophils with at least six lobes and an elevated MPXI on the Siemens H.1 counter.

Differential diagnosis

The differential diagnosis includes other causes of macrocytosis (see Table 3.2) and, in severe cases with rapid onset, other causes of bone marrow failure. An increased RDW [8] and increased MPXI [86] have been found of some use in separating megaloblastic

anaemia from other causes of macrocytosis in which these parameters are less often abnormal. Blood film features are also useful. In macrocytosis due to liver disease and chronic alcohol abuse, macrocytes are round rather than oval, hypersegmented neutrophils are absent and there may be other abnormalities (see below). In macrocytosis due to MDS there may be dysplastic neutrophils (hypogranular or hypolobated) or a population of hypochromic microcytes consequent on sideroblastic erythropoiesis; in a minority of patient there is thrombocytosis. In chronic haemolytic anaemia macrocytosis may be marked but polychromasia is usually apparent. The blood film features are very important in the identification of congenital dyserythropoietic anaemia as a cause of macrocytosis (see below). In patients with severe megaloblastic anaemia with marked red cell fragmentation and thrombocytopenia, there is a possibility of misdiagnosis as thrombotic thrombocytopenic pur-pura (TTP) [82].

Further tests
The peripheral blood features of severe megaloblas-tic anaemia are so characteristic that the diagnosis is often obvious from the blood film and count. A bone marrow aspiration is confirmatory, but is often not necessary. Tests that are useful in distinguish-ing between vitamin B_{12} and folic acid deficiency are serum B_{12} and red cell folate assays. The serum vitamin B_{12} concentration is reduced in about 97% of patients with clinical evidence of vitamin B_{12} deficiency [87]. Serum vitamin B_{12} assay is usually normal in children with vitamin B_{12} deficiency due to transcobalamin deficiency. It should also be noted that some assay methods give invalid measurements of serum vitamin B_{12} in the presence of intrinsic factor antibodies, sometimes leading to a deficiency being missed. Assay of serum holotranscobalamin (i.e. of cobalamin bound to transcobalamin – previ-ously known as transcobalamin II) may detect some further patients with vitamin B_{12} deficiency in whom the concentration of total serum B_{12} is normal, but this assay is not yet established in routine use. Serum folate assay is a more sensitive indicator of negative folate balance than red cell folate, but red cell folate assay is more specific for significant tissue deficiency. Increased plasma homocysteine concentration is a sensitive indicator of vitamin B_{12} deficiency [87] (sensitivity of 96%) [88], but increased levels may also be found in folic acid deficiency, alcohol abuse and renal insufficiency; the need for rapid pro-cessing of the blood sample lessens the clinical use-fulness. Serum methylmalonic acid concentration is at least as sensitive as a homocysteine assay (sensi-tivity 98%) [88] and is more specific for vitamin B_{12} deficiency; however, concentration is also increased in renal insufficiency and the assay is more difficult. The Schilling test, measuring B_{12} excretion with and without intrinsic factor after administration of oral radio-labelled B_{12}, was previously diagnostically very valuable, identifying B_{12} malabsorption and distin-guishing between a gastric and an intestinal cause, but unfortunately reagents are no longer available.

Tests for intrinsic factor antibodies are useful in confirming the diagnosis of pernicious anaemia, the commonest cause of vitamin B_{12} deficiency, and

when positive can replace the Schilling test; they are detected in about two-thirds of patients. It should be noted that false positive results may occur if the serum B_{12} is high, so assays should not be performed within 24 hours of a vitamin B_{12} injection [89]. Parie-tal cell antibodies are also usually present in per-nicious anaemia, but are less specific than intrinsic factor antibodies. As tests for malabsorption of food-B_{12} are not readily available, this is usually a diag-nosis of exclusion. Elevated serum gastrin is useful in the diagnosis of pernicious anaemia, being elevated in about 90% of patients; however, it is also increased in about a third of patients with food-B_{12} malabsorption [90]. If coeliac disease is suspected as a cause of folic acid deficiency or, less often, vitamin B_{12} deficiency, the most useful serological test is for antibody to tissue transglutaminase; it is usual to test for immu-noglobulin (Ig) A antibodies and in patients with coexisting IgA deficiency (increased in frequency in patients with coeliac disease) this test will therefore be negative. If the test is negative it is therefore essen-tial to be sure that the patient is not IgA deficient; deficient patients should be tested for IgG antibodies. The definitive test for coeliac disease is a small bowel biopsy.

In thiamine-responsive megaloblastic anaemia (Fig. 8.35) and Wolfram syndrome, bone marrow aspir-ation shows erythropoiesis to be sideroblastic as well as megaloblastic.

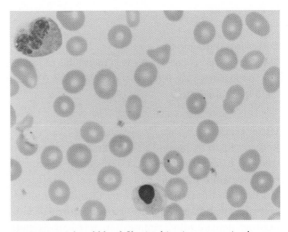

Fig. 8.35 Peripheral blood film in thiamine-responsive haemo-lytic anaemia showing macrocytosis, mild poikilocytosis and a circulating erythroblast, which is mildly megaloblastic. By cour-tesy of Dr Abbas Hashim Abdulsalam, Baghdad.

Macrocytic anaemia associated with excess alcohol intake and liver disease

Both excess alcohol intake and chronic liver disease can cause macrocytic anaemia. The two aetiologies often coexist. Associated leucopenia and thrombocytopenia are common, caused either by the effect of alcohol on the bone marrow or by hypersplenism associated with chronic liver disease. Patients may suffer from bruising or symptoms of anaemia, but often the other effects of alcohol excess or liver disease are more evident than the haematological effects.

Blood film and count

The blood film shows macrocytosis, with the macrocytes being predominantly round rather than oval. Anisocytosis and poikilocytosis are less marked than in megaloblastic anaemia and there may be associated target cells and stomatocytes. There may be leucopenia and thrombocytopenia, but hypersegmented neutrophils are not a feature. In chronic liver disease, rouleaux formation is increased as a result of increased concentration of immunoglobulins. Patients with acute alcoholic liver disease may also suffer from haemolytic anaemia with spherocytes (or, more likely, irregularly contracted cells) and associated hyperlipidaemia (Zieve syndrome). Patients with advanced liver failure from any cause may suffer 'spur cell haemolytic anaemia', characterised by acanthocytosis.

The Hb, RBC and Hct are reduced. The MCV and MCH are increased. The MCHC is normal and the RDW is often normal.

Differential diagnosis

The major differential diagnosis is megaloblastic anaemia, particularly that due to dietary folate deficiency in 'Skid Row' alcoholics.

Other tests

Red cell folate is normal or low. Serum vitamin B_{12} concentration is increased as a result of release of transcobalamin from the damaged liver. A prothrombin time and liver function tests, including γ glutamyl transpeptidase assay, are useful. A normal bone marrow deoxyuridine suppression test can exclude significant deficiency of vitamin B_{12} or folic acid in alcoholics with macrocytosis, but this test is not routinely available.

Macrocytic anaemia due to a myelodysplastic syndrome

Macrocytic anaemia is common in MDS, which is discussed in more detail in Chapter 9.

Blood film and count

The blood film shows macrocytes and often anisocytosis and poikilocytosis. In patients with sideroblastic anaemia, the film is dimorphic with hypochromic microcytes in addition to well-haemoglobinised macrocytes. There may be neutropenia and thrombocytopenia and dysplastic feature in other lineages.

The Hb, RBC and Hct are reduced. The MCV, MCH and RDW are increased. Red cell cytograms on Siemens Advia series instruments demonstrate a particular pattern that has been found to be predictive of the presence of ring sideroblasts (Fig 8.36). There is scattering of signals over eight of the nine areas of the cytogram (all except hyperchromic macrocytes) with a particular increase in microcytic cells (to the left of the left-hand vertical threshold) and of hypochromic cells (below the lower horizontal threshold); the shape of the scatter plot differs from that of iron deficiency and thalassaemia [91]. The pattern is reasonably sensitive in the detection of sideroblastic erythropoiesis (32/38 cases) and is predictive (20/21 cases) [91]. Patients with sideroblastic erythropoiesis have a normal reticulocyte haemoglobin content (CHr) in contrast to the low levels seen in iron deficiency [91].

Differential diagnosis

The differential diagnosis is with other macrocytic anaemias. In addition, a distinction must be made from idiopathic macrocytosis (idiopathic dysplasia of undetermined significance), a condition that is, by definition, of unknown cause but may be a prelude to MDS [92].

Other tests

The investigation of suspected MDS requires bone marrow aspiration and cytogenetic analysis (see Chapter 9).

Congenital haemolytic anaemias

Congenital haemolytic anaemias usually result from inherited abnormalities of the red cell membrane, haemoglobin or red cell enzymes. Enzyme deficiencies

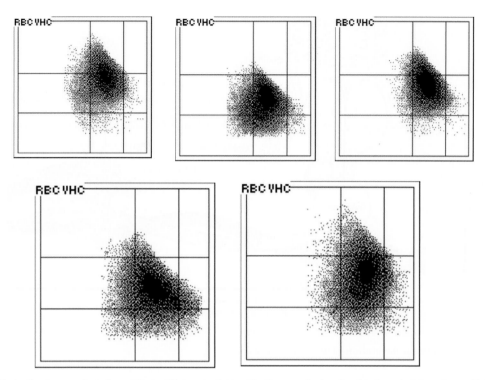

Fig. 8.36 Red cell cytograms from five patients with acquired sideroblastic anaemia showing the characteristic pattern with increased hypochromic and microcytic cells and usually also an increase in hypochromic and normochromic macrocytes. By courtesy of Dr Alicia Rovó, Basel.

are mainly those of the glycolytic pathway, which are concerned with the energy requirements of the cell, and those of the pentose shunt, which protect the cell from oxidant damage. Congenital haemolytic anaemias of these types persist throughout life. Congenital haemolytic anaemia can also be acquired *in utero*, e.g. haemolytic disease of the newborn caused by ABO or Rh incompatibility, in which case it is a transient disorder. Haemolysis associated with abnormal haemoglobins has been discussed above. Red cell membrane and enzyme abnormalities will be discussed here. The structure of the normal red cell membrane, which is a lipid bilayer supported by a cytoskeleton, is illustrated in Fig. 8.37.

Hereditary spherocytosis and variants
Hereditary spherocytosis
The condition designated hereditary spherocytosis is actually a heterogeneous group of disorders [93]. Hereditary spherocytosis occurs in various ethnic groups including Caucasian, North African, Indian subcontinent and Japanese subjects and rarely in those

of sub-Saharan African ethnic origin. The prevalence in Northern European Caucasians is at least 1 in 2000 [94]. About three-quarters of cases show an autosomal dominant inheritance, the remainder either being sporadic new mutations or showing an autosomal recessive inheritance [94]. Of the cases not showing dominant inheritance, the majority result from new mutations and the minority from recessively inherited disease [95]. The underlying genetic defect in the common autosomal dominant form of the disease is a mutation in the ankyrin (*ANK1*) gene in about 50% of cases, in the β spectrin (*SPTB*) gene in about 30%, in the gene for the red cell membrane protein, band 3 (*SLC4A1* or *EPB3*), in 15–20% [94] and in the α spectrin gene (*SPTA*) or the protein 4.2 (palladin) gene (*EPB42*) in a small minority. The rate of synthesis of α spectrin is usually three to four times greater than the rate of synthesis of β spectrin, so that hereditary spherocytosis is likely to be associated only with homozygosity or compound heterozygosity for *SPTA* mutations but with heterozygosity for *SPTB* mutations. Mutations in the band 3 gene that can

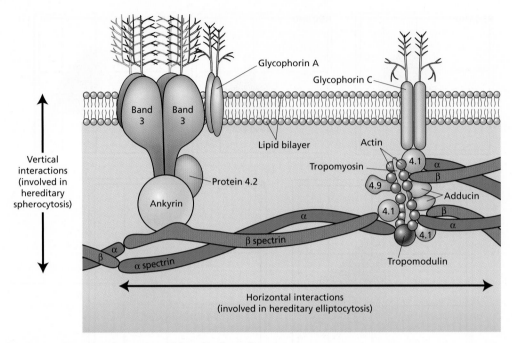

Fig. 8.37 Diagram illustrating the structure of the red cell membrane.

cause hereditary spherocytosis either lead to a reduced synthesis of band 3 or to synthesis of a protein that is unstable or that shows reduced binding to protein 4.2 or ankyrin [96]. The uncommon autosomal recessive forms of hereditary spherocytosis have been associated particularly with compound heterozygosity or homozygosity for α spectrin mutations [97], but also with mutations of the genes encoding band 3 [96], β spectrin and protein 4.2 [98,99]. Mutations of *EPB42* have been reported mainly in Japanese individuals [98]. Rarely, mutations in the *SLC4A1* gene resulting in a complete absence of band 3 cause distal renal tubular acidosis and hereditary spherocytosis, but in other kindreds mutation leads to the occurrence of one or other condition [93] or to renal tubular acidosis with acanthocytic or ovalocytic haemolytic anaemia. Homozygosity for such mutations (e.g. band 3 Coimbra) can cause renal tubular acidosis with severe hereditary spherocytosis and hydrops fetalis and is generally incompatible with life [100]. The mechanism of spherocytosis in most cases of hereditary spherocytosis is that a deficiency of spectrin, either primary or secondary to an abnormality of ankyrin, leads to reduced density of the cytoskeleton, lack of binding of the cytoskeleton to band 3 and consequent instability of unsupported areas of the lipid bilayer. There is

then loss of lipid, as vesicles, from the destabilised membrane, *in vitro* and probably *in vivo*, leading to spherocytosis. A reduction in band 3 protein has a similar effect. It appears likely that in protein 4.2 deficiency there is impairment of binding of spectrin through ankyrin and band 3 to the membrane protein, CD47 [99]. Mutations associated with hereditary spherocytosis are listed on the Human Gene Mutation Database [101] and Online Mendelian Inheritance in Man [102].

Hereditary spherocytosis may be asymptomatic and only diagnosed incidentally or there may be symptomatic anaemia and intermittent jaundice. The spleen is sometimes enlarged. Because of the chronic haemolysis there is increased production of bilirubin and the incidence of gallstones is increased. Symptomatic anaemia may occur only when there is intercurrent bacterial infection, parvovirus B19 infection or folic acid deficiency. Haemolysis may worsen, causing symptomatic anaemia as a result of repeated vigorous exercise in athletes [103]. Hereditary spherocytosis may be ameliorated by coinheritance of β thalassaemia trait [96].

Babies with hereditary spherocytosis usually have a normal Hb at birth. Neonatal jaundice is common and they may require phototherapy and, sometimes, exchange transfusion. Babies with hereditary spherocytosis are prone to develop a transient but severe anaemia around 20 days of age [104]. Blood transfusion is often needed at this stage. Splenomegaly is common during the first year of life.

Blood film and count

Depending on the specific genetic abnormality, there may be either anaemia or compensated haemolysis. The blood film (Fig. 8.38) shows variable numbers of spherocytes and less easily recognised spherostomatocytes. There are also some cells with normal central pallor. Scanning electron microscopy has shown that generally only a minority of the cells are spherical, the majority being discocytes, stomatocytes or spherostomatocytes [105]. In mild cases of hereditary spherocytosis it is sometimes very difficult to be certain, on examining the blood film, whether or not spherocytes are present and confirmatory tests are needed. In severe cases there is obvious spherocytosis, polychromasia and polychromatic macrocytes and sometimes the presence of other poikilocytes. The reticulocyte percentage and absolute count are elevated. After splenectomy the usual post-splenectomy features are seen but target cells are not a feature; spheroacanthocytes may be very numerous (Fig. 8.39). Ultrastructural studies show that splenectomy leads to the disappearance of a minor population

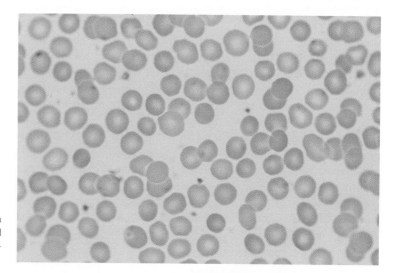

Fig. 8.38 The blood film of a patient with hereditary spherocytosis who had mild chronic haemolysis without anaemia showing moderately numerous spherocytes.

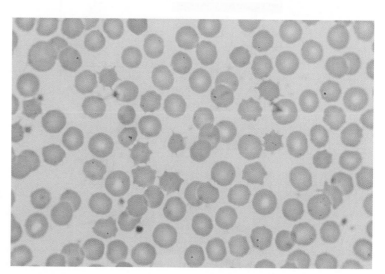

Fig. 8.39 The blood film of a patient with hereditary spherocytosis (the father of the patient shown in Fig. 8.37) who has been splenectomised, showing spheroacanthocytes.

of microspherocytes [105]. Diagnosis can be difficult in the neonatal period, with a third of babies not showing a significant number of spherocytes [106].

Certain characteristic morphological features are associated with specific mutations [107–112]: the presence of both spherocytes and acanthocytes or sphero-echinocytes has been associated with a mutant β spectrin with defective binding to protein 4.1 and with certain other mis-sense and null mutations of the β spectrin gene, including a mutation leading to truncation of β spectrin [109] and a mutation of the initiation codon [111]; band 3 deficiency is associated with pincered or mushroom-shaped cells (see Fig. 3.59), which are lost after splenectomy; band 4.2[Nippon] and band 4.2[Komatsu] can be associated with stomatocytes, ovalocytes and sphero-ovalocytes in homozygotes [98]; protein 4.2 deficiency is associated with ovalospherocytes and pincer cells [99]; severe spectrin and ankyrin deficiency has irregular spherocytes, some of which resemble the cells of hereditary pyropoikilocytosis. Heterozygosity for band 3[Coimbra] causes typical hereditary spherocytosis, whereas the rare homozygous state is associated with a total absence of band 3 and very severe hereditary spherocytosis with spherocytosis and marked poikilocytosis, the poikilocytes including erythrocytes with stalk-like elongations [112].

The blood count in hereditary spherocytosis shows a normal or reduced Hb and a normal MCV and MCH, although the MCV is low if account is taken of the young age of the cells. With impedance counters, the MCHC is towards the upper limit of normal or somewhat increased. With Siemens H.1 and Advia series instruments, the MCHC is increased in the majority of patients who also show an increased RDW and HDW and, on the histograms, a tail of microcytes and a tail of hyperchromic cells [113]. Red cell cytograms (Figs 8.40 & 8.41) show a characteristic increase of hyperchromic or hyperdense cells and, if there is significant macrocytosis, an increase of hypochromic macrocytes. An increased percentage of hyperdense cells is not specific for spherocytosis, but examination of the blood film allows spherocytes to be distinguished from other hyperdense cells such as sickle cells and irregularly contracted cells. Post-splenectomy the Hb rises, usually to normal, and the RDW and HDW usually return to normal. Microcytes are less consistently present, but increased numbers of hyperchromic cells are usually still present [113]. With the Beckman–Coulter Gen S and LH750 instrument a mean sphered cell volume (MSCV) (see Chapter 2) that is substantially less than the MCV has been found to have a high sensitivity and reasonable specificity for hereditary spherocytosis [114,115].

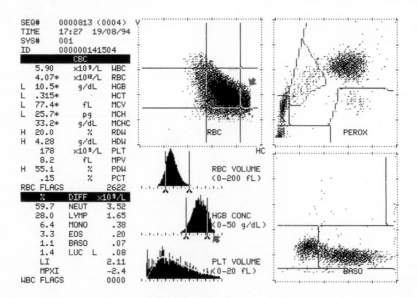

Fig. 8.40 Bayer H.2 scatter plots and histograms of a patient with hereditary spherocytosis. Both the red cell cytogram and the haemoglobin histogram show a large number of dense cells, which are the spherocytes (green arrows).

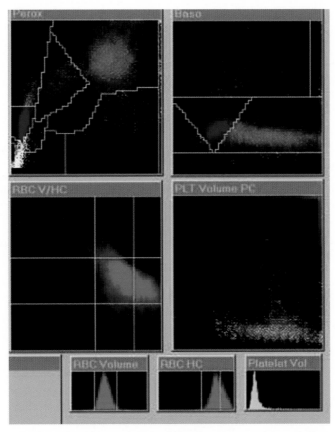

Fig. 8.41 Bayer Advia 120 scatter plots and histograms of a patient with hereditary spherocytosis. By courtesy of Ms Sue Mead, Woodley.

Findings are usually normal in autoimmune haemolytic anaemia [115].

Sudden worsening of anaemia in hereditary sphero-cytosis may be caused by: (i) megaloblastic anaemia resulting from folate deficiency; (ii) 'anaemia of chronic disease' developing during acute infection; or (iii) red cell aplasia induced by parvovirus B19 infection or, less often, resulting from infection by another virus (e.g. influenza virus) [116]. Because of the shortened red cell lifespan, the anaemia develops acutely. In megaloblastic anaemia, polychromasia is diminished in comparison with the stable state and some macrocytes, oval macrocytes and hypersegmented neutrophils are present (Fig. 8.42). In 'anaemia of chronic disease', e.g. resulting from acute or chronic infection, polychromasia also diminishes and red cells become less spherocytic, some developing central pallor. The blood film may be dimorphic (Fig. 8.43). If the patient is not known to suffer from hereditary spherocytosis, the diagnosis may be difficult to make at this stage. In pure red cell aplasia, cells remain sphero-cytic but polychromasia disappears and the reticulocyte count is close to zero. Previously undiagnosed hereditary spherocytosis may be unmasked by parvovirus infection and also by infectious mononucleosis, which aggra-vates the haemolysis. Diagnosis is more difficult during recovery from parvovirus-induced red cell aplasia, as young red cells newly released from the bone marrow are not spherocytic. Haemolytic episodes can also be induced by exercise or precipitated by pregnancy. The predispo-sition to gallstones means that patients with hereditary spherocytosis have an increased likelihood of develop-ing obstructive jaundice. When this occurs, more lipid is taken up into the red cell membrane and consequently spherocytosis and haemolysis lessen. Iron deficiency is also associated with a reduction of spherocytosis and sometimes a dimorphic blood film.

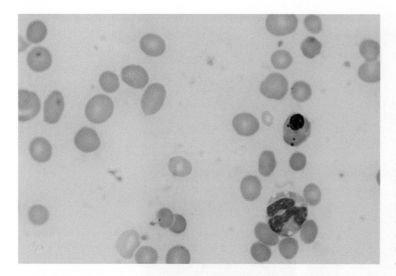

Fig. 8.42 The blood film of a patient with hereditary spherocytosis who has developed a megaloblastic anaemia consequent on inadequate dietary intake of folate in the face of increased requirements caused by chronic haemolysis. The film shows macrocytes, oval macrocytes, occasional spherocytes and a megaloblast containing Howell–Jolly bodies.

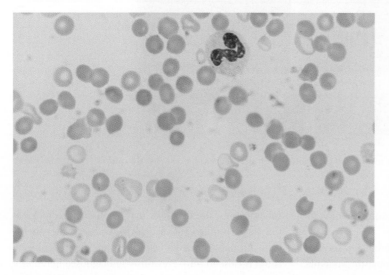

Fig. 8.43 The blood film of a patient with hereditary spherocytosis (the same patient as shown in Fig. 8.41) during an episode of 'anaemia of chronic disease' associated with intercurrent infection. Some cells have central pallor and are hypochromic and microcytic. The film is dimorphic.

Differential diagnosis

The main differential diagnosis is warm autoimmune haemolytic anaemia (see below). The blood films are often indistinguishable, and thus family history and a direct antiglobulin test are needed. Other causes of spherocytosis that may have to be considered in the differential diagnosis are shown in Table 3.3. Often the diagnosis is readily evident from the clinical history, but laboratory features can help. In the mild, compensated haemolytic anaemia associated with the Rh deficiency syndrome (see Table 8.4), there are some stomatocytes as well as spherocytes and there is reduced or absent expression of Rh antigens on red cell membranes. In Zieve syndrome, an acute haemolytic anaemia associated with alcoholic liver disease, there are irregularly contracted cells as well as spherocytes. In *Clostridium perfringens* sepsis the red cell membrane may be so damaged that numerous ghosts are seen. Further lysis occurring in the blood specimen *in vitro* can cause artefactual elevation of the MCH and MCHC.

In the neonatal period, the differential diagnosis includes haemolytic disease of the newborn, particularly that due to ABO incompatibility (see below). It should, however, be noted that clinically evident ABO incompatibility is commoner in babies who are subsequently found to have hereditary spherocytosis.

Further tests

The direct antiglobulin test is negative. The diagnosis has traditionally been confirmed by an osmotic fragility test. This test confirms the presence of osmotically fragile cells, but does not distinguish between hereditary spherocytosis and warm autoimmune haemolytic anaemia or other causes of spherocytosis. In mild cases, an osmotic fragility test after the incubation of red cells at 37°C for 24 hours may be necessary to demonstrate the presence of abnormal cells. In very mild cases, the osmotic fragility may be normal, even after incubation. The osmotic fragility may be normal in hereditary spherocytosis in the presence of iron deficiency, obstructive jaundice or post-aplasia reticulocytosis. Post-splenectomy, the osmotic fragility test remains abnormal but a small population of very fragile cells may have disappeared; this population probably represents very abnormal cells resulting from damage within the spleen. When an automated counter that detects hyperdense cells is available, the need for an osmotic fragility test is much diminished and the detection of a MSCV/MCV discrepancy may play a similar role. Flow cytometry showing uptake of eosin-5-maleimide (which binds to membrane band 3, Rh protein, Rh glycoprotein and CD47, all of which are reduced in hereditary spherocytosis) may obviate the need for an osmotic fragility test [116–118]: the majority of patients with hereditary spherocytosis show a reduction of mean fluorescence (whereas in autoimmune haemolytic anaemia results are normal or increased); contrary to earlier observations, this test is abnormal whether hereditary spherocytosis is due to a deficiency of band 3, spectrin or ankyrin [119]. Abnormal results are not specific for hereditary spherocytosis, being observed also in hereditary pyropoikilocytosis, South-East Asian ovalocytosis, type II congenital dyserythropoietic anaemia, cryohydrocytosis, in some patients with hereditary elliptocytosis [116,117] and in homozygotes for an *SLC4A1* mutation that leads to an acanthocytic haemolytic anaemia [120]. However, assessment of eosin-5-maleimide (EMA) uptake together with the blood film features permits the correct diagnosis to be made. The glycerol lysis, acidified glycerol lysis and cryohaemolysis tests are abnormal in hereditary spherocytosis. Positive results with a glycerol lysis test are also seen in spherocytosis from other causes, hereditary persistence of fetal haemoglobin, pyruvate kinase deficiency and severe glucose-6-phosphate dehydrogenase (G6PD) deficiency and also in a third of pregnant women and some patients with MDS or who are on dialysis for chronic renal failure [116]. Positive cryohaemolysis tests are also seen in South-East Asian ovalocytosis and congenital dyserythropoietic anaemia type II [121]. The definitive test for hereditary spherocytosis, although not often needed, is quantification of spectrin and other proteins of the red cell membrane. Membrane spectrin is normal in autoimmune haemolytic anaemia. The most relevant genetic studies can be predicted from the defect demonstrated in membrane proteins: (i) spectrin and ankyrin deficient – investigate *ANK1* gene; (ii) spectrin deficient – investigate *SPTB* and *SPTA* genes; (iii) protein 3 deficient – investigate *SLC4A1*gene.

With the increasing availability of an EMA binding test, the importance of the osmotic fragility test has decreased considerably. A comparison of the tests customarily used in the diagnosis of hereditary spherocytosis in 150 patients with various genetic defects found that EMA binding had a sensitivity of 93% and a specificity of 98% [118]. An acidified glycerol lysis test had a sensitivity of 95%. The osmotic fragility test had a sensitivity of 68% on fresh blood and 81% on incubated blood [118]. The authors therefore recommended a combination of EMA binding and an acidified glycerol lysis test [118]. The British Committee for Standards in Haematology (BCSH) considers that no further testing is necessary when there are typical clinical and laboratory features and a positive family history; when features are atypical, EMA binding and a cryohaemolysis test are advised [122].

Hereditary elliptocytosis and ovalocytosis
Hereditary elliptocytosis

The condition designated hereditary elliptocytosis is actually a heterogeneous group of inherited conditions characterised by elliptocytic red cells. The presence of at least 25% elliptocytes or ovalocytes has been suggested as a diagnostic criterion. However, subjects with mutations capable of leading to hereditary elliptocytosis can have from 0 to 100% elliptocytes, so the selection of any cut-off point for diagnosis is arbitrary. Inheritance is usually autosomal dominant. Many ethnic groups are affected including individuals of African origin, northern European Caucasians, Chinese, Japanese and Indians. The incidence is highest in West and Central Africa where the prevalence is at least 6 per 1000, and in Benin and some parts of Central Africa it is as high as 1% [106]. In Caucasians the prevalence is about 1 in 5000. Hereditary elliptocytosis results from a variety of genetic abnormalities that affect the integrity of the red cell cytoskeleton [93,107,108,123]. Most mutations leading to hereditary elliptocytosis affect the structure of α or β spectrin, causing either a truncated β spectrin chain or a defect in either the α or the β chain near the sites that are involved in the self-assembly of the spectrin heterodimers into tetramers, i.e. the NH$_2$-terminus of the α spectrin chain or the COOH-terminus of the β spectrin chain. As a result, the normal lattice of interconnected spectrin tetramers is disrupted. Overall, about 80% of cases of hereditary elliptocytosis are caused by a mutation in the α spectrin gene (*SPTA1*), about 15% by a mutation in the protein 4.1 gene (*EPB41*) and about 5% by a mutation in the β spectrin gene (*SPTB*) [94]. *SPTA* mutations predominate in Africans, whereas *EPB41* mutations are common in Arabs [124]. Less commonly, there is a mutation in the glycophorin C gene (*GYPC*), giving the rare Leach phenotype (lack of expression of Gerbich blood group antigens, glycophorin C and glycophorin D in association with elliptocytosis) [125]. Ovalocytosis in the Wosera region of Papua New Guinea has been associated with Gerbich negativity and a deletion in the *GYPC* gene [126]. There is also a gene on the X chromosome, mutation of which can give rise to elliptocytosis associated with Alport syndrome [94]. Mutations associated with hereditary elliptocytosis are listed on the Human Gene Mutation Database [101] and Online Mendelian Inheritance in Man [102].

The majority of patients with hereditary elliptocytosis are asymptomatic and the diagnosis is made incidentally. In a minority there is symptomatic anaemia. Sometimes there is more severe anaemia with transient poikilocytosis in infancy (see below); transfusion can be needed up during the first year of life [127].

Blood film and count

The severity of hereditary elliptocytosis is very variable, ranging from a morphological abnormality without any shortening of the red cell lifespan, through mild or moderate compensated haemolysis to severe intermittent or severe chronic haemolytic anaemia. The majority of patients, however, are not anaemic. The blood film (Fig. 8.44) shows predominantly elliptocytes or, in some patients with the same genetic defect, ovalocytes [123]. Haemoglobinisation of cells is normal. When there is anaemia, there is also polychromasia; more severe cases sometimes have a variety of other poikilocytes, including fragments and spherocytes. A variant with sphero-elliptocytes has been associated with β spectrin variants, β spectrin Rouen [128] and β spectrin Prague [129]. Other cases of dominantly inherited spherocytic elliptocytosis (characterised by the presence of elliptocytes, spherocytes, micro-elliptocytes and microspherocytes) are of unknown molecular basis [124]. Spherocytes as well as elliptocytes can also be seen in patients with glycophorin C mutations [124]. Morphological abnormalities are greater in those who have inherited the low expression α spectrin allele, α spectrin^{Lely}, in *trans* to the hereditary elliptocytosis mutation [130]; such

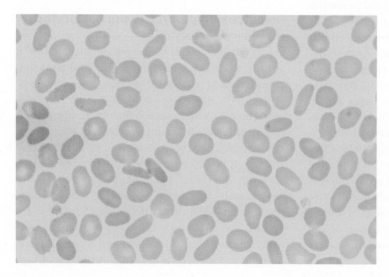

Fig. 8.44 The blood film of a patient with hereditary elliptocytosis showing elliptocytes and ovalocytes. The patient had a normal Hb and reticulocyte count.

patients may have poikilocytes and fragments, in addition to elliptocytes, and sometimes have the clinicopathological features of hereditary pyropoikilocytosis (see below [131]). Conversely, the α spectrin[Lely] mutation occurring in *cis* to a hereditary elliptocytosis mutation lessens the phenotypic abnormality.

The Hb and red cell indices are usually normal. The reticulocyte count is normal or increased. Cases with haemolytic anaemia have an increased RDW. Siemens H.1 and Advia series red cell cytograms are usually normal but, in cases with haemolysis, increased numbers of hyperdense and hypodense cells may be detected and the volume histograms may show two populations of red cells, normocytic and microcytic. The proportion of microcytes correlates with the severity of haemolysis [132].

In hereditary elliptocytosis, there is considerable variation in the severity of the defect between individuals who have the same genotype; the phenotype in heterozygotes for some defects varies from an asymptomatic state, with less than 2% elliptocytes, to mild or moderately severe hereditary elliptocytosis [107,108,123]. In subjects with the same genotype there is a correlation between the degree of abnormality of red cell shape and the severity of haemolysis. However, the genotypes that most often cause severe haemolysis are not those in which the cells are most elliptocytic or in which the percentage of elliptocytes is highest [123]. Despite the variable expression, some generalisations can be made with regard to the usual phenotypic expression of different genetic abnormalities

[107,108,123]. Glycophorin C deficiency causes no significant abnormality in heterozygotes, while homozygotes have mild hereditary elliptocytosis. Protein 4.1 deficiency and several α spectrin variants cause a minimal or mild abnormality in heterozygotes and severe hereditary elliptocytosis in homozygotes [108,133,134]. The most severe elliptogenic mutations generally cause the phenotype of hereditary elliptocytosis in heterozygotes, while homozygotes and certain compound heterozygotes have the phenotype of hereditary pyropoikilocytosis (see below).

Exacerbations of haemolysis are sometimes seen during infections, during pregnancy [135], in the postpartum period and when the microcirculation is compromised or there is reticuloendothelial hyperplasia, e.g. in disseminated intravascular coagulation, TTP, malaria or infectious mononucleosis [107,123,124]. Parvovirus B19 infection can cause significant anaemia [136].

Patients with haemolysis severe enough to require splenectomy may thereafter have marked poikilocytosis, in addition to the usual post-splenectomy features; the poikilocytes include prominent spherocytes, microelliptocytes and fragments (Fig. 8.45). Patients with mild disease in whom splenectomy is carried out for other reasons, e.g. following trauma, can also have bizarre films post-splenectomy.

In general, subjects with hereditary elliptocytosis have very few elliptocytes at birth. However, some who in later life have typical hereditary elliptocytosis with only mild haemolysis may, in the neonatal

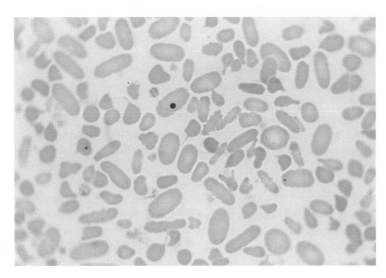

Fig. 8.45 The blood film of a patient with severe hereditary elliptocytosis who required splenectomy for haemolysis, showing marked poikilocytosis with the poikilocytes including elliptocytes, ovalocytes and fragments. One ovalocyte contains a Howell–Jolly body. By courtesy of Dr Raina Liesner, London.

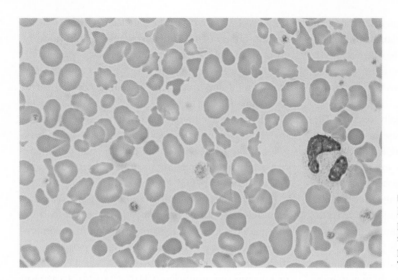

Fig. 8.46 The blood film of a neonate with hereditary elliptocytosis and neonatal poikilocytosis showing marked poikilocytosis with a mixture of elliptocytes and other poikilocytes. By courtesy of Dr Marilyn Treacy, London.

period when haemoglobin F is high, have severe haemolysis and a blood film showing marked poikilocytosis with the presence not only of elliptocytes but also of fragments, irregularly contracted cells and microspherocytes [137,138] (Fig. 8.46). The likely explanation of the more marked abnormality in the neonatal period is that haemoglobin F has a lower affinity for 2,3-diphosphoglycerate (2,3-DPG) than does haemoglobin A and the free 2,3-DPG destabilises the spectrin–actin–protein 4.1 interaction, thus exacerbating the abnormality.

Differential diagnosis

When the blood film shows a high proportion of elliptocytes or ovalocytes the diagnosis of hereditary elliptocytosis is very probable. Rare patients with developing primary myelofibrosis [139] or MDS [140] have shown similar numbers of elliptocytes, and this may be attributable to an acquired deficiency of protein 4.1. The differential diagnosis of cases of hereditary elliptocytosis with marked neonatal poikilocytosis is hereditary pyropoikilocytosis. Follow-up beyond the neonatal period permits the two conditions to be distinguished; alteration of the phenotype can take from 4 months to 2 years [124].

Further tests

Osmotic fragility is normal except in those with severe haemolysis. Family studies are useful in confirming the inherited nature of the condition. A definitive diagnosis can be made by biochemical investigation of red cell membranes in a reference laboratory. Testing for Gerbich red cell antigens is useful in recognition of the Leach phenotype. Both normal [117] and abnormal [141] results for EMA binding have been reported.

Hereditary pyropoikilocytosis

The condition designated hereditary pyropoikilocytosis is a heterogeneous group of inherited haemolytic anaemias characterised by recessive inheritance and bizarre poikilocytes, including red cell fragments and microspherocytes. It has been described in Caucasian, Black and Arab populations. The condition is defined by enhanced red cell fragmentation on *in vitro* heating, which occurs at a lower temperature than with normal red cells. This feature is indicated in the name 'pyropoikilocytosis'. Hereditary elliptocytosis shows a similar but milder defect on heat exposure. Red cell membranes often show two defects, a partial spectrin deficiency and a defect of self-assembly of spectrin dimers into tetramers, the latter as a result of an elliptogenic mutation. It may be the spectrin deficiency (absent in typical hereditary elliptocytosis) that leads to the presence of spherocytes as well as elliptocytes in patients with hereditary pyropoikilocytosis [124]. The underlying genetic defects are various [142]. There may be homozygosity or compound heterozygosity for a mutant spectrin that has a defect affecting dimer self-assembly and is also degraded rapidly. Alternatively, there may be compound heterozygosity for a mutant spectrin (α or β chain) and for a polymorphism leading to a reduced rate of synthesis of α spectrin, α spectrin[Lely] occurring in *trans*. Parents of patients with hereditary pyropoikilocytosis may both have morphologically normal red cells or one or occasionally both parents may have typical hereditary elliptocytosis.

Patients with hereditary pyropoikilocytosis have a severe haemolytic anaemia. Anaemia tends to be more severe in the neonatal period, since haemoglobin F binds 2,3-DPG less well than does haemoglobin A and the free 2,3-DPG weakens spectrin–actin interactions.

Blood film and count

There is anaemia and the blood film (Figs 8.47 & 8.48) shows gross anisocytosis and poikilocytosis, with the poikilocytes including microspherocytes, cells with bud-like projections and fragments; elliptocytes may be a minor or a major component. Sometimes they are absent. The reticulocyte count is increased. The Hb is reduced. The MCV and MCH are markedly reduced. The MCV is usually 50–60 fl and may be as low as 25 fl [106]. The RDW and HDW are increased. Morphological abnormalities may be particularly marked in the neonatal period.

Differential diagnosis

In the neonatal period some cases of hereditary elliptocytosis have marked poikilocytosis (see above) and therefore resemble hereditary pyropoikilocytosis. Patients with homozygosity for protein 4.1 deficiency also have a severe anaemia and fragmenting

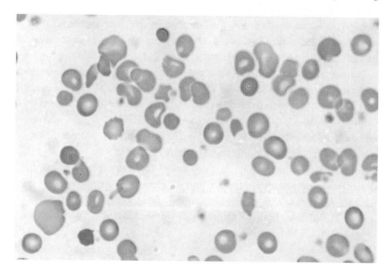

Fig. 8.47 The blood film of a patient with hereditary pyropoikilocytosis showing numerous spherocytes, other poikilocytes and polychromatic macrocytes. By courtesy of Professor Irene Roberts, Oxford.

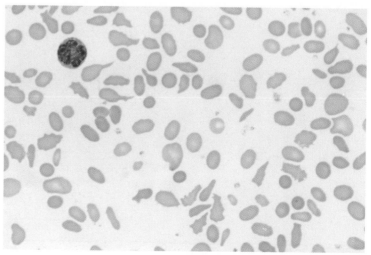

Fig. 8.48 The blood film of a patient with hereditary pyropoikilocytosis showing marked poikilocytosis and polychromatic macrocytes; among the poikilocytes, elliptocytes and spherocytes are prominent. By courtesy of Professor Irene Roberts.

elliptocytes, but have normal thermal stability [124]. Haemoglobin H disease and the congenital dyserythropoietic anaemias also sometimes show a similar degree of poikilocytosis, but they lack the microspherocytes and budding cells. Hereditary pyropoikilocytosis can be simulated by accidental *in vitro* heating of a blood specimen [143].

Further tests
Osmotic fragility and autohaemolysis are increased. The diagnosis is confirmed by demonstration of fragmentation on *in vitro* exposure to heat and by biochemical analysis of red cell membranes. EMA binding is reduced (even more than in hereditary spherocytosis) [144].

South-East Asian ovalocytosis
South-East Asian ovalocytosis, also sometimes referred to as hereditary ovalocytosis of Melanesians, Melanesian elliptocytosis or stomatocytic elliptocytosis, is a distinct and homogeneous disorder that occurs in Melanesians in Papua and New Guinea, the Solomon and Torres Strait Islands, in Malaysian aboriginals, in southern Thailand, Cambodia, Borneo and some populations in Indonesia and the Philippines. The condition has been recognised among the South African Cape Coloured population [145]. A single case has been described in a Mauritian Indian and single affected African American and Caucasian families have been reported [96]. Inheritance is autosomal dominant. In some of the affected ethnic groups, as many as 20–30% of the population are affected [146]. The underlying genetic defect is deletion of nine codons in the gene for band 3 (*SLC4A1*), which results in tight binding of band 3 to ankyrin, reduced lateral mobility and rigidity of the membrane. A polymorphic point mutation in the same gene, the Memphis polymorphism, usually occurs in *cis* to the deletion responsible for this condition. South-East Asian ovalocytosis has a cation leak at low temperatures that shows the same characteristics as that present in cryohydrocytosis [147].

Heterozygotes for South-East Asian ovalocytosis are usually completely asymptomatic, but epidemiological studies suggest that homozygosity for this mutation is incompatible with fetal survival.

Blood film and count
In the vast majority of cases there is neither anaemia nor compensated haemolysis. The exception is in the neonatal period when a significant haemolytic anaemia can occur and persist into infancy [148]. A greater fall of Hb during intercurrent *Plasmodium falciparum* malaria has been observed in heterozygotes for this condition in comparison with subjects with normal red cell membranes [149]. Red cells are round or oval and include stomatocytes. There is a minor population of macro-ovalocytes, many of which are stomatocytic (Fig. 8.49). Stomas may be longitudinal, transverse, V-shaped or Y-shaped or there may be two stomas per cell. Some

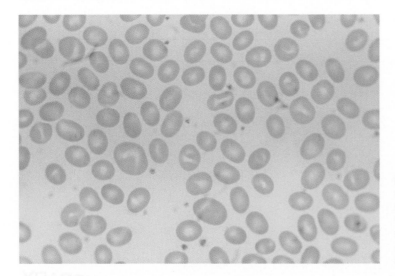

Fig. 8.49 The blood film of a patient with South-East Asian ovalocytosis showing several macro-ovalocytes one of which has a V-shaped stoma and the other an eccentric transverse stoma. Many of the smaller cells are either stomatocytes, ovalocytes or stomato-ovalocytes.

cases, diagnosed by molecular genetic analysis, have lacked ovalocytes but have shown stomatocytes or red cells with multiple irregular or linear pale areas [149]. The reticulocyte count is normal. The Hb, MCV, MCH and MCHC are normal.

Differential diagnosis

The blood film in the majority of patients is so distinctive that as long as the characteristic features are known, it is unlikely to be confused with any other condition.

Further tests

The blood film is usually pathognomonic so that further tests are unnecessary. However, molecular genetic analysis is possible. There is reduced expression of many red cell antigens including Rh D, so that subjects may type as D^U [150]. EMA binding is abnormal, whereas it is generally normal in hereditary elliptocytosis [117]. Osmotic fragility is reduced [124].

Hereditary stomatocytosis and related conditions

Hereditary stomatocytosis and related disorders are a heterogeneous group of rare dominantly inherited haemolytic anaemias and related conditions characterised by stomatocytes in blood films, an increased cation flux through red cell membranes or both. In the majority of cases there is increased intracellular sodium and decreased intracellular

potassium. These disorders can be further categorised as shown in Table 8.3.

Hereditary stomatocytosis

The term hereditary stomatocytosis describes a heterogeneous group of rare inherited haemolytic anaemias characterised by a red cell membrane defect that leads to the formation of overhydrated stomatocytic cells. An alternative designation is hereditary stomatocytosis, overhydrated variant, or 'hydrocytosis'. There is a very marked increase in cation flux. In the majority of affected families the condition is due to a mutation in the *RHAG* gene [156]. The red cell membrane shows reduced expression of stomatin, Rhesus-associated glycoprotein (RHAG) expression is slightly reduced and an electrophoretically abnormal RHAG protein is present [156]. In families where stomatocytosis is part of a syndrome that also includes neurological abnormalities, this gene is not involved [156].

Haemolysis is often severe and patients are chronically jaundiced. When splenectomy has been performed, post-splenectomy thrombosis has sometimes been a problem. Intercurrent parvovirus B19 infection can lead to life-threatening and even fatal anaemia [161].

Blood film and count

Haemolysis may be compensated or there may be anaemia that is mild, moderate or severe. The blood

Table 8.3 Hereditary stomatocytosis and related conditions [151–160]

Condition	Blood film	Other characteristics	Mutated gene
Hereditary stomatocytosis, overhydrated variant	Stomatocytes	Mild to severe haemolytic anaemia	*RHAG* at 6q12.3 [156]
Hereditary xerocytosis or hereditary stomatocytosis, dehydrated variant	Target cells and sometimes also stomatocytes	Haemolytic anaemia or compensated haemolysis, may have perinatal oedema and ascites	*PIEZO1* at 16q24.3 [157,158]
Familial pseudohyperkalaemia	Normal blood film	Fully compensated mild haemolytic anaemia; loss of potassium at room temperature	*PIEZO1* at 16q24.3 [157,158]
Cryohydrocytosis	Stomatocytes	Mild to moderate haemolytic anaemia with loss of potassium at low temperatures	*SLC4A1* at 17q21.31 in most cases [159]
Stomatin-deficient cryohydrocytosis	Stomatocytosis (2 cases)	Haemolytic anaemia with increased anion leak, cryohydrocytosis, cataracts and neurodevelopmental delay	*SLC2A1* at 1p34.2 [160]

film shows a variable number of stomatocytes, usually 10–30% (Fig. 8.50). There are also macrocytes, echinocytes and target cells [156].

There is an increased MCV and decreased MCHC. Red cell cytograms show increased normochromic and, in particular, hypochromic macrocytes. The HDW is increased. Typical red cell indices have been given as Hb 80–100 g/l, MCV 120 fl, MCHC 280 g/l and reticulocyte count 10–30% [124]. A change in red cell indices *ex vivo* can be diagnostically useful; overnight storage, whether at room temperature or at 4°C, can lead to an increase from an MCV of 95–98 fl to 110–120 fl, with a corresponding fall in the MCHC [127].

Differential diagnosis

The differential diagnosis includes other inherited conditions characterised by stomatocytes and also the much more frequent cases of acquired stomatocytosis (see Chapter 3). Rh deficiency disease (see Table 8.4) has many characteristics in common with hereditary stomatocytosis. Blood films show similar numbers of stomatocytes together with a few spherocytes. Cation flux is abnormal. There is a mild haemolytic anaemia or well-compensated haemolysis. The demonstration of a total lack of Rh antigens allows the diagnosis to be made. Stomatocytes are also a feature of Mediterranean stomatocytosis/macrothrombocytopenia (see below) [162].

Further tests

Osmotic fragility is increased. There may be pseudohyperkalaemia resulting from leakage of potassium from cells if there is delay in processing blood specimens; this abnormality can be sought when stomatocytosis is suspected. Blood grouping is indicated to exclude Rh null disease. EMA binding is increased [127].

Hereditary xerocytosis

Hereditary xerocytosis, also referred to as the dehydrated variant of hereditary stomatocytosis, is a rare inherited haemolytic anaemia characterised by increased cation flux, normal or increased cellular cation content and loss of red cell water. Inheritance is autosomal dominant with variable penetrance. Pseudohyperkalaemia can occur. Fetal ascites and neonatal ascites and peripheral oedema have been reported [163]. This condition is now recognised as being the same as that initially described under the designation 'high phosphatidyl choline haemolytic anaemia' [155,164]. It is both milder and more common than the overhydrated variant of hereditary stomatocytosis. Hereditary xerocytosis and related syndromes result from a mutation in the *PIEZO1* gene, which encodes a component of a cation channel [157,158]. When splenectomy has been performed, post-splenectomy thrombosis has sometimes occurred [155].

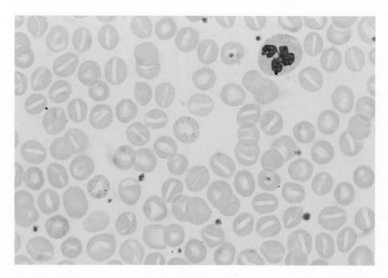

Fig. 8.50 The blood film of a patient with hereditary stomatocytosis showing basophilic stippling and numerous stomatocytes. By courtesy of Dr Carol Barton, Reading.

Blood film and count

Some patients are anaemic and some have compensated haemolysis. The blood film (Figs 8.51 & 8.52) shows target cells, sometimes a small number of stomatocytes, echinocytes, irregularly contracted cells and cells with the haemoglobin apparently 'puddled' at the periphery or on one or two edges of the cell [165]. There is polychromasia and the reticulocyte count is increased. Stomatocytes may be more prominent on wet preparations.

The MCV is normal or high and the MCHC may be elevated. The RDW and HDW are increased. Typical red cell indices have been given as Hb 110–140 g/l, MCV 110–120 fl, MCHC 360–370 g/dl and reticulocyte count 5–10% [124]. Red cell cytograms produced by the Siemens instruments may show a population of hyperdense cells.

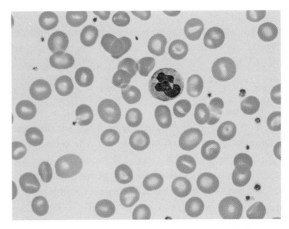

Fig. 8.52 Blood film of a patient with hereditary xerocytosis showing both stomatocytes and several dense cells with little or no central pallor. By courtesy of Dr Mark Layton, London.

Differential diagnosis

The differential diagnosis includes other causes of haemolytic anaemia, particularly those conditions that usually have some stomatocytes or target cells.

Further tests

The osmotic fragility is decreased although there may be a small tail of fragile cells. The demonstration of a population of cells with an increased MCHC is diagnostically useful. Patients may exhibit pseudohyperkalaemia if there is delay in measuring plasma

potassium, as a result of leakage of potassium from the red cells. The acid glycerol lysis time is normal and EMA binding is normal or increased [127].

Familial pseudohyperkalaemia

This term refers to a heterogeneous group of inherited red cell membrane defects that lead to increased cation flux with loss of potassium from red cells at room temperature [155,166]. Diagnosis of this condition usually follows observation of a falsely elevated

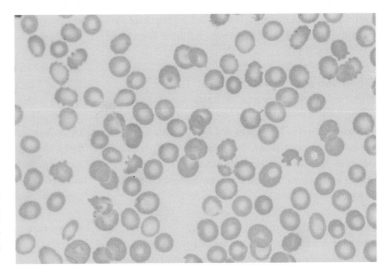

Fig. 8.51 The blood film of a patient with hereditary xerocytosis showing target cells, poikilocytes and several cells with haemoglobin distributed unevenly in the cell or 'puddled'. By courtesy of Dr Joan Luis Vives Corrons, Barcelona.

plasma potassium concentration. In some kindreds the abnormality is due to a *PIEZO* mutation, indicating a close relationship to hereditary xerocytosis. In other kindreds it is probably a mild variant of hereditary cryohydrocytosis [124].

Blood film and count
There is fully compensated haemolysis so that the haemoglobin concentration is normal. The reticulocyte count may be slightly elevated. The blood film does not show any stomatocytes. There may be mild macrocytosis and the MCV may rise markedly on room temperature or cold storage [167].

Differential diagnosis
The differential diagnosis includes hereditary stomatocytosis and other defects leading to pseudohyperkalaemia. The normal or near normal blood film and the mildness of the haemolysis distinguish this condition from related disorders.

Cryohydrocytosis
This term refers to a very rare group of disorders with increased erythrocyte cation flux, loss of potassium from the red cell and red cell lysis at low temperatures [168]. On storage in the cold, red cells swell so that the MCV rises and the MCHC falls. Splenectomy is not of benefit, but has not been reported to have any deleterious effects [169]. This condition is usually due to a mutation in *SLC4A1* (encoding anion exchanger 1, band 3) [159]. Other patients with mutations in this gene also have a low temperature cation leak, but have spherocytosis rather than stomatocytosis and it can be regarded as a variant of hereditary spherocytosis resulting from band 3 deficiency [159].

Blood film and count
There is either haemolytic anaemia or compensated haemolysis. The blood film shows stomatocytes and macrospherocytes [169]. The MCHC is increased when measured without delay, but decreases with storage, whereas the MCV rises with storage [155]. Storage effects are aggravated if storage is in the cold rather than at room temperature.

Differential diagnosis
The differential diagnosis includes other types of hereditary stomatocytosis and other defects leading to pseudo-

hyperkalaemia. Misdiagnosis as hereditary spherocytosis may occur because storage in the cold leads to the appearance of increased numbers of macrospherocytes and increasing osmotic fragility [169] and, in addition, EMA binding may be reduced [127].

Further tests
Plasma potassium may be increased. Overnight storage at 4°C causes lysis and a rise of extracellular potassium concentration.

Stomatin-deficient cryohydrocytosis
This very rare condition has a phenotype intermediate between that of overhydrated stomatocytosis (stomatin-deficient stomatocytic red cells) and cryohydrocytosis (cells sensitive to cold). It is due to a mutation in the *SLC2A1* gene [160]. There is moderate haemolytic anaemia with episodic crises. There are associated neurological abnormalities (mild or severe mental retardation, seizures), growth retardation, cataracts and massive hepatosplenomegaly [160,170].

In one reported patient with the same neurological syndrome and mutated *SLC2A1*, there was echinocytosis rather than stomatocytosis [171].

Sitosterolaemia
Sitosterolaemia (also known as phytosterolaemia) is an autosomal recessive disorder resulting from mutation in *ABCG5* or *ABCG8* at 2p21, in which there is unselective and unrestricted absorption of dietary cholesterol and plant-derived cholesterol-like molecules (phytosterols) [172]. Serum phytosterols are increased and serum cholesterol may be increased. In addition to the haematological manifestations, short stature and xanthomas are typically present and there may also be splenomegaly. This condition has been observed in Northern and Eastern Europeans, in Chinese, in Japanese and in an Indian family [162,172].

A similar condition described in Australians of Greek or Balkan origin (Adelaide and Perth only), prior to 1975, and designated Mediterranaen stomatocytosis/macrothrombocytosis appears likely to have been an acquired condition; it has been speculated that a contaminant of olive oil could have been responsible [173].

Blood film and count
There is mild haemolysis with marked stomatocytosis. The platelet count is reduced and platelets are large.

Differential diagnosis

The differential diagnosis includes other causes of stomatocytosis and others causes of thrombocytopenia with large platelets.

Other defects of the erythrocyte membrane

Other rare inherited defects of the red cell membrane leading to haemolytic anaemia are summarised in Table 8.4. In addition, familial hypercholesterolaemia is associated with a red cell membrane abnormality and a reduced red cell survival in the absence of any morphological abnormality [180]. When such patients are treated by plasmapheresis, haemolysis increases and iron deficiency anaemia subsequently develops.

Red cell enzyme abnormalities

The red cell contains many enzymes that are crucial for maintaining the integrity of the cell. The most important enzymatic pathways are the glycolytic pathway, which provides energy for the cell, and the pentose shunt, which protects the red cell from oxidant damage. These pathways are shown in Figs 8.53 & 8.54.

Table 8.4 Other rare hereditary haemolytic anaemias caused by red cell membrane defects [171,174–179].

Defect	Antigenic or biochemical defect and genetic abnormality (when known)	Haematological features	Associated abnormalities
McLeod phenotype [174]	Lack of Kx antigen encoded by *KX* gene at Xp21; Kell antigens are generally reduced	Acanthocytosis, compensated haemolysis	Late onset of muscular and neurological abnormalities (neuropathy and choreiform movements), cardiomyopathy; when caused by a large deletion may occur in association with chronic granulomatous disease, Duchenne muscular dystrophy or retinitis pigmentosa
Neuro-acanthocytosis [175]	Normal Kell and Kx antigens, mutation in *CHAC* gene or *JP3* gene	Acanthocytosis	Dystonic and choreiform movements (atypical Huntington disease)
Acanthocytosis with red cell anion leak [176,177]	*SLC4A1* mutation	Acanthocytosis with increased red cell anion leak	
Echinocytosis with cation leak	*SLC2A1* mutation	Echinocytosis, cation leak in red cells	Exertion-induced dyskinesia [171]
Inherited CD59 deficiency [178]	Autosomal recessive inheritance of CD59 deficiency	Chronic haemolytic anaemia resembling acquired paroxysmal nocturnal haemoglobinuria	
Rh deficiency syndrome [179]	Rh$_{null}$ Lack of all Rh and LW antigens and also Fy5 antigen, reduced expression of CD47, Ss and U, caused either by homozygosity for a silent allele at the *RH* locus or homozygosity for an autosomal suppressor gene X^or, an allele at the *RHAG* (Rh-associated glycoprotein) locus Rh$_{mod}$ Reduced expression of Rh antigens caused by mutations in the *RHAG* gene	Chronic haemolytic anaemia or compensated haemolysis with spherocytes and stomatocytes; increased osmotic fragility	

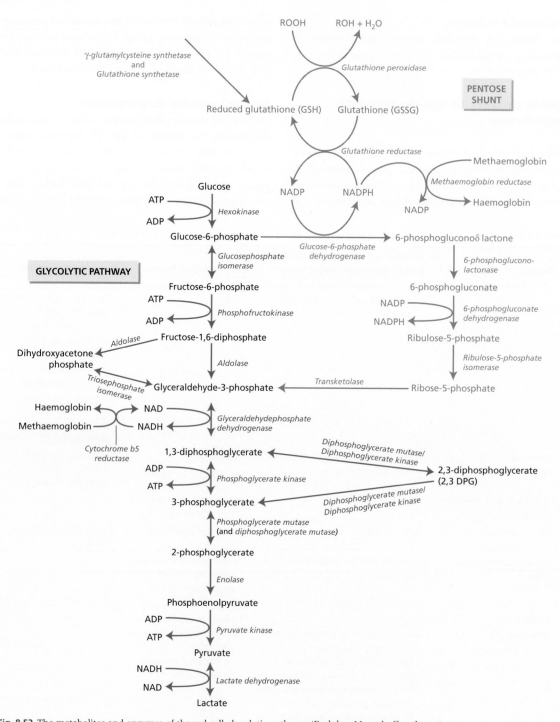

Fig. 8.53 The metabolites and enzymes of the red cell glycolytic pathway (Embden-Meyerhoff pathway).

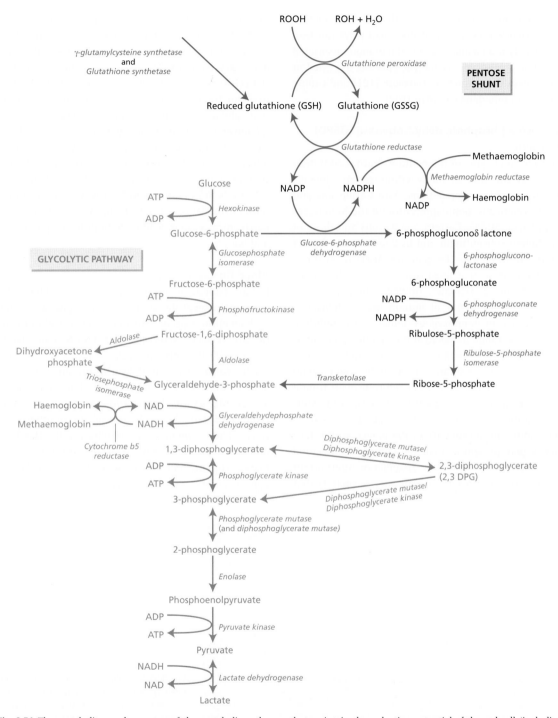

Fig. 8.54 The metabolites and enzymes of the metabolic pathways that maintain the reduction potential of the red cell (including the pentose shunt).

Other enzymes are concerned with nucleotide metabolism. Deficiencies in any of these pathways can lead to haemolytic anaemia. Individual mutations associated with non-spherocytic haemolytic anaemia are listed in the Human Gene Mutation Database [101] and Online Mendelian Inheritance in Man [102].

Glucose-6-phosphate dehydrogenase (G6PD) deficiency

G6PD is an enzyme of the pentose shunt. G6PD deficiency is common in many ethnic groups, including many African populations, Afro-Caribbeans and Black Americans, populations around the Mediterranean basin, Middle-Eastern populations and those of the Indian subcontinent and in South-East Asia and Papua New Guinea. The gene for G6PD is on the X chromosome so that most cases of G6PD deficiency are in hemizygous males. However, in populations with a high incidence of mutant genes, deficiency also occurs in homozygous females. In addition, because of random inactivation of one X chromosome, deficiency is sometimes seen in heterozygous females. Haemolysis can also occur in women who have had a haemopoietic stem cell transplant from a G6PD-deficient male. In parts of Greece and the Middle East the prevalence in males is as high as 35–40%. Depending on the severity of the defect, G6PD deficiency may present as neonatal jaundice, congenital non-spherocytic haemolytic anaemia or intermittent haemolysis triggered by oxidant stress, such as that caused by intercurrent infection, by eating broad beans (fava beans) or by exposure to naphthalene or oxidant drugs. Mediterranean subjects with G6PD deficiency have a mild reduction of the steady-state red cell survival, reduced from a normal of 120 days to about 100 days, together with reduction of plasma haptoglobin [181] and a mean Hb averaging about 15 g/l lower than that in non-deficient subjects [182]. Neonatal jaundice occurs in as many as a third of affected males, being attributable to impaired liver function more than to haemolysis [183]; when medical care is unavailable, kernicterus may result. Intermittent oxidant-induced haemolysis is acute and partly intravascular, leading to both haemoglobinuria and jaundice.

Blood film and count

In most patients with G6PD deficiency, the blood film is normal except during haemolytic episodes. When such an episode occurs, the morphological abnormalities are very characteristic (Figs 8.55 & 8.56). There are irregularly contracted cells, some of which have small protrusions caused by the presence of Heinz bodies. Keratocytes, often called 'bite cells', have an irregular gap in their outline, probably caused by removal of Heinz bodies by the spleen. In other cells, referred to as hemighosts or blister cells, the haemoglobin appears to have retracted to form a dense mass occupying half the cell while the rest of the cell appears empty. When haemolysis is very acute, a few

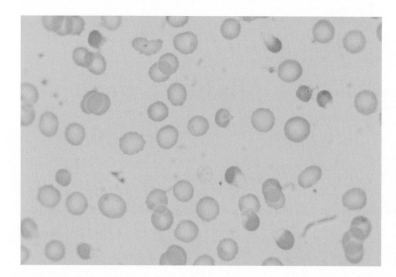

Fig. 8.55 The blood film of an Afro-Caribbean child with G6PD deficiency who had suffered an episode of acute haemolysis, showing anaemia, irregularly contracted cells, a hemighost, a complete ghost, and a cell with a protrusion attributable to a Heinz body; the Heinz body preparation was positive.

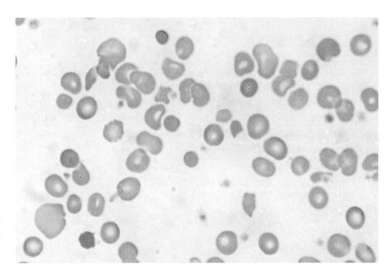

Fig. 8.56 The blood film of a patient with acute haemolysis associated with G6PD deficiency showing a 'bite cell' and a cell with haemoglobin retracted from the cell margin.

complete ghosts may be present. At the height of a haemolytic episode there is leucocytosis and neutrophilia and the features of hyposplenism can appear as a result of reticuloendothelial overload. In the few days following an episode of oxidant stress there may be a further fall in the Hb as damaged cells are cleared by the spleen. Subsequently, polychromatic macrocytes appear.

When there is chronic haemolytic anaemia due to severe G6PD deficiency, the blood film (Fig. 8.57) may show anisocytosis, poikilocytosis, basophilic stippling, macrocytosis and polychromasia without any specific diagnostic features. Patients with chronic non-spherocytic haemolytic anaemia caused by G6PD deficiency can have their haemolysis exacerbated by infection or other oxidant stress.

G6PD deficient patients with chronic non-spherocytic haemolytic anaemia have a reduced Hb, RBC and Hct and an increased MCV and MCH. Those with episodic haemolysis have a reduced Hb, RBC and Hct during attacks together with an increased RDW, a population of cells with an increased haemoglobin concentration and, if haemolysis is very acute, an increased MCHC. When recovery starts, there is

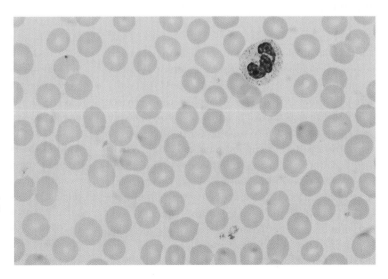

Fig. 8.57 The blood film of a patient with congenital non-spherocytic haemolytic anaemia caused by G6PD deficiency showing macrocytosis and slight polychromasia. By courtesy of Professor Lucio Luzzatto, Florence.

a further increase in the RDW and the MCV, MCH and HDW also increase. In these patients the steady-state Hb in hemizygous males is somewhat reduced, a mean of 141.2 g/l in comparison with 156.8 g/l in normal subjects being observed in one study [182]; the mean RBC and Hct are similarly significantly reduced. The mean steady-state MCV is slightly but significantly increased reflecting the slight increase in reticulocytes, 90.16 fl in comparison with 87.54 fl in the same study [182]. Heterozygous females show a slight but significant decrease in the RBC and Hct and a slight but significant increase in the MCV and MCH [182].

Differential diagnosis

In the neonatal period, the differential diagnosis includes other causes of neonatal jaundice, particularly haemolytic disease of the newborn with an immune basis. In cases with chronic haemolysis, the differential diagnosis includes other causes of congenital non-spherocytic haemolytic anaemia (see below). In patients with intermittent haemolysis the differential diagnosis is other much less common defects of the pentose shunt and haemolytic anaemia due to exposure to oxidant drugs or chemicals in a patient with no underlying enzyme deficiency; when there is oxidant damage to red cells the blood films are indistinguishable whether or not there is an underlying enzyme defect. To a lesser extent other causes of irregularly contracted cells, such as unstable haemoglobins, should be included in the differential diagnosis.

Further tests

There is haemoglobinuria and free haemoglobin may be present in the plasma during haemolytic episodes. Haptoglobin is greatly reduced or absent. Unconjugated bilirubin is increased. Diagnosis can be based on screening tests for G6PD deficiency or on an assay. Screening tests are very suitable for population surveys. During haemolytic episodes, the high reticulocyte count can cause screening tests and sometimes even assays to be normal. This is particularly so in individuals of African ancestry who often have a G6PD mutation associated with relatively high enzyme levels in reticulocytes. It can also occur in female heterozygotes who suffer haemolysis, since the deficient cells will be selectively lysed, leaving cells with a more normal G6PD content in the circulation [184]. If G6PD deficiency is suspected, on the basis of the clinical history and the blood count and film, and the assay is normal, it should be repeated after the reticulocyte count has returned to normal.

In some countries with a high prevalence of G6PD deficiency, neonatal screening is performed on cord blood.

Pyruvate kinase deficiency

Pyruvate kinase deficiency is the most common of the congenital non-spherocytic haemolytic anaemias resulting from a glycolytic pathway enzyme deficiency. Its prevalence is about one in 20 000 [185], similar to that of non-spherocytic haemolytic anaemia due to G6PD deficiency. There is a high prevalence among the Amish population. Pyruvate kinase deficiency is recessive, so that affected individuals are either homozygotes or, more often, compound heterozygotes. This diagnosis should be suspected when there is either neonatal jaundice associated with haemolysis or chronic haemolysis in older children or adults without any specific morphological abnormality. Anaemia is very variable in severity, with rare patients being transfusion dependent. Hydrops fetalis has occurred [185]. Extramedullary haemopoiesis can lead to spinal cord compression [185]. Leg ulcers occasionally occur [186]. Anaemia may be aggravated by intercurrent infection, oxidant stress, pregnancy and possibly by administration of oral contraceptives [187]. Sudden worsening of anaemia may also result from pure red cell aplasia caused by parvovirus B19 infection. Iron overload sometimes occurs, particularly in individuals who are also heterozygous for familial haemochromatosis.

Pyruvate kinase deficiency is associated with increased levels of 2,3-DPG and therefore milder symptoms than would be expected for the degree of anaemia.

Blood film and count

There is chronic anaemia, varying from very severe to mild, or compensated haemolysis. The blood film (Fig. 8.58) usually shows only non-specific features such as anisocytosis, macrocytosis and polychromasia. There may be occasional ovalocytes and elliptocytes and small numbers of densely staining spiculated cells; in one study 3–30% of spiculated cells

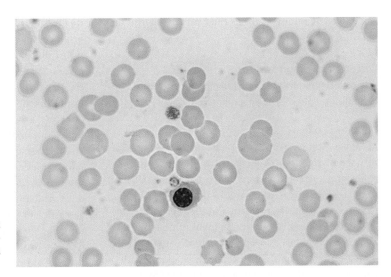

Fig. 8.58 The blood film of a patient with pyruvate kinase deficiency showing aniso-cytosis, macrocytosis, polychromasia and an NRBC.

were seen in 15% of 61 patients [185]. It has been postulated that these spiculated cells are adenosine triphosphate (ATP)-depleted erythrocytes at the end of their lifespan. Elliptocytes have been attributed to associated dyserythropoiesis, but the presence of appreciable numbers may indicate a coexisting membrane defect [188]. The reticulocyte count is increased but, because of the increased concentration of 2,3-DPG, less than might have been expected from the Hb. Some patients have leucopenia consequent on hypersplenism.

After splenectomy, the Hb usually rises by 10–30 g/l and the MCV and MCH may rise. Following splenectomy, some but not all cases have very frequent spiculated cells, resembling acanthocytes or abnormal echinocytes [189] (Fig. 8.59); there may be a paradoxical rise in the reticulocyte count to 40–70% despite improvement in the haemolysis, the likely explanation being that prior to splenectomy some highly defective newly produced cells were removed rapidly by the spleen and also that reticulocytes are selectively sequestered in the spleen. When

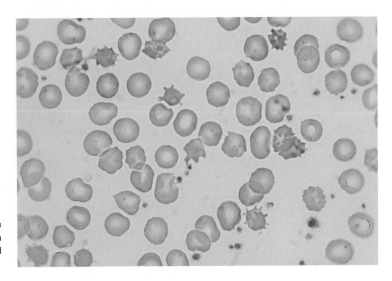

Fig. 8.59 The blood film of a patient with pyruvate kinase deficiency who has been splenectomised showing macrocytosis and acanthocytosis.

8

the spleen is removed these cells survive in the circulation.

Differential diagnosis

The differential diagnosis includes other causes of congenital non-spherocytic anaemia (see below).

Further tests

Pyruvate kinase deficiency is characterised by signs of haemolysis, such as increased non-conjugated bilirubin and increased lactate dehydrogenase (LDH). In some cases there is intravascular haemolysis, leading to reduced serum haptoglobin and the presence of urinary haemosiderin. Osmotic fragility is normal in three-quarters and reduced in one-quarter of patients [185]. Increased autohaemolysis is seen in only about a fifth of patients and is therefore not a useful test [185]. Definitive diagnosis requires a pyruvate kinase assay.

Congenital nonspherocytic haemolytic anaemia resulting from other red cell enzyme deficiencies

A variety of inherited congenital haemolytic anaemias consequent on a red cell enzyme deficiency have no characteristic abnormality of red cell shape and are grouped together under the designation 'congenital non-spherocytic haemolytic anaemia'. There may be echinocytes and, in defects of glutathione synthesis, irregularly contracted cells. The two most common causes of congenital non-spherocytic haemolytic anaemia are pyruvate kinase deficiency and G6PD deficiency. All others are rare or very rare. They should be suspected when there is either neonatal jaundice associated with haemolysis or chronic haemolysis in older children or adults. Neonatal jaundice, which is mainly hepatic in origin, is particularly a feature of G6PD deficiency. The underlying defect may be in enzymes of the: (i) glycolytic pathway; (ii) pentose shunt and glutathione synthesis and metabolism; or (iii) nucleotide metabolism. The inheritance and associated clinical features of these defects are summarised in Tables 8.5–8.7. In addition, an association of haemolytic anaemia with glyceraldehyde-3-phosphate dehydrogenase deficiency has been suspected but not firmly established [186]. Deficiencies of a single enzyme are heterogeneous; the mutations differ and they occur in a variety of ethnic groups spread over a wide geographical area. Most enzyme

Table 8.5 Associated clinical features and inheritance of glycolytic pathway enzyme deficiencies, most of which cause congenital non-spherocytic anaemias [101,186,190–204].

Enzyme	Frequency	Inheritance	Associated features
Hexokinase [196,197]	Rare; at least 17 known families	AR* HK1 gene at 10q22.1; at least 7 known mutations	Multiple congenital abnormalities, latent diabetes mellitus or psychomotor retardation in some cases; intrauterine periventricular leucomalacia reported in a compound heterozygote and a homozygote with lethal haemolytic anaemia
Glucose phosphate isomerase [198]	Third most common enzyme deficiency causing haemolytic anaemia; at least 50 known families among Caucasians, Afro-Americans, Turks, Japanese and Jews	AR GPI gene at 19q13.11; at least 29 known mutations	Five mutations have been associated with non-haematological abnormalities including myopathy, mental retardation, neurological symptoms and granulocyte dysfunction
Phosphofructokinase† [195,199]	Rare; at least 39 known families in Caucasians, Japanese and Jews (a third of known families with PFKM mutations are Jewish)	AR mutation in PFKM gene at 12q13 (at least 15 known) or in the PFKL gene at 21q22.3	Myopathy (type VII glycogen storage disease) in about half (those with a mutation in the PFKM gene); myopathy can also occur without haemolysis; some individuals with deficiency are asymptomatic
Aldolase [195,200,201]	Very rare, at least six cases in five kindreds	AR mutations in ALDOA gene at 16q22-23	Mental retardation, multiple congenital abnormalities, type VI glycogen storage disease in 1 kindred; myopathy in two cases (rhabdomyolysis can occur)

Enzyme	Frequency	Inheritance	Associated features
Triosephosphate isomerase [195,202,203]	Rare, at least 35 known cases; however heterozygosity is unexpectedly common among Afro-Americans	AR at least 14 known mutations in *TPI1* gene at 12p13	Progressive neuromuscular and cardiac dysfunction in the great majority of cases; sometimes mental retardation; increased susceptibility to infection; death *in utero* or early childhood
Phosphoglycerate kinase [195,199]	Rare, at least 29 known families	X-linked recessive *PGK1* gene at Xq21.1; at least 17 known variants; female heterozygotes may have mild haemolytic anaemia	No associated defect or various combinations of myopathy with exercise-induced rhabdomyolysis, growth retardation, mental retardation and progressive neurological dysfunction; myopathy, neurological dysfunction or both can occur without haemolysis
2,3 diphosphoglycerate mutase [195][‡]	Rare, about 20 cases known	AR *BPGM* gene at 7q33	
Enolase [195]	Very rare, 3 known families with deficiency and haemolysis but there may not be a causal relationship	? AD *ENO1* gene at 1q36.23 but no mutations identified	In these families enolase of about half normal is seen in individuals with hereditary spherocytosis with AD inheritance
Pyruvate kinase [195,204]	Similar frequency to G6PD deficiency as a cause of chronic haemolytic anaemia, prevalence among Caucasians 50/10[6], more than 500 cases reported	AR *PKLR* gene at 1q22; more than 160 known mutations	
Lactate dehydrogenase[§] [195]	Very rare	AR *LDHA* gene at 11p15.1 or *LDHB* gene at 12p12.1	

*AD in two families with unusual morphological features
† Can be associated with haemolytic anaemia, compensated haemolysis or mild polycythaemia
‡ Causes polycythaemia rather than anaemia because of decreased 2,3 DPG; compensated haemolysis has been described but a causal association has not been shown [186]
§ Reduced enzyme level but no anaemia (although haemolysis is seen in deficient mice) [186]
AD, autosomal dominant; AR, autosomal recessive; G6PD, glucose-6-phosphate dehydrogenase

Table 8.6 Clinical features and inheritance of deficiencies or excesses of enzymes involved in nucleotide metabolism, most of which cause congenital non-spherocytic anaemias [101,186,192–194,205–210].

Enzyme	Frequency	Inheritance	Associated features
Adenylate kinase* [195,205,206]	Rare	AR *AK1* gene at 9q34.11; at least 7 mutations known	Mental retardation in some patients
Pyrimidine 5' nucleotidase[†] [37,207–209]	Rare; about 64 known cases in 54 families	AR *NT5C3A* at 7p14.3 [208]	Possible association with learning difficulties, seen in 7 cases [208,209]
Adenosine deaminase excess[‡]	Rare	AD *ADA* gene at 20q13.2, possible increased translation of mRNA	[210]

*Association with anaemia is inconsistent [186]
† Correctly designated pyrimidine 5' nucleotidase 1
‡ Deficiency causes immune deficiency but not anaemia
AD, autosomal dominant; AR, autosomal recessive; mRNA, messenger ribonucleic acid

Table 8.7 Clinical features and inheritance of deficiencies of enzymes of the hexose monophosphate shunt and enzymes concerned in glutathione synthesis and metabolism that can cause congenital non-spherocytic anaemias [101,192–195,211–217].

Enzyme	Frequency	Inheritance	Associated features
Glucose-6-phosphate dehydrogenase [211]	Similar frequency to pyruvate kinase deficiency as a cause of chronic haemolytic anaemia; occurs sporadically in many ethnic groups	X-linked, *G6PD* gene at Xq28	Neonatal jaundice
γ-glutamyl cysteine synthetase* [212,213]	Rare; Caucasian, Japanese, Moroccan and mixed Caucasian-American Indian	AR, mutations described in *GCLC* gene at 6p12.1	Spinocerebellar disease or neuropathy and mental retardation in 4 of 9 reported patients, aminoaciduria in 2
Glutathione synthetase [214,215]	Rare	AR *GSS* gene at 20q11.22	Mental retardation, ataxia and metabolic acidosis with 5-oxoprolinuria in some cases with generalised rather than red cell restricted deficiency; may have intermittent neutropenia
Glutathione peroxidase [195,216]	Rare: English, Polish, Syrian, Jewish, Mediterranean, Black	Autosomal *GPX1* at 3p21.31	Neonatal jaundice and drug-induced haemolysis in heterozygotes, compensated haemolysis in homozygotes
Glutathione reductase[†] [195,217]	Rare	AR *GSR* gene at 8p12	Cataracts, favism, neonatal jaundice not caused by haemolysis

*Enzymes required for glutathione synthesis
[†] Enzyme that favours maintaining glutathione in reduced state; acquired deficiency has been associated with haemolysis, panmyelopathy and a neurological disorder and is mainly caused by riboflavin deficiency
AR, autosomal recessive

deficiencies show an autosomal recessive inheritance, with affected individuals being homozygotes or, more often, compound heterozygotes. Exceptions are phosphoglycerate kinase and G6PD deficiency, which have an X-linked recessive inheritance, enolase deficiency, which is probably autosomal dominant, and the very rare haemolytic anaemia associated with adenosine deaminase excess, which is autosomal dominant. Heterozygotes do not suffer haemolysis, with the exception of some female heterozygotes for phosphoglycerate kinase deficiency [193]. Anaemia may be aggravated by intercurrent infection or pregnancy. In defects in the pentose shunt or glutathione synthesis, haemolysis may be aggravated by infection, drugs or ingestion of fava beans [214]. Sudden worsening of anaemia can also result from pure red cell aplasia caused by parvovirus B19 infection. Iron overload sometimes occurs, particularly in individuals who are also heterozygous for familial haemochromatosis. In one kindred with pyrimidine 5′ nucleotidase deficiency there was intravascular haemolysis leading to iron deficiency [208].

It should be noted that deficiencies of enzymes early in the glycolytic pathway lead to reduced synthesis of 2,3-DPG, which in turn causes a left shift of the oxygen dissociation curve, aggravates the symptoms of anaemia and provides a hypoxic drive to erythropoiesis. This may, paradoxically, lead to polycythaemia, as has been observed for individuals with diphosphoglycerate mutase deficiency and some with phosphofructokinase deficiency. Conversely, deficiency of enzymes involved late in the glycolytic pathway is associated with increased levels of 2,3-DPG and milder symptoms than would be expected for the degree of anaemia.

Blood film and count

There is chronic anaemia, varying from very severe to mild, or compensated haemolysis. The blood film (see Fig. 8.57) usually shows non-specific features such as anisocytosis, macrocytosis, polychromasia and basophilic stippling. Sometimes there are echinocytes [190] or other poikilocytes, usually in small numbers. Echinocytes have been noted in some cases of triose phosphate isomerase deficiency (Fig. 8.60) [218], aldolase deficiency [219], phosphoglycerate kinase deficiency [220] and glucose phosphate isomerase deficiency (Fig. 8.61). Small numbers of irregularly contracted cells have been noted in triose phosphate isomerase deficiency [221] and stomatocytes [222] in glucose phosphate isomerase deficiency. Irregularly contracted cells can also be a feature of defects of glutathione biosynthesis, and are prominent during haemolytic episodes (Fig. 8.62). Adenylate kinase deficiency has been associated with small numbers of elliptocytes, spherocytes,

schistocytes and stomatocytes [223,224]. Glutathione synthetase deficiency has been associated with teardrop poikilocytes [214]. One kindred with deficiency of 2,3-diphosphoglycerate mutase had occasional microspherocytes [225]. Enolase deficiency is unusual in that in the three reported kindreds it has been associated with the presence of spherocytes [193,195], but for convenience it is discussed here with other enzyme deficiencies. Only in pyrimidine 5′-nucleotidase deficiency is the blood film distinctive. In this condition there is very prominent basophilic stippling (Fig. 8.63), best

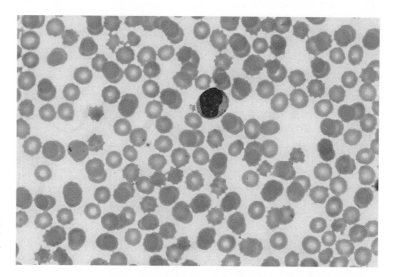

Fig. 8.60 The blood film of a patient with triose phosphate isomerase deficiency showing echinocytosis. By courtesy of Dr Joan Luis Vives Corrons.

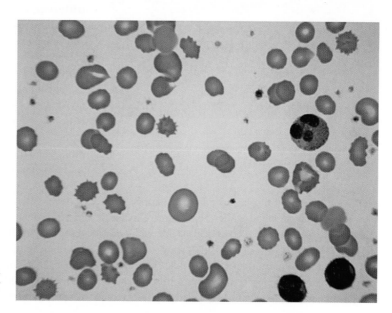

Fig. 8.61 The blood film of a patient with glucose phosphate isomerase deficiency showing echinocytosis.

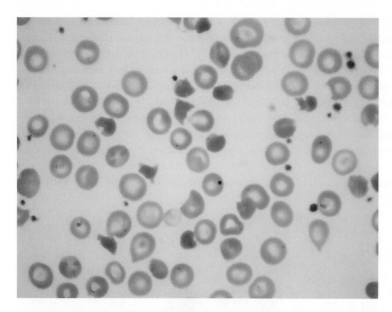

Fig. 8.62 The blood film of a patient with glutathione peroxidase deficiency during an acute haemolytic episode showing irregularly contracted cells, polychromasia and an erythrocyte containing a Howell–Jolly body. The latter is attributable to functional hyposplenism resulting from splenic overload during acute haemolysis. By courtesy of Dr Mark Layton.

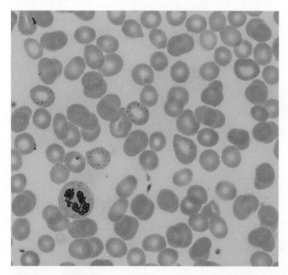

Fig. 8.63 The blood film of a patient with pyrimidine 5′ nucleotidase deficiency showing prominent basophilic stippling. By courtesy of Dr Joan Luis Vives Corrons.

seen when the blood film is made from heparinised or non-anticoagulated blood rather than from ethylenediaminetetra-acetic acid (EDTA)-anticoagulated blood. Basophilic stippling disappears if EDTA-anticoagulated blood is stored for more than four hours [37]. In addition to basophilic stippling, it is common for there to be a low percentage of spherocytes or spiculated spherocytes

(but with the osmotic fragility test usually being normal) [207]. The reticulocyte count is increased. Some cases have leucopenia as a result of hypersplenism.

After splenectomy, the Hb usually rises by 10–30 g/l and the MCV and MCH may rise. If there is a poor response to splenectomy, thrombocytosis may be very marked. Splenectomy is not usually useful in pyrimidine 5′-nucleotidase deficiency [207].

Differential diagnosis

The differential diagnosis of pyruvate kinase deficiency and other enzyme deficiencies includes: (i) congenital haemolytic anaemias due to membrane abnormalities but with only minor morphological abnormalities such as congenital xerocytosis and some cases of congenital stomatocytosis; (ii) certain porphyrias; and (iii) lead poisoning. Congenital erythropoietic porphyria causes chronic haemolysis with or without anaemia. The blood film in this condition shows anisocytosis, poikilocytosis, basophilic stippling and polychromasia [226]; Howell–Jolly bodies are often present. Slender purple-violet crystals, often radially arranged, have been observed in erythrocytes (see Fig. 3.63); they are likely to represent crystallised porphyrins [227]. Hypersplenism is common with resultant leucopenia and thrombocytopenia [226]. One case of the very rare harderoporphyria showed basophilic stippling [228] but, in general, cases of porphyria with haemolysis have not shown any specific morphological features. Lead poisoning enters particularly into the differential diagnosis of pyrimidine 5′-nucleotidase deficiency, since it can cause a haemolytic anaemia with prominent basophilic stippling; the stippling is the result of an acquired deficiency of the same enzyme. In cases presenting beyond the neonatal period, the differential diagnosis also includes Wilson disease, congenital erythropoietic porphyria and acquired haemolytic anaemias. Wilson disease can cause acute haemolysis with minimal morphological abnormalities in advance of any obvious evidence of liver disease.

Further tests

Congenital nonspherocytic anaemia is characterised by signs of haemolysis, such as increased unconjugated bilirubin. In some cases there is intravascular haemolysis, leading to reduced serum haptoglobin and the presence of urinary haemosiderin. The demonstration of normal osmotic fragility with or without increased autohaemolysis is consistent with a red cell enzyme deficiency. However, definitive diagnosis requires biochemical assays, which can generally only be performed in a reference laboratory. Congenital erythropoietic porphyria can be confirmed by demonstrating fluorescence in a proportion of erythrocytes and in the nuclei of any circulating erythroblasts when the blood is examined under ultraviolet light.

Acquired haemolytic anaemias

Acquired haemolytic anaemias with an immune mechanism

Warm autoimmune haemolytic anaemia

Most cases of autoimmune haemolytic anaemia (AIHA) are caused by warm-acting antibodies, usually IgG, which are directed at red cell membrane antigens. The phagocytic cells of the spleen, and to a lesser extent the liver, remove both whole cells and parts of the red cell membrane to which immunoglobulin and sometimes also complement have been bound. Removal of pieces of the red cell membrane leads to spherocyte formation. Autoimmune haemolytic anaemia may be primary, one feature of an autoimmune disease such as systemic lupus erythematosus (SLE) or the autoimmune lymphoproliferative syndrome or secondary to other diseases such as chronic lymphocytic leukaemia (CLL),

non-Hodgkin lymphoma, Hodgkin lymphoma, carcinoma of the ovary or diGeorge syndrome; in one study, 3 of 13 patients with either AIHA or Evans syndrome (autoimmune haemolytic anaemia plus autoimmune thrombocytopenic purpura) had a population of peripheral blood cells with a CLL phenotype, suggesting that monoclonal B lymphocytosis may also predispose to AIHA [229]. Rarely, AIHA has been induced by a drug – in the past most often α-methyl dopa but occasionally levodopa, mefenamic acid, interferon alpha [230] or other drugs. One case has been reported in association with infection by a novel micro-organism provisionally designated *Candidatus Mycoplasma haemohominis* [231]. Autoimmune haemolytic anaemia can occur as a complication of Wiskott–Aldrich syndrome and when it occurs early in life is prognostically adverse and an indication for transplantation [232].

Warm AIHA can occur in recent recipients of allogeneic haemopoietic stem cell and solid organ transplants, as a result of disordered cellular immune responses. In the case of stem cell transplantation there are donor antibodies against donor-derived erythrocytes, whereas in the case of solid organ transplants there are recipient antibodies against recipient erythrocytes [233].

Blood film and count

The blood film (Fig. 8.64) shows spherocytosis and sometimes also polychromasia and polychromatic macrocytes.

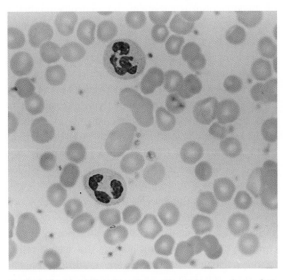

Fig. 8.64 The blood film of a patient with autoimmune haemolytic anaemia showing spherocytes and polychromatic macrocytes.

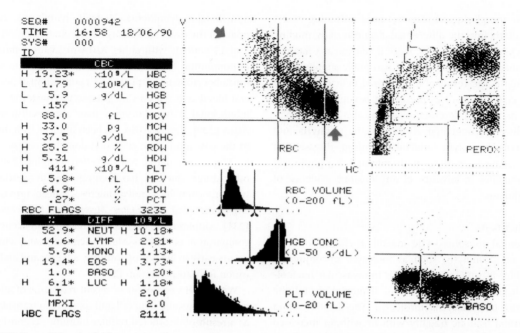

```
SEQ#      0000942
TIME      16:58  18/06/90
SYS#      000
ID
              CBC
H  19.23*    x10 9/L   WBC
L   1.79     x10 12/L  RBC
L   5.9       g/dL     HGB
L   .157               HCT
    88.0       fL      MCV
H  33.0       pg       MCH
H  37.5      g/dL      MCHC
H  25.2       %        RDW
H   5.31     g/dL      HDW
H  411*      x10 9/L   PLT
L   5.8*      fL       MPV
    64.9*      %       PDW
    .27*       %       PCT
RBC FLAGS            3235
    %         DIFF    10 9/L
    52.9*    NEUT  H  10.18*
L   14.6*    LYMP      2.81*
     5.9*    MONO  H   1.13*
H   19.4*    EOS   H   3.73*
     1.0*    BASO      .20*
H    6.1*    LUC   H   1.18*
    LI                 2.04
    MPXI                2.0
WBC FLAGS           2111
```

RBC

HC

RBC VOLUME
(0–200 fL)

HGB CONC
(0–50 g/dL)

PLT VOLUME
(0–20 fL)

PERO:

BASO

Fig. 8.65 Bayer H.2 red cell histograms and cytogram from a patient with autoimmune haemolytic anaemia showing dense cells, which are spherocytes, and hypochromic macrocytes, which are mainly reticulocytes (green arrows). There is also eosinophilia evident in the peroxidase channel.

There may be phagocytosis of erythrocytes by neutrophils and monocytes, but such phagocytic cells are sufficiently infrequent that they are only readily noted of a buffy coat preparation. In severe cases, granulocyte precursors and NRBC are present and there may be features of hyposplenism consequent on reticuloendothelial overload. In occasional patients, teardrop poikilocytes have been prominent and have disappeared after splenectomy [234]. Some patients have an associated immune thrombocytopenia. More rare is immune pancytopenia in which there is also neutropenia. The blood film may show features of an underlying disease such as CLL, large granular lymphocyte leukaemia, non-Hodgkin lymphoma or angioimmunoblastic T-cell lymphoma.

The Hb, RBC and Hct are reduced. The MCH and MCV may be normal or elevated. The MCHC is elevated when measured by an instrument that is sensitive to changes in this variable. The RDW and HDW are increased. The reticulocyte count is increased. Some automated instruments indicate the presence of hyperchromia. Red cell cytograms plotting size against cellular haemoglobin concentration are not distinguishable from those of hereditary spherocytosis but, because haemolysis is often more severe, there may be a prominent population of hypochromic and normochromic macrocytes, which represent reticulocytes and other young red cells (Fig. 8.65).

Differential diagnoses

The differential diagnosis includes hereditary spherocytosis and other causes of immune haemolytic anaemia. Occasionally, there are specific blood film features suggestive of immune haemolysis, such as small red cell agglutinates, red cell phagocytosis by monocytes, rosetting of red cells around neutrophils (as an *in vitro* phenomenon) [235] or thrombocytopenia. More often the peripheral blood features are indistinguishable from those of hereditary spherocytosis. Other immune haemolytic anaemias that can also be confused with autoimmune haemolytic anaemia if sufficient weight is not given to the clinical history are: (i) paroxysmal cold haemoglobinuria; (ii) drug-induced immune haemolytic anaemia; and (iii) alloimmune haemolytic anaemia (see below), including delayed transfusion reactions. In delayed transfusion reactions, examination of a blood film permits a diagnosis, since only transfused cells are affected and the film is dimorphic (see Fig. 3.30).

When ABO incompatible plasma or immunoglobulin is transfused, the spherocytosis is generalised so that the film appearances do not differ from those of AIHA. Spherocytosis may persist for weeks [236] so that confusion with AIHA is possible. Immediate transfusion reactions are unlikely to be confused with AIHA since most of the donor cells are destroyed and spherocytosis is not prominent.

Chronic haemolytic anaemia mediated by a cold agglutinin (see below) can usually be readily distinguished from warm AIHA on the blood film. The blood film of acute cold antibody-induced haemolytic anaemia is more likely to cause confusion but, in comparison with warm AIHA, red cell agglutinates are more prominent and spherocytes are not so numerous.

Paroxysmal cold haemoglobinuria and drug-induced immune haemolytic anaemias (see below) can sometimes cause confusion since some spherocytes are present, but consideration of the history should suggest the correct diagnosis.

Further tests
A positive direct antiglobulin test (Coombs' test) is critical in distinguishing AIHA from hereditary spherocytosis. There may also be free autoantibody in the plasma, detected by an indirect antiglobulin test. The direct antiglobulin test is positive in 99% of cases; a negative result in a patient with AIHA may be the result of the autoantibody being IgA or IgM or because an IgG autoantibody has low affinity [237]. Some patients have, in addition, other autoantibodies such as anti-DNA antibodies or antinuclear factor. An osmotic fragility test is positive in both hereditary spherocytosis and AIHA, so is not of use in distinguishing between these two conditions. EMA binding, however, is normal in AIHA, which aids the distinction from hereditary spherocytosis. In children, Evans syndrome may be the initial presentation of the autoimmune lymphoproliferative syndrome; immunophenotyping to detect CD4-negative CD8-negative cells has therefore been advised [238].

Cold antibody-induced haemolytic anaemia
Haemolysis may be induced by autoantibodies that have maximal activity at low temperatures. Cold antibodies are often IgM antibodies that can cause both red cell agglutination and complement-mediated haemolysis. Clinical features may be mainly due to

haemolysis or mainly due to red cell agglutination in small peripheral vessels following exposure to cold. Cold antibody production may be an acute phenomenon when polyclonal antibodies are produced following infections such as infectious mononucleosis, *Mycoplasma pneumoniae* infection, rubella, varicella, cytomegalovirus (CMV) infection, human immunodeficiency virus (HIV) infection, Legionnaires' disease [239] or brucellosis [240]. In these cases acute haemolysis is the dominant clinical feature. Cold antibody production can also be chronic, when a clone of neoplastic lymphocytes produces a monoclonal cold agglutinin, the syndrome being known as chronic cold haemagglutinin disease. The dominant clinical features are those of peripheral cyanosis (acrocyanosis) and ischaemia following cold exposure, but there may also be haemolysis and features, such as lymphadenopathy, suggestive of a lymphoproliferative disease.

Cold antibodies produced following infections such as measles and other viral infections can also cause a distinct clinical syndrome known as paroxysmal cold haemoglobinuria (see below).

Blood film and count
In acute cold antibody-induced haemolytic anaemia the peripheral blood film (Fig. 8.66) shows red cell agglutinates, variable numbers of spherocytes and, subsequently, polychromasia and the presence of polychromatic macrocytes. Erythrophagocytosis is occasionally present. Variable numbers of atypical lymphocytes are present when haemolysis is caused by infectious mononucleosis and, less often, when it is caused by other infections. In chronic cold agglutinin disease, the dominant peripheral blood feature is red cell agglutination, which may be massive (see Fig. 3.2). Some cases also have lymphocytosis and there may be plasmacytoid lymphocytes. The presence of a cold agglutinin is often first suspected from the automated FBC as the red cell agglutinates cause a factitious elevation in the MCV, MCH and MCHC with impedance counters such as Coulter instruments and, to a lesser extent, with light-scattering instruments such as the Siemens H.I and Advia series. Histograms and cytograms may show two populations of red cells, the apparent macrocytes being red cell agglutinates. The presence of a cold agglutinin is easily verified by warming the blood specimen and repeating the FBC.

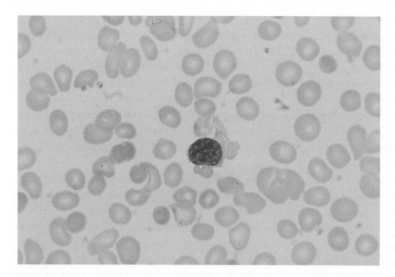

Fig. 8.66 The blood film of a patient with acute haemolytic anaemia caused by anti-i autoantibodies occurring as a complication of infectious mononucleosis. There are several spherocytes, a single small agglutinate and an atypical lymphocyte.

Differential diagnosis

The differential diagnosis includes other causes of acute haemolysis, spherocytosis and red cell agglutination. The blood film in acute paroxysmal cold haemoglobinuria can be confused with that of other types of acute cold antibody-induced haemolytic anaemia.

Further tests

Confirmation that haemolysis or ischaemia is caused by a cold haemagglutinin is by a direct antiglobulin test, which is positive for complement but not IgG, and by the detection of a cold agglutinin. This is usually IgM. It most often has anti-I specificity and less often anti-i or other specificity. In mycoplasma infections, anti-I specificity is usual and in infectious mononucleosis anti-i. Cold agglutinins are not uncommon in healthy subjects, but in patients with relevant clinical features they are present at a high titre and/or have a wide thermal amplitude.

Paroxysmal cold haemoglobinuria

The term 'paroxysmal cold haemoglobinuria' (PCH) covers two distinct syndromes, both of which are caused by a biphasic antibody referred to as a Donath–Landsteiner antibody. A biphasic antibody is one that is bound to red cells at low temperature but causes potent complement activation on warming to 37°C. The antibody is usually IgG with anti-P specificity. In chronic PCH, there is episodic haemolysis, hence the designation 'paroxysmal'. In acute transient PCH,

there is a single episode of haemolysis; the term 'paroxysmal cold haemoglobinuria' is therefore inappropriate but no more suitable alternative has been suggested. Chronic PCH is very rare and may be idiopathic or secondary to syphilis or other infections. Rarely it is consequent on non-Hodgkin lymphoma, the autoantibody being secreted by the lymphoma cells [241]. Acute transient PCH usually follows a non-specific febrile illness but can also follow specific infections, either bacterial or viral (e.g. measles, mumps, chicken pox, CMV infection, infectious mononucleosis, *Mycoplasma pneumoniae* infection, *Haemophilus influenzae* infection or *Klebsiella pneumoniae* infection) [239]. Haemolysis in PCH is intravascular so that haemoglobinuria is a feature.

Blood film and count

In acute transient PCH the Hb, RBC and Hct are reduced, often severely. The reticulocyte count is usually increased but some patients have reticulocytopenia [239]. There are small red cell agglutinates and spherocytes (Fig. 8.67). Erythrophagocytosis by neutrophils (Fig. 8.68) is often prominent and large round vacuoles in neutrophils are also seen [242]. Red cell rosetting around neutrophils can occcur [243]. In chronic PCH there are no specific blood film features. Associated features sometimes present in PCH include leucopenia, neutropenia, leucocytosis, neutrophilia, left shift, eosinopenia, monocytopenia and a lesser degree of lymphopenia [239,244]. The platelet count is normal or increased.

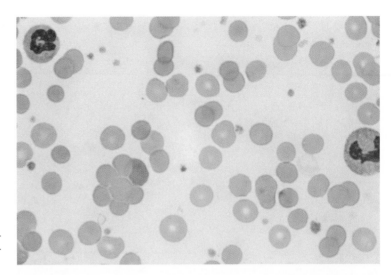

Fig. 8.67 The blood film in acute paroxysmal cold haemoglobinuria showing spherocytosis and red cell agglutination.

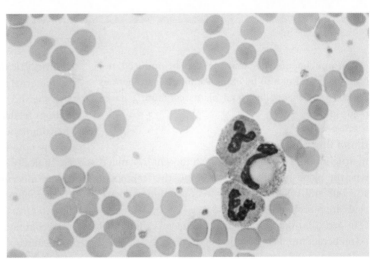

Fig. 8.68 The blood film in acute paroxysmal cold haemoglobinuria showing erythrophagocytosis (same case as Fig. 8.66).

Further tests

The diagnosis of PCH is confirmed by demonstration of the Donath–Landsteiner antibody, usually anti-P, which causes biphasic haemolysis, i.e. haemolysis on rewarming a previously chilled blood sample.

Combined cold and warm autoimmune haemolytic anaemia

Uncommonly a patient meets the serological criteria for warm autoimmune haemolytic anaemia and also has a high thermal amplitude cold agglutinin [239]. Haemolysis is usually severe but responsive to corticosteroids. Chronicity is common. There is an association with SLE and with lymphoma [245].

Immune haemolytic anaemia induced by drugs and other exogenous antigens

Drugs are now a rare but still important cause of haemolytic anaemia. Antibodies are produced that damage red cells only in the presence of the drug. Haemolysis is acute and severe when the red cell is an 'innocent bystander', damaged by drug–antibody complexes. The most common cause of immune complex-mediated drug-induced haemolytic anaemia is now third-generation cephalosporins, particularly cefotetan and ceftriaxone [246]. When the antibody is directed at a drug bound to the red cell membrane ('hapten mechanism'), as in penicillin-induced haemolysis, haemolysis is usually less acute and less severe.

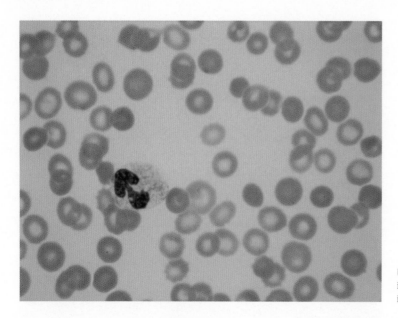

Fig. 8.69 The blood film in cephalosporin-induced immune haemolytic anaemia showing a moderate number of spherocytes.

Immune haemolytic anaemia can be induced not only by drugs but also by exposure to other exogenous antigens such as pollens and plants containing flavonoids [247].

Blood film and count
In drug-induced haemolysis of the 'innocent bystander' type the blood film usually shows only the features of anaemia and spherocytes are rare. Sometimes spherocytes are more numerous (Fig. 8.69).

In penicillin-induced haemolytic anaemia there may be moderate numbers of spherocytes.

Differential diagnosis
The differential diagnosis includes other causes of acute haemolysis and other causes of spherocytosis.

Further tests
Suspected drug-induced haemolysis can be confirmed serologically. With penicillin-induced haemolysis the direct antiglobulin test is positive in the absence of the drug and the patient's serum immunoglobulins bind to penicillin-coated cells. When there is haemolysis with an innocent-bystander mechanism, the antiglobulin test is usually positive as complement is bound to the red cells. Serological tests using normal red cells, the patient's serum and the causative drug are positive.

Haemolytic disease of the fetus and newborn
IgG maternal alloantibodies cross the placenta and those with specificity for antigens on fetal red cells can cause hydrops fetalis and haemolytic disease of the newborn. The commonest form of haemolytic disease of the newborn is now that caused by anti-A or anti-B antibodies; clinically significant ABO haemolytic disease of the newborn occurs in one in 3000 pregnancies in the UK. Rh haemolytic disease of the fetus and newborn, caused by anti-D or other Rh antibodies, is now the second most common cause. Occasionally, haemolytic disease of the newborn is caused by antibodies of other systems such as Kell.

Blood film and count
Anaemia varies from mild to severe. The blood film in ABO haemolytic disease of the newborn shows prominent spherocytosis (Fig. 8.70), whereas in Rh haemolytic disease of the newborn the degree of spherocytosis is usually much less (Fig. 8.71). There is polychromasia and the number of NRBC is increased. Erythrophagocytosis by monocytes had been observed in Rh haemolytic disease [248]. There may be associated neutropenia, lymphopenia, monocytopenia and thrombocytopenia [249,250]. The reticulocyte count is generally elevated.

In Kell haemolytic disease of the newborn, the evidence of a bone marrow response to haemolysis (reticulocytosis and circulating NRBC) is not

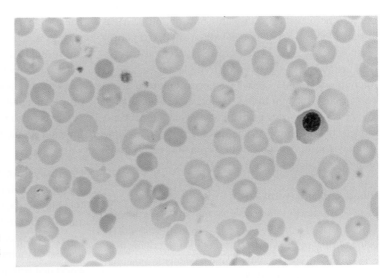

Fig. 8.70 The blood film of a baby with ABO haemolytic disease of the newborn showing marked spherocytosis and an NRBC.

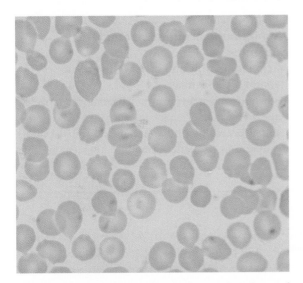

Fig. 8.71 The blood film of a baby with Rh haemolytic disease of the newborn showing that the degree of spherocytosis is much less than that which is seen in ABO haemolytic disease of the newborn (see Fig. 8.69).

increased appropriately to the degree of anaemia as there is also an element of bone marrow suppression [251], attributable to suppression of proliferation of erythroid progenitors by antibodies to Kell group antigens [252]. Marked thrombocytopenia is also a particular feature of Kell haemolytic disease of the newborn and is attributable to inhibition of proliferation of megakaryocyte progenitors by antibodies to Kell group antigens [252].

Differential diagnosis

The main differential diagnosis is hereditary spherocytosis.

Further tests

The diagnosis is confirmed by a positive direct antiglobulin test in the baby and detection of an IgG antibody in maternal serum with specificity against a fetal red cell antigen. In the case of ABO haemolytic disease of the newborn, a high titre IgG antibody will be demonstrated.

Other alloimmune haemolytic anaemias

Beyond the neonatal period, alloimmune haemolytic anaemia is uncommon. Delayed transfusion reactions following transfusion of incompatible red cells are alloimmune in nature, as is immune haemolysis following transfusion of incompatible plasma, cryoprecipitate, high-dose intravenous immunoglobulin or other blood products containing immunoglobulin, such as some factor VIII or IX concentrates. Alloimmune haemolysis can result from administration of anti-D in the treatment of autoimmune thrombocytopenic purpura [253]; uncommonly there may be acute haemoglobinaemia and haemoglobinuria with a sudden marked fall in the Hb. Transient alloimmune haemolysis can follow transplantation of ABO-incompatible bone marrow, e.g. A or B marrow transplanted into an O recipient as a result of preformed anti-A or anti-B antibodies. If peripheral blood is used as a source of stem cells, severe haemolysis can also occur with a transplant showing minor ABO incompatibility (e.g. O donor with A or B recipient), presumably because of the greater content of donor lymphocytes with this type of transplantation [254]. Alloimmune haemolysis can even occur following solid organ transplantation from O donors as a result of passenger B lymphocytes in the graft. Mixed chimaerism can lead to alloimmune haemolysis following transplantation when surviving recipient B lymphocytes produce antibodies against donor-derived erythrocytes.

Blood film and count

In delayed transfusion reactions, only a proportion of red cells are spherocytic, the patient's own cells either being normal or showing features of the underlying disease. In other types of alloimmune haemolytic anaemia spherocytosis is generalised.

Differential diagnosis

The differential diagnosis includes other causes of spherocytosis with a positive direct antiglobulin test, particularly autoimmune and immune drug-induced haemolytic anaemia.

Further tests

The direct antiglobulin test is positive, as are tests indicative of intravascular haemolysis; there may be

haemoglobinaemia and haemoglobinuria (when haemolysis is acute and severe), a positive Schumm's test, low serum haptoglobin and presence of urinary haemosiderin. Otherwise the clinical history is of more importance than laboratory tests in elucidating the nature of the anaemia. Alloimmune haemolysis is sometimes severe enough to precipitate renal failure, so that renal function should be monitored.

Haemolysis in familial autoimmune/lymphoproliferative syndrome

Haemolysis with either a positive or negative direct antiglobulin test, a poor reticulocyte response and associated dyserythropoiesis has been reported in the familial autoimmune/lymphoproliferative syndrome associated with mutations in the *FAS* gene and impaired Fas-mediated apoptosis [255].

Non-immune acquired haemolytic anaemias
Microangiopathic and other schistocytic haemolytic anaemias

The term microangiopathic haemolytic anaemia refers to haemolytic anaemia caused by red cell fragmentation resulting from endothelial damage, fibrin deposition in capillaries or both. Causes are multiple

Table 8.8 Some causes of red cell fragmentation.

Microangiopathic haemolytic anaemia
Congenital, inherited and familial

Familial thrombotic thrombocytopenic purpura resulting from deficiency of von Willebrand factor-cleaving protease (ADAMTS13) [256,257]; familial haemolytic–uraemic syndrome (some caused by autosomal recessively inherited deficiency of complement factor H [258] or of other complement-regulatory proteins such as membrane cofactor protein and factor I [259]); haem oxygenase 1 deficiency [260]; associated with congenital cobalamin C defect [261]

Epidemic or sporadic haemolytic–uraemic syndrome, thrombotic thrombocytopenic purpura and related thrombotic microangiopathies
Following infection by Shigella, verotoxin-producing *E.coli*, *Campylobacter jejuni*, *Legionella pneumophila* [262], *Rickettsia rickettsii* [263], *Borrelia burgdorferi* [264], *Streptococcus pneumoniae* [265], *Aeromonas hydrophilia* [266], *Campylobacter upsaliensis* [266], *Campylobacter canimorsus* [266], *Mycoplasma pneumoniae*, *Staphylococcus epidermidis* (bacterial endocarditis with vegetations) [267], brucellosis [268], leptospirosis [269], viruses (including HIV, HTLV-1, CMV, varicella zoster, adenovirus and possibly human herpesvirus 6 [270]), fungi [271–275] or following vaccination (influenza, polio, measles, smallpox, triple antigen or typhoid-paratyphoid) [276]

Associated with pregnancy (including HELLP syndrome), oral contraceptive intake or the postpartum state
Drug toxicity [277] including due to quinine [278], mitomycin C, bleomycin, pentostatin [279], daunorubicin [280], gemcitabine [281], methyl-CCNU [282], tamoxifen [282], atorvastatin [282], penicillin, rifampicin [280], sulphonamides [280], quinolones [280], aciclovir [280], valaciclovir [280], penicillamine [272], ciclosporin, tacrolimus [283], sirolimus [282], simvastatin [284], ticlopidine [285], clopidogrel [280,286], risperidone [280], OKT3 [287], interferon β [266], interferon α therapy in CML [288], heroin [266], traditional African medicine ('Pitocine') [289], quinine hypersensitivity [290], arsenic [282], iodine [282], 'crack' cocaine [282], anti-CD22 recombinant immunotoxin [291], treatment of acute promyelocytic leukaemia with all-*trans* retinoic acid [292], bevacizumab [293], abuse of oxymorphone slow-release tablets by intravenous injection [294]

Other pathological processes involving small vessels in the kidney (with or without extra-renal vascular lesions)
  Pregnancy-associated hypertension
  Malignant hypertension
  Renal cortical necrosis
  Microscopic polyarteritis nodosa
  Acute glomerulonephritis
  Renal involvement by systemic lupus erythematosus (may precede other manifestations of the disease) [295]
  Renal involvement by systemic sclerosis (scleroderma) [296]
  Granulomatosis with polyangiitis (Wegener's granulomatosis)
  Renal irradiation
  Rejection of transplanted kidney
  POEMS syndrome [281]
  Anti-phospholipid antibody syndrome [281]
  Dysfibrinogenaemia and other prothrombotic states [281]
Diabetic angiopathy [297]
Following haemopoietic stem cell transplantation
Associated with pancreatitis [298]
Light chain deposition disease (one case) [299]
Secondary oxalosis (one case) [300]
Systemic amyloidosis
Disseminated intravascular coagulation (including that associated with malignant disease, aortic aneurysm, renal vein thrombosis and snake bite)
Therapeutic defibrination (occasionally)
Atrial myxoma [301]
Disseminated carcinoma (particularly mucin-secreting carcinoma, particularly carcinoma of the stomach)
Following arteriography [302]
Reaction to bee sting [272]
Bone marrow transplantation
Thymoma-associated (1 case) [303]

Associated with vascular malformations and other large vessel and valvular lesions
Haemangioma
Haemangioendothelioma of the liver or spleen
Haemangioendotheliosarcoma
Plexiform pulmonary lesions of pulmonary hypertension
Plexiform pulmonary lesions of cirrhosis [304]
Giant cell arteritis [305]
Umbilical vein varix (in a fetus) [306]
Prosthetic valves (aortic more than mitral, much more common when there is regurgitation around a valve)
Homograft, xenograft (porcine) and fascia lata autograft valves (less likely than with prosthetic valves)
Acute rheumatic valvulitis [307]
Prosthetic patches, e.g. for ventricular septal defect
Endoluminal closure of patent ductus arteriosus [308]
Severe aortic stenosis (very uncommon)
Severe mitral valve disease and following valvuloplasty for mitral valve disease (rare)
Cardiac myxoma
Aortic coarctation (rare)
Use of subclavian dialysis catheters [309]

Associated with extracorporeal circulation (associated with thrombosis in the apparatus) [309] **and long-term extracorporeal membrane oxygenation in neonates** [310]

Drug-induced thrombotic microangiopathy may be either idiosyncratic (e.g. with quinine and ticlopidine) or dose-related (as with cytotoxic chemotherapeutic agents) [277]

CML, chronic myelogenous leukaemia; CMV, cytomegalovirus; HELLP, **H**aemolysis, **E**levated **L**iver enzymes and **L**ow **P**latelet syndrome; HIV, human immunodeficiency virus; HTLV-1, human T-cell lymphotropic virus type 1; POEMS, **P**olyneuropathy, **O**rganomegaly, **E**ndocrinopathy, **M** protein, **S**kin changes syndrome.

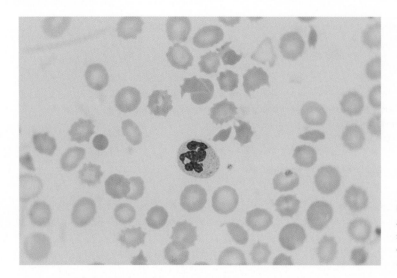

Fig. 8.72 The blood film of an adult patient at presentation with haemolytic–uraemic syndrome, showing both fragments and echinocytes. By courtesy of Dr Ayed Eden, Southend-on-Sea.

(Table 8.8). In childhood the commonest cause is enteric infection, most often by a verocytotoxin-secreting *Escherichia coli* (serotype O157:H7), resulting in haemolytic–uraemic syndrome. In adults the commonest causes are probably idiopathic TTP, pregnancy-associated hypertension and carcinoma. An outbreak of adult cases of haemolytic–uraemic syndrome in 2011, centred on Germany, was due to *E. coli* serotype O104:H4; women were particularly affected [311]. Schistocytic haemolytic anaemia can also occur with large vessel or valvular lesions and with prosthetic cardiac valves. In some of these instances there is thrombosis on an abnormal surface and in others there is red cell damage resulting from turbulent flow or from mechanical damage to red cells by components of a malfunctioning prosthetic valve.

Blood film and count

The blood film shows microspherocytes, keratocytes and schistocytes and often polychromasia and polychromatic macrocytes. When there is associated platelet consumption, thrombocytopenia and large platelets are apparent. In the post-diarrhoeal haemolytic–uraemic syndrome of childhood there is often leucocytosis and neutrophilia, the severity of which correlates with associated renal damage; the degree of elevation of the WBC and the duration of leucocytosis are both of prognostic significance [312]. Prolonged thrombocytopenia is associated with long-term renal sequelae [266]. Occasionally there is also marked echinocytosis (Figs 8.72 & 8.73). In microangiopathic haemolytic anaemia there is often associated thrombocytopenia, but otherwise the blood films of microangiopathic haemolytic anaemia (Figs 8.74 & 8.75) and of haemolytic anaemia caused by large vessel or valvular diseases or prostheses (Fig. 8.76) cannot be readily distinguished. Haemolysis in the microangiopathic and mechanical haemolytic anaemias is intravascular and when it is severe and chronic the resultant haemoglobinuria can lead to complicating

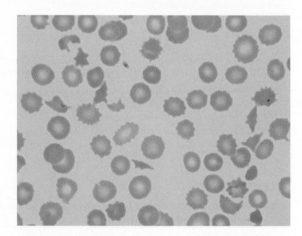

Fig. 8.73 The blood film of a hyposplenic adult patient with the haemolytic–uraemic syndrome induced by gemcitabine showing schistocytes, crenation (attributable to acute kidney injury), a cell containing a Howell–Jolly body and thrombocytopenia. Some of the schistocytes are crenated.

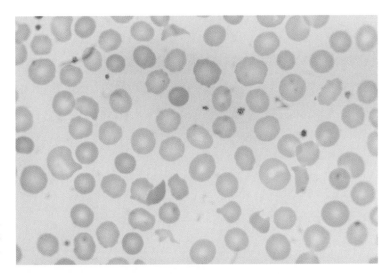

Fig. 8.74 The blood film of an adult with the haemolytic–uraemic syndrome showing fragments, several spherocytes and several polychromatic macrocytes.

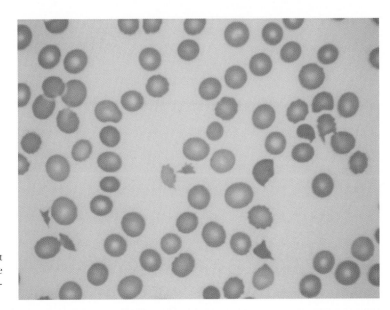

Fig. 8.75 The blood film of an adult patient with the haemolytic–uraemic syndrome induced by peginterferon showing schistocytes and thrombocytopenia.

iron deficiency, the features of which are then apparent on the blood film (Fig. 8.77).

It should be noted that, although red cell fragmentation is often a feature of chronic disseminated intravascular coagulation (DIC), it is quite uncommon in acute DIC. Examination of a blood film is therefore not often a useful screening test if this diagnosis is suspected [313]. Conversely, blood film examination is very important if TTP or the HELLP (**h**aemolysis, **e**levated **l**iver enzymes and **l**ow **p**latelet count) syndrome

is suspected. It should, however, be noted that in TTP, schistocytes are sometimes lacking in the first few days after presentation [314].

The International Council for Standardization in Haematology (ICSH) has recommended that, for the purposes of counting schistocytes in suspected microangiopathic haemolytic anaemia, the following forms should be included: fragments with sharp angles and straight borders, small crescents, helmet cells, keratocytes and microspherocytes (if other

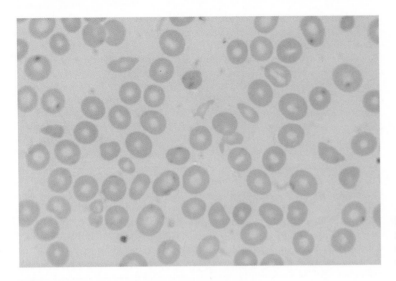

Fig. 8.76 The blood film of a patient with mechanical haemolytic anaemia, due to a defective prosthetic mitral valve, showing numerous fragments.

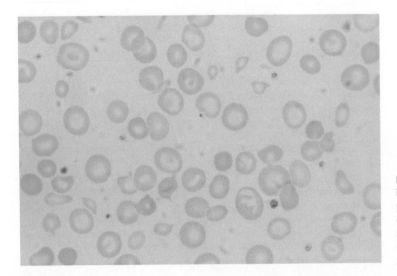

Fig. 8.77 The blood film of an Afro-Caribbean patient with iron deficiency as a complication of mechanical haemolysis from a defective prosthetic valve. The film shows fragments, hypochromia, microcytosis and one target cell. The patient also had haemoglobin C trait.

typical forms are also present) [315]. The presence of more than 1% of schistocytes defined in this manner, 1000 cells having been counted, is diagnostically significant if fragmentation is the dominant abnormality present [315]. A higher threshold of 4% has been used for the diagnosis of post-transplant microangiopathy [315].

The FBC shows a reduced Hb, increased RDW, sometimes an increased MCV and HDW (consequent on reticulocytosis) and sometimes a low platelet count with an increased MPV. There may be 'flagging' indicating the presence of both microcytes and macrocytes. If there are large numbers of schistocytes there may be 'flagging' indicating poor separation of red cells and platelets and the possibility of factitious elevation of the platelet count. Some instruments (Siemens Advia and Sysmex XE-2100) are able to specifically flag and enumerate schistocytes, a normal value having a high negative predictive value for schistocytes in the blood film (but with some false negatives in specimens with an MCV above 105 fl) [316]. Red cell histograms and cytograms (Figs 8.78 & 8.79) may show hyperchromic cells, normochromic and hyperchromic microcytes and hypochromic macrocytes.

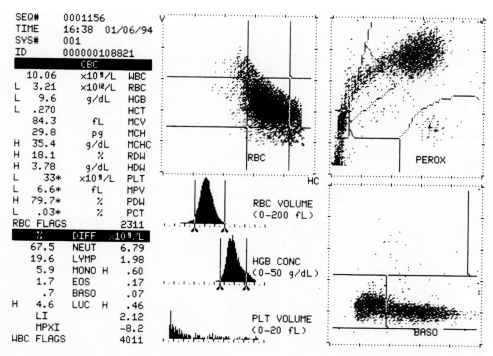

Fig. 8.78 Bayer H.2 red cell and platelet histograms and cytograms from a patient with microangiopathic haemolytic anaemia. There are many hyperchromatic cells (spherocytes and microspherocytes) and normochromic microcytic cells (other fragments). The platelet histogram illustrates that in this patient the platelet count was very low.

Differential diagnosis

The blood film of schistocytic haemolytic anaemias is distinctive and usually there is no diagnostic difficulty. However, it should be noted that the blood film of severe megaloblastic anaemia may have prominent schistocytes and has been confused with microangiopathic haemolytic anaemia.

Further tests

The speedy recognition of haemolytic–uraemic syndrome by the laboratory is of critical importance for optimal management. In addition to appropriate management of the renal failure, early stool culture is indicated and therapy that may aggravate the condition, e.g. antibiotics and agents to reduce gut motility, should be avoided [266]. Death associated with delay in diagnosis has been reported when a blood film was not examined [317]. Speedy diagnosis of TTP is likewise critical, since plasmapheresis should be instituted promptly, but it must be remembered that initial absence of fragments does not exclude the diagnosis. Patients presenting with the clinicopathological features of TTP should be tested for HIV.

Bilirubin and LDH estimations and a reticulocyte count are useful in assessing the severity of the haemolysis. In cases with chronic mild haemolysis and few fragments, the detection of haemosiderin in urinary sediment is useful in demonstrating that intravascular haemolysis has occurred.

Oxidant-induced haemolytic anaemia

Exposure to sufficiently potent oxidants, either drugs or chemicals, can cause haemolytic anaemia even in individuals in whom G6PD and other enzymes of the pentose shunt are normal. Neonates, especially premature neonates, are particularly susceptible to oxidant-induced haemolysis. Oxidants can cause both acquired methaemoglobinaemia, resulting from oxidation of haemoglobin, and acute or chronic haemolytic anaemia, resulting from oxidation of both haemoglobin and membrane components. When haemolysis is acute, oxidised haemoglobin precipitates as Heinz bodies, hence the name 'Heinz-body haemolytic anaemia'. Heinz bodies are cleared by the spleen, but when haemolysis is acute they may be detected in circulating red cells.

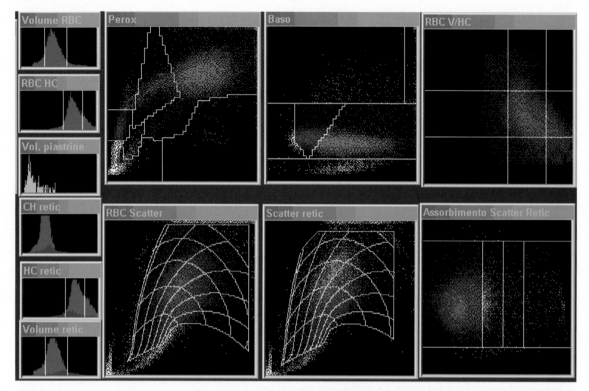

Fig. 8.79 Siemens Advia series cytogram and histograms from a patient with thrombotic thrombocytopenic purpura. The FBC was: WBC 19.17×10^9/l, RBC 1.45×10^{12}/l, Hb 42 g/l, Hct 0.12 l/l, MCH 28.9 pg, MCHC 344 g/l, CHCM 361 g/l, RDW 25.6%, platelets 17×10^9/l, reticulocyte count 7.9%, 114×10^9/l. The red cell cytogram and haemoglobin concentration histogram (RBC HC) show an increase in cells with an increased haemoglobin concentration (to the right of the right-hand vertical threshold) and there was a +++ hyperchromia flag. There was also a flag indicating the presence of NRBC. Red cell fragments were 2.75%. By courtesy of Professor Gina Zini.

Oxidant-induced haemolysis is most often caused by drugs, particularly dapsone and sulfasalazine. It can also result from nitrate contamination of drinking water or from accidental or deliberate exposure to agricultural and industrial chemicals. Copper sulphate, taken with suicidal intent, is a common cause in some countries.

It should be noted that if patients have methaemoglobinaemia as well as oxidant-induced haemolysis, their symptoms are often more severe than would be expected from the degree of anaemia. This is because methaemoglobin does not function in oxygen transport and, in addition, causes a left shift of the oxygen dissociation curve, further reducing the capacity of haemoglobin to deliver oxygen to tissues.

Blood film and count

When the haemolysis is acute the blood film (Fig. 8.80) is similar to that of G6PD deficiency during acute haemolytic episodes. Heinz bodies may produce a visible

protrusion of the surface of the red cell, the reason for this being apparent from electron microscopy [318]. Heinz bodies do not merely bind to the red cell membrane but protrude through it (Fig. 8.81). When haemolysis is milder and more chronic, there are variable numbers of irregularly contracted cells and sometimes also macrocytosis with polychromatic macrocytes.

Differential diagnosis

The differential diagnosis includes G6PD deficiency, unstable haemoglobins and other causes of irregularly contracted cells (see Chapter 3).

Further tests

The diagnosis can usually be made from the clinical history and the blood film. A Heinz body preparation is positive in acute cases. In some patients it may be necessary to confirm that the G6PD activity is normal after the episode of haemolysis has passed.

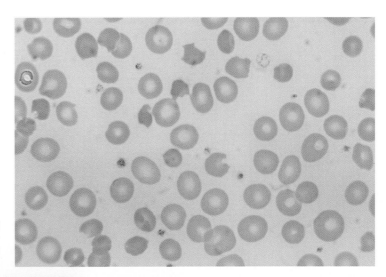

Fig. 8.80 The blood film of a patient taking dapsone for a skin condition showing macrocytosis, irregularly contracted cells and several bite cells.

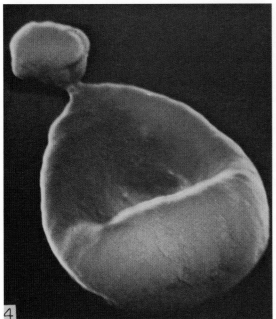

Fig. 8.81 Scanning electron micrograph of an erythrocyte with a projecting Heinz body. By courtesy of Dr M. Amare and colleagues, Kansas City.

Neonatal glutathione peroxidase deficiency

Glutathione peroxidase deficiency can occur transiently in the neonatal period as a result of deficiency of selenium, an essential cofactor.

Blood film and count

The blood film shows irregularly contracted cells and other features similar to those of oxidant damage.

Renal disease

Red cell survival is usually reduced in acute renal failure. The features of a microangiopathic haemolytic anaemia are commonly present. Reduced red cell survival is one of the mechanisms, although not the principal one, in anaemia of chronic renal failure. Small numbers of keratocytes and other fragments may be present. Occasionally there are echinocytes. In chronic renal failure the oxygen dissociation curve is often right shifted, improving oxygen delivery to tissues and reducing the erythropoietic drive [319].

Liver disease

Liver disease is associated with several haemolytic syndromes. In Zieve syndrome there is acute alcoholic liver disease associated with hyperlipidaemia and acute haemolysis. Zieve [320] and others [321] have described the abnormal cells as 'spherocytes' and in one case Zieve suspected an inherited haemolytic anaemia. However, illustrations have shown irregularly contracted cells [321] and these are sometimes prominent (Fig. 8.82). A distinct syndrome initially called 'spur cell haemolytic anaemia', which is characterised by numerous acanthocytes (Fig. 8.83), is caused by liver failure of any aetiology.

Wilson disease

Wilson disease can cause both acute haemolytic anaemia with no morphological abnormality and an acute Heinz-body haemolytic anaemia consequent on sudden release of copper from a gravely damaged liver [322] (Fig. 8.84). It is important to think of previously undiagnosed Wilson disease when an acute haemolytic

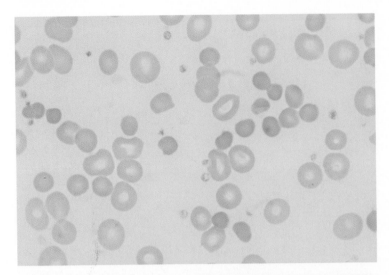

Fig. 8.82 The blood film of a patient with Zieve syndrome as a complication of acute alcoholic liver disease showing irregularly contracted cells and polychromatic macrocytes.

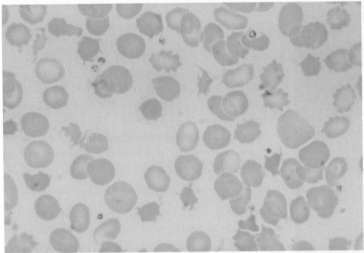

Fig. 8.83 The blood film of a patient with terminal liver disease of unknown aetiology showing numerous acanthocytes ('spur cell' haemolytic anaemia).

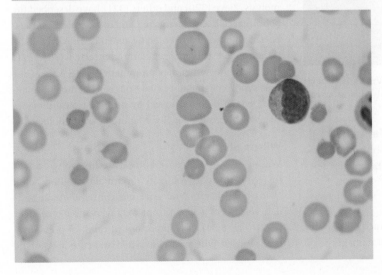

Fig. 8.84 The blood film in a patient with terminal liver failure as a complication of Wilson disease showing irregularly contracted cells and polychromatic macrocytes.

anaemia is unexplained, since this may be the presenting feature of a condition that is fatal if left untreated.

Diabetes mellitus

Compensated haemolysis without anaemia or morphological abnormalities appears to be common in diabetes mellitus [323].

Vitamin E deficiency and infantile pyknocytosis

Vitamin E deficiency can cause haemolysis, particularly in neonates and particularly when iron-supplemented milk is used for feeding. This may be the initial presentation of cystic fibrosis [324]. The blood film shows 'pyknocytes' – irregularly contracted spiculated cells, resembling acanthocytes. Other cases of infantile pyknocytosis may be the result of oxidant stress without vitamin E deficiency [325]. Plots of cell density, e.g. on Siemens automated instruments, show two populations representing normal and abnormal cells, whereas reticulocytes have a normal density distribution [325].

Phosphate depletion

Phosphate depletion, leading to reduced ATP, is a rare cause of haemolytic anaemia. This is the likely mechanism of haemolytic anaemia reported in association with hypophosphataemia during refeeding of a patient with anorexia nervosa [326].

Bacterial and parasitic infections

Bartonellosis, malaria and babesiosis characteristically cause haemolytic anaemia. Rarely this is also seen in patients with Whipple disease who have been splenectomised. Bacterial and viral infections can be associated with microangiopathic haemolytic anaemia. Clostridial toxins can cause a severe spherocytic haemolytic anaemia. *Bacillus cereus* infection, mainly in immunodeficient patients, can cause hyperacute haemolysis with red cell ghosts and, probably, spherocytes. Bacterial infections can also alter red cell membrane antigens to cause T activation. Anti-T antibodies in the plasma can then bind to red cells causing spherocytosis and haemolysis. This has been observed with infection by *Staphylococcus aureus*, *Escherichia coli* and pneumococcus and in necrotising enteritis caused by *Clostridium perfringens*. Acute haemolysis can follow transfusion of normal blood, which contains anti-T antibodies, and this type of haemolysis can therefore be confused with other types of haemolytic transfusion reaction [327].

Snake and insect bites

Bites of a number of snakes (Fig. 8.85) and insects can cause an acute spherocytic or microangiopathic haemolytic anaemia, sometimes with associated DIC and thrombocytopenia [328].

March haemoglobinuria

March haemoglobinuria describes haemolytic anaemia observed in soldiers on forced marches. Although haemolysis is mechanical, resulting from damage of red cells in blood vessels in the feet, it is rare for any fragments or other specific features to be observed. A similar type of haemolysis can be induced by jogging on hard surfaces,

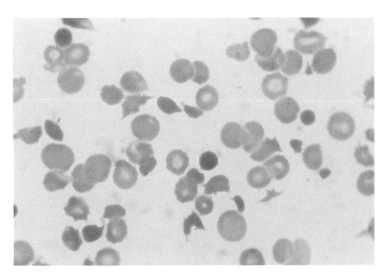

Fig. 8.85 The blood film of a Sri Lankan patient who had suffered a viper bite showing fragments and microspherocytes. By courtesy of Dr Sudharma Vidyatilake, Colombo.

tennis playing, karate, drumming with the hands and even swimming. These conditions should be sought by specific questioning whenever there is mild unexplained anaemia in an apparently fit, usually young, person. (There may be factors other than haemolysis operating in some cases of exercise-induced anaemia, e.g. exercise-induced gastrointestinal haemorrhage.)

Haemolysis caused by infusion of hypotonic fluid

Acute intravascular haemolysis with no morphological abnormality can be caused by inadvertent intravenous infusion of hypotonic fluid.

Paroxysmal nocturnal haemoglobinuria

Paroxysmal nocturnal haemoglobinuria (PNH) is a clonal haemopoietic stem cell disorder in which red cells with a specific membrane defect are abnormally sensitive to complement-induced lysis. This results from an acquired somatic mutation in the phosphatidylinositol-glycan complementation class A (*PIGA*) gene that leads to a deficiency of glycosylphosphatidylinositol (GPI) and therefore of the numerous membrane proteins that are anchored to GPI [329]. A tendency to bone marrow hypoplasia or aplasia must also be present so that the PNH clone is favoured. Some but not all patients give a history of nocturnal haemolysis, i.e. of the first urine specimen passed in the morning being red. A diagnosis of PNH should be considered when there is an unexplained haemolytic anaemia, particularly if associated with leucopenia or thrombocytopenia. Acute myeloid

leukaemia (AML) and MDS may develop during the course of PNH.

It should be noted that very rarely the phenotype of PNH results from an inherited deficiency of CD59 (membrane inhibitor of reactive lysis, MIRL) [330].

Blood film and count

There are no specific blood film features. Polychromatic macrocytes may be present (Fig. 8.86) {previously 8.73}. Eighty percent of patients have neutropenia or thrombocytopenia [329].

Differential diagnosis

The differential diagnosis includes other causes of normocytic anaemia and pancytopenia.

Further tests

The diagnosis can be confirmed by flow cytometry using monoclonal antibodies directed at GPI-anchored antigens such as CD55 and CD59 on red cells or neutrophils. The absence of such antigens can also be demonstrated by a modification of the gel technology used for blood grouping. If this technology is not available, the diagnosis can also be confirmed by a Ham test showing lysis of red cells following exposure to acidified serum.

Miscellaneous causes of acquired haemolytic anaemia

Haemolytic anaemia with a negative direct and indirect anti-globulin test and with no specific morphological

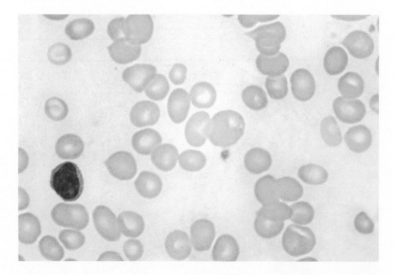

Fig. 8.86 The blood film of a patient with paroxysmal nocturnal haemoglobinuria (PNH) showing polychromatic macrocytes.

features has been described as a transient phenomenon, sometimes accompanied by thrombocytopenia, in patients with hepatitis C infection [331].

Haemolysis as a contributing factor to anaemia

A shortened red cell lifespan can also contribute to anaemia when haemolysis is not the primary mechanism, e.g. in iron deficiency anaemia [19], in protein-calorie malnutrition [332] and in leishmaniasis (possibly immune mediated) [333].

Dyserythropoietic anaemias
Congenital dyserythropoietic anaemias (CDA)

The congenital dyserythropoietic anaemias are inherited disorders characterised by ineffective and dysplastic erythropoiesis, shortened red cell lifespan and anaemia with marked poikilocytosis. There are three well-characterised types, the features of which are summarised in Tables 8.9 and 8.10. There are also cases that appear to conform to these types but have a different inheritance and therefore presumably a different underlying defect. There are autosomal dominant cases resembling type I and apparently autosomal recessive cases resembling type III. In addition there are individual cases or families with distinctive features. These include congenital megaloblastic anaemia independent of vitamin B_{12} or folate deficiency and cases with various red cell inclusions [334]. Variants have been described with microcytosis attributable to sideroblastic erythropoiesis [340] and with prominent ovalocytosis [341]. Two cases have been described with features resembling those

Table 8.9 Inheritance pattern, ethnic distribution and associated features in the congenital dyserythropoietic anaemias [334–338].

Type	Inheritance	Reported cases	Gene	Ethnic origin and associated features
Type I	AR	More than 150	*CDAN1* at 15q15.1–15.3; some cases not linked to chromosome 15	Caucasians (including Germans, Swiss, Yugoslavs, Russians), Turks, Israeli Bedouins, Lebanese, Kuwaitis, Saudi Arabians, North Africans, Indians, Japanese, Polynesians; associated constitutional abnormalities such as facial dysmorphism and abnormalities of distal limbs are common
Type II (HEMPAS)	AR	More than 300	*SEC23B* at 20q11.2 in 90%, unknown in others	Caucasians, particularly Italian, Indian and North African; red cell life span reduced
Type III	AD in 2 families (Swedish and American)	Rare	*KIF23* at 15q23 in Swedish and US families	Swedish, American, Filipino and Argentinean families; Swedish family shows association with retinal abnormalities and plasma cell neoplasia; intravascular haemolysis
Type IV	AD	Rare	*KLF1* at19p13.2	One Danish case

AD, autosomal dominant; AR, autosomal recessive; HEMPAS, hereditary erythroid multinuclearity with positive acidified-serum lysis test

Table 8.10 Peripheral blood features in the congenital dyserythropoietic anaemias [334,335,339].

Type	Red cell size	Other blood film features
Type I	Usually macrocytic	Round and oval macrocytes, marked anisocytosis, marked poikilocytosis including elliptocytes and teardrop poikilocytes, basophilic stippling, irregularly contracted cells, polychromasia
Type II (HEMPAS)	Normocytic	Moderate anisocytosis, variable anisochromasia, moderate poikilocytosis including 'pincer cells' [339], teardrop cells and irregularly contracted cells, occasional spherocytes, basophilic stippling, some NRBC, polychromasia
Type III	Normocytic or slightly macrocytic	Marked anisocytosis with some large macrocytes, marked poikilocytosis including fragments and irregularly contracted cells, basophilic stippling, polychromasia; some patients have superimposed iron deficiency
Type IV	Normocytic normochromic	Basophilic stippling, erythroblastosis, irregular nuclear outline, reticulocyte count may be elevated

HEMPAS, hereditary erythroid multinuclearity with positive acidified-serum lysis test; NRBC, nucleated red blood cells

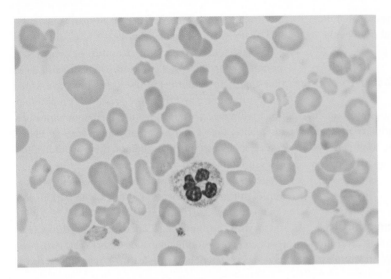

Fig. 8.87 The blood film of a patient with type I congenital dyserythropoietic anaemia showing marked anisocytosis, poikilocytosis and some macrocytes.

of type II CDA but with spherocytosis and a negative acid lysis test [342]. Cases with X-linked inheritance and coexisting thrombocytopenia result from *GATA1* mutation [343,344]. Provisional categorisation of some atypical forms as CDA, types IV to VII, has been proposed when at least three unrelated families have been described [334,336]. It has been suggested that cases of congenital ineffective erythropoiesis without significant erythroid dysplasia should also be included in the category of CDA [334].

The genes implicated in the three major forms of CDA have now been identified. Type I is due to a mutation in *CDAN1*, encoding codanin, type II to a mutation in *SEC23B* and type III to a mutation in *KIF23* [345]. A *KLF1* mutation has been identified in CDA type IV [338]. Some cases, particularly of type I CDA, have other associated congenital abnormalities. Patients typically present with anaemia, hepatomegaly, splenomegaly and intermittent jaundice. Cases of type III are typically milder than cases of types I and II. Coexisting β thalassaemia trait has been observed to aggravate type II. In a patient CDA type IV, the condition was severe enough to cause hydrops fetalis [338].

Since interferon alpha has been found to be of considerable therapeutic benefit in type I CDA, the laboratory diagnosis of these rare conditions is becoming increasingly important. Correct diagnosis may also lead to therapeutic measures to reduce iron overload and consequent organ damage.

Blood film and count

In a minority of cases the anaemia is severe. Usually it is mild or moderate. Some cases have macrocytic red cells and others normocytic. There is usually marked anisocytosis and striking poikilocytosis (Figs 8.87 & 8.88), but in CDA type II the peripheral blood abnormality may be minor (Fig. 8.89). Haemoglobinisation is generally normal, but some cells may be poorly haemoglobinised. The absolute reticulocyte count is normal. Some cases have had circulating NRBC, which become very numerous after splenectomy [346]. Erythroblastosis is striking in CDA associated with *KLF1* mutation [338]. The RDW and HDW are increased, the RDW markedly so, and this is reflected in the red cell cytograms and histograms (Fig. 8.90).

A sudden fall of Hb with a very low reticulocyte count as a result of pure red cell aplasia has been reported following parvovirus B19 infection in patients with CDA type II [347]. In CDA resulting from mutation of the *GATA1* gene there is thrombocytopenia with large platelets. Acanthocytes, which are not often a feature of CDA, have been noted in this syndrome [343,344]. The platelet count is also reduced in some cases of type II CDA.

Differential diagnosis

The differential diagnosis includes haemolytic anaemias with marked morphological abnormalities, particularly hereditary poikilocytosis and haemoglobin H disease. In both these conditions the reticulocyte count is elevated

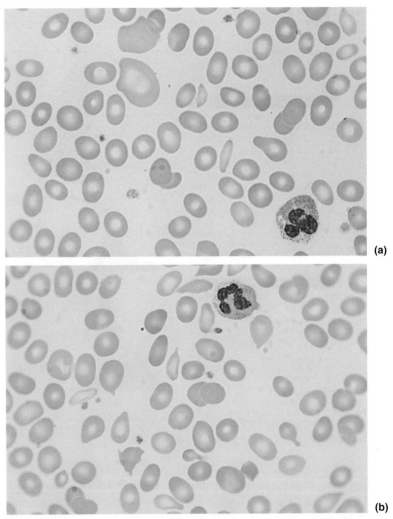

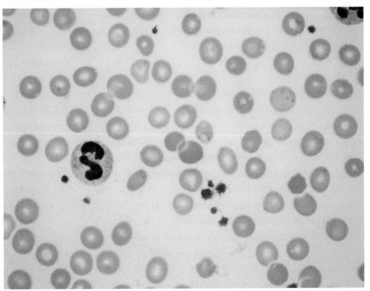

Fig. 8.88 (a,b) The blood film of a patient with type III congenital dyserythropoietic anaemia showing anisocytosis and poikilocytosis. Courtesy of the late Professor Sunitha Nimal Wickramasinghe.

Fig. 8.89 The blood film in type II congenital dyserythropoietic anaemia showing only mild anisocytosis and poikilocytosis.

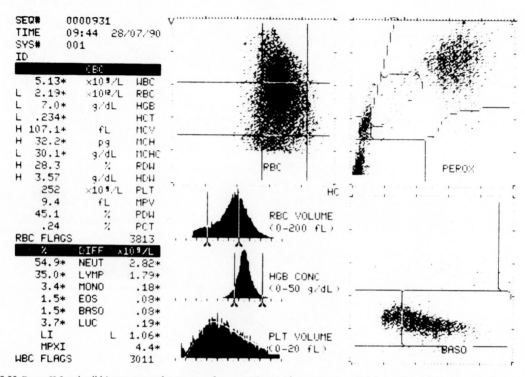

Fig. 8.90 Bayer H.2 red cell histograms and cytograms from a patient with type I congenital dyserythropoietic anaemia (same patient as in Fig. 8.85) showing a marked variation in red cell size (as reflected in the increased RDW) and a lesser degree of variation in red cell haemoglobinisation (as reflected in the increased HDW).

and in haemoglobin H disease there is hypochromia and microcytosis. Cases presenting beyond childhood need to be distinguished from MDS and other conditions causing acquired dyserythropoiesis. Cases of CDA usually lack significant dysplastic features in non-erythroid lineages.

Further tests

A provisional diagnosis can be made from the blood film. Confirmation of the diagnosis requires bone marrow examination with ultrastructural examination being particularly useful. In type I CDA there may be an increased percentage of haemoglobin A_2 and a slight reduction in red cell membrane protein 4.1 [93]. In the case of suspected type II CDA, the demonstration of a positive acid lysis (Ham) test is useful; this may require testing with multiple fresh sera. Type II CDA also shows increased expression of the i antigen and on SDS-polyacrylamide gel electrophoresis red cell membrane band 3, which is hypoglycosylated, shows an abnormal migration

pattern. In type II CDA, EMA binding can be normal or reduced [117,127], osmotic fragility may be increased and the acidified glycerol lysis time is sometimes shortened [127]. Thymidine kinase is increased in type III CDA. CDA due to *KLF1* mutation is associated with markedly increased haemoglobin F, persistence of haemoglobin Portland, absent erythroid expression of CD44 and reduced expression of AQP1 [338].

Bilirubin and LDH concentrations are generally increased and serum haptoglobin is decreased. In more severe cases there may be significant haemosiderinuria.

Acquired dyserythropoietic anaemias

Dyserythropoiesis as an acquired phenomenon can be secondary to severe protein–calorie malnutrition, acute severe illness, autoimmune disease, HIV infection or exposure to drugs (such as cytotoxic drugs) or to toxic substances (such as alcohol or arsenic). It can also be a manifestation of MDS (see Chapter 9) or of other haemopoietic neoplasms. Severe dyserythropoiesis has been observed in peripartum women with pregnancy-associated hypertension and parvovirus B19 infection [348].

Blood film and count

Red cells may show anisocytosis, poikilocytosis, macrocytosis or basophilic stippling and there may be a population of hypochromic microcytes. Neutrophils may show hypogranularity and defects of nuclear lobulation. The FBC may show anaemia, neutropenia or thrombocytopenia. Red cell histograms and cytograms may show an increased MCV, RDW and HDW.

Differential diagnosis

The differential diagnosis includes congenital dyserythropoietic anaemias and other causes of anaemia with or without other cytopenia.

Further tests

Which further tests are indicated is dependent on the clinical setting and the specific cytological abnormalities present.

Aplastic anaemias and pure red cell aplasia
Inherited aplastic anaemia

There are various inherited syndromes in which haemopoietic stem cells are abnormal, leading to the onset of aplastic anaemia during childhood or adolescence. The least uncommon of these is Fanconi anaemia, a genetically diverse group of disorders in which there are often associated constitutional abnormalities; these may include mental retardation, abnormalities of skin pigmentation, urogenital abnormalities and abnormalities of limbs and digits. There appear to be at least 16 different genes, mutation of which can lead to the phenotype of Fanconi anaemia. Inheritance is autosomal recessive. Fanconi anaemia may progress to MDS and AML. In Fanconi anaemia, improvement in blood counts can occur as a result of gene conversion or another second mutation that compensates for the inherited abnormality [349].An even more rare inherited condition leading to aplastic anaemia is dyskeratosis congenita, characterised also by prominent abnormalities of skin and nails. Inheritance can be autosomal dominant, autosomal recessive or X-linked recessive. Most cases result from mutation in *DKC1*, *TERC*, *TERT* or *TINF2*, but a total of nine genes have been implicated.

Blood film and count

There is thrombocytopenia, which is often the presenting feature. Anaemia is often macrocytic and is accompanied by reticulocytopenia. Sometimes anisocytosis and poikilocytosis are marked. With progression, there is pancytopenia.

Differential diagnosis

The differential diagnosis includes acquired aplastic anaemia and other causes of anaemia or pancytopenia.

Further tests

Diagnosis of aplastic anaemia requires bone marrow aspiration and a trephine biopsy. Diagnosis of Fanconi anaemia is traditionally by demonstration of increased chromosomal breaks on exposure to clastogenic agents (diepoxybutane or mitomycin C), but it should be noted that about 10% of patients do not show sensitivity to clastogenic agents [33]. Sometimes results are abnormal on skin fibroblasts although normal on lymphocytes. A more economical screening test is measurement of serum alpha-fetoprotein; it is elevated in the majority of patients and is not elevated in other bone marrow failure syndromes [350]. Demonstration of a block in G2 on cell cycle analysis is also a sensitive diagnostic test. Haemoglobin F may be increased in Fanconi anaemia. Diagnosis of dyskeratosis congenita can be facilitated by demonstration of shortened telomeres in peripheral blood lymphocytes, by a polymerase chain reaction (PCR), flow cytometry or Southern blotting. DNA analysis can be used for confirmation in both syndromes.

Acquired aplastic anaemia

Aplastic anaemia may be: (i) a dose-related effect of irradiation or certain drugs or chemicals (e.g. chemotherapeutic agents or benzene); (ii) an idiosyncratic reaction to a drug (e.g. chloramphenicol or sulphonamides and related drugs including anti-thyroid drugs); or (iii) possibly the result of infection by certain viruses, possibly non-A, non-B, non-C hepatitis and certainly, in patients with defective immunity, the Epstein–Barr virus. In many cases the cause cannot be ascertained so that the condition is classified as idiopathic. Aplastic anaemia may lead to death from infection or haemorrhage. In patients who survive, e.g. following immunosuppressive treatment, PNH, MDS and AML may subsequently emerge.

Blood film and count

There is pancytopenia with a markedly reduced reticulocyte count. Red cells are normochromic and either normocytic or macrocytic. Poikilocytosis is sometimes marked. The neutrophils may show heavy granulation. Platelet size is normal on the blood film and MPV is not increased. In contrast to pancytopenia resulting from bone marrow infiltration, circulating granulocyte precursors and nucleated red blood cells are absent.

Differential diagnosis

The differential diagnosis included inherited causes of aplastic anaemia (particularly when there is a late onset and other constitutional abnormalities are minor or absent), an aplastic presentation of acute lymphoblastic leukaemia, hypoplastic AML and MDS, HIV infection and other causes of pancytopenia.

Further tests

Bone marrow aspiration and a trephine biopsy are required for diagnosis. Cytogenetic analysis is indicated, although the detection of an abnormal clone does not necessarily indicate that there will be rapid progression to MDS or AML. Young patients, e.g. under the age of 35 years, should be tested for Fanconi anaemia, even in the absence of evident constitutional abnormalities. This is particularly important if stem cell transplantation is being considered. Detection of a minor PNH clone by peripheral blood flow cytometry is possible in more than 60% of patients and is predictive or response to immunosuppressive treatment and better failure-free survival [351].

Inherited pure red cell aplasia

Diamond–Blackfan anaemia is a haemopoietic stem cell disorder of which the earliest manifestation is pure red cell aplasia. Later, neutropenia and thrombocytopenia may also develop. Inheritance is usually autosomal dominant but in some families is autosomal recessive. The condition results from mutation or deletion of one of a considerable number of genes encoding ribosomal proteins, among which the most often implicated are *RPS19*, *RPS26* and *RPL11*. Phenotypic expression of mutations is variable. In addition to red cell aplasia, there are some individuals in affected families in whom a mutated gene has no apparent effect; in others it causes only macrocytosis, an elevated red cell adenosine deaminase activity or both. Intrauterine anaemia

severe enough to cause hydrops fetalis has been reported [352]. About 40% of patients have associated congenital abnormalities [353]. The incidence of AML is increased [33].

The prevalence is 5–7/100 000 live births [353].

Blood film and count

Initially there is anaemia and macrocytosis with a low reticulocyte count. The neutrophil count is normal or slightly reduced. The platelet count is normal or increased. With disease progression, there may be neutropenia or thrombocytopenia progressing to pancytopenia.

Differential diagnosis

The differential diagnosis includes transient erythroblastopenia of childhood and persistent parvovirus B19 infection.

Further tests

Serum soluble transferrin receptor is greatly reduced in all types of pure red cell aplasia. Erythrocyte adenosine deaminase activity is increased in 40–80% of patients with Diamond–Blackfan syndrome whereas it is normal in transient erythroblastopenia of childhood [353]; among patients with inherited bone marrow failure syndromes, its specificity is 95% [354]. Haemoglobin F may be increased. Bone marrow examination usually shows reduction of proerythroblasts and marked reduction of later erythroblasts. In a minority of patients, proerythroblast numbers are normal. Cells of other lineages are initially normal. In transient erythroblastopenia, the haemoglobin A_{1c} may be elevated, as a result of the increased mean age of the red cells, whereas in Diamond–Blackfan syndrome the haemoglobin A_{1c} would be expected to be normal as the decline in erythropoiesis has been very gradual [355]. The diagnosis can be confirmed by DNA analysis in approaching 90% of patients [356].

Acquired pure red cell aplasia

Acquired pure red cell aplasia may be transient or persistent. Transient pure red cell aplasia is often caused by parvovirus B19 infection and, unless the patient has, coincidentally, a shortened red cell life span, is so brief that it often goes undiagnosed. More prolonged pure red cell aplasia occurs in transient erythroblastopenia of childhood, which results, in some cases, from human herpesvirus 6 infection. Chronic pure red cell aplasia may result from persistent parvovirus B19 infection in patients with impaired immunity, e.g. in HIV infection or following immunosuppressive therapy. Red cell aplasia may be immunological in origin, as when it is associated with thymoma, autoimmune disease, large granular lymphocyte leukaemia or CLL. A significant proportion of cases represent the most prominent manifestation of MDS.

Blood film and count

There is a macrocytic or normocytic anaemia with marked reticulocytopenia. Depending on the aetiology, there may be dysplastic features in cells of other lineages or an increase in large granular lymphocytes. In those with an underlying haemolytic anaemia there may be spherocytes or elliptocytes. Transient erythroblastopenia of childhood is associated with a normal MCV, with a neutrophil count of less than $1 \times 10^9/l$ in up to a fifth of patients and with thrombocytopenia in about 5% [357].

Differential diagnosis

The differential diagnosis includes other causes of a normocytic or macrocytic anaemia.

Further tests

Bone marrow examination is diagnostic. Depending on the clinical context, other indicated tests may include serological tests for herpesvirus 6 and parvovirus B19, tests for parvovirus DNA, screening for autoantibodies, chest radiology, immunophenotypic analysis of lymphocytes or cytogenetic analysis.

Polycythaemia

Polycythaemia refers to an increased RBC, Hb and Hct/PCV. It may be relative, resulting from a decreased plasma volume, or absolute, caused by an increase in the total volume of red cells in the circulation.

Relative polycythaemia

Relative or apparent or pseudo-polycythaemia may be the result of acute plasma loss, as in burns and dehydration. The explanation will be readily apparent from the clinical history and no further diagnostic tests are required. Relative polycythaemia also occurs as a chronic condition, which is sometimes attributable to cigarette smoking but is usually unexplained. The blood film appears 'packed' but is otherwise normal. The blood film cannot be distinguished from that in idiopathic erythrocytosis (see below), the distinction being made by radioisotopic estimations of total plasma volume and total red cell volume (traditionally referred to as 'red cell mass'). Measurement of the Hb is not reliable in distinguishing a true from a relative polycythaemia. Even Hbs of over 200 g/l may be observed in relative polycythaemia [358].

True polycythaemia

True polycythaemia refers to an increase in the total volume of circulating red cells ('red cell mass') above that which is predicted for the individual's height and weight. The total plasma volume is often increased but may be normal or decreased. True polycythaemia may result from: (i) chronic hypoxia such as that caused by living at altitude, cyanotic heart disease and chronic hypoxic lung disease; (ii) increased secretion of erythropoietin as from renal cysts and tumours or other tumours; (iii) idiopathic erythrocytosis (an unexplained condition); or (iv) polycythaemia vera. All these conditions cause a high RBC, Hb and Hct/PCV and the blood film appears 'packed'. With the exception of polycythaemia vera (see below), the blood film and count are usually otherwise normal.

Polycythaemia vera

Polycythaemia vera (PV), previously often known as polycythaemia rubra vera (PRV) and sometimes as primary proliferative polycythaemia, is a myeloproliferative neoplasm (MPN) in which there is increased production of red cells and sometimes also of granulocytes and platelets. It is largely a disease of the middle-aged and elderly, although occasional cases are seen in younger adults and very rare cases in children. Common clinical features are those resulting from the hyperviscosity of the polycythaemic blood, such as cerebrovascular accidents and peripheral gangrene, and those indicative of an MPN, such as hepatomegaly, splenomegaly and pruritus. Presentation can also be with splanchnic vein thrombosis or Budd–Chiari syndrome, with the MPN being occult. A high platelet count with normal Hb and Hct can represent occult or prepolycythaemic PV.

PV may eventually enter a 'burnt-out' phase or may be complicated by the development of post-polycythaemic myelofibrosis or AML.

Blood film and count

The peripheral blood film in polycythaemia of any aetiology shows a 'packed film' appearance since the viscosity of the blood means that the film of blood is not spread as thinly as normal (Fig. 8.91). The WBC, neutrophil and basophil counts are increased in the majority of cases. A WBC greater than 15×10^9/l correlates with an increased risk of thrombosis [359] and a white cell count greater than 13×10^9/l with worse overall survival [360]. Monocyte and eosinophil counts are much less often increased. The platelet count is elevated in about two-thirds of cases and platelet size is increased. There may be small numbers of circulating nucleated red blood cells or granulocyte precursors. Red cells can be normocytic and normochromic or, if hyperplastic erythropoiesis has led to exhaustion of

iron stores, they can be hypochromic and microcytic. If complicating iron deficiency occurs there can be anaemia (Fig. 8.92), but the underlying polycythaemia is revealed if the patient is given iron. Less often PV is masked by complicating vitamin B_{12} or folate deficiency.

The FBC usually shows an elevated RBC, Hb and Hct and normal or reduced MCV and MCH. However, early in the disease course the RBC, Hb and Hct may be normal despite the total red cell volume being increased [361]. The platelet count may be increased, sometimes in the absence of an increased Hb. The MPV is raised in relation to the platelet count. In PV complicated by iron deficiency, the red cell indices are very similar to those of thalassaemia trait, but the MCHC is reduced and the RDW is increased.

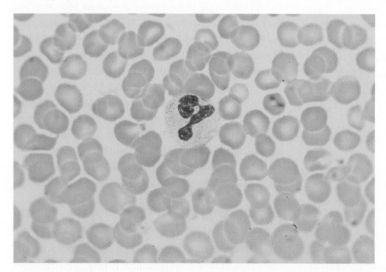

Fig. 8.91 A 'packed film' consequent on post-transplant polycythaemia. The Hb was 200 g/l and the Hct 0.59. The MCV was increased to 114 fl as a result of azathioprine therapy.

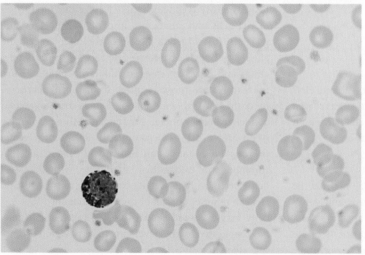

Fig. 8.92 The blood film of a patient with polycythaemia vera complicated by iron deficiency, showing anaemia and thrombocytosis and some hypochromic and microcytic cells. There was an increased basophil count and there is one basophil in the field. FBC (Coulter S Plus IV) was: WBC 6.7 × 10^9/l, RBC 4.38 × 10^{12}/l, Hb 106 g/l, Hct 0.33 l/l, MCV 75 fl, MCH 24.2 pg, MCHC 323 g/l, RDW 24.9%, platelet count 1056 × 10^9/l.

Differential diagnosis

The differential diagnosis includes other causes of poly-cythaemia (see Table 6.1). In particular, it is necessary to distinguish PV from essential erythrocytosis. This term means that there is unexplained polycythaemia with-out clinical or laboratory features diagnostic of an MPN; some but not all of these patients are now found to have molecular evidence of PV so that this diagnosis is now less often made.

Neutrophilia, an increased basophil count, thrombo-cytosis, giant platelets and an elevated MPV favour a diagnosis of PV. An increased basophilia count is par-ticularly useful in the differential diagnosis since it is not seen in secondary polycythaemia.

Further tests

Polycythaemia should be confirmed by obtaining a repeat blood specimen, with minimal stasis, before proceeding to further investigations. The plasma erythropoietin concen-tration should be measured; it is often decreased whereas it is more likely to be normal in relative polycythaemia. A low serum erythropoietin has a high specificity but only mod-erate sensitivity [362], being normal in 20% of patients at presentation in one series [361]. However, it should also be noted that 30–50% of patients with essential throm-bocythaemia (ET) show a reduced erythropoietin concen-tration [362,363] and this test therefore cannot be used to distinguish between these two conditions; a low level can also be seen in idiopathic erythrocytosis [364]. Deter-mination of total red cell and plasma volume by radio-iso-topic dilution studies excludes relative polycythaemia, but this is no longer a first-line test. The World Health Organi-zation (WHO) 2008 classification of MPN suggests that measurement of the red cell mass is unnecessary if the Hb is greater than 185 g/l in a man or greater than 165 g/dl in a woman [365], although in one comparison of true and relative polycythaemia, the Hb exceeded these levels in 14% of men with relative polycythaemia and in 35% of women [358]. A lower Hb concentration (> 170 and > 150 g/l for men and women respectively) is accepted if there has been a documented rise of 20 g/l [365]. It has similarly been suggested that a red cell mass is not necess-ary if Hct exceed 0.52, but otherwise should be performed if the Hct is greater than 0.45 in a woman or greater than 0.48 in a man [366]. The British Committee for Standards in Haematology guidelines suggest that confirmation of polycythaemia is not required if the Hct is greater than 0.60 in a man or greater than 0.56 in a woman [364]. When the

diagnosis is suspected but the Hb and Hct do not meet diag-nostic criteria, a bone marrow aspirate and trephine biopsy provide an alternative to red cell mass and plasma vol-ume determination for confirmation of the diagnosis. The trephine biopsy both confirms the diagnosis of an MPN and, since megakaryocyte morphology differs, permits a distinction between ET and the prepolycythaemic phase of PV; it should be supplemented by cytogenetic analysis (since a clonal chromosomal abnormality is confirmatory of a haematological neoplasm). Molecular analysis for the *JAK2* V617F mutation should be performed on periph-eral blood. This mutation is found in the great majority of patients with PV and in a quarter to a third of patients it is homozygous. Its detection confirms that there is an MPN but does not distinguish PV from ET. If *JAK2* V617F is not detected, a *JAK2* exon 12 mutation should be sought. The serum ferritin is often low. Serum vitamin B_{12} is often ele-vated as a result of an increase of B_{12}-binding proteins in the plasma. Growth of erythropoietin-independent eryth-roid colonies from peripheral blood or bone marrow sug-gests PV, although a significant proportion of cases of idio-pathic erythrocytosis also show this phenomenon; this test is not widely used, but a simplified method could make it more widely applicable [367]. The neutrophil alkaline phosphatase (NAP) score is often increased and is much less likely to be increased in secondary polycythaemia; this test is not, however, of diagnostic importance if molecular analysis is available.

Secondary polycythaemia

A diagnosis of secondary polycythaemia can often be made by consideration of the blood count and film in the light of the clinical features. If it is not clear whether the patient has a secondary polycythaemia or PV, inves-tigations as above are indicated. Some patients with sec-ondary polycythaemia have neutrophilia or thrombocy-tosis, but an increased basophil count (confirmed on a blood film) and giant platelets are strongly suggestive of PV. A raised serum erythropoietin has a high specificity but is observed in around 50% of patients; occasional patients even have a reduced concentration [362].

Other tests

Arterial blood gas measurements should be performed to identify pulmonary causes of secondary polycythae-mia. Ultrasound or computed tomography examination of the abdomen is indicated to detect relevant renal lesions.

Relative polycythaemia

This condition is generally asymptomatic, the diagnosis being made incidentally.

Blood film and count

The RBC, Hb and Hct are increased. The white cell count and platelet count are normal. The blood film may appear 'packed', as a result of increased blood viscosity. Otherwise it is normal.

Differential diagnosis

The differential diagnosis is true polycythaemia and, particularly, essential erythrocytosis.

Further tests

Distinction from true polycythaemia is made by studies of total red cell and plasma volume. Bone marrow aspiration and trephine biopsy show no abnormality [368], although these tests are not necessary if blood volume studies are available. No *JAK2* mutation is detected. The serum erythropoietin concentration is usually normal but is occasionally low [362,368].

Disorders of platelets

Thrombocytopenia
Congenital and neonatal thrombocytopenias

Congenital thrombocytopenia may be inherited or due to a pathological process, e.g. infection or exposure to an antibody or a toxic substance, occurring during intrauterine life. It may be caused by failure of production or increased consumption or destruction of platelets. Neonatal thrombocytopenia can result from intrauterine or neonatal events [369].

Congenital thrombocytopenia may be an isolated abnormality or may be associated with abnormalities of granulopoiesis or erythropoiesis, with constitutional abnormalities or with immune deficiency. In congenital amegakaryocytic thrombocytopenia resulting from a mutation in the *MPL* gene (the thrombopoietin receptor), there is slow progression to pancytopenia [370]. The rare syndrome of amegakaryocytic thrombocytopenia with radio-ulnar synostosis, resulting from *HOXA11* mutation, can show progression to hypoplastic anaemia or pancytopenia [371,372]. Patients with Fanconi anaemia and dyskeratosis congenita can also present with isolated thrombocytopenia, only later showing progression to pancytopenia. Wiskott–Aldrich syndrome, an X-linked syndrome resulting from mutation in the *WAS* gene, is characterised by thrombocytopenia, eczema, immune deficiency and sometimes neutropenia; female heterozygotes are sometimes affected. Wiskott–Aldrich syndrome may be complicated by severe refractory thrombocytopenia (platelet count 10×10^9/l or less), probably immune in nature; when this occurs early in life it is prognostically adverse and an indication for transplantation [232]. Constitutional syndromes and other inherited causes of thrombocytopenia are summarised in Tables 8.11–8.13 and causes of neonatal thrombocytopenia in Table 8.14. Other congenital thrombocytopenias have been described in single families or small numbers of

Table 8.11 Inherited and other constitutional abnormalities leading to thrombocytopenia with small platelets [373–377].

Defect	Inheritance	Platelet functional defect	Associated abnormalities	References
Wiskott–Aldrich syndrome	Sex-linked recessive (*WAS* gene at Xp11.23)*	Yes (reduced dense granules and reduced expression of GpIIb/IIIa and IV)	Eczema and defective cell-mediated immunity	[374,375]
X-linked thrombocytopenia including intermittent X-linked thrombocytopenia with small platelets	Sex-linked recessive (*WAS* gene at Xp11. 23)	Yes (reduced dense granules and reduced expression of GpIIb/IIIa and IV)	Isolated thrombocytopenia (although there is a mutation in the same gene as causes Wiskott–Aldrich syndrome)	[375,376]
Autosomal dominant thrombocytopenia with micro-thrombocytes	AD	Normal function		[377]

*Occasional cases occur in females, either because of extreme Lyonisation or because of failure of the mechanism that usually ensures that in heterozygotes there is preferential proliferation/survival of cells expressing the paternal wild type *WAS* [374]

AD, autosomal dominant

Table 8.12 Inherited and other constitutional abnormalities leading to thrombocytopenia with normal sized platelets [373,378–392].

Defect	Inheritance	Platelet functional defect	Associated abnormalities	References
Fanconi anaemia	AR		Progression to pancytopenia; reduced stature, abnormal digits and other dysmorphic features	
Thrombocytopenia with absent radii	AR due to coinheritance of a noncoding polymorphism and a null allele of *RBM8A* at 1q21.1, rarely AD		Absent radii, sometimes other congenital abnormalities, thrombocytopenia improves with age; occasional cases have developed acute leukaemia	[378]
Amegakaryocytic thrombocytopenia	AR, mutation in *MPL* gene (encoding thrombopoietin receptor) at 1p34.2		Slow progression to pancytopenia due to aplastic anaemia; propensity to MDS and AML	[371,372,379, 380,381]
Amegakaryocytic thrombocytopenia with radio-ulnar synostosis	AD, *HOXA11* gene at 7p15.2		Radio-ulnar fusion (synostosis); progression to pancytopenia due to aplastic anaemia, possible sensorineural deafness	[371,372,380]
Autosomal dominant thrombocytopenia	AD, *MASTL* (previously *FLJ14813*) gene at 10p12.1			[382]
Autosomal dominant thrombocytopenia with palely staining platelets	AD, *ANKRD26* at 10p12.1	No consistent defect observed; glycoprotein Ia and α granules may be reduced	There may be lecucocytosis and a high Hb; propensity to develop AML; WBC often increased	[383,384,385]
Familial platelet disorder with a propensity to develop AML	AD, *RUNX1* at 21q22.12, either haploinsufficiency or dominant negative mutation	Very abnormal platelet function, storage pool defect and greatly reduced aggregation with all agents	Propensity to develop AML	[386]
Quebec platelet disorder (previously known as factor V Quebec)	AD, gain of function mutation in *PLAU* at 10q22.2, encoding urokinase plasminogen activator	Abnormal epinephrine-induced aggregation, delayed bleeding; falsely normal on Lumi aggregometry		[387]
Dysmegakaryopoietic thrombocytopenia	AR	Normal or increased numbers of small dysmorphic megakaryocytes		[388]
Mild autosomal dominant thrombocytopenia	AD, mutation of *CYCS* at 7p15.3 encoding mitochondrial cytochrome c	Premature release of platelets in marrow space instead of in sinusoids	None	[389]
Autosomal dominant thrombocytopenia with platelet anisocytosis	AD, activating mutation of *ITGB3* gene, encoding platelet glycoprotein IIIa, at 17q21.32	Reduced aggregation with ADP and collagen, normal agglutination with ristocetin		[390]
Mild thrombocytopenia in heterozygotes in a Micronesian family	AD, mutation or deletion of *THPO* at 3q27.1		Aplastic anaemia in homozygotes	[391]
Paris-Trousseau thrombocytopenia	A contiguous gene syndrome due to microdeletion of 11q23-24; deletion of *FLI1* at 11q24.3 is responsible for thrombocytopenia	Platelets have abnormally large α granules and sometimes deficiency of dense granules, platelet count improves over time	Features of Jacobsen syndrome: psychomotor retardation, facial dysmorphism and cardiac defects	[379,381,392]
ACTN1-related thrombocytopenia	AD, mutation in *ACTN1* at 14q24			[385]

AD, autosomal dominant; ADP, adenosine diphosphate; AML, acute myeloid leukaemia; AR, autosomal recessive; Hb, haeomglobin concentration; MDS, myelodysplastic syndrome/s; WBC, white blood cell count.

Table 8.13 Inherited and other constitutional abnormalities leading to thrombocytopenia with large platelets [172,343,344,378, 379,381,393–414].

Defect	Inheritance	Platelet functional defect	Associated abnormalities	References
Bernard–Soulier syndrome	AR, homozygosity or compound heterozygosity for mutations in the *GP1BA* gene (17p13.2), *GP1BB* gene (22q11.21) or *GP9* gene (3q21.3)	Abnormal glycoprotein Ib/IX/V complex with marked defect in von Willebrand factor-dependent and ristocetin-induced aggregation	Nil	
Monoallelic Bernard–Soulier syndrome; large platelets with or without thrombocytopenia	AD, dominant negative mutations in the *GP1BA* gene (17p13.2) or *GP1BB* gene (22q11.21)	Usually normal; ristocetin-induced aggregation sometimes reduced	Nil	[381,385, 393,394]
DiGeorge and velocardiofacial syndrome	AD, a contiguous gene syndrome due to microdeletion; loss of *GP1BB* gene at 22q11.21	Carriers of Bernard–Soulier syndrome with large platelets and reduced ristocetin aggregation; Bernard–Soulier syndrome occurs when there is mutation in the other *GP1BB* allele	Cardiac, parathyroid and thymus abnormalities, cognitive impairment in velocardiofacial syndrome, also facial dysmorphism; autoimmune cytopenias	[381,395]
Macrothrombocytopenia due to *ITGB3* mutation	AD, activating mutation of *ITGB3* gene, encoding platelet glycoprotein IIIa, at 17q21.32	Normal		[396]
Macrothrombocytopenia due to *ITGA2B* mutation*	AD, activating mutation of *ITGA2B* gene, encoding platelet glycoprotein IIb, at 17q21.31	Reduced aggregation with ADP and collagen		[397]
Mediterranean stomatocytosis/macrothrombocytopenia (phytosterolaemia)	AR, mutation in *ABCG5* at 2p21 or *ABCG8* gene at 2p21	Abnormal with ristocetin; variable abnormalities with other agonists	Short stature, hyperphytosterolaemia, variable hypercholesterolaemia	[172]
Grey platelet syndrome	AR, mutation in *NBEAL2* at 3p21.31; heterozygotes have large platelets and reduced α granules	α granule defect with hypogranular platelets and mild functional defect; combined α and δ granule deficiency	Severely hypogranular neutrophils in some families [398]; myelofibrosis and splenomegaly	[398]
GFI1B-related thrombocytopenia	AD due to mutation of *GFI1B* at 9q34.13 (two families)	α granule defect	Anisopoikilocytosis in one family	[385]
White platelet syndrome	AD	α granule defect, prominent Golgi complexes, defective aggregation with epinephrine and adenosine diphosphate		[399]
Arthrogryphosis, renal dysfunction and cholestasis (ARC) syndrome	AR, *VPS33B* at 15q26.1 or *VIPAR* at 14q24.3	Normal platelet count or mild thrombocytopenia, large pale platelets, decreased α granule proteins	Joint contractures, renal tubular acidosis, cholestasis	

Defect	Inheritance	Platelet functional defect	Associated abnormalities	References
York platelet syndrome	Unknown		Thrombocytopenia and mitochondrial myopathy, variable lack of α and δ granules, giant electron-dense organelles in platelets	[400]
Medich giant platelet syndrome	Unknown	Large agranular platelets with distinctive ultrastructure		
MYH9-related disease: May–Hegglin anomaly	AD, MYH9 (non-muscle myosin heavy chain 9 gene) at 22q12.3	Reduced glycoprotein Ib/IX/V complex	Neutrophil inclusions	[401,402]
MYH9-related disease: Fechtner syndrome	AD, MYH9 at 22q12.3	Glycoprotein Ib/IX/V may be reduced	Neutrophil inclusions, Alport-like syndrome – nephritis, sensorineural deafness, cataracts	[378,403,404]
MYH9-related disease: Epstein syndrome	AD, MYH9 at 22q12.3	Glycoprotein Ib/IX/V may be reduced	Alport-like syndrome – nephritis, sensorineural deafness, cataracts – but no neutrophil inclusions	[378,404]
MYH9-related disease: Sebastian syndrome	AD, MYH9 at 22q12.3	Reduced glycoprotein Ib/IX/V complex	Neutrophil inclusions	[401,403,404]
Homozygous Pelger–Huët anomaly	AD, LBR gene at 1q42.12		Lack of lobulation in granulocytes and monocytes; developmental delay, epilepsy, skeletal abnormalities in some families	[405]
X-linked thrombocytopenia, with abnormal erythropoiesis (occasionally a mild syndrome in female heterozygotes)	X-linked, mutation in GATA1 at Xp11.23	Grey platelets – reduced α granules, abnormal glycoproteins Ibβ and IX, abnormal ristocetin-induced aggregation, may have severe functional defect	Macrocytosis, dyserythropoiesis or dyserythropoietic anaemia in some families, β thalassaemia in some families, occasionally congenital erythropoietic porphyria	[343,344,379, 406,407]
Thrombocytopenia with neutropenia	Unknown but presumably inherited	Reduced glycoprotein Ib	Neutropenia with reduced sialyl-Lewis X on neutrophils	[408]
Thrombocytopenia with large platelets in West Bengal, Bangladesh, Bhutan and Nepal (Harris platelet syndrome)	Unknown	Normal		[409]
Giant platelets with mitral valve insufficiency	Unknown	Reduced glycoproteins Ia, Ic and IIa, reduced aggregation with ADP and epinephrine	Mitral insufficiency	[410]

(continued)

Table 8.13 *(continued)*

Defect	Inheritance	Platelet functional defect	Associated abnormalities	References
Giant platelets with ineffective thrombopoiesis	AD	Increased platelet glycoprotein Ib and IIb/IIIa	Nil	[411]
Platelet-type von Willebrand disease	AD, *GP1BA* (encoding GpIbα) at 17p13.2	Increased aggregation with ristocetin		
Type IIB von Willebrand disease (including 'Montreal platelet syndrome')	AD, gain of function mutation of *VWF* at 12p13.31	Spontaneous platelet aggregation of resting or stirred platelets	Rarely platelet aggregates are present in the circulation	[412]
Macrothrombocytopenia due to *TUBB1* mutation	AD, *TUBB1* at 20q13.32	β1 tubulin 50% of normal levels		[413]
Macrothrombocytes, with or without thrombocytopenia	X-linked dominant, *FLNA* at Xq28	Impaired interaction of von Willebrand factor with platelet glycoproteins	Isolated platelet defect or associated with periventricular nodular heterotopia	[414]

*It is probable that homozygosity causes a syndrome resembling Glanzmann thrombasthenia
AD, autosomal dominant; ADP, adenosine diphosphate; AR autosomal recessive

Table 8.14 Causes of neonatal thrombocytopenia (most common causes are bold) (modified from reference 369)

Onset within first 72 hours of life	Onset after 72 hours of life
Chronic fetal hypoxia	**Neonatal sepsis**
Perinatal asphyxia	**Necrotising enterocolitis**
Perinatal bacterial infection	Congenital infection
Alloimmune thrombocytopenia	Maternal autoimmune thrombocytopenia
Maternal autoimmune thrombocytopenia	Kasabach–Merritt syndrome
Congenital infection (toxoplasmosis, cytomegalovirus, HIV, rubella)	Inherited metabolic disorders
Thrombosis of aorta or renal vein	Inherited thrombocytopenia (thrombocytopenia with absent radius, congenital amegakaryocytic thrombocytopenia)
Congenital leukaemia	
Kasabach–Merritt syndrome	
Inherited metabolic disorders	
Inherited thrombocytopenia (thrombocytopenia with absent radius, congenital amegakaryocytic thrombocytopenia)	

HIV, human immunodeficiency virus

families, e.g. autosomal dominant macrothrombocytopenia without any bleeding tendency and with reduced glycosylation of platelet glycoprotein IV, enhanced aggregation with ADP, epinephrine and collagen, and ristocetin-induced platelet agglutination at lower than normal ristocetin concentration [415] and autosomal dominant macrothrombocytopenia with reduced aggregation with adrenaline and arachidonic acid, platelet expression of glycophorin, and late onset hearing loss [416]. Intermittent thrombocytopenia

has also been described in patients with severe congenital neutropenia resulting from a mutation in the *G6PC3* gene [417]. It should be noted that the Bernard–Soulier syndrome is a severe bleeding disorder with giant platelets and abnormal platelet function as well as marked thrombocytopenia, whereas heterozygosity for certain dominant negative Bernard–Soulier mutations leads to a milder form of the syndrome. The syndromes resulting from mutation in the *MHY9* gene, which encodes the heavy chain of non-muscle

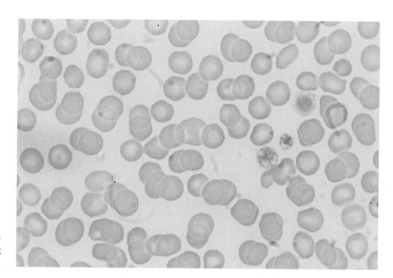

Fig. 8.93 The blood film of a patient with the Bernard–Soulier syndrome showing thrombocytopenia and three giant platelets.

myosin heavy chain 9, differ in associated features and in the ultrastructure of any neutrophil inclusions [418]. There are other rare congenital syndromes in which thrombocytopenia has been described. The von Voss-Cherstvoy or DK-phocomelia syndrome is a syndrome of multiple congenital abnormalities, which may have associated thrombocytopenia and is often fatal in the perinatal period [419]; bone marrow megakaryocytes are reduced. Congenital thrombocytopenia has also been associated with agenesis of the corpus callosum and distinctive facies [420]. Another autosomal dominant syndrome associates deformity of the upper limb, hearing loss, external ophthalmoplegia and thrombocytopenia [421]. Fetal and congenital thrombocytopenia can also be a feature of Down syndrome, trisomy 13, trisomy 18, Turner syndrome and triploidy [369].

Congenital thrombocytopenia can be immune in origin and transient, resulting from transplacental passage of maternal autoantibodies or alloantibodies (including anti-glycoprotein IV – anti-CD36). It can be a feature of severe Rh haemolytic disease of the fetus and newborn [369]. Other congenital abnormalities may indicate either an inherited syndrome or exposure to a teratogenic substance *in utero*.

The most likely cause of neonatal thrombocytopenia varies with whether the onset is within the first 72 hours of life or later. The great majority of cases occurring after 72 hours are due to necrotising enterocolitis or sepsis [369].

Blood film and count

The blood film should be examined for morphology of erythrocytes and leucocytes as well as platelets. Platelets may be small, normal in size or large. Small platelets are uncommon but are seen in the Wiskott–Aldrich syndrome (see Fig. 3.157). Platelets of normal size are seen when there is bone marrow or megakaryocytic hypoplasia. Large platelets are common in various inherited causes of thrombocytopenia, e.g. Bernard–Soulier syndrome (Fig. 8.93) and *MYH9*-related disease including the May–Hegglin anomaly (see Fig. 3.93) and a number of other more rare conditions. In Bernard–Soulier syndrome there is marked thrombocytopenia with giant platelets. In heterozygosity for the Bernard Soulier syndrome the platelet count may be as low as 40–50 × 10^9/l but in some individuals is normal; all have giant platelets [393]. In most disorders the platelets show normal granulation, but in the rare grey platelet syndrome they appear agranular or hypogranular (Fig. 8.94) and in Paris-Trousseau thrombocytopenia (Jacobsen syndrome) platelets have giant granules. In thrombocytopenia associated with a *GATA1* mutation there are large hypogranular platelets [378]. Neutrophils should be examined for abnormal inclusions, which are detectable in many cases, but not invariably, in a heterogeneous group of disorders that are now grouped together as *MYH9*-related disease (including May–Hegglin anomaly and Fechtner, Sebastian and Epstein syndromes). Inclusions may be spindle-shaped or irregular [418]. These inclusions result

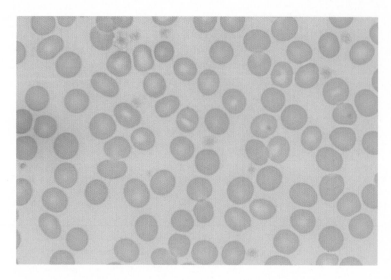

Fig. 8.94 The blood film of a patient with the grey platelet syndrome showing six agranular platelets.

from abnormal localisation of *MYH9* in association with ribosomes, [418,422]. Ultrastructurally there may be clusters of ribosomes, segments of rough endoplasmic reticulum and parallel longitudinal filaments or cross-striated inclusions [418,423]. The neutrophil inclusions in *MYH9*-related disease may be below the level of resolution of the light microscope, although they can be demonstrated either by immunofluorescence to show the distribution of *MYH9* or by ultrastructural examination [423]. In another rare congenital syndrome, the Upshaw–Schulman syndrome, there is episodic thrombocytopenia associated with microangiopathic haemolytic anaemia; this syndrome, which is responsive to plasma infusion, has been shown to result from a congenital deficiency of von Willebrand factor cleaving protease, ADAMTS13 [424]. Red cells should be examined for anisocytosis, poikilocytosis and macrocytosis, which may be indicative of a mutation in the *GATA1* gene affecting both erythropoiesis and thrombopoiesis [344]. In babies with Down syndrome, the blood film should be examined for features of transient abnormal myelopoiesis (see Chapter 9), which may cause thrombocytopenia. Rarely, in other thrombocytopenic babies, the blood film shows features of congenital leukaemia.

The platelet count is low, but when a large proportion of platelets are very large the count on an automated instrument may be an underestimate of the true count. In one study the underestimation was greater with an impedance counter than with a counter based on light scattering [425]. Depending on the aetiology of the thrombocytopenia, the MPV may be low, normal or high. In *MYH9*-related disorders and in Bernard–Soulier syndrome an MPV of 12.4 fl has been found to be a suitable cut-off point for separating these inherited thrombocytopenias from autoimmune thrombocytopenic purpura [425]. In inherited thrombocytopenia with large platelets, the percentage of reticulated platelets is normal or slightly elevated, whereas in autoimmune thrombocytopenic purpura the percentage is often considerably increased [426].

Differential diagnosis
The differential diagnosis of congenital thrombocytopenia includes all the causes of congenital thrombocytopenia listed in Tables 6.27 and 8.11–8.13. A rare cause of thrombocytopenia that could be confused with the Bernard–Soulier syndrome is pseudo-Bernard–Soulier syndrome resulting from a drug-induced anti-platelet autoantibody [427].

Further tests
Whether further tests are needed and the choice of any further tests depends on the aetiology that is suspected on the basis of the clinical features and blood film and count. Useful tests may include study of platelet membrane antigens by immunological techniques, testing of the mother's serum for antibodies

to Kell group antigens or specific antiplatelet antibodies, bone marrow examination, cytogenetic analysis (for the detection of a constitutional abnormality or a leukaemia-related clonal abnormality) and platelet function studies (e.g. showing aggregation only with ristocetin in Bernard–Soulier syndrome). Investigation of other family members may be useful. Ultrastructural examination of platelets or neutrophils is sometimes useful. If fetomaternal alloimmune thrombocytopenia is suspected, the tests indicated are HPA typing on baby and mother and investigation of maternal serum for platelet alloantibodies, most often anti-HPA-1a and less often anti-HPA-5b [428]. If Wiskott–Aldrich syndrome is suspected, assessment of immunological status is indicated. This diagnosis can also be confirmed by genetic analysis or by demonstration of absent or abnormal WAS protein [429]. Coagulation factors and Von Willebrand factor multimer distribution require investigation if von Willebrand disease or pseudo-von Willebrand disease is suspected. Inclusions may be detected by immunofluorescence for *MYH9* protein in patients with *MYH9*-related disorders who lack neutrophil inclusions on light microscopy; in these particular patients the inclusions do not contain polyadenylated ribonucleic acid (RNA) [430].

Autoimmune ('idiopathic') thrombocytopenic purpura (ITP)

Autoimmune or 'idiopathic' thrombocytopenic purpura is an acquired condition in which platelet survival is reduced by the presence of platelet-directed autoantibodies. Autoimmune thrombocytopenia can also occur as one feature of a more generalised autoimmune disease such as SLE or the rare autoimmune lymphoproliferative syndrome associated with Fas deficiency [255]. There is an increased incidence in diGeorge syndrome. Autoimmune thrombocytopenia is a common complication of CLL and a less common complication of other lymphoproliferative disorders. In one study, 3 of 20 patients with either autoimmune thrombocytopenic purpura or Evans syndrome were found to have a population of peripheral blood lymphocytes with a CLL phenotype, suggesting that monoclonal B lymphocytosis as well as CLL can predispose to ITP [229]. Idiopathic autoimmune thrombocytopenic purpura has generally been regarded as particularly likely to occur in young women, but in one population-based survey the incidence in adults was 1.6/100 000/year overall, was similar in men and women and was higher above the age of 60 years [431]. In another survey the incidence was estimated at 8.1/100 000/year in children and 12.1/100 000/year in adults [432]. Incidence rose with age and was higher in females than males up to the age of 70 years [432].

Blood film and count

The blood film shows thrombocytopenia and, unless the onset is very acute, increased platelet size (Fig. 8.95). Usually other cell lineages are normal, but occasionally there is associated AIHA or evidence of an underlying causative condition such as CLL, lymphoma or large granular lymphocyte leukaemia.

The platelet count is reduced and, unless the onset is very acute, the MPV and the platelet distribution width (PDW) are increased. The percentage of reticulated platelets (see Chapter 2) is often considerably increased. Whether this is a useful variable for distinguishing increased platelet destruction from a failure of platelet production is not clear, since conflicting results have been reported [426,433].

Among childhood cases of ITP, less than a fifth develop chronic disease [434]. Those with the lowest platelet counts are least likely to develop chronic ITP [434].

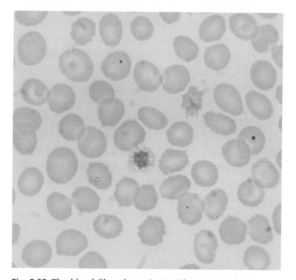

Fig. 8.95 The blood film of a patient with autoimmune thrombocytopenic purpura, post-splenectomy, showing thrombocytopenia, a single giant platelet and Howell–Jolly bodies.

Differential diagnosis

The differential diagnosis includes thrombocytopenia following rubella and other viral infections, drug-induced thrombocytopenia and TTP. Cytomegalovirus infection, infectious mononucleosis and other viral infections can also present with severe thrombocytopenia as the major manifestation. Symptomatic thrombocytopenia may be the presenting feature of HIV infection. Hepatitis C infection is common in patients who would otherwise meet the diagnostic criteria for ITP, so testing for hepatitis C should be done in all patients; hepatitis C-related cases often have cryoglobulinaemia and anticardiolipin antibodies [435]. *Helicobacter pylori* infection has also been related to what would otherwise be categorised as ITP. Some cases have a rise in the platelet count in response to the elimination of helicobacter, but how often this occurs is disputed. It is important to exclude congenital thrombocytopenia, which has sometimes been misdiagnosed and treated inappropriately as ITP.

Further tests

Before any other investigations are performed the blood film must be examined to confirm thrombocytopenia and, unless the patient has obvious petechiae or purpura, the thrombocytopenia must be confirmed on a second carefully taken blood specimen. The blood film should also be examined for spherocytes, red cell fragments, polychromasia, atypical lymphocytes, lymphoma cells and cryoglobulin deposits. The features of specific types of congenital thrombocytopenia should be specifically sought in platelets and neutrophils. Other tests that are indicated depend on the diagnosis suspected on the basis of the clinical features and the blood film examination. For example, if ITP seems the most likely diagnosis no further tests are usually required. However, in adults a bone marrow examination is considered indicated if: (i) there are atypical features; (ii) the patient is aged above 60 years; (iii) the patient has relapsed; or (iv) splenectomy is required [436]. Similarly, bone marrow aspiration is advised in children who (i) have atypical features; (ii) relapse; or (iii) require corticosteroid therapy [436]. Tests for antinuclear antibodies and DNA binding should also be carried out, since ITP may be the initial presentation of SLE. The presence of antiphospholipid antibodies also supports the diagnosis of immune-mediated thrombocytopenia. If atypical lymphocytes are detected, a Paul–Bunnell screening test for infectious mononucleosis and specific serology for Epstein–Barr virus (EBV) and CMV may be useful and, if HIV infection appears possible, a specific test for HIV infection should generally be performed. Serology for chronic hepatitis C infection is indicated, particularly in countries with a high prevalence of this virus [437], since this diagnosis has therapeutic implications. Investigation for *H. pylori* infection should be considered in countries with a high prevalence of this infection, e.g. Italy and Japan; however, it is uncertain to what extent this is a worthwhile test since there are conflicting reports as to the likelihood of improvement following eradication of the bacterium [438,439]. The BCSH recommends testing patients who relapse for *H. pylori* [436]. If red cell fragments are present, investigations relevant to TTP should be initiated as a matter of urgency.

Post-infection immune thrombocytopenic purpura

Immune thrombocytopenic purpura, in many ways resembling autoimmune thrombocytopenic purpura, can occur following various infections (e.g. rubella) or following vaccination, e.g. vaccination for rubella, influenza, measles, hepatitis B, poliomyelitis, mumps and triple vaccine for diphtheria, polio and tetanus [440]. Post-infection thrombocytopenia is particularly common in children.

Thrombotic thrombocytopenic purpura (TTP)

TTP is a systemic disorder, usually resulting from autoantibodies to ADAMTS13 (von Willebrand factor cleaving protease), in which microthrombi in multiple organs lead to platelet consumption and renal and cerebral manifestations. The thrombocytopenia may lead to haemorrhage. A minority of cases follow identifiable infections such as *Escherichia coli* O157:H7 [441] or Legionnaires' disease. TTP can occur during the course of HIV infection and can relapse following interruption of effective antiretroviral therapy [442]. Ticlopidine [443] and clopidogrel therapy can cause TTP and occasional cases have been linked to abuse of cocaine or Ecstasy [444] or to interferon therapy [445].

The incidence has been variously estimated at 1, 1.7, 3.7 and 3.8/1 000 000/year [314,446]. The classic pentad of disease features is thrombocytopenia, microangiopathic haemolytic anaemia, renal impairment, neurological abnormalities and fever. However, since urgent treatment by plasma exchange is required, it is recommended that a provisional diagnosis be made and treatment be started if a patient has thrombocytopenia and microangiopathic haemolytic anaemia for which there is no other apparent explanation [277].

Blood film and count

The blood film shows the features of a microangiopathic haemolytic anaemia (fragments and polychromasia) together with thrombocytopenia with platelet anisocytosis. Fragments comprising more than 1% of red cells have been found to be strongly suggestive of TTP [447]. However, red cell fragments may initially be quite infrequent [314] or absent [448] and if there is a strong clinical suspicion of this diagnosis blood films should be kept under very regular review and ADAMTS13 should be assayed. The RDW, MPV and PDW may be increased. The percentage of reticulated platelets is likely to be increased. Once treatment has commenced, the platelet count is the most important laboratory test for monitoring progress [277].

Differential diagnosis

The differential diagnosis includes other causes of red cell fragmentation, particularly those that can also cause thrombocytopenia. The possibility of familial TTP (atypical haemolytic–uraemic syndrome) should be considered.

Further tests

TTP is usually the result of an autoantibody to von Willebrand factor cleaving protease (ADAMTS13); the definitive test is as assay of ADAMTS13, which is found to be less than 10% of normal. Tests for the relevant autoantibody can be performed in patients with a reduced concentration. A biopsy confirmation of capillary thrombi confirms the diagnosis but is not generally indicated. HIV testing is important, since TTP may be the initial presentation of HIV infection and patients require antiretroviral therapy in addition to plasma exchange. Particularly in young patients, consideration should be given to genetic testing for familial atypical haemolytic–uraemic syndrome. LDH is often greatly elevated.

Thrombocytosis
Familial thrombocytosis

Familial thrombocytosis is a rare condition, usually with an autosomal dominant inheritance. It can result from a mutation in the promoter of *THPO*, the gene that encodes thrombopoietin, the mutation leading to an aberrantly stable messenger RNA. It can also result from a dominant activating mutation in the *MPL* gene that encodes the thrombopoietin receptor [449]. Germline *JAK2* V617I has also been associated with hereditary thrombocytosis [450]. Apparently recessive inheritance was reported in one family, but the genetic basis was not elucidated [451].

Blood film and count

The platelet count is increased. Platelet size is usually normal and cells of other lineages are usually normal. One family with autosomal dominant thrombocytosis with small platelets has been reported [452]. A prolonged leukaemoid reaction in infancy was reported in one infant [453].

Differential diagnosis

The differential diagnosis is reactive thrombocytosis and essential thrombocythaemia. Familial thrombocytosis should be suspected and family studies should be performed when unexplained thrombocytosis is detected in a child or young adult.

Further tests

Genetic analysis is indicated, if available, both to confirm the diagnosis and to exclude a diagnosis of essential thrombocythaemia.

Essential thrombocythaemia

Essential thrombocythaemia is an MPN characterised by increased platelet production. In the WHO classification it is defined as a Ph-negative, *BCR-ABL1*-negative condition. Essential thrombocythaemia is predominantly a disease of the middle-aged and elderly population, but cases also occur in young adults and even in children. Clinical features are either caused directly by the thrombocytosis or reflect the abnormal proliferation of myeloid cells. They include microvascular obstruction, bleeding and, less often, splenomegaly and itch. However, the majority of patients are now diagnosed at a presymptomatic stage as a result of the increasing performance of blood counts for a variety of reasons. Since automated counters now generally in use include a platelet count in the FBC, the incidental detection of thrombocytosis is not infrequent.

Essential thrombocythaemia progresses, uncommonly, to myelofibrosis and less often transforms to AML. These stages of the disease may be preceded by the development of dysplastic features.

Blood film and count

According to the WHO 2008 classification, the diagnosis can be made when the platelet count reaches $450 \times 10^9/l$ and other criteria are met. In many cases the count is in excess of $1000 \times 10^9/l$. The blood film shows increased platelet anisocytosis and usually a significant proportion of giant platelets (Fig. 8.96). Some of the platelets may be hypogranular. Neutrophilia is present in about one third of patients (and correlates with a higher risk of thrombosis [454]). The basophil count is often elevated, but does not usually exceed 3%. A basophil count of more than 5% suggests that the patient may be Philadelphia positive. Occasional NRBC and immature granulocytes may be present. There may be features of iron deficiency as a result of bleeding. Rarely, there are features of hyposplenism following earlier splenic infarction. During the accelerated phase of the disease, dysplastic features may be present (Fig. 8.97).

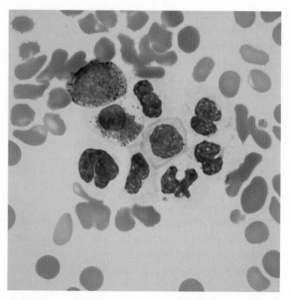

Fig. 8.97 The blood film of a patient with essential thrombocythaemia in accelerated phase showing development of dysplastic features in granulocytes. Neutrophils are hypogranular with nuclei of abnormal shapes. An eosinophil is nonlobated and the number of granules is reduced. Thrombocytopenia has now supervened.

The platelet count, MPV and PDW are elevated, whereas in reactive thrombocytosis the MPV and PDW are not usually increased. Splenectomy or hyposplenism can, however, cause thrombocytosis with an increased MPV and PDW.

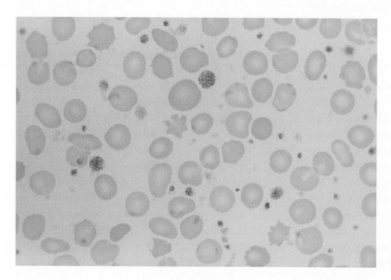

Fig. 8.96 The blood film of a patient with essential thrombocythaemia showing thrombocytosis with platelet anisocytosis and giant platelets. There is also red cell anisocytosis and poikilocytosis.

Differential diagnosis

The differential diagnosis includes many of the other causes of thrombocytosis (see Table 6.15), particularly those conditions that can cause reactive thrombocytosis without clear clinical features suggesting the underlying disease, e.g. occult neoplasms and connective tissue disorders. In iron deficient patients, uncomplicated iron deficiency should be included in the differential diagnosis since iron deficiency alone can cause a platelet count of $450 \times 10^9/l$ or even higher. Patients with iron deficiency may also have an occult neoplasm, occult haemorrhage or both as a cause of thrombocytosis. It can also be difficult to distinguish iron deficient PV and prepolycythaemic PV from ET. Up to 15% of patients with PV present with features that mimic ET.

Further tests

A suspicion of ET is an indication for molecular analysis for *JAK2* V617F. If this mutation is not found, a *CALR* or *MPL* mutation should be sought. *JAK2* V617F is found in about two-thirds of patients and correlates with a higher Hb [455–457] and WBC [454,456], more bone marrow erythropoiesis and granulopoiesis [454,456], lower serum erythropoietin and serum ferritin [456], more frequent microcytosis, a greater likelihood of evolving into overt PV [455,456] and, for pregnant women, a worse fetal outcome [458]. A *CALR* mutation is found in about a quarter of patients [459] and an *MPL* mutation in 5–10%. Using X-linked polymorphism analysis, it previously appeared that a significant proportion of patients with essential thrombocythaemia had polyclonal haemopoiesis; with the discovery of the *JAK2* V617F mutation, monoclonality can be demonstrated in a significant proportion of such patients (4 of 8 in one study) [460]. Cytogenetic analysis is particularly indicated whenever it is not clear that the patient has an MPN and if there are atypical disease characteristics – such as myelodysplastic features, circulating blast cells or a markedly elevated basophil count – which suggest either Philadelphia positivity or another unfavourable karyotype that would influence management. However, with the availability of effective tyrosine kinase inhibitor therapy for Ph-positive conditions, it is now important to undertake cytogenetic or molecular genetic analysis (for the *BCR-ABL1* fusion gene) whenever ET is suspected in order to identify any Ph-positive patients and treat them appropriately. If t(9;22)(q34;q11.2) or a *BCR-ABL1* fusion gene is found, the diagnosis is chronic myelogenous leukaemia (CML), even if the WBC is not increased. In the absence of tyrosine kinase therapy, cases of so-called Ph-positive ET, in comparison with true ET, have an increased probability of developing MDS, myelofibrosis or blastic transformation. Prepolycythaemic and occult PV should be distinguished from ET using the tests described above. A bone marrow aspirate and trephine biopsy provide evidence of an MPN and help to distinguish ET from PV and from prefibrotic myelofibrosis. Megakaryocytes are increased in number, large, well lobulated and clustered, whereas the megakaryocytes in PV are more pleomorphic. Reticulin is not increased. It should be noted that iron deficiency alone can cause thrombocytosis, marked erythroid hyperplasia and quite a marked increase in megakaryocytes, so that the diagnosis of essential thrombocythaemia should be made with caution in iron deficient patients. A low serum erythropoietin is seen in as many as a third of patients with ET, so does not help in making a distinction from PV [362]. Plasma thrombopoietin may be normal or decreased but is not elevated. Detection of splenomegaly on ultrasonography supports a diagnosis of ET and makes reactive thrombocytosis very unlikely [461]. Various laboratory tests, such as an elevated plasma fibrinogen, elevated C-reactive protein or an elevated ESR, can provide indirect evidence of an occult neoplasm or connective tissue disorder and thus support a diagnosis of reactive thrombocytosis rather than essential thrombocythaemia. The NAP score is low in a minority of patients, elevated in some and normal in the majority; it is not useful in differentiating Philadelphia-positive and Philadelphia-negative cases and is no longer considered a useful test.

Primary myelofibrosis

Primary myelofibrosis, also known as chronic idiopathic myelofibrosis and myelofibrosis with myeloid metaplasia, is a haematological neoplasm characterised by extramedullary haemopoiesis together with bone marrow fibrosis that is reactive to the underlying proliferation of myeloid cells. The discovery of the *JAK2* V617F mutation has revealed that PV, ET and primary myelofibrosis comprise a cluster of closely related conditions that are distinct from other MPN. Myelofibrosis following either PV or ET is similar to primary myelofibrosis. Polycythaemia occasionally develops during the clinical course of primary myelofibrosis.

Blood film and count

The blood film is leucoerythroblastic and shows anisocytosis and poikilocytosis, particularly the presence of teardrop poikilocytes (Fig. 8.98). There are also short elliptocytes ('stubby' elliptocytes) [462]. In the early stages of the disease there may be leucocytosis and thrombocytosis. Later in the course there is pancytopenia. Often there are some giant platelets, hypogranular platelets and occasional circulating micromegakaryocytes or megakaryocyte nuclei (Fig. 8.99). In multivariate analysis, the severity of the anaemia and the degree of elevation of the WBC are of independent prognostic significance [463].

Therapy with cytoreductive agents such as hydroxycarbamide leads to macrocytosis, stomatocytosis and reduction of the WBC and platelet count. Treatment with thalidomide may increase the WBC, Hb and platelet count [464].

Differential diagnosis

The differential diagnosis includes other causes of a leucoerythroblastic blood film and other causes of pancytopenia (see Tables 6.19 and 6.30). In patients with thrombocytosis, the differential diagnosis includes ET and CML.

Further tests

Molecular genetic analysis for *JAK2* V617F is indicated. This mutation is found in around a half of patients; it is much more common in myelofibrosis following PV than

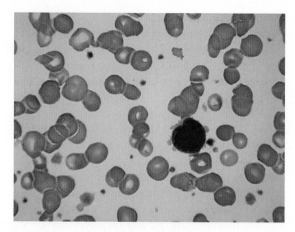

Fig. 8.99 Blood film in primary myelofibrosis showing a circulating megakaryocyte.

in primary myelofibrosis [465]. The prevalence in post-ET myelofibrosis may be intermediate. In cases of primary myelofibrosis, there is a correlation between *JAK2* V617F and a higher Hb. If a *JAK2* mutation is not found, a *CALR* or *MPL* mutation should be sought, being found in about a third and in 10–15% of patients respectively. If none of these mutations is found, molecular analysis for *BCR-ABL1* may be informative.

A bone marrow trephine biopsy is required for diagnosis and for distinguishing early, prefibrotic or hypercellular phase primary myelofibrosis from ET. Cytogenetic analysis can be useful, particularly to exclude the presence of the Philadelphia chromosome. A clonal cytogenetic abnormality is sometimes demonstrated.

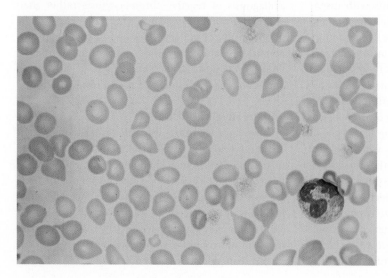

Fig. 8.98 Blood film in primary myelofibrosis showing anisocytosis and poikilocytosis with prominent teardrop poikilocytes.

TEST YOUR KNOWLEDGE

Visit the companion website for MCQs and EMQs
on this topic:
www.wiley.com/go/bain/bloodcells

References

1 Hershko C, Ronson A, Souroujon M, Maschler I, Heyd J and
Patz J (2006) Variable hematologic presentation of autoimmune gastritis: age-related progression from iron deficiency
to cobalamin depletion. *Blood*, **107**, 1673–1679.

2 Pellegrino RM, Coutinho M, D'Ascola D, Lopes AM, Palmieri A, Carnuccio F *et al.* (2012) Two novel mutations in the
tmprss6 gene associated with iron-refractory iron-deficiency
anaemia (irida) and partial expression in the heterozygous
form. *Br J Haematol*, **158**, 670–671.

3 Thomas DW, Hinchliffe RF, Briggs C, Macdougall IC, Littlewood T and Cavill I on behalf of British Committee for
Standards in Haematology (2013) Guideline for the laboratory diagnosis of functional iron deficiency. *Br J Haematol*,
161, 639–648.

4 Harrington AM, Ward PCJ and Kroft SH (2008) Iron
deficiency anemia, β-thalassemia minor, and anemia of
chronic disease. *Am J Clin Pathol*, **129**, 466–471.

5 Jolobe OMP (2000) Prevalence of hypochromia (without
microcytosis) vs microcytosis (without hypochromia) in
iron deficiency. *Clin Lab Haematol*, **22**, 79–80.

6 Patton WN, Cave RJ and Harris RI (1991) A study of
changes in red cell volume and haemoglobin concentration during phlebotomy induced iron deficiency and
iron repletion using the Technicon H1. *Clin Lab Haematol*,
13, 153–161.

7 Jolobe OMP (2011) Mean corpuscular haemoglobin, refer-
enced and resurrected. *J Clin Pathol*, **64**, 833–834.

8 Bessman JD, Gilmer PR and Gardner FH (1983) Improved
classification of the anemias by MCV and RDW. *Am J Clin
Pathol*, **80**, 322–326.

9 Schleper B and Stuerenburg HJ (2001) Copper deficiency-
associated myelopathy in a 46-year-old woman. *J Neurol*,
248, 705–706.

10 Intragumtornchai T, Rojnukkarin P, Swasdikul D and
Israsena S (1998) The role of serum ferritin in the diagnosis
of iron deficiency anemia in patients with liver cirrhosis. *J
Intern Med*, **243**, 233–241.

11 Guyatt GH, Oxman AD, Ali M, Willan A, Mcilroy W and
Patterson C (1992) Laboratory diagnosis of iron-deficiency
anemia: an overview. *J Gen Intern Med*, **7**, 145–153.

12 Corte TJ and Tattersall S (2006) Iron deficiency anaemia:
a presentation of idiopathic pulmonary haemosiderosis. *Int
Med J*, **36**, 207–208.

13 Rüfer A, Howell JP, Lange AP, Yamamoto R, Heuscher
J, Gregor M and Wuillemin WA (2011) Hereditary
hyperferritinemia-cataract syndrome (HHCS) presenting
with iron deficiency anemia associated with a new mutation
in the iron responsive element of the L ferritin gene in a
Swiss family. *Eur J Haematol*, **87**, 274–278.

14 7 Punnonen K, Irjala K and Rajamaki A (1997) Serum
transferrin receptor and its ratio to serum ferritin in the
diagnosis of iron deficiency. *Blood*, **89**, 1052–1057.

15 Cermak J and Brabec V (1998) Transferrin receptor-ferritin
index: a useful parameter in differential diagnosis of iron
deficiency and hyperplastic erythropoiesis. *Eur J Haematol*,
61, 210–212.

16 Rimon E, Levy S, Sapir A, Gelzer G, Peled R, Ergas D and
Sthoeger ZM (2002) Diagnosis of iron deficiency anemia in
the elderly by transferrin receptor-ferritin index. *Arch Intern
Med*, **162**, 445–449.

17 Cook JD, Flowers CH and Skikne BS (2003) The quantitative assessment of body iron. *Blood*, **101**, 3359–3364.

18 Witte DL, Kraemer DF, Johnson GF, Dick FR and Hamilton
H (1986) Prediction of bone marrow iron findings from
tests performed on peripheral blood. *Am J Clin Pathol*, **85**,
202–206.

19 Loría A, Sánchez-Medal L, Lisker R, de Rodríguez E and
Labardini J (1967) Red cell life span in iron deficiency anaemia. *Br J Haematol*, **13**, 294–302.

20 Howard MR, Morley P, Turnbull AJ, Hollier P, Webb R,
Wilkinson H and Clarke A (2000) A prospective study of
screening for coeliac disease in laboratory defined iron and
folate deficiency. *Hematol J*, **1**, Suppl. 1, 41.

21 Weiss G and Goodnough LT (2005) Anemia of chronic
disease. *N Engl J Med*, **353**, 1011–1023.

22 Marsh WL, Bishop JW and Darcy TP (1987) Evaluation of
red cell volume distribution width (RDW). *Hematol Pathol*, **1**,
117–123.

23 Cazzola M, May A, Bergamaschi G, Cerani P, Rosti V and
Bishop DF (2000) Familial-skewed X-chromosome inactivation as a predisposing factor for late-onset X-linked
sideroblastic anemia in carrier females. *Blood*, **96**, 4363–
4365.

24 Pagon RA, Bird TD, Detter JC and Pierce I (1985) Hereditary
sideroblastic anaemia and ataxia: an X linked recessive disorder. *J Med Genet*, **22**, 267–273.

25 Kaneko K, Furuyama K, Fujiwara T, Kobayashi R, Ishida
H, Harigae H and Shibahara S (2014) Identification of
a novel erythroid-specific enhancer for the *ALAS2* gene
and its loss-of-function mutation which is associated
with congenital sideroblastic anemia. *Haematologica*, **99**,
252–261.

26 Kannengiesser C, Sanchez M, Sweeney M, Hetet G, Kerr B,
Moran E *et al.* (2011) Missense *SLC25A38* variations play an
important role in autosomal recessive inherited sideroblastic
anemia. *Haematologica*, **96**, 808–813.

27 Camaschella C, Campanella A, De Falco L, Boschett, L,
Merlini R, Silvestri L *et al.* (2007) The human counterpart of

zebrafish shiraz shows sideroblastic-like microcytic anemia and iron overload. *Blood*, **110**, 1353–1358.

28 Cazzola M and Invernizzi R (2011) Ring sideroblasts and sideroblastic anemias. *Haematologica*, **96**, 789–792.

29 Maguire A, Hellier K, Hammans S and May A (2001) X-linked cerebellar ataxia and sideroblastic anaemia associated with a missense mutation in the *ABC7* gene predicting V411L. *Br J Haematol*, **315**, 910–917.

30 Wiseman DH, May A, Jolles S, Connor P, Powell C, Heeney MM *et al.* (2013) A novel syndrome of congenital sideroblastic anemia, B-cell immunodeficiency, periodic fevers, and developmental delay (SIFD). *Blood*, **122**, 112–123.

31 Holme SA, Worwood M, Anstey AV, Elder GH and Badminton MN (2007) Erythropoiesis and iron metabolism in dominant erythropoietic protoporphyria. *Blood*, **110**, 4108–4110.

32 Grandchamp B, Hetet G, Kannengiesser C, Oudin C, Beaumont C, Rodrigues-Ferreira S *et al.* (2011) A novel type of congenital hypochromic anemia associated with a nonsense mutation in the *STEAP3/TSAP6* gene. *Blood*, **118**, 6660–6666.

33 Sieff CA, Nisbet-Brown E and Nathan DG (2000) Congenital bone marrow failure syndromes. *Br J Haematol*, **111**, 30–37.

34 Borgna-Pignatti C, Marradi P, Pinelli L, Monetti N and Patrini C (1989) Thiamine-responsive anemia in DIDMOAD syndrome. *J Pediatr*, **114**, 405–410.

35 Tuckfield A, Ratnaike S, Hussein S and Metz J (1997) A novel form of hereditary sideroblastic anaemia with macrocytosis. *Br J Haematol*, **97**, 279–285.

36 Aguiar E, Freitas I and Barbot J (2014) Different haematological picture of congenital sideroblastic anaemia in a hemizygote and a heterozygote. *Br J Haematol*, **166**, 469.

37 Vives i Corrons LJ-L (2000) Chronic non-spherocytic haemolytic anaemia due to congenital pyrimidine 5′ nucleotidase deficiency: 25 years later. *Bailière's Clin Haematol*, **13**, 103–118.

38 Mazza U, Saglio G, Cappio FC, Camaschella C, Neretto G and Gallo E (1976) Clinical and haematological data in 254 cases of beta-thalassaemia trait in Italy. *Br J Haematol*, **33**, 91–99.

39 d'Onofrio G, Zini G, Ricerca BM, Mancini S and Mango G (1992) Automated measurement of red blood cell microcytosis and hypochromia in iron deficiency and β-thalassaemia trait. *Arch Pathol Lab Med*, **116**, 84–89.

40 Weatherall DJ and Clegg JB (1981) *The Thalassaemia Syndromes*. Blackwell Scientific Publications, Oxford.

41 Mentzer WC (1973) Differentiation of iron deficiency from thalassaemia trait. *Lancet*, **i**, 882.

42 England JM and Fraser PM (1973) Differentiation of iron deficiency from thalassaemia trait by routine blood count. *Lancet*, **i**, 449–452.

43 England JM, Bain BJ and Fraser PM (1973) Differentiation of iron deficiency from thalassaemia trait. *Lancet*, **i**, 1514.

44 Srivastava PC (1973) Differentiation of thalassaemia minor from iron deficiency. *Lancet*, **ii**, 154–155.

45 Shine I and Lal S (1977) A strategy to detect β thalassaemia trait. *Lancet*, **I**, 692–694.

46 Green R and King R (1989) A new red cell discriminant incorporating volume dispersion for differentiating iron deficiency anemia from thalassemia minor. *Blood Cells*, **15**, 481–495.

47 Jiminez CV, Minchinela J and Ros J (1995) New indices from H2 analyzer improve differentiation between heterozygous β and δβ thalassaemia. *Clin Lab Haematol*, **17**, 151–155.

48 Bain BJ (2006) *Haemoglobinopathy Diagnosis*, 2nd edn, Blackwell Publishing, Oxford.

49 Bain BJ (1988) Screening of antenatal patients in a multiethnic community for β-thalassaemia trait. *J Clin Pathol*, **41**, 481–485.

50 Polliack A and Rachmilewitz EA (1983) Ultrastructural studies in β-thalassaemia major. *Br J Haematol*, **24**, 319–326.

51 Dozy AM, Kan YW, Embury SH, Mentzer WC, Wang WC, Lubin B *et al.* (1979) α-globin gene organization in blacks precludes the severe form of α-thalassaemia. *Nature*, **280**, 605–607.

52 Serjeant GR, Serjeant BE, Forbes M, Hages RJ, Higgs DR and Lehmann H (1986) Haemoglobin gene frequencies in the Jamaican population: a study of 100,000 newborns. *Br J Haematol*, **64**, 253–262.

53 Falusi AG, Esan GJF, Ayyub H and Higgs DR (1987) Alpha-thalassaemia in Nigeria: its interaction with sickle-cell disease. *Eur J Haematol*, **38**, 370–375.

54 Tzotzos S, Kavavakis E, Metaxotou-Mavromati A and Kattamis C (1986) The molecular basis of haemoglobin H disease in Greece. *Br J Haematol*, **63**, 263–271.

55 Serjeant GR (1974) *The Clinical Features of Sickle Cell Disease*. North Holland Publishing Company, Amsterdam.

56 Wong W-Y, Zhou Y, Operskalski EA, Hassett J, Powars DR, Mosley JW and the Transfusion Safety Study Group (1996) Hematologic profile and lymphocyte subpopulations in hemoglobin SC disease: comparison with hemoglobin SS and black controls. *Am J Hematol*, **52**, 150–154.

57 Davis LR (1976) Changing blood picture in sickle cell anaemia from shortly after birth to adolescence. *J Clin Pathol*, **29**, 898–901.

58 Serjeant GR, Grandison Y, Lowrie Y, Mason K, Phillips J, Serjeant BE and Vaidya S (1981) The development of haematological changes in homozygous sickle cell disease: a cohort study from birth to 6 years. *Br J Haematol*, **48**, 533–543.

59 Vichinsky EP, Neumayr LD, Earles AN, Williams R, Lennette ET, Dean D *et al.* (2000) Causes and outcomes of the acute chest syndrome in sickle cell disease. *N Engl J Med*, **342**, 1855–1865.

60 Islam MS and Chia L (2010) Hyperhemolysis syndrome in a patient with sickle cell disease with erythrophagocytosis in peripheral blood. *Eur J Haematol*, **84**, 188.

61 Lesesve J-F and Perrin J (2012) Association of homozygous sickle cell anemia and glucose-6-phosphate dehydrogenase deficiency. *Eur J Haematol*, **88**, 370.

62 Glader BE, Propper RD and Buchanan GR (1979) Microcytosis associated with sickle cell anemia. *Am J Clin Pathol*, **72**, 63–64.

63 Mohandas N, Kim YR, Tycko DH, Orlik J, Wyatt J and Groner W (1986) Accurate and independent measurement of volume and hemoglobin concentration of individual red cells by laser light scattering. *Blood*, **68**, 506–513.

64 Ballard SK and Smith ED (1992) Red blood cell changes during the evolution of the sickle cell painful crisis. *Blood*, **79**, 2154–2163.

65 Monplaisir N, Merault G, Poyart C, Rhoda MD, Craescu CT, Vidaud M *et al.* (1987) Hb-S-Antilles ($\alpha_2\beta_2$Glu Val, 23Va1 Ile): a new variant with lower solubility than Hb S and producing sickle cell disease in heterozygotes. *Acta Haematol*, **78**, 222.

66 Wilson CI, Hopkins PL, Cabello-Inchausti B, Melnick SJ and Robinson MJ (2000) The peripheral blood smear in patients with sickle cell trait: a morphologic observation. *Lab Med*, **31**, 445–447.

67 Mowafy N (2005) *Hematomorphology*. XXXth Congress of the International Society of Hematology, Istanbul.

68 Sheehan RG and Frenkel EP (1983) Influence of hemoglobin phenotype on the mean erythrocyte volume. *Acta Haematol*, **69**, 260–265.

69 Mears JG, Lachman HM, Labie D and Nagel RL (1983) Alpha-thalassaemia trait is related to prolonged survival in sickle cell anemia. *Blood*, **62**, 286–290.

70 Beutler E and West C (2005) Hematologic differences between African-Americans and whites; the role of iron deficiency and α-thalassemia on hemoglobin levels and mean corpuscular volume. *Blood*, **106**, 740–745.

71 Serjeant GR and Serjeant BE (1972) A comparison of erythrocyte characteristics in sickle cell syndromes in Jamaica. *Br J Haematol*, **23**, 205–213.

72 Serjeant GR, Sommereux A, Stevenson M, Mason K and Serjeant BE (1979) Comparison of sickle cell-β^0-thalassaemia with homozygous sickle cell disease. *Br J Haematol*, **41**, 83–93.

73 Bain BJ (1992) Blood film features of sickle cell–haemoglobin C disease. *Br J Haematol*, **83**, 516–518.

74 Diggs LW and Bell A (1965) Intraerythrocytic hemoglobin crystals in sickle cell-hemoglobin C disease. *Blood*, **25**, 218–223.

75 Lawrence C, Hirsch RE, Fataliev NA, Patel S, Fabry ME and Nagel RL (1997) Molecular interactions between Hb α-G Philadelphia, HbC and HbS: phenotypic implications for SC α-G Philadelphia disease. *Blood*, **90**, 2819–2825.

76 Ballas SK, Larner J, Smith ED, Surrey S, Schwartz E and Rappaport EF (1987) The xerocytosis of SC disease. *Blood*, **69**, 124–130.

77 Lachant NA (1987) Hemoglobin E: an emerging hemoglobinopathy in the United States. *Am J Hematol*, **25**, 449–462.

78 Bunyaratvej A, Sahaphong S, Bhamarapravati N and Wasi P (1985) Quantitative changes in red blood cell shapes in relation to clinical features in β-thalassemia/HbE disease. *Am J Clin Pathol*, **83**, 555–559.

79 Rieder RF and Bradley TB (1968) Hemoglobin Gun Hill: an unstable protein associated with chronic hemolysis. *Blood*, **32**, 355–369.

80 Whitehead VM, Rosenblatt DS and Cooper DA (2003) Megaloblastic anemia. In: NathanDG, OrkinSH, GinsburgD and LookAT (eds), *Nathan and Oski's Hematology of Infancy and Childhood*, 6th edn, Saunders, Philadelphia.

81 van der Zee SP, Schretlen ED and Monnens LA (1968) Megaloblastic anaemia in the Lesch-Nyhan syndrome. *Lancet*, **i**, 1427.

82 Andrès E, Affenberger S, Zimmer J, Vinzio S, Grosu D, Pistol G *et al.* (2006) Current hematological findings in cobalamin deficiency. A study of 201 consecutive patients with documented cobalamin deficiency. *Clin Lab Haematol*, **28**, 50–56.

83 Bhatnagar N, Wechalekar A and McNamara C (2012) Pancytopenia due to severe folate deficiency. *Int Med J*, **42**, 1063–1064.

84 Taylor C and Bain BJ (1991) Technicon H.1 automated white cell parameters in the diagnosis of megaloblastic erythropoiesis. *Eur J Haematol*, **46**, 248–249.

85 Bessman JD, Williams LJ and Gilmer PR (1982) Platelet size in health and hematologic disease. *Am J Clin Pathol*, **78**, 150–153.

86 Bain BJ and Taylor C (1991) *L'uso dei parametri leucocitari automatizzati nella diagnosi dell'anemia megaloblastica*. Atti del V Incontro del Club Utilizzatori Sistemi Ematologici Bayer-Technicon, Montecatini Terme, Giugno.

87 Lindenbaum J, Savage DG, Stabler SP and Allen RH (1990) Diagnosis of cobalamin deficiency: II. Relative sensitivities of serum cobalamin, methylmalonic acid, and total homocysteine concentrations. *Am J Hematol*, **34**, 99–107.

88 Savage DG, Lindenbaum J, Stabler SP and Allen RH (1994) Sensitivity of serum methylmalonic acid and total homocysteine determinations for diagnosis of cobalamin and folate deficiencies. *Am J Med*, **96**, 239–246.

89 Muckerheide MM, Wolfman JA, Rohde DA and McManamy GE (1984) Studies on a radioassay for intrinsic factor antibody: comparison of methods and false positive results due to elevated serum B12 levels. *Am J Clin Pathol*, **82**, 300–304.

90 Carmel R (2008) How I treat cobalamin (vitamin B_{12}) deficiency. *Blood*, **112**, 2214–2221.

91 Rovó A, Stüssi G, Meyer-Monard S, Favre G, Tsakiris D, Heim D *et al.* (2010) Sideroblastic changes of the bone marrow can be predicted by the erythrogram of peripheral blood. *Int J Lab Hematol*, **32**, 339–325.

92 Valent P, Bain BJ, Bennett JM, Wimazal F, Sperr WR, Mufti G and Horny HP (2011) Idiopathic cytopenia of undetermined significance (ICUS) and idiopathic dysplasia of uncertain significance (IDUS), and their distinction from low risk MDS. *Leuk Res*, **36**, 1–5.

93 Delaunay J (2002) Molecular basis of red cell membrane disorders. *Acta Haematol*, **108**, 210–218.

94 Tse WT and Lux SE (1999) Red blood cell membrane disorders. *Br J Haematol*, **104**, 2–13.

95 Miraglia del Giudice E, Nobili B, Francese M, d'Urso L, Iolascon A, Eber S and Perrotta S (2001) Clinical and molecular evaluation of non-dominant hereditary spherocytosis. *Br J Haematol*, **112**, 42–47.

96 Bruce LJ and Tanner MJA (2000) Erythroid band 3 variants and disease. *Baillière's Clin Haematol*, **12**, 637–654.

97 McMullin M (1999) The molecular basis of disorders of the red cell membrane. *J Clin Pathol*, **52**, 245–248.

98 Yawata Y (2001) Genotyping and phenotyping characteristics in hereditary red cell membrane disorders. *Gene Funct Dis*, **2**, 113–121.

99 Bruce LJ, Ghosh S, King MJ, Layton M, Mawby WJ, Stewart GJ *et al.* (2002) Absence of CD47 in protein 4.2-deficient hereditary spherocytosis in man: an interaction between the Rh complex and the band 3 complex. *Blood*, **100**, 1878–1885.

100 Ribeiro ML, Alloisio N, Almeida H, Gomes C, Texier P, Lemos C *et al.* (2000) Severe hereditary spherocytosis and distal renal tubular acidosis associated with the total absence of band 3. *Blood*, **96**, 1602–1604.

101 http://www.hgmd.org/ (accessed April 2014).

102 www.omim.org/ (accessed April 2014).

103 Godal HC and Refsum HE (1979) Haemolysis in athletes due to hereditary spherocytosis. *Scand J Haematol*, **22**, 83–86.

104 Delhommeau F, Cynober T, Schischmanoff PO, Rohrlich P, Delaunay J, Mohandas N and Tchernia G (2000) Natural history of hereditary spherocytosis during the first year of life. *Blood*, **95**, 393–397.

105 Sugihara T, Miyashima K and Yawata Y (1984) Disappearance of microspherocytes in peripheral circulation and normalization of decreased lipids in plasma and in red cells of patients with hereditary spherocytosis after splenectomy. *Am J Hematol*, **17**, 129–139.

106 Gallagher PG and Lux SE (2003) Disorders of the erythrocyte membrane. In: Nathan DG, Orkin SH, Ginsburg D and Look AT (eds), *Nathan and Oski's Hematology of Infancy and Childhood*, 6th edn, Saunders, Philadelphia.

107 Palek J and Jarolim P (1993) Clinical expression and laboratory detection of red blood cell membrane protein mutations. *Semin Hematol*, **30**, 249–283.

108 Palek J and Sahr K (1992) Mutations of the red blood cell membrane proteins: from clinical evaluation to detection of the underlying genetic defect. *Blood*, **80**, 308–330.

109 Hassoun H, Vassiliadis JN, Murray J, Yi SJ, Hanspal M, Johnson CA and Palek J (1997) Hereditary spherocytosis with spectrin deficiency due to an unstable truncated β spectrin. *Blood*, **87**, 2538–2545.

110 Hassoun H, Vassiliadis JN, Murray J, Njolstad PR, Rogas JJ, Ballas SH *et al.* (1997) Characterisation of the underlying molecular defect in hereditary spherocytosis associated with spectrin deficiency. *Blood*, **90**, 398–406.

111 Bassères DS, Vincentim DL, Costa FF and Saad STO (1998) β-spectrin Promissão: a translation initiation codon mutation of the β-spectrin gene (ATG→GTG) associated with hereditary spherocytosis and spectrin deficiency in a Brazilian family. *Blood*, **91**, 368–369.

112 Ribeiro ML, Alloisio N, Almeida H, Gomez C, Texier P, Lemos C *et al.* (2000) Severe hereditary spherocytosis and distal renal tubular acidosis associated with total absence of band 3. *Blood*, **96**, 1602–1604.

113 Pati AR, Patten WN and Harris RI (1989) The use of the Technicon H1 in the diagnosis of hereditary spherocytosis. *Clin Lab Haematol*, **11**, 27–30.

114 Chiron M, Cynober T, Mielot F, Tchernia G and Croisolle L (1999) The GEN-S: a fortuitous finding of a routine screening test for hereditary spherocytosis. *Hemato Cell Ther*, **Spring**, 113–116.

115 Broséus J, Visomblain B, Guy J, Maynadié M and Girodon F (2010) Evaluation of mean sphered corpuscular volume for predicting hereditary spherocytosis. *Int J Lab Hematol*, **32**, 519–523.

116 Bolton-Maggs PH, Stevens RF, Dodd NJ, Lamont G, Tittensor P and King MJ; General Haematology Task Force of the British Committee for Standards in Haematology (2004) Guidelines for the diagnosis and management of hereditary spherocytosis. *Br J Haematol*, **126**, 455–474.

117 King M-J, Behrens J, Rogers C, Flynn C, Greenwood D and Chambers K (2000) Rapid flow cytometric test for the diagnosis of membrane cytoskeleton-associated haemolytic anaemia. *Br J Haematol*, **111**, 924–933.

118 Bianchi P, Fermo E, Vercellati C, Marcello AP, Porretti L, Cortelezzi A *et al.* (2012) Diagnostic power of laboratory tests for hereditary spherocytosis: a comparison study on 150 patients grouped according to the molecular and clinical characteristics. *Haematologica*, **97**, 516–523.

119 Girodon F, Garçon L, Bergoin E, Largier M, Delaunay J, Fénéant-Thibault M *et al.* (2008) Usefulness of the eosin-5′-maleimide cytometric method as a first-line screening test for the diagnosis of hereditary spherocytosis: comparison with ektacytometry and protein electrophoresis. *Br J Haematol*, **140**, 468–470.

120 Fawaz NA, Beshlawi IO, Al Zadjali S, Al Ghaithi HK, Elnaggari MA, Elnour I *et al.* (2012) dRTA and hemolytic anemia: first detailed description of *SLC4A1* A858D mutation in homozygous state. *Eur J Haematol*, **88**, 350–355.

121 King M-J (2000) Diagnosis of red cell membrane disorders. *CME Bull Haematol*, **3**, 39–41.

122 Bolton-Maggs PH, Langer JC, Iolascon A, Tittensor P and King MJ; General Haematology Task Force of the British Committee for Standards in Haematology (2010) Guidelines for the diagnosis and management of hereditary spherocytosis–2011 update. *Br J Haematol*, **126**, 455–474.

123 Lecomte MC, Garbarz M, Gautero H, Bournier A, Galand C, Boivin P and Dhermy D (1993) Molecular basis of clinical and morphological heterogeneity in hereditary elliptocytosis (HE) with spectrin I variants. *Br J Haematol*, **85**, 584–595.

124 Iolascon A, Perrotta S and Stewart GW (2003) Red blood cell membrane defects. *Rev Clin Exp Hematol*, **7**, 22–56.

125 Reid ME (1993) Associations of red blood cell membrane abnormalities with blood group phenotype. In: Garratty G (ed.) *Immunobiology of Transfusion Medicine*, Marcel Dekker, New York.

126 Patel SS, Mehlotra RK, Kastens W, Mgone CS, Kazura JW and Zimmerman PA (2001) The association of the glycophorin C exon 3 deletion with ovalocytosis and malaria susceptibility in the Wosera, Papua New Guinea. *Blood*, **98**, 3489–3491.

127 King M-J and Zanella A (2013) Hereditary red cell membrane disorders and laboratory diagnostic testing. *Int J Lab Hematol*, **35**, 237–243.

128 Lecomte MC, Gautero H, Boumier O, Galand C, Lahary A, Vannier JP *et al.* (1992) Elliptocytosis-associated spectrin Rouen ($\beta^{220/218}$) has a truncated but still phosphorylatable β chain. *Br J Haematol*, **80**, 242–250.

129 Jarolim P, Wichterle H, Hasnpal M, Murray J, Rubin HL and Palek J (1995) β spectrin^{PRAGUE}: a truncated β spectrin producing β spectrin deficiency, defective spectrin heterodimers association and a phenotype of spherocytic elliptocytosis. *Br J Haematol*, **91**, 502–510.

130 Bassères DS, Pranke PHL, Vincentim DL, Costa FF and Saad STO (1998b) Expression of spectrin αI/50 hereditary elliptocytosis and its association with the α^{LELY} allele. *Acta Haematol*, **100**, 32–38.

131 Bain BJ, Swirsky D, Bhavnani M, Layton M, Parker N, Makris M *et al.* (2001) British Society for Haematology Slide Session, Annual Scientific Meeting of BSH, Bournemouth, 2000. *Clin Lab Haematol*, **23**, 1–5.

132 Silveira P, Cynober T, Dhermy D, Mohandas N and Tchernia G (1997) Red blood cell abnormalities in hereditary elliptocytosis and their relevance to variable clinical expression. *Am J Clin Pathol*, **108**, 391–399.

133 Conboy JG, Mohandas N, Tchernia G and Kan YW (1986) Molecular basis of hereditary elliptocytosis due to protein 4.1 deficiency. *N Engl J Med*, **315**, 680–685.

134 Alloisio N, Morlé L, Pothier B, Roux A-F, Maréchal J, Ducluzeau M-T *et al.* (1988) Spectrin Oran ($\alpha^{II/21}$), a new spectrin variant concerning the αII domain and causing severe elliptocytosis in the homozygous state. *Blood*, **71**, 1039–1047.

135 Pajor A and Lehozky D (1996) Hemolytic anemia precipitated by pregnancy in a patient with hereditary elliptocytosis. *Am J Hematol*, **52**, 240–241.

136 Castleton A, Burns A, King M-J and McNamara C (2007) Acute anaemia in a renal transplant patient. *Int Med J*, **37**, 419–420.

137 Austin RF and Desforges JF (1969) Hereditary elliptocytosis: an unusual presentation of hemolysis in the newborn associated with transient morphologic abnormalities. *Pediatrics*, **44**, 189–200.

138 Coetzer T, Lawler J, Prchal JT and Palek J (1987) Molecular determinants of clinical expression of hereditary elliptocytosis and pyropoikilocytosis. *Blood*, **70**, 766–772.

139 Djaldetti M, Cohen A and Hart J (1982) Elliptocytosis preceding myelofibrosis in a patient with polycythemia vera. *Acta Haematol*, **72**, 26–28.

140 Rummens IL, Verfaillie C, Criel A, Hidajat M, Vanhoof A, van den Berghe H and Louwagie A (1986) Elliptocytosis and schistocytosis in myelodysplasia: report of two cases. *Acta Haematol*, **75**, 174–177.

141 Kedar PS, Colah RB, Kulkarni S, Ghosh K and Mohanty D (2003) Experience with eosin-5′-maleimide as a diagnostic tool for red cell membrane cytoskeleton disorders. *Clin Lab Haematol*, **26**, 373–376.

142 Palek J and Lambert S (1990) Genetics of the red cell membrane skeleton. *Semin Hematol*, **27**, 290–332.

143 Bain BJ and Liesner R (1996) Pseudopyropoikilocytosis: a striking artefact. *J Clin Pathol*, **49**, 772–773.

144 King MJ, Telfer P, MacKinnon H, Langabeer L, McMahon C, Darbyshire P and Dhermy D (2008) Using the eosin-5-maleimide binding test in the differential diagnosis of hereditary spherocytosis and hereditary pyropoikilocytosis. *Cytometry B Clin Cytom*, **74**, 244–250.

145 Coetzer TL, Beeton L, van Zyl D, Field SP, Agherdien A, Smart E and Daniels GL (1996) Southeast Asian ovalocytosis in a South African kindred with hemolytic anemia. *Blood*, **87**, 1656–1657.

146 Liu S-C, Zhai S, Palek J, Golan DE, Amato D, Hassan K *et al.* (1990) Molecular defect of the band 3 protein in Southeast Asian ovalocytosis. *N Engl J Med*, **323**, 1530–1538.

147 Guizouarn H, Borgese F, Gabillat N, Harrison P, Goede JS, McMahon C *et al.* (2011) South-east Asian ovalocytosis and the cryohydrocytosis form of hereditary stomatocytosis show virtually indistinguishable cation permeability defects. *Br J Haematol*, **152**, 655–664.

148 Laosombat V, Viprakasit V, Dissaneevate S, Leetanaporn R, Chotsampancharoen T, Wongchanchailert M *et al.* (2010) Natural history of Southeast Asian Ovalocytosis during the first 3 years of life. *Blood Cells Mol Dis*, **45**, 29–32.

149 O'Donnel A, Allen SJ, Mgone CS, Martinson JJ, Clegg JB and Weatherall DJ (1998) Red cell morphology and malaria anaemia in children with Southeast Asian ovalocytosis and band 3 in Papua and New Guinea. *Br J Haematol*, **101**, 407–412.

150 Booth PB, Serjeantson S, Woodfield DG and Amato D (1977) Selective depression of blood group antigens associated with hereditary ovalocytosis among Melanesians. *Vox Sang*, **32**, 99–110.

151 Stewart GW, Hepworth-Jones BE, Keen JN, Dash BCJ, Argent AC and Casimir CM (1992) Isolation of cDNA coding for a ubiquitous membrane protein deficient in high Na^+, low K^+ stomatocytic erythrocytes. *Blood*, **79**, 1593–1661.

152 Yawata Y, Kanzaki A, Sugihara T, Inoue T, Yawata A, Kaku M *et al.* (1996) Band 4.2 doublet Nagano: a trait with 72 kD and 74 kD peptides of red cell band 4.2 in equal amount and with increased red cell membrane cholesterol and phosphatidyl choline. *Br J Haematol*, **93**, Suppl. 2, 199.

153 Yawata Y, Kanzaki A, Inoue T, Yawata A, Kaku M, Takezono M *et al.* (1996b) Partial deficiency of band 4.2 due to its impaired binding to a mutated band 3 in a homozygote of band 3 Fukuoka (133 GGA→AGA:Gly→Arg). *Br J Haematol*, **93**, Suppl. 2, 199.

154 Mohandas N and Gascard P (2000) What do mouse gene knockouts tell us about the structure and function of the red cell membrane? *Baillière's Clin Haematol*, **12**, 605–620.

155 Stewart GW and Turner EJH (2000) The hereditary stomatocytoses and allied disorders of erythrocyte membrane permeability to Na and K. *Baillière's Clin Haematol*, **12**, 707–727.

156 Bruce LJ, Guizouarn H, Burton NM, Gabillat N, Poole J, Flatt JF *et al.* (2009) The monovalent cation leak in overhydrated stomatocytic red blood cells results from amino acid substitutions in the Rh-associated glycoprotein, *Blood*, **113**, 1350–1357.

157 Zarychanski R, Schulz VP, Houston BL, Maksimova Y, Houston DS, Smith B *et al.* (2012) Mutations in the mechanotransduction protein PIEZO1 are associated with hereditary xerocytosis. *Blood*, **120**, 1908–1915.

158 Andolfo I, Alper SL, De Franceschi L, Auriemma C, Ruisso T, De Falco L *et al.* (2013) Multiple clinical forms of dehydrated hereditary stomatocytosis arise from mutations in PIEZO1. *Blood*, **121**, 3295–3935.

159 Bruce LJ, Robinson HC, Guizouarn H, Borgese F, Harrison P, King M-J *et al.* (2005) Monovalent cation leaks in human red cells caused by single amino-acid substitutions in the transport domain of the band 3 chloride-bicarbonate exchanger, AE1. *Nat Genet*, **37**, 1258–1263.

160 Flatt JF, Guizouarn H, Burton NM, Borgese F, Tomlinson RJ, Forsyth RJ *et al.* (2011) Stomatin-deficient cryohydrocytosis results from mutations in *SLC2A1*: a novel form of GLUT1 deficiency syndrome. *Blood*, **118**, 5267–5277.

161 Barton CJ, Chowdhury V and Marin D (2003) Hereditary haemolytic anaemias and parvovirus infections in Jehovah's witnesses. *Br J Haematol*, **121**, 675–676.

162 Jackson JM, Stanley ML, Crawford IG, Barr AL and Hilton HB (1978) The problem of Mediterranean stomatocytosis. *Aust NZ J Med*, **8**, 216–217.

163 Grootenboer S, Schischmanhoff PO, Cynober T, Rodrigue J-C, Delaunay J, Tchernia G and Dommergues J-P (1998) A genetic syndrome associating dehydrated hereditary stomatocytosis, pseudohyperkalaemia and perinatal oedema. *Br J Haematol*, **103**, 383–386.

164 Clark MR, Shohet SB and Gottfried EL (1993) Hereditary hemolytic disease with increased red blood cell phosphatidylcholine and dehydration: one, two, or many disorders? *Am J Hematol*, **42**, 25–30.

165 Vives Corrons JL, Besson I, Merino A, Monteagudo J, Reverter JC, Aguilar JL and Enrich C (1991) Occurrence of hereditary leaky red cell syndrome and partial coagulation factor VII deficiency in a Spanish family. *Acta Haematol*, **86**, 194–199.

166 Stewart GW, Corrall RJM, Fyffe JA, Stockdill GM and Strong JA (1979) Familial pseudohyperkalaemia: a new syndrome. *Lancet*, **ii**, 175–177.

167 Haines PG, Crawley C, Chetty MC, Jarvis H, Coles SE, Fisher J *et al.* (2001) Familial pseudohyperkalaemia Chiswick: a novel congenital thermotropic variant of K and Na transport across the human red cell membrane. *Br J Haematol*, **112**, 469–474.

168 Coles SE, Chetty MC, Ho MM, Nicolaou A, Kearney JW, Wright SD and Stewart GW (1999) Two British families with variants of the 'cryohydrocytosis' form of hereditary stomatocytosis. *Br J Haematol*, **105**, 1055–1065.

169 Haines PG, Jarvis HG, King S, Noormohamed FH, Chetty MC, Coles SE *et al.* (2001) Two further British families with the 'cryohydrocytosis' form of hereditary stomatocytosis. *Br J Haematol*, **113**, 932–937.

170 Fricke B, Jarvis HG, Reid CD, Aguilar-Martinez P, Robert A, Quitted P *et al.* (2004) Four new cases of stomatin-deficient hereditary stomatocytosis syndrome: association of the stomatin-deficient cryohydrocytosis variant with neurological dysfunction. *Br J Haematol*, **125**, 796–803.

171 Weber YG, Storch A, Wuttke TV, Brockmann K, Kempfle J, Maljevic S *et al.* (2008) GLUT1 mutations are a cause of paroxysmal exertion-induced dyskinesias and induce hemolytic anemia by a cation leak. *J Clin Invest*, **118**, 2157–2168.

172 Rees DC, Iolascon A, Carella M, O'Marcaigh AS, Kendra JR, Jowitt SN *et al.* (2005) Stomatocytic haemolysis and macrothrombocytopenia (Mediterranean stomatocytosis/macrothrombocytopenia) is the haematological presentation of phytosterolaemia. *Br J Haematol*, **130**, 297–309.

173 Stewart GW, Lloyd J and Pegel K (2006) Mediterranean stomatocytosis/macrothrombocytopenia: update from Adelaide, Australia. *Br J Haematol*, **132**, 651–661.

174 Redman CM, Russo D and Lee S (2000) Kell, Kx and the McLeod phenotype. *Baillière's Clin Haematol*, **12**, 621–635.

175 Hardie RJ (1989) Acanthocytosis and neurological impairment—a review. *Q J Med*, **71**, 291–306.

176 Kay MM, Bosman GJ and Lawrence C (1988) Functional topography of band 3: specific structural alteration linked to functional aberrations in human erythrocytes. *Proc Nat Acad Sci*, **85**, 492–496.

177 Bruce LJ, Kay MM, Lawrence C and Tanner MJ (1993) Band 3 HT, a human red-cell variant associated with acanthocytosis and increased anion transport, carries the mutation pro868-to-leu in the membrane domain of band 3. *Biochem J*, **293**, 317–320.

178 Yamashima M, Ueda E, Kinoshita T, Takami T, Ojima A, Ono H *et al.* (1990) Inherited complete deficiency of 20-kilodalton homologous restriction factor (CD59) as a cause of paroxysmal nocturnal hemoglobinuria. *N Engl J Med*, **328**, 1184–1189.

179 Cartron J-P (2000) *RH* blood group system and molecular basis of Rh-deficiency. *Baillière's Clin Haematol*, **12**, 655–689.

180 Wood L, Jacobs P, Byrne M, Marais D and Jackson G (1997) Iron deficiency as a consequence of serial plasma exchange for the management of familial hypercholesterolaemia. *Proceedings of the 37th Annual Congress of the South African Societies of Pathology*, 160.

181 Bernini L, Latte B, Siniscalco M, Piomelli S, Spada U, Adinolfi M and Mollison PL (1964) Survival of ^{51}Cr-labelled red cells in subjects with thalassaemia-trait or G6PD deficiency or both abnormalities. *Br J Haematol*, **10**, 171–180.

182 Piomelli S and Siniscalco M (1969) The haematological effects of glucose-6-phosphate dehydrogenase deficiency and thalassaemia trait: interaction between the two genes at the phenotype level. *Br J Haematol*, **16**, 537–549.

183 Mehta A, Mason PJ and Vulliamy TJ (2000) Glucose-6-phosphate dehydrogenase deficiency. *Baillière's Clin Haematol*, **13**, 21–38.

184 Lim F, Vulliamy T and Abdalla SH (2005) An Ashenkenazi Jewish woman presenting with favism. *J Clin Pathol*, **58**, 317–319.

185 Zanella A, Fermo E, Bianchi P and Valentini G (2005) Red cell pyruvate kinase deficiency: molecular and clinical aspects. *Br J Haematol*, **130**, 11–25.

186 Mentzer WC (2003) Pyruvate kinase deficiency and disorders of glycolysis. In: NathanDG, OrkinSH, GinsburgD and LookAT (eds), *Nathan and Oski's Hematology of Infancy and Childhood*, 6th edn, Saunders, Philadelphia.

187 Mainwaring CJ, James CM, Butcher J and Clarke S (2001) Haemolysis and the combined oral contraceptive pill. *Br J Haematol*, **115**, 710–714.

188 Branca R, Costa E, Rocha S, Coelho H, Quintanilha A, Cabeda JM *et al.* (2004) Coexistence of congenital red cell pyruvate kinase and band 3 deficiency. *Clin Lab Haematol*, **26**, 297–300.

189 Leblond PF, Lyonnais J and Delage J-M (1978) Erythrocyte populations in pyruvate kinase deficiency anaemias following splenectomy. *Br J Haematol*, **39**, 55–61.

190 Brecher G and Bessis M (1972) Present status of spiculated red cells and their relationship to the discocyte-echinocyte transformation: a critical review. *Blood*, **40**, 333–344.

191 van Wijk R and van Solinge WW (2005) The energy-less red blood cell is lost: erythrocyte enzyme abnormalities of glycolysis. *Blood*, **106**, 4034–4042.

192 Fujii H and Miwa S (1990) Recent progress in the molecular genetic analysis of erythroenzymopathy. *Am J Hematol*, **34**, 301–310.

193 Tanaka KR and Zerez CR (1990) Red cell enzymopathies of the glycolytic pathway. *Semin Hematol*, **27**, 165–185.

194 McMullin M (1999) The molecular basis of disorders of red cell enzymes. *J Clin Pathol*, **52**, 241–244.

195 Jacobasch G (2000) Biochemical and genetic basis of red cell enzyme deficiencies. *Baillière's Clin Haematol*, **13**, 1–20.

196 Kanno H (2000) Hekokinase: gene structure and mutations. *Baillière's Clin Haematol*, **13**, 83–88.

197 Kanno H, Murakami K, Hariyama Y, Ishikawa K, Miwa S and Fujii H (2002) Homozygous intragenic deletion of type I hexokinase gene causes lethal hemolytic anemia of the affected fetus. *Blood*, **100**, 1930.

198 Kugler W and Lakomek M (2000) Glucose-6-phosphate isomerase deficiency. *Baillière's Clin Haematol*, **13**, 89–102.

199 Fujii H and Miwa S (2000) Other erythrocyte enzyme deficiencies associated with non-haematological symptoms: phosphoglycerate kinase and phosphofructokinase deficiency. *Baillière's Clin Haematol*, **13**, 141–148.

200 Kreuder J, Borkhardt A, Repp R, Pekrun A, Gottsche B, Gottschalk U *et al.* (1996) Brief report: inherited metabolic myelopathy and hemolysis due to a mutation in aldolase A. *N Engl J Med*, **334**, 1100–1104.

201 Yao DC, Tolan DR, Murray MF, Harris DJ, Darras BT, Geva A and Neufeld EJ (2004) Hemolytic anemia and severe rhabdomyolysis caused by compound heterozygous mutations of the gene for erythrocyte/muscle isozyme of aldolase, ALDOA(Arg303X/Cys338Tyr). *Blood*, **103**, 2401–2403.

202 Schneider A (2000) Triosephosphate isomerase deficiency: historical perspectives and molecular aspects. *Baillière's Clin Haematol*, **13**, 119–140.

203 Valentin C, Pissard S, Martin J, Héron D, Labrune P, Livet M-O *et al.* (2000) Triose phosphate isomerase deficiency in 3 French families: two novel null alleles, a frameshift mutation (TPI Altfortville) and an alteration in the initiation codon (TPI Paris) *Blood*, **96**, 1130–1135.

204 Zanella A and Bianchi P (2000) Red cell pyruvate kinase deficiency: from genetics to clinical manifestations. *Baillière's Clin Haematol*, **13**, 57–82.

205 Bianchi P, Zappa M, Bredi E, Vercellati C, Pelissero G, Barraco F and Zanella A (1999) A case of complete adenylate kinase deficiency due to a nonsense mutation in *AK-1* gene (Arg 107→Stop, CGA→TGA) associated with chronic haemolytic anaemia. *Br J Haematol*, **105**, 75–79.

206 Toren A, Brok-Simoni F, Ben-Bassat I, Holtzman F, Mandel M, Neumann Y *et al.* (1994) Congenital haemolytic anaemia associated with adenylate kinase deficiency. *Br J Haematol*, **87**, 376–380.

207 Bianchi P, Fermo E, Alfinito F, Vercellati C, Baserga M, Ferraro F *et al.* (2003) Molecular characterization of six unrelated Italian patients affected by pyrimidine 5′-nucleotidase deficiency. *Br J Haematol*, **122**, 847–851.

208 Rees DC, Duley DA and Marinaki AM (2003) Pyrimidine 5′ nucleotidase deficiency. *Br J Haematol*, **120**, 375–383.

209 Zanella A, Bianchi P, Fermo E and Valentini G (2006) Hereditary pyrimidine 5′ nucleotidase deficiency; from genetics to clinical manifestations. *Br J Haematol*, **133**, 113–123.

210 Chottiner EG, Ginsburg D, Tartaglia AP and Mitchell BS (1989) Erythrocyte adenosine deaminase overproduction in hereditary haemolytic anemia. *Blood*, **74**, 448–453.

211 Fiorelli G, Martinez di Montmuros F and Cappellini MD (2000) Chronic non-spherocytic haemolytic disorders associated with glucose-6-phosphate dehydrogenase variants. *Baillière's Clin Haematol*, **13**, 39–55.

212 Ristoff E, Augustson C, Geissler J, de Rijk T, Carlsson K, Luo J-L *et al.* (2000) A missense mutation in the heavy subunit of γ-glutamylcysteine synthetase gene causes hemolytic anemia. *Blood*, **95**, 2193–2197.

213 Mañú Pereira M, Gelbart T, Ristoff E, Crain KC, Bergua JM, López Lafuente A *et al.* (2007) Chronic non-spherocytic hemolytic anemia associated with severe neurological disease due to γ-glutamylcysteine synthetase deficiency in a patient of Moroccan origin. *Haematologica*, **92**, e102–e105.

214 Vives Corrons J-L, Alvarez R, Pujades A, Zarza R, Oliva E, Lasheras G *et al.* (2001) Hereditary non-spherocytic haemolytic anaemia due to red blood cell glutathione synthetase deficiency in four unrelated patients from Spain: clinical and molecular studies. *Br J Haematol*, **112**, 475–482.

215 Boxer LA, Oliver JM, Spielberg SP, Allen JM and Schulman JD (1979) Protection of granulocytes by vitamin E in glutathione synthetase deficiency. *N Engl J Med*, **310**, 901–905.

216 Necheles TF, Steinberg MH and Cameron D (1970) Erythrocyte glutathione peroxidase deficiency. *Br J Haematol*, **19**, 605–612.

217 Kamerbeek NM, van Zwieten R, de Boer M, Morren G, Vuil H, Bannink N *et al.* (2007) Molecular basis of glutathione reductase deficiency in human blood cells. *Blood*, **109**, 3560–3566.

218 Schneider A, Westwood B, Yim C, Prchal J, Berkow R, Labotka R *et al.* (1995) Triosephosphate isomerase deficiency: repetitive occurrence of a point mutation in amino acid 104 in multiple apparently unrelated families. *Am J Hematol*, **50**, 263–268.

219 Miwa S, Fujii H, Tani K, Takahashi K, Takegawa S, Fujinami N *et al.* (1981) Two cases of red cell aldolase deficiency associated with hereditary hemolytic anemia in a Japanese family. *Am J Hematol*, **11**, 425–437.

220 Feo CJ, Tchernia G, Subtil E and Leblond PF (1978) Observations of echinocytosis in eight patients: a phase contrast and SEM study. *Br J Haematol*, **40**, 519–526.

221 Valentine WN, Schneider AS and Baughan MA (1966) Hereditary hemolytic anemia with triosephosphate isomerase deficiency. Studies in kindreds with coexisting sickle cell trait and erythrocyte glucose-6-phosphate dehydrogenase deficiency. *Am J Med*, **41**, 27–41.

222 Vives Corrons JL, Camera A, Triginer J, Kahn A and Rozman C (1974) Anemia hemolitica por déficit congénito en fosfohexosaisomerasa—descripcíon de una nueva variante (PHI Barcelon) con estomatocitosis y disminucíon de la resistencia osmotica eritrocitaria. *Sangre*, **20**, 197–206.

223 Qualtieri A, Pedoce V, Bisconte MG, Bria M, Gulino B, Andreoli V and Brancati C (1997) Severe erythrocyte adenylate kinase deficiency due to homozygous A→G substitution at codon 164 of human AK1 gene associated with chronic haemolytic anaemia. *Br J Haematol*, **99**, 770–776.

224 Fermo E, Bianchi P, Vercellati C, Micheli C, Marcello AP, Portaleone D and Zanella A (2004) A new variant of adenylate kinase (delG138) associated with severe hemolytic anemia. *Blood Cells Mol Dis*, **33**, 146–149.

225 Travis SF, Martinez J, Garvin J, Atwater J and Gillmer P (1978) Study of a kindred with partial deficiency of red cell 2,3-diphoshoglycerate mutase (2,3-DPGM) and compensated hemolysis. *Blood*, **51**, 1107–1116.

226 Desnick RJ and Astrin KH (2002) Congenital erythropoietic porphyria: advances in pathogenesis and treatment. *Br J Haematol*, **117**, 779–795.

227 Merino A, To-Figueras J and Herrero C (2006) Atypical red cell inclusions in congenital erythropoietic porphyria. *Br J Haematol*, **132**, 124.

228 Lamoril J, Puy H, Gouya L, Rosipal R, da Silva V, Grandchamp B *et al.* (1998) Neonatal hemolytic anemia due to inherited harderoporphyria: clinical characteristics and molecular basis. *Blood*, **91**, 1453–1457.

229 Mittal S, Blaylock MG, Culligan DJ, Barker RN and Vickers MA (2008) A high rate of CLL phenotype lymphocytes in autoimmune hemolytic anemia and immune thrombocytopenic purpura. *Haematologica*, **93**, 151–152.

230 Stavroyianni N, Stamatopoulos K, Viniou M, Vaiopoulos G and Yataganas X (2001) Autoimmune haemolytic anemia during α-interferon treatment in a patient with chronic myelogenous leukemia. *Leuk Res*, **25**, 1097–1098.

231 Steer JA, Tasker S, Barker EN, Jensen J, Mitchell J, Stocki T *et al*. (2011) A novel hemotropic mycoplasma (hemoplasma) in a patient with hemolytic anemia and pyrexia. *Cin Infect Dis*, **53**, e147–e151.

232 Mahlaoui N, Pellier I, Mignot C, Jais JP, Bilhou-Nabéra C, Moshous D *et al*. (2013) Characteristics and outcome of early-onset, severe forms of Wiskott-Aldrich syndrome. *Blood*, **121**, 1510–1516.

233 Packman CH (2008) Hemolytic anemia due to warm autoantibodies. *Blood Rev*, **22**, 17–31.

234 Farolino DL, Rustagi PK, Currie MS, Doeblin TD and Logue GL (1986) Teardrop-shaped red cells in autoimmune hemolytic anemia. *Am J Hematol*, **21**, 415–418.

235 Pettit JE, Scott J and Hussein S (1976) EDTA dependent red cell neutrophil rosetting in autoimmune haemolytic anaemia. *J Clin Pathol*, **29**, 345–346.

236 Ervin DM, Christian RM and Young L (1950) Dangerous universal donors. *Blood*, **5**, 553–567.

237 Garratty G and Petz LD (2007) Direct antiglobulin test negative autoimmune haemolytic anaemia associated with fludarabine/cyclophosphamide/rituximab therapy. *Br J Haematol*, **139**, 622–623.

238 Teachey DT, Manno CS, Axsom KM, Andrews T, Choi JK, Greenbaum BH *et al*. (2005) Unmasking Evans syndrome: T-cell phenotype and apoptotic response reveal autoimmune lymphoproliferative syndrome (ALPS). *Blood*, **105**, 2443–2448.

239 Petz LD (2008) Cold antibody autoimmune haemolytic anemias. *Blood Rev*, **22**, 1–15.

240 Wehbe E and Moore TA (2008) Cold agglutinin-associated hemolytic anemia due to brucellosis: first case report. *Am J Hematol*, **83**, 685–686.

241 Sivakumaran M, Murphy PT, Booker DJ, Wood JK, Stampo R and Sohol RJ (1999) Paroxysmal cold haemoglobinuria caused by non-Hodgkin's lymphoma. *Br J Haematol*, **105**, 278–279.

242 Bharadwaj V, Chakravorty S and Bain BJ (2011) The cause of sudden anemia revealed by the blood film. *Am J Hematol*, **87**, 520.

243 Gregory GP, Opat S, Quach H, Shortt J and Tran H (2011) Failure of eculizumab to correct paroxysmal cold hemoglobinuria. *Ann Hematol*, **90**, 989–990.

244 Jordan WS, Prouty RL, Heinle RW and Dingle JH (1952) The mechanism of hemolysis in paroxysmal cold hemoglobinuria. *Blood*, **7**, 387–403.

245 Sokol RJ, Hewitt S and Stamps BK (1983) Autoimmune hemolysis: mixed warm and cold antibody type. *Acta Haematol*, **69**, 266–274.

246 Arndt OA and Garratty G (2005) The changing spectrum of drug-induced immune hemolytic anemia. *Semin Hematol*, **42**, 137–144.

247 Bauer P, Bellou A and El Kouch S (1998) Acute intravascular haemolysis after pollen ingestion. *Ann Intern Med*, **129**, 72–73.

248 Radhakrishnan K, Tan C and Gallo J (2008) Erythrophagocytosis in haemolytic disease of the newborn. *Am J Hematol*, **83**, 679.

249 Koenig JM and Christensen RD (1989). Neutropenia and thrombocytopenia in infants with Rh hemolytic disease. *J Pediatr*, **114**, 625–631.

250 Davies NP, Buggins AGS, Snijders AJM, Noble PN, Layton DM and Nicolaides KH (1992) Fetal leucocyte count in rhesus disease. *Arch Dis Child*, **67**, 404–406.

251 Vaughan JI, Manning M, Warwick RM, Letsky EA, Murray NA and Roberts IAG (1998) Inhibition of erythroid progenitor cells by anti-Kell antibodies in fetal alloimmune anemia. *N Engl J Med*, **338**, 798–803.

252 Wagner T, Bernaschek G and Geissler G (2000) Inhibition of megakaryopoiesis by Kell-related antibodies. *N Engl J Med*, **343**, 72.

253 Gaines AR (2000) Acute hemoglobinemia and/or hemoglobinuria and sequelae following $Rh_0(D)$ immune globulin intravenous administration in immune thrombocytopenic purpura patients. *Blood*, **95**, 2523–2529.

254 Bolan CD, Childs RW, Proctor JL, Barrett JA and Leitman SF (2001) Massive immune haemolysis after allogeneic peripheral blood stem cell transplantation with minor ABO incompatibility. *Br J Haematol*, **112**, 787–795.

255 Bader-Meunier B, Croisille L, Ledeist F, Rince P, Miélot F, Fabre M *et al*. (1997) Dyserythropoiesis and hemolytic anemia as initial presentation of Fas deficiency conditions. *Blood*, **90**, Suppl 1, 316a.

256 Schulman I, Pierce M, Lukens A and Currimbhoy Z (1960) Studies on thrombopoiesis I. A factor in normal human plasma required for platelet production, chronic thrombocytopenia due to its deficiency. *Blood*, **16**, 943–957.

257 Upshaw JD (1978) Congenital deficiency of a factor in normal plasma that reverses microangiopathic hemolysis and thrombocytopenia. *N Engl J Med*, **298**, 1350–1352.

258 Remuzzi G, Ruggenenti P, Codazzi D, Noris M, Caprioli J, Locatelli G and Gridelli B (2003) Combined kidney and liver transplantation for familial haemolytic uraemic syndrome. *Lancet*, **359**, 1671–1672.

259 Caprioli J, Noris M, Brioschi S, Pianetti G, Castelletti F, Bettinaglio P *et al*. (2006) Genetics of HUS: the impact of MCP, CFH, and IF mutations on clinical presentation, response to treatment, and outcome. *Blood*, **108**, 1267–1279.

260 Yachie A, Niida Y, Wada T, Igarashi N, Kaneda H, Toma T *et al*. (1999) Oxidative stress causes enhanced endothelial cell injury in human heme oxygenase-1 deficiency. *J Clin Invest*, **103**, 129–135.

261 Geraghty MT, Perlman EJ, Martin LS, Hayflick SJ, Casella JF, Rosenblatt DS and Valle D (1992) Cobalamin C defect

associated with hemolytic-uremic syndrome. *J Pediatr*, **120**, 934–937.

262 Riggs SA, Wray NP, Waddell CC, Rossen RD and Gyorkey F (1982) Thrombotic thrombocytopenic purpura complicating Legionnaires' disease. *Arch Intern Med*, **142**, 2275–2280.

263 Case Records of the Massachusetts General Hospital (1997) A 43-year-old woman with rapidly changing pulmonary infiltrates and markedly increased intracranial pressure. *N Engl J Med*, **337**, 1149–1156.

264 Schröder St, Spyridopoulos I, König J, Jaschonek KG, Luft D and Seif FJ (1995) Thrombotic thrombocytopenic purpura (TTP) associated with a *Borrelia burgdorferi* infection. *Am J Hematol*, **50**, 72–73.

265 Communicable Disease Report (2000) Active surveillance for rare and serious diseases in children. *CDR Weekly*, **10**, 349 and 352.

266 Allford SL, Hunt BJ, Rose P and Machin SJ, on behalf of the Haemostasis and Thrombosis Task Force of the British Committee for Standards in Haematology (2003) Guidelines on the diagnosis and management of the thrombotic microangiopathic haemolytic anaemias. *Br J Haematol*, **120**, 556–573.

267 Selleng K, Warkentin TE, Greinacher A, Morris AM, Walker IR, Heggtveit HA *et al.* (2007) Very severe thrombocytopenia and fragmentation hemolysis mimicking thrombotic thrombocytopenic purpura associated with a giant intracardiac vegetation infected with Staphylococcus epidermidis: role of monocyte procoagulant activity induced by bacterial supernatant. *Am J Hematol*, **82**, 766–771.

268 Kuperman AA, Baidousi A, Nasser M, Braester A and Nassar F (2010) Microangiopathic anemia of acute brucellosis. *Mediterr J Hematol Infect Dis*, **2**, e2010031.

269 Quinn DK, Quinn J, Conlon PJ and Murphy PT (2013) A case of leptospirosis presenting as TTP. *Am J Hematol*, **88**, 337.

270 Matsuda Y, Hara J, Miyoshi H, Osugi Y, Fujisaki H, Takai K *et al.* (1999) Thrombotic microangiopathy associated with reactivation of human herpesvirus 6 following high-dose chemotherapy with autologous bone marrow transplantation in young children. *Bone Marrow Transplant*, **24**, 919–923.

271 Turner RC, Chaplinski TI and Adams HG (1986) Rocky Mountain spotted fever presenting as thrombotic thrombocytopenic purpura. *Am J Med*, **81**, 153–157.

272 Kwaan HC (1987) Miscellaneous secondary thrombotic microangiopathy. *Semin Hematol*, **24**, 141–147.

273 Nishiura T, Miyazaki Y, Oritani K, Tominaga N, Tomiyama Y, Katagiri S *et al.* (1986) *Aspergillus* vegetative endocarditis complicated with schizocytic hemolytic anemia in a patient with acute lymphocytic leukemia. *Acta Haematol*, **76**, 60–62.

274 Meir BM, Amital H, Levy Y, Kneller A and Bar-Dayan Y (2000) *Mycoplasma-pneumoniae*-induced thrombotic thrombocytopenic purpura. *Acta Haematol*, **103**, 112–115.

275 Fassas AB-T, Buddharaju LN, Rapoport A, Cottler-Fox M, Drachenberg C, Meisenberg B and Tricot G (2001) Fatal disseminated adenoviral infection associated with thrombotic thrombocytopenic purpura after allogeneic bone marrow transplantation. *Leuk Lymphoma*, **42**, 801–804.

276 Brown RC, Blecher TE, French EA and Toghill PJ (1973) Thrombotic thrombocytopenic purpura after influenza vaccination. *BMJ*, **ii**, 303.

277 George JN (2000) How I treat patients with thrombotic thrombocytopenic purpura-hemolytic uremic syndrome. *Blood*, **96**, 1223–1229.

278 Koujouri K, Vesely SK and George JN (2001) Quinine-associated thrombotic thrombocytopenic purpura-hemolytic uremic syndrome: frequency, clinical features, and long-term outcomes. *Ann Intern Med*, **135**, 1047–1051.

279 Leach JW, Pham T, Diamandidis D and Georg JN (1999) Thrombotic thrombocytopenia purpura—hemolytic uremic syndrome (TTP-HUS) following treatment with deoxycoformycin in a patient with cutaneous T-cell lymphoma (Sézary syndrome): a case report. *Am J Hematol*, **61**, 268–270.

280 Hankey GT (2000) Clopidogrel and thrombotic thrombocytopenic purpura. *Lancet*, **356**, 269–270.

281 Humphreys BD, Sharman JP, Henderson JM, Clark JW, Marks PW, Rennke HG *et al.* (2004) Gemcitabine-associated thrombotic microangiopathy. *Cancer*, **100**, 2664–2670.

282 Kwaan HC and Gordon LI (2001) Thrombotic microangiopathy in the cancer patient. *Acta Haematol*, **106**, 52–56.

283 Mach-Pascual S, Samii K and Beris P (1996) Microangiopathic hemolytic anemia complicating FK506 (tacrolimus) therapy. *Am J Hematol*, **52**, 310–312.

284 McCarthy LJ, Porcu P, Fausel CA, Sweeney CJ and Danielson CFM (1998) Thrombotic thombocytopenic purpura and simvastatin. *Lancet*, **352**, 1284–1285.

285 Kupfer Y and Tessler S (1997) Ticlopidine and thrombotic thrombocytopenic purpura. *N Engl J Med*, **337**, 1245.

286 Bennett CL, Connors JM, Carwile JM, Moake JL, Bell WR, Tarantolo SR *et al.* (2000) Thrombotic thrombocytopenic purpura associated with clopidogrel. *N Engl J Med*, **342**, 1773–1777.

287 Case Records of the Massachusetts General Hospital (1999) A 54-year-old woman with acute renal failure and thrombocytopenia. *N Engl J Med*, **340**, 1900–1909.

288 Lipton JH and Minden M (1995) CML may not be part of HUS. *Am J Hematol*, **49**, 100–101.

289 Masokoane SI (2000) Dangers of uninformed use of "African Pitocine". 24th World Congress of Medical Technology, Vancouver, Canada.

290 Maguire RB, Stroncek DF and Campbell AC (1993) Recurrent pancytopenia, coagulopathy, and renal failure

associated with multiple quinine-dependent antibodies. *Ann Intern Med*, **119**, 215–217.

291 Kreitman RJ, Wilson WH, Bergeron K, Raggio M, Stetler-Stevenson M, Fitzgerald DJ and Pastan I (2001) Efficacy of the anti-CD22 recombinant immunotoxin BL22 in chemotherapy-resistant hairy cell leukemia. *N Engl J Med*, **345**, 241–247.

292 Fujita H, Takemura S, Hyo R, Tanaka M, Koharazawa H, Fujisawa S *et al.* (2003) Pulmonary embolism and thrombotic thrombocytopenic purpura in acute promyelocytic leukemia treated with all-*trans* retinoic acid. *Leuk Lymphoma*, **44**, 1627–1629.

293 Eremina V, Jefferson JA, Kowalewska J, Hochster H, Haas M, Weisstuch J *et al.* (2008) VEGF inhibition and renal thrombotic microangiopathy. *N Engl J Med*, **358**, 1129–1136.

294 Amjad AI and Parikh RA (2013) Opana-ER used the wrong way: intravenous abuse leading to microangiopathic hemolysis and a TTP-like syndrome. *Blood*, **122**, 3403.

295 Musa MA, Nounou R, Sahovic E, Seth P, Qadi A and Aljurf M (2000) Fulminant thrombotic thrombocytopenic purpura in two patients with systemic lupus erythematosus and phospholipid autoantibodies. *Eur J Haematol*, **64**, 433–435.

296 Salyer WR, Salyer DC and Heptinstall RH (1973) Scleroderma and microangiopathic hemolytic anemia. *Ann Intern Med*, **78**, 895–897.

297 Brunning RD, Jacob HS, Brenckman WD, Jimenez-Pasqau F and Goetz FC (1976) Fragmentation hemolysis in patients with severe diabetic angiopathy. *Br J Haematol*, **34**, 283–289.

298 Silva VA (1995) Thrombotic thrombocytopenic purpura/hemolytic uremic syndrome secondary to pancreatitis. *Am J Clin Pathol*, **103**, 519.

299 Cho YU, Chi HS, Park CJ, Jang S, Cho YM and Park JS (2009) A case of light chain deposition disease involving kidney and bone marrow with microangiopathic hemolytic anemia. *Korean J Lab Med*, **29**, 384–389.

300 Stepien KM, Prinsloo P, Hitch T, McCulloch TA and Sims R (2011) Acute renal failure, microangiopathic haemolytic anemia, and secondary oxalosis in a young female patient. *Int J Nephrol*, 2011, 679160.

301 Kaplon M, Karnad A, Mehata J and Krishnan J (1999) Left atrial myxoma complicated by microangiopathic haemolytic anemia (MAHA). *Blood*, **94**, Suppl. 1, Part 2, 6b.

302 Fairley S and Ihle BU (1986) Thrombotic microangiopathy and acute renal failure associated with arteriography. *BMJ*, **293**, 922–923.

303 Rauch AE, Tartaglia AP, Kaufman B and Kausel H (1984) RBC fragmentation and thymoma. *Arch Intern Med*, **144**, 1280–1282.

304 Paré PD, Chan-Yan C, Wass H, Hooper R and Hogg JC (1983) Portal and pulmonary hypertension with microangiopathic hemolytic anemia. *Am J Med*, **74**, 1093–1096.

305 Zauber NP and Echikson AB (1982) Giant cell arteritis and microangiopathic hemolytic anemia. *Am J Med*, **73**, 928–930.

306 Batton D, Amanullah A and Cornstock C (2000) Fetal schistocytic hemolytic anemia and umbilical vein varix. *J Pediatr Hematol Oncol*, **22**, 259–261.

307 Gudena M, Schmotzer J, Dopriak M, Novoa R and Morgan R (2004) Microangiopathic haemolytic anemia (MHA) associated with acute rheumatic valvulitis. *Blood*, **104**, 5b–6b.

308 Hayes AM, Redington AN and Rigby ML (1992) Severe haemolysis after transcatheter duct occlusion: a non-surgical remedy. *Br Heart J*, **67**, 321–322.

309 Nand S, Bansal VK, Kozeny G, Vertuno L, Remlinger KA and Jordan JV (1985) Red cell fragmentation syndrome with the use of subclavian hemodialysis catheters. *Arch Intern Med*, **145**, 1421–1423.

310 Steinhorn RH, Isham-Schopt B, Smith C and Green TP (1989) Hemolysis during long-term extracorporeal membrane oxygenation. *J Pediatr*, **115**, 625–630.

311 Frank C, Werber D, Cramer JP, Askar M, Faber M, an der Heiden M *et al.*; HUS Investigation Team (2011) Epidemic profile of Shiga-toxin-producing Escherichia coli O104:H4 outbreak in Germany. *N Engl J Med*, **365**, 1771–1780.

312 Green DA, Murphy WG and Uttley WS (2000) Haemolytic uraemic syndrome: prognostic factors. *Clin Lab Haematol*, **22**, 11–14.

313 Visudhiphan S, Piankijagum A, Sathayapraseart P and Mitrchai N (1983) Erythrocyte fragmentation in disseminated intravascular coagulation and other disease. *N Engl J Med*, **309**, 113.

314 Allford SA and Machin SJ (1999) Thrombotic thrombocytopenic purpura: current concepts. *CME Bull Haematol*, **2**, 80–84.

315 Zini G, d'Onofrio G, Briggs C, Erber W, Jou JM, Lee SH *et al.*; International Council for Standardization in Haematology (ICSH) (2012) ICSH recommendations for identification, diagnostic value, and quantitation of schistocytes. *Int J Lab Hematol*, **34**, 107–116.

316 Lesesve JF, Asnafi V, Braun F and Zini G (2012) Fragmented red blood cells automated measurement is a useful parameter to exclude schistocytes on the blood film. *Int J Lab Hematol*, **34**, 566–576.

317 Casebook of the Medical Protection Society.

318 Amare M, Lawson B and Larsen WE (1972) Active extrusion of Heinz bodies in drug-induced haemolytic anaemia. *Br J Haematol*, **23**, 215–219.

319 Mitchell TR and Pegrum GD (1972) The oxygen affinity of haemoglobin in chronic renal failure. *Br J Haematol*, **21**, 463–472.

320 Zieve L (1958) Jaundice, hyperlipidemia and hemolytic anemia: a heretofore unrecognized syndrome associated with alcoholic fatty liver and cirrhosis. *Ann Intern Med*, **48**, 471–496.

321 Melrose WD, Bell PA, Jupe DML and Baikie MJ (1990) Alcohol-associated haemolysis in Zieve's syndrome: a clinical and laboratory study of five cases. *Clin Lab Haematol*, **12**, 159–169.

322 Bain BJ (1999) Images in haematology: Heinz body haemolytic anaemia in Wilson's disease. *Br J Haematol*, **104**, 647.

323 Hudson PR, Tandy SC, Child DF, Williams CP and Cavill I (2001) Compensated haemolysis: a consistent feature of diabetes mellitus. *Br J Haematol*, **113**, Suppl. 1, 47.

324 Swann IL and Kendra JR (1998) Anaemia, vitamin E deficiency and failure to thrive in an infant. *Clin Lab Haematol*, **20**, 61–63.

325 Eyssette-Guerreau S, Bader-Meunier B, Garcon L, Guitton C and Cynober T (2006) Infantile pyknocytosis: a cause of haemolytic anaemia of the newborn. *Br J Haematol*, **133**, 439–442.

326 Kaiser U and Barth N (2001) Haemolytic anaemia in a patient with anorexia nervosa. *Acta Haematol*, **106**, 133–135.

327 Placzek MM and Gorst DW (1987) T activation haemolysis and death after blood transfusion. *Arch Dis Child*, **62**, 743–744.

328 Isbister GK, Little M, Cull G, McCoubrie D, Lawton P, Szabo F *et al.* (2007) Thrombotic microangiopathy from Australian brown snake (Pseudonaja) envenoming. *Intern Med J*, **37**, 523–528.

329 Hillmen P and Richards SJ (2000) Implications of recent insights into the pathophysiology of paroxysmal nocturnal haemoglobinuria. *Br J Haematol*, **108**, 470–479.

330 Yamashima M, Ueda E and Kinoshita T (1990) Inherited complete deficiency of 20-kilodalton homologous restriction factor (CD59) as a cause of paroxysmal nocturnal hemoglobinuria. *N Engl J Med*, **323**, 1184–1189.

331 Schreiber ZA (1999) Hemolytic anemia associated with hepatitis C infection. *Blood*, **94**, Suppl. 1, 7b.

332 Lanzkowsky P, McKenzie D, Katz S, Hoffenberg R, Friedman R and Black E (1967) Erythrocyte abnormality induced by protein malnutrition. II. 51-chromium labelled erythrocyte studies. *Br J Haematol*, **13**, 639–649.

333 Woodruff AW, Topley E, Knight R and Downie CGB (1971) The anaemia of Kala Azar. *Br J Haematol*, **22**, 319–329.

334 Wickramasinghe SN (1997) Dyserythropoiesis and congenital dyserythropoietic anaemias. *Br J Haematol*, **98**, 788–787.

335 Delaunay J and Iolascon A (2000) The congenital dyserythropoietic anaemias. *Baillière's Clin Haematol*, **12**, 691–705.

336 Wickramasinghe SN and Wood WG (2005) Advances in the understanding of the congenital dyserythropoietic anaemias. *Br J Haematol*, **131**, 431–436.

337 Parsons SF, Jones J, Anstee DJ, Judson PA, Gardner B, Wiener E *et al.* (1994) A novel form of congenital dyserythropoietic anemia associated with deficiency of erythroid CD44 and a unique blood group phenotype [In(a-b-), Co(a-b-)]. *Blood*, **83**, 860–868.

338 Arnaud L, Saison C, Helias V, Lucien N, Steschenko D, Giarratana MC *et al.* (2010) A dominant mutation in the gene encoding the erythroid transcription factor KLF1 causes a congenital dyserythropoietic anemia. *Am J Hum Genet*, **87**, 721–727.

339 McCann SR, Firth R, Murray N and Temperley IJ (1980) Congenital dyserythropoietic anaemia type II (HEMPAS): a family study. *J Clin Pathol*, **33**, 1197–1201.

340 Brien WF, Mant MJ and Etches WS (1985) Variant congenital dyserythropoietic anaemia with ringed sideroblasts. *Clin Lab Haematol*, **7**, 231–237.

341 Jankovic M, Sansone G, Comer V, Iolascon A and Masera G (1993) Atypical hereditary ovalocytosis associated with dyserythropoietic anemia. *Acta Haematol*, **89**, 35–37.

342 Bianchi P, Pelissero G, Bredi E, Zappa M, Vercellati C, Boscetti C *et al.* (1998) Two cases of atypical congenital dyserythropoietic anemia (type II) presenting with laboratory features of hereditary spherocytosis. *Br J Haematol*, **102**, 300.

343 Nichols KE, Crispino JD, Poncz M, White JG, Orkin SH, Maris JM and Weiss MJ (2000) Familial dyserythropoietic anemia and thrombocytopenia due to an inherited mutation in *GATA1*. *Nat Genet*, **24**, 266–270.

344 Freson K, Devriendt K, Matthijs G, Van Hoof A, De Vos R, Thys C *et al.* (2001) Platelet characteristics in patients with X-linked macrothrombocytopenia because of a novel *GATA1* mutation. *Blood*, **98**, 85–92.

345 Liljeholm M, Irvine AF, Vikberg AL, Norberg A, Month S, Sandström H *et al.* (2103) Congenital dyserythropoietic anemia type III (CDA III) is caused by a mutation in kinesin family member, *KIF23*. *Blood*, **121**, 4791–4799.

346 Bethlenfalvay NC, Hadnagy CS and Heimpel H (1985) Unclassified type of congenital dyserythropoietic anaemia (CDA) with prominent peripheral erythroblastosis. *Br J Haematol*, **60**, 541–550.

347 Heimpel H, Wilts H, Hirschmann WD, Hofman WK, Siciliano RD, Steinke B and Weschler JG (2007) Aplastic crisis as a complication of congenital dyserythropoietic anemia type II. *Acta Haematol*, **117**, 115–118.

348 Yeh SP, Chiu CF, Lee CC, Peng CT, Kuan CY and Chow KC (2004) Evidence of parvovirus B19 infection in patients of pre-eclampsia and eclampsia with dyserythropoietic anaemia. *Br J Haematol*, **126**, 428–433.

349 Gross M, Hanenberg H, Lobitz S, Friedl R, Herterich S, Dietrich R *et al.* (2002) Reverse mosaicism in Fanconi anemia: natural gene therapy via molecular self-correction. *Cytogenet Genome Res*, **98**, 126–135.

350 Cassinat B, Guardiola P, Chevret S, Schlageter M-H, Tobert M-E, Rain J-D and Gluckman E (2000) Constitutive elevation of serum alpha-fetoprotein in Fanconi anemia. *Blood*, **96**, 859–863.

351 Sugimori C, Chuhjo T, Feng X, Yamazaki H, Takami A, Teramura M *et al.* (2006) Minor population of CD55-CD59-blood cells predicts response to immunosuppressive therapy and prognosis in patients with aplastic anemia. *Blood*, **107**, 1308–1314.

352 Da Costa L, Chanoz-Poulard G, Simansour M, French M, Bouvier R, Prieur F *et al.* (2013) First de novo mutation in

RPS19 gene as the cause of hydrops fetalis in Diamond-Blackfan anemia. *Am J Hematol*, **88**, 160.

353 Freedman MH (2000) Diamond–Blackfan anaemia. *Baillière's Clin Haematol*, **13**, 591–606.

354 Fargo JH, Kratz CP, Giri N, Savage SA, Wong C, Backer K *et al.* (2013) Erythrocyte adenosine deaminase: diagnostic value for Diamond-Blackfan anaemia. *Br J Haematol*, **160**, 547–554.

355 Karsten J, Anker AP and Odink RJ (1996) Glycosylated haemoglobin and transient erythroblastopenia of childhood. *Lancet*, **347**, 273.

356 Gerrard G, Valgañón M, Foong HE, Kasperaviciute D, Iskander D, Game L *et al.* (2013) Target enrichment and high-throughput sequencing of 80 ribosomal protein genes to identify mutations associated with Diamond-Blackfan anaemia. *Br J Haematol*, **162**, 530–536.

357 Alter B (2003) Inherited bone marrow failure syndromes. In: NathanDG, OrkinSH, GinsburgD and LookAT (eds), *Nathan and Oski's Hematology of Infancy and Childhood*, 6th edn, Saunders, Philadelphia.

358 Johansson PL, Safai-Kutti S and Kutti J (2005) An elevated venous haemoglobin concentration cannot be used as a surrogate marker for absolute erythrocytosis: a study of patients with polycythaemia vera and apparent polycythaemia. *Br J Haematol*, **129**, 701–705.

359 Landolfi R, Di Gennaro L, Barbui T, De Stefano V, Finazzi G, Marfisi R-M *et al.* (2007) Leukocytosis as a major thrombotic risk factor in patients with polycythemia vera. *Blood*, **109**, 2446–2452.

360 Bonicelli G, Abdulkarim K, Mounier M, Johansson P, Rossi C, Jooste V *et al.* (2013) Leucocytosis and thrombosis at diagnosis are associated with poor survival in polycythaemia vera; a population-based study of 327 patients. *Br J Haematol*, **160**, 251–254.

361 Silver RT, Chow W, Orazi A, Arles SP and Goldsmith SJ (2013) Evaluation of WHO criteria for diagnosis of polycythemia vera: a prospective analysis. *Blood*, **122**, 1881–1886.

362 Messinezy M, Westwood NB, El-Hemaidi I, Marsden JT, Sherwood RS and Pearson TC (2002) Serum erythropoietin values in erythrocytoses and in primary thrombocythaemia. *Br J Haematol*, **117**, 47–53.

363 Carneskog J, Kutti J, Wadenvik H, Lundberg P-A and Lindstedt G (1998) Plasma erythropoietin by high detectability immunoradiometric assay in untreated patients with polycythaemia rubra vera and essential thrombocythaemia. *Eur J Haematol*, **60**, 278–282.

364 McMullin MF, Bareford D, Campbell P, Green AR, Harrison C, Hunt B *et al.*, On behalf of the General Haematology Task Force of the British Committee for Standards in Haematology (2005) Guidelines for the diagnosis, investigation and management of polycythaemia/erythrocytosis. *Br J Haematol*, **130**, 166–173.

365 Thiele J, Kvasnicka HM, Orazi A, Tefferi A and Birgegard G (2008) Polycythaemia vera. In: Swerdlow SH, Campo E, Harris NL, Jaffe ES, Pileri SA, Stein H *et al.* (eds), *WHO Classification of Tumours of Haematopoietic and Lymphoid Tissues*, IARC, Lyon.

366 Alvarez-Larrán A, Ancochea A, Angona A, Pedro C, García-Pallarols F, Martínez-Avilés L *et al.* (2012) Red cell mass measurement in patients with clinically suspected diagnosis of polycythemia vera or essential thrombocythemia. *Haematologica*, **97**, 1704–1707.

367 Tey S-K, Cobcroft R, Grimmett K, Marlton P, Gill D and Mills A (2004) A simplified endogenous erythroid colony assay for the investigation of polycythaemia. *Clin Lab Haematol*, **26**, 115–122.

368 Carneskog J, Safai-Kutti S, Suurküla M, Wadenvik H, Bake B, Lindstedt G and Kutti J (1998) The red cell mass, plasma erythropoietin and spleen size in apparent polycythaemia. *Eur J Haematol*, **62**, 43–48.

369 Roberts I, Stanworth S and Murray NA (2008) Thrombocytopenia in the neonate. *Blood Rev*, **22**, 173–186.

370 Germeshausen M, Ballmaier M and Welte K (2001) Implications of mutations in hematopoietic growth factor receptor genes in congenital cytopenias. *Ann NY Acad Sci*, **938**, 305–320.

371 Thompson AA and Nguyen LT (2000) Amegakaryocytic thrombocytopenia and radio-ulnar synostosis are associated with *HOXA11* mutation. *Nat Genet*, **26**, 397–398.

372 Thompson AA, Woodruff K, Feig SA, Nguyen LT and Schanen NC (2001) Congenital thrombocytopenia and radio-ulnar synostosis: a new familial syndrome. *Br J Haematol*, **113**, 866–870.

373 Balduini CL, Cattaneo M, Fabris F, Gresele P, Iolascon A, Pulcinelli FM and Savoia A (2003) Inherited thrombocytopenias: a proposed diagnostic algorithm from the Italian Gruppo di Studio delle Piastrine. *Haematologica*, **89**, 325–329.

374 Lutskiy MI, Sasahara Y, Kenney DM, Rosen FS and Remold-O'Donnell E (2002) Wiskott-Aldrich syndrome in a female. *Blood*, **100**, 2763–2768.

375 Ho LL, Ayling J, Prosser I, Kronenberg H, Iland H and Joshua D (2001) Missense C168T in the Wiskott-Aldrich syndrome protein gene is a common mutation in X-linked thrombocytopenia. *Br J Haematol*, **112**, 76–80.

376 Notarangelo LD, Mazza C, Gilliani S, d'Aria C, Gandellini F, Locatelli MG *et al.* (2002) Missense mutations of the *WASP* gene cause intermittent X-linked thrombocytopenia. *Blood*, **99**, 2268–2269.

377 Jackson N, Mohammad S, Zainal N, Jamaluddin N and Hishamuddin M (1995) Autosomal dominant thrombocytopenia with microthrombocytes: a family study. *Med J Malaysia*, **50**, 421–424.

378 Geddis AE (2005) Congenital cytopenias. The molecular basis of congenital thrombocytopenias: insights into megakaryopoiesis. *Hematology*, **10**, Suppl. 1, 299–305.

379 Geddis AE (2013) Inherited thrombocytopenias: an approach to diagnosis and management. *Int J Lab Hematol*, **35**, 14–25.

380 Ballmaier M, Germeshausen M, Schulze H, Cherkaoui K, Lang S, Gaudig A *et al.* (2001) c-*mpl* mutations are the cause of congenital amegakaryocytic thrombocytopenia. *Blood*, **97**, 139–146.

381 Drachman JG (2004) Inherited thrombocytopenia: when a low platelet count does not mean ITP. *Blood*, **103**, 390–398.

382 Gandhi ML, Cummings CL and Drachman JG (2003) *FLJ14813*: a candidate for autosomal dominant thrombocytopenia on chromosome 10. *Hum Hered*, **55**, 66–70.

383 Savoia A, Del Vecchio M, Totaro A, Perrotta S, Amendola G, Moretti A *et al.* (1999) An autosomal dominant thrombocytopenia gene maps to chromosomal region 10p. *Am J Hum Genet*, **65**, 1401–1405.

384 Noris P, Perrotta S, Seri M, Pecci A, Gnan C, Loffredo G *et al.* (2011) Mutations in *ANKRD26* are responsible for a frequent form of inherited thrombocytopenia: analysis of 78 patients from 21 families. *Blood*, **117**, 6673–6680.

385 Pecci A and Balduini CL (2014) Lessons in platelet production from inherited thrombocytopenias. *Br J Haematol*, **165**, 179–192.

386 Buijs A, Poddighe P, van Wijk R, van Solinge W, Borst E, Verdonck L *et al.* (2001) A novel *CBFA2* single-nucleotide mutation in familial platelet disorder with propensity to develop myeloid malignancies. *Blood*, **98**, 2856–2858.

387 Hayward CP, Cramer EM, Kane WH, Zheng S, Bouchard M, Masse JM and Rivard GE (1997) Studies of a second family with the Quebec platelet disorder: evidence that the degradation of the alpha-granule membrane and its soluble contents are not secondary to a defect in targeting proteins to alpha-granules. *Blood*, **89**, 1243–1253.

388 van den Oudenrijn S, Bruin M, Folman CC, Bussel J, de Haas M, von dem Borne AEGK (2002) Three parameters, plasma thrombopoietin levels, plasma glycocalicin levels and megakaryocyte culture, distinguish between different causes of congenital thrombocytopenia. *Br J Haematol*, **117**, 390–398.

389 Morison IM, Cramer Bordé EM, Cheesman EJ, Cheong PL, Holyoake AJ, Fichelson S *et al.* (2008) A mutation of human cytochrome *c* enhances the intrinsic apoptotic pathway but causes only thrombocytopenia. *Nature Genet*, **40**, 387–389.

390 Kobayashi Y, Matsui H, Kanai A, Tsumura M, Okada S, Miki M *et al.* (2013) Identification of the integrin β3 L718P mutation in a pedigree with autosomal dominant thrombocytopenia with anisocytosis. *Br J Haematol*, **160**, 521–529.

391 Dasouki MJ, Rafi SK, Olm-Shipman AJ, Wilson NR, Abhyankar S, Ganter B *et al.* (2013) Exome sequencing reveals a thrombopoietin ligand mutation in a Micronesian family with autosomal recessive aplastic anemia. *Blood*, **122**, 3440–3449.

392 Favier R, Jondeau K, Boutard P, Grossfeld P, Reinert P, Jones C *et al.* (2003) Paris-Trousseau syndrome: clinical, hematological, molecular data of ten new cases. *Thromb Haemost*, **90**, 893–897.

393 Savoia A, Balduini CL, Savino M, Noris P, del Vecchio M, Perrotta S *et al.* (2001) Autosomal dominant macrothrombocytopenia in Italy is most frequently a type of heterozygous Bernard-Soulier syndrome. *Blood*, **97**, 1330–1335.

394 Noris P, Perrotta S, Bottega R, Pecci A, Melazzini F, Civaschi E *et al.* (2012) Clinical and laboratory features of 103 patients from 42 Italian families with inherited thrombocytopenia derived from the monoallelic Ala156Val mutation of GPIbα (Bolzano mutation). *Haematologica*, **97**, 82–88.

395 Davies JK, Telfer P, Cavenagh JD, Foot N and Neat M (2003) Autoimmune cytopenias in the 22q11.2 deletion syndrome. *Clin Lab Haematol*, **25**, 195–197.

396 Ghevaert C, Salsmann A, Watkins NA, Schaffner-Reckinger E, Rankin A, Garner SF *et al.* (2008) A nonsynonymous SNP in the *ITGB3* gene disrupts the conserved membrane-proximal cytoplasmic salt bridge in the alphaIIbbeta3 integrin and cosegregates dominantly with abnormal proplatelet formation and macrothrombocytopenia. *Blood*, **111**, 3407–3414.

397 Kunishima S, Kashiwagi H, Otsu M, Takayama N, Eto K, Onodera M *et al.* (2011) Heterozygous *ITGA2B* R995W mutation inducing constitutive activation of the αIIbβ3 receptor affects proplatelet formation and causes congenital macrothrombocytopenia. *Blood*, **117**, 5479–5484.

398 Drouin A, Favier R, Massé J-M, Debili N, Schmitt A, Elbin C *et al.* (2001) Newly recognized cellular abnormalities in the gray platelet syndrome. *Blood*, **98**, 1382–1391.

399 White JG (2006) Localization of a lysosomal enzyme in platelets from patients with the White platelet syndrome. *Platelets*, **17**, 231–249.

400 White JG, Pakzad K and Meister L (2012) The York platelet syndrome: a fourth case with unusual pathologic features. *Platelets*, **24**, 44–50.

401 Di Pumpo M, Noris P, Pecci A, Savoia A, Seri M, Ceresa IF and Balduini CL (2005) Defective expression of GPIb/IX/V complex in platelets from patients with May-Hegglin anomaly and Sebastian syndrome. *Haematologica*, **87**, 943–947.

402 Kunishima S, Kojima T, Matsushita T, Tanaka T, Tsurusawa M, Furukawa Y *et al.* (2001) Mutations in the NMMHC-A gene cause autosomal dominant macrothrombocytopenia with leukocyte inclusions (May-Hegglin anomaly/Sebastian syndrome). *Blood*, **97**, 1147–1149.

403 Bellucci S (1997) Megakaryocytes and inherited thrombocytopenias. *Baillière's Clin Haematol*, **10**, 149–162.

404 Toren A, Rozenfeld-Granot G, Rocca B, Epstein CJ, Amariglio N, Laghi F *et al.* (2000) Autosomal-dominant giant platelet syndromes: a hint of the same genetic defect as in Fechtner syndrome owing to a similar genetic linkage to chromosome 22q11-13. *Blood*, **96**, 3447–3451.

405 Erice JG, Perez JM and Pericas FS (1999) Homozygous form of the Pelger-Huet anomaly. *Haematologica*, **84**, 748.

406 Phillips JD, Steensma DP, Pulsipher MA, Spangrude GJ and Kushner JP (2007) Congenital erythropoietic porphyria

due to a mutation in *GATA1*: the first trans-acting mutation causative for a human porphyria. *Blood*, **109**, 2618–2621.

407 Yu C, Niakan KK, Martsushita M, Stamatoyannopoulos G, Orkin SH and Raskind WH (2002) X-linked thrombocytopenia with thalassaemia from a mutation in the amino finger of GATA-1 affecting DNA binding rather than FOG-1 interaction. *Blood*, **100**, 2040–2045.

408 Willig T-N, Breton-Gorius J, Elbim C, Mignotte V, Kaplan C, Mollicone R *et al.* (2001) Macrothrombocytopenia with abnormal demarcation membranes in megakaryocytes and neutropenia with a complete lack of sialyl-Lewis-X antigens on leukocytes. *Blood*, **97**, 826–828.

409 Harris VK, Nair SC, Dolley D, Amelia SM and Chandy M (2002) Asymptomatic constitutional macrothrombocytopenia among West Bengal blood donors. *Br J Haematol*, **117**, Suppl. 1, 88.

410 Becker PS, Clavell LA and Beardsley DS (1998) Giant platelets with abnormal surface glycoproteins: a new familial disorder associated with mitral valve insufficiency. *J Pediatr Hematol Oncol*, **20**, 69–73.

411 Fabris F, Fagioli F, Basso G and Girolami A (2002) Autosomal dominant macrothrombocytopenia with ineffective thrombopoiesis. *Haematologica*, **87**, ELT27.

412 Nurden P, Gobbi G, Nurden A, Enouf J, Youlyouz-Marfak I, Carubbi C *et al.* (2010) Abnormal VWF modifies megakaryocytopoiesis: studies of platelets and megakaryocyte cultures from patients with von Willebrand disease type 2B. *Blood*, **115**, 2649–2656.

413 Kunishima S, Kobayashi R, Itoh TJ, Hamaguchi M and Saito H (2009) Mutation of the β1-tubulin gene associated with congenital macrothrombocytopenia affecting microtubule assembly. *Blood*, **113**, 458–461.

414 Nurden P, Debili N, Coupry I, Bryckaert M, Youlyouz-Marfak I, Solé G *et al.* (2011) Thrombocytopenia resulting from mutations in filamin A can be expressed as an isolated syndrome. *Blood*, **118**, 5928–5937.

415 Yufu Y, Ideguchi H, Narishige T, Suematsu E, Toyoda K, Nishimura J *et al.* (1990) Familial macrothrombocytopenia associated with decreased glycosylation of platelet membrane glycoprotein IV. *Am J Hematol*, **33**, 271–273.

416 Gilman AL, Sloand E, White JG and Sacher R (1995) A novel hereditary macrothrombocytopenia. *J Pediatr Hematol Oncol*, **17**, 296–305.

417 Boztug K, Appaswamy G, Ashikov A, Schäffer AA, Salzer U, Diestelhorst J *et al.* (2009) A syndrome with congenital neutropenia and mutations in *G6PC3*. *N Engl J Med*, **360**, 32–43.

418 Pujol-Moix N, Kelley MJ, Hernandez A, Muniz-Diaz E and Espanol I (2004) Ultrastructural analysis of granulocyte inclusions in genetically confirmed MYH9-related disorders. *Haematologica*, **89**, 330–337.

419 Lubinsky MS, Kahler SG, Speer IE, Hoyme HE, Kirillova IA and Lurie IW (1994) von Voss-Cherstvoy syndrome: a variable perinatally lethal syndrome of multiple congenital anomalies. *Am J Med Genet*, **52**, 272–278.

420 Braddock SR and Carey JC (1994) A new syndrome: congenital thrombocytopenia, Robin sequence, agenesis of the corpus callosum, distinctive facies and developmental delay. *Clin Dysmorphol*, **3**, 75–81.

421 Arias S, Penchaszadeh VB, Pinto-Cisternas J and Larrauri S (1980) The IVIC syndrome: a new autosomal dominant complex pleiotropic syndrome with radial ray hypoplasia, hearing impairment, external ophthalmoplegia, and thrombocytopenia. *Am J Med Genet*, **6**, 25–59.

422 Pecci A, Noris P, Invernizzi R. Savoia A, Seri M, Ghiggeri GM *et al.* (2002) Immunocytochemistry for the heavy chain of the non-muscle myosin IIA as a diagnostic tool for *MYH9*-related disorders. *Br J Haematol*, **117**, 164–157.

423 Sun XH, Wang ZY, Yang HY, Cao LJ, Su J, Yu ZQ *et al.* (2013) Clinical, pathological, and genetic analysis of ten patients with MYH9-related disease. *Acta Haematol*, **129**, 106–113.

424 Yagi H, Matumoto M, Ishizashi H, Kinoshita S, Konno M, Matsui T *et al.* (2000) Plasmas with Upshaw-Schulman syndrome, a congenital deficiency of von Willebrand factor-cleaving protease, augment the aggregation of normal washed platelets under high-shear-stress. *Blood*, **96**, 630a.

425 Noris P, Klersy C, Zecca M, Arcaini L, Pecci A, Melazzini F *et al.* (2009) Platelet size distinguishes between inherited macrothrombocytopenias and immune thrombocytopenia. *J Thromb Haemost*, **7**, 2131–2136.

426 Fabris F, Cordiano I, Steffan A, Ramon R, Scandellari R, Nichol JL and Girolami A (2000) Indirect study of thrombopoiesis (TPO, reticulated platelets, glycocalicin) in patients with hereditary macrothrombocytopenia. *Eur J Haematol*, **64**, 151–156.

427 Devine DV, Currie MS, Rosse WF and Greenberg CS (1987) Pseudo-Bernard-Soulier syndrome: thrombocytopenia caused by autoantibody to platelet glycoprotein Ib. *Blood*, **70**, 428–431.

428 Murphy MF and Williamson LM (2000) Antenatal screening for fetomaternal alloimmune thrombocytopenia: an evaluation using the criteria of the UK National Screening Committee. *Br J Haematol*, **111**, 726–732.

429 Qasim W, Gilmour KC, Heath S, Ashton E, Cranston T, Thomas A *et al.* (2001) Protein assays for diagnosis of Wiskott-Aldrich syndrome and X-linked thrombocytopenia. *Br J Haematol*, **113**, 861–863.

430 Kunishima S, Yoshinari M, Nishio H, Ida K, Miura T, Matsushita T *et al.* (2007) Haematological characteristics of *MYH9* disorders due to *MYH9* R702 mutations. *Eur J Haematol*, **78**, 220–226.

431 Neylon AJ, Saunders PWG, Howard MR, Proctor SJ and Taylor PRA on behalf of the Northern Region Haematology Group (2003) Clinically significant newly presenting autoimmune thrombocytopenic purpura in adults: a prospective study of a population-based cohort of 245 patients. *Br J Haematol*, **122**, 966–974.

432 Terrell DR, Beebe LA, Neas BR, Vesely SK, Segal JB and George JN (2012) Prevalence of primary immune thrombocytopenia in Oklahoma. *Am J Hematol*, **87**, 848–852.

433 Koh K-R, Yamane T, Ohta K, Hino M, Takubo T and Tatsumi N (1999) Pathophysiological significance of simultaneous measurement of reticulated platelets, large platelets and serum thrombopoietin in non-neoplastic thrombocytopenic disorders. *Eur J Haematol*, **63**, 295–301.

434 Rosthøj S, Hedlund-Treutiger I and Zeller B on behalf of the Nordic Society for Paediatric Haematology and Oncology Idiopathic Thrombocytopenic Purpura Working Group (2005) Factors predicting development of chronic disease in Nordic children with acute onset of idiopathic thrombocytopenic purpura. *Br J Haematol*, **130**, 148–149.

435 Rajan SK, Espina BM and Liebman HA (2005) Hepatitis C virus-related thrombocytopenia: clinical and laboratory characteristics compared with chronic immune thrombocytopenic purpura. *Br J Haematol*, **129**, 818–824.

436 British Committee for Standards in Haematology General Haematology Task Force (2003) Guidelines for the investigation and management of idiopathic thrombocytopenic purpura in adults, children and in pregnancy. *Br J Haematol*, **120**, 574–596.

437 Garcia-Suárez J, Burgaleta C, Hernanz N, Albarran F, Tobaruela P and Alvarez-Mon M (2000) HCV-associated thrombocytopenia: clinical characteristics and platelet response after recombinant α2b-interferon therapy. *Br J Haematol*, **110**, 98–103.

438 Kuga T, Kohda K, Koike K, Matsunaga T, Kogawa K, Kanisawa Y *et al.* (2001) Effect of *Helicobacter pylori* eradication on platelet recovery in chronic idiopathic thrombocytopenic purpura and secondary autoimmune thrombocytopenic purpura. *Blood*, **98**, 520a.

439 Jarque I, Andrea R, Llopis I, de la Rubia J, Gomis F, Senent L *et al.* (2001) Absence of platelet response after eradication of *Helicobacter pylori* infection in patients with chronic idiopathic thrombocytopenic purpura. *Br J Haematol*, **115**, 1002–1003.

440 Petrov V, Vdovin V and Svirin P (2004) Vaccine-associated immune thrombocytopenic purpura in childhood. *Br J Haematol*, **125**, Suppl. 1, 50.

441 Su C and Brandt LJ (1995) *Escherichia coli* O157: H7 infection in humans. *Ann Intern Med*, **123**, 698–714.

442 Scully M, Miller R, Cohen H, Roedling S, Starke R, Edwards S *et al.* (2005) Treatment of HIV associated thrombotic thrombocytopenic purpura – importance of prompt diagnosis. *Br J Haematol*, **129**, Suppl. 1, 12.

443 Weinberg PD, Bennett CL, Rozenberg-Ben-Drot K, Kwaan HC and Green D (1997) Ticlopidine associated thrombotic thrombocytopenic purpura. *Blood*, **90**, Suppl. 1, 462a.

444 Schirron CA, Berghaus TM and Sackmann M (1999) Thrombotic thrombocytopenic purpura after Ecstasy-induced acute liver failure. *Ann Intern Med*, **130**, 163.

445 Rachmani R, Avigdor A, Youkla M, Raanani P, Zilber M, Ravid M and ben-Bassat I (1998) Thrombotic thrombocytopenic purpura complicating chronic myelogenous leukemia treated with interferon-α. *Acta Haematol*, **100**, 204–206.

446 Schech SD, Brinker A, Shatin D and Burgess M (2006) New-onset and idiopathic thrombotic thrombocytopenic purpura: incidence, diagnostic validity, and potential risk factors. *Am J Hematol*, **81**, 657–663.

447 Burns ER, Lou Y and Pathak A (2004) Morphologic diagnosis of thrombotic thrombocytopenic purpura. *Am J Hematol*, **75**, 18–21.

448 Idowu M and Reddy P (2013) Atypical thrombotic thrombocytopenic purpura in a middle-aged woman who presented with a recurrent stroke. *Am J Hematol*, **88**, 237–239.

449 Ding J, Komatsu H, Wakita A, Kato-Uranishi M, Ito M, Satoh A *et al.* (2004) Familial essential thrombocythaemia associated with a dominant-positive activating mutation of the *c-MPL* gene, which encodes for the receptor for thrombopoietin. *Blood*, **103**, 4198–4200.

450 Mead AJ, Rugless MJ, Jacobsen SE and Schuh A (2012) Germline *JAK2* mutation in a family with hereditary thrombocytosis. *N Engl J Med*, **366**, 967–969.

451 Stuhrmann M, Bashawri L, Ahmed MA, Al-Awamy BH, Kühnau W, Schmidtke J and El-Harith EA (2001) Familial thrombocytosis as a recessive, possibly X-linked trait in an Arab family. *Br J Haematol*, **112**, 616–620.

452 Cohen N, Almoznino-Sarafian D, Weissgarten J, Alon I, Zaidenstein R, Dishi V *et al.* (1997) Benign familial microcytic thrombocytosis with autosomal dominant transmission. *Clin Genet*, **52**, 47–50.

453 van Dijken PJ, Woldendorp KH and van Wouwe JP (1996) Familial thrombocytosis in infancy presenting with a leukaemoid reaction. *Acta Paediatr*, **85**, 1132–1134.

454 Carobbio A, Finazzi G, Guerini V, Spinelli O, Delaini F, Marchioli R *et al.* (2007) Leukocytosis is a risk factor for thrombosis in essential thrombocythemia: interaction with treatment, standard risk factors, and Jak2 mutation status. *Blood*, **109**, 2310–2313.

455 Wolanskyj AP, Lasho TL, Schwager SM, McClure RF, Wadleigh M, Lee SJ *et al.* (2005) *JAK2*^{V617F} mutation in essential thrombocythaemia: clinical associations and long-term prognostic relevance. *Br J Haematol*, **131**, 208–213.

456 Green A, Campbell P, Scott L, Buck G, Wheatley K, East C *et al.* (2005) JAK2 V617F mutation identified a biologically distinct subtype of essential thrombocythaemia which resembles polycythaemia vera. *Blood*, **106**, 77a.

457 Cheung B, Radia D, Pantelidis P, Yadegarfar G and Harrison C (2006) The presence of the *JAK2* V617F mutation is associated with a higher haemoglobin and increased risk of thrombosis in essential thrombocythaemia. *Br J Haematol*, **132**, 244–245.

458 Passamonti F, Randi ML, Rumi E, Pungolino E, Elena C, Pietra D *et al.* (2007) Increased risk of pregnancy complications in patients with essential thrombocythemia carrying the JAK2 (617V>F) mutation. *Blood*, **110**, 485–489.

459 Klampfl T, Gisslinger H, Harutyunyan AS, Nivarthi H, Rumi E, Milosevic JD *et al.* (2013) Somatic mutations of

calreticulin in myeloproliferative neoplasms. *N Engl J Med*, **369**, 2379–2390.

460 Kiladjian J-J, Elkassar N, Hetet G, Balitrand N, Conejero C, Girauduer S *et al.* (2005) Analysis of JAK2 mutation is essential thrombocythaemia (ET) patients with monoclonal and polyclonal X-chromosome inactivation patterns (XCIPs). *Blood*, **106**, 732a.

461 Picardi M, Martinelli V, Ciancia R, Soscia E, Morante R, Sodano A *et al.* (2002) Measurement of spleen volume by ultrasound scanning in patients with thrombocytosis: a prospective study. *Blood*, **99**, 4228–4230.

462 Quigley M, Linfesty RL, Bethel K and Sharpe R (2007) Stubby elliptocytes are an invariable feature of leukoerythroblastosis. *Blood*, **109**, 2666.

463 Arora B, Sirhan S, Hoyer JD, Mesa RA and Tefferi A (2005) Peripheral blood CD34 count in myelofibrosis with myeloid metaplasia: a prospective evaluation of prognostic value in 94 patients. *Br J Haematol*, **128**, 42–48.

464 Tefferi A and Elliott MA (2000) Serious myeloproliferative reactions associated with the use of thalidomide in myelofibrosis with myeloid metaplasia. *Blood*, **96**, 4007.

465 Tefferi A, Lasho TL, Schwager SM, Steensma DP, Mesa RA, Li CY *et al.* (2005) The *JAK2*^{V617F} tyrosine kinase mutation in myelofibrosis with myeloid metaplasia: lineage specificity and clinical correlates. *Br J Haematol*, **131**, 320–328.

CHAPTER 9
Disorders of white cells

Acquired disorders primarily involving white cells may be either reactive, to a primary usually non-haematological disease, or neoplastic. Neoplastic disorders result from the clonal proliferation of a haemopoietic stem cell, either myeloid, lymphoid or pluripotent, that has undergone mutation. Numerical changes in white cells are summarised in Chapter 6. Here the typical peripheral blood changes in reactive leucocyte disorders are described, followed by the characteristic features of haematological neoplasms.

Reactive changes in white cells

Bacterial infection
Acute and chronic bacterial infection
Blood film and count
In an adult, the usual response to a bacterial infection is a neutrophil leucocytosis with a left shift, toxic granulation, Döhle bodies and, when infection is severe, cytoplasmic vacuolation (Fig. 9.1). Occasionally, bacteria are seen within neutrophils. In severe infections there may be myelocytes, promyelocytes and even a few blast cells in the peripheral blood. The lymphocyte and eosinophil counts are reduced. A rise in the monocyte count occurs later than the rise in the neutrophil count. During recovery, there is a rise in the eosinophil count, sometimes to above normal. If infection persists, a normocytic normochromic anaemia develops and, if the infection becomes chronic, red cells may become hypochromic and microcytic. There is an increase in rouleaux formation and in background staining. The platelet count is often elevated during acute or severe chronic infection, but is sometimes reduced. Sometimes bacterial infections are associated with pancytopenia as a result of haemophagocytosis.

In overwhelming sepsis, particularly in alcoholics and neonates, infection can be associated with paradoxical leucopenia and neutropenia. A left shift and toxic changes nevertheless occur. Neutropenia in bacteraemic patients is indicative of a worse prognosis [1]. Neutropenia in the course of infections that more often cause neutrophilia may be the result of increased margination of neutrophils, impaired granulopoiesis or migration of peripheral blood neutrophils to tissues more rapidly than they can be replenished by a bone marrow with

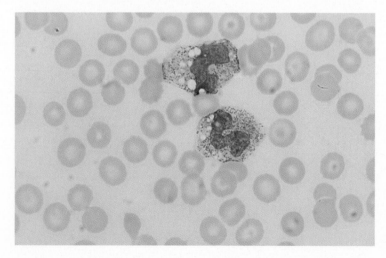

Fig. 9.1 Blood film in reactive neutrophilia; both cells are band forms showing vacuolation and marked toxic granulation.

Blood Cells A Practical Guide, Fifth Edition. By Barbara J. Bain © 2015 John Wiley & Sons, Ltd. Published 2015 by John Wiley & Sons, Ltd.
Companion Website: www.wiley.com/go/bain/bloodcells

an inadequate reserve capacity. In some studies in neonates, an increased proportion of band cells has been found more useful than neutrophilia in identifying infected infants. However, others have found an increased band count to be no more sensitive in predicting a positive blood culture than an increase in the absolute neutrophil count [2].

Although neutrophilia is the characteristic response to bacterial infection, this is not invariable. Certain infections are characterised by either a normal white blood cell count (WBC) or even leucopenia and neutropenia, e.g. typhoid fever, brucellosis and rickettsial infections. Typhoid fever can also cause anaemia, isolated thrombocytopenia, bicytopenia or pancytopenia. Brucellosis occasionally causes isolated thrombocytopenia. Lymphocytosis is characteristic of pertussis (whooping cough). Infants and young children sometimes also respond to other bacterial infections with lymphocytosis rather than neutrophilia.

In addition to the elevated WBC, automated instruments may indicate a left shift, the presence of immature granulocytes or increased peroxidase activity of neutrophils.

Differential diagnosis

The differential diagnosis of neutrophil changes suggestive of infection includes other causes of neutrophilia (see Chapter 6). Toxic granulation and Döhle bodies are not specific for infection, being seen also in pregnancy, in inflammatory and autoimmune diseases, following administration of cytokines and when there is tissue damage or death, e.g. as a result of surgery, trauma or infarction. The presence of neutrophil vacuolation is more specific for infection, very commonly indicating septicaemia [3]. The observation of bacteria within neutrophils in a film made without delay may indicate colonisation of an indwelling venous line (if the blood specimen is obtained directly from the line), but otherwise is specific for bacteraemia. However, this finding is rare. Neutrophilia resulting from granulocyte colony-stimulating factor (G-CSF) therapy) is associated with dysplastic features (Fig 9.2). Neutrophilia as a leukaemoid reaction to multiple myeloma is associated with toxic granulation (Fig. 9.3).

In the neonatal period, neutrophilia may be caused not only by infection but also by hypoxia or stressful labour, intrapartum oxytocin administration, maternal fever or seizures, neonatal hypoglycaemia and haemolytic disease of the newborn [4] (see Chapter 6). Even crying can cause an increase in WBC and the proportion of band cells [5].

Further tests

Characteristic peripheral blood features are often present in bacterial infection but, since they are neither specific nor invariably present, a definitive diagnosis

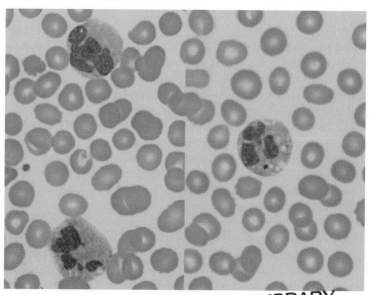

Fig. 9.2 Composite image of the blood film of a patient with neutrophilia resulting from granulocyte colony-stimulating factor (G-CSF) therapy showing dysplastic features, abnormal nuclear shapes (left) and a detached nuclear fragment (right).

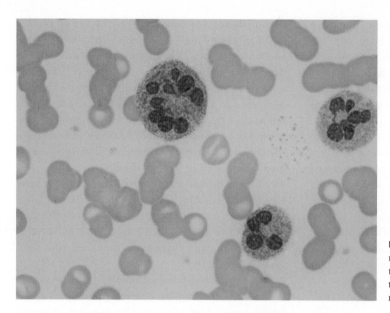

Fig. 9.3 Blood film of a patient with multiple myeloma (note increased rouleaux formation) and a neutrophilic leukaemoid reaction. There is one macropolycyte and all the neutrophils show toxic granulation.

necessitates consideration of clinical features and specific bacteriological tests. In patients with known bacterial infection, the neutrophil count can be used to monitor the progress of the disease.

Tuberculosis

The haematological manifestations of tuberculosis are protean, although some of the abnormalities attributed to tuberculosis in the past are likely to have been caused by the coexistence of tuberculosis and a disease such as hairy cell leukaemia or primary myelofibrosis.

Blood film and count

Pulmonary tuberculosis causes a normocytic normochromic anaemia with increased rouleaux formation and an increased erythrocyte sedimentation rate (ESR). When the disease is severe, leucocytosis and neutrophilia are common [6]. Lymphocytosis is present in about one quarter of patients and lymphopenia in one fifth. Although monocytosis has been regarded as characteristic of tuberculosis, it is present in only about one quarter of patients while about one half have monocytopenia. Thrombocytosis is common. Automated blood counts show a low haemoglobin concentration (Hb), normal or reduced mean cell volume (MCV) and increased red cell distribution width (RDW).

Patients with miliary tuberculosis [7] are usually anaemic. In contrast to acute pulmonary tuberculosis,

leucocytosis is uncommon and leucopenia is common. Monocytosis occurs in about one quarter of patients. Lymphopenia is usual. A minority of patients have pancytopenia (which is sometimes the result of haemophagocytosis).

Differential diagnosis

The haematological manifestations of tuberculosis are so variable that many infective, inflammatory and neoplastic conditions enter into the differential diagnoses.

Further tests

Bone marrow aspiration and trephine biopsy can be useful in the diagnosis of miliary tuberculosis. However, blood cultures are also often positive so that bone marrow examination can be avoided.

Viral infections
Infectious mononucleosis

Infectious mononucleosis is an acute clinicopathological syndrome resulting from primary infection by the Epstein–Barr virus (EBV). In developed countries it is predominantly a disease of adolescents and young adults, occurring in one quarter to three-quarters of those suffering a primary EBV infection. It is rare in underdeveloped countries, where primary EBV infection usually occurs in childhood. Common clinical features are fever, pharyngitis, lymphadenopathy (hence the common designation 'glandular fever'), spleno-megaly and hepatitis. Haematologically, the disease is characterised by 'atypical mononuclear cells' or 'atypical lymphocytes', which are mainly activated T lymphocytes produced as part of the immunological response to EBV-infected B lymphocytes.

Blood film and count

There is often lymphocytosis and leucocytosis as a result of the presence of atypical lymphocytes, representing mainly activated cytotoxic T cells. Suggested criteria alerting laboratory staff to the possibility of infectious mononucleosis are lymphocytes comprising at least 50% of peripheral blood leucocytes and atypical lymphocytes comprising at least 10% of circulating lymphocytes [8]; in one study the former observation had a sensitivity of 66% and the latter a sensitivity of 75% for heterophile-positive disease among patients with suspected infectious mononucleosis [9]. Some patients are thrombocytopenic and a minority are anaemic. Atypical lymphocytes are highly pleomorphic (Figs 9.4 & 9.5). Many are large, with diameters up to 15–30 μm, and have abundant strongly basophilic cytoplasm. Some have large central nucleoli and resemble immunoblasts (i.e. they have the same cytological features as lymphocytes stimulated *in vitro* by mitogens); others resemble the blasts of acute lymphoblastic leukaemia (ALL). Nuclei can be round, oval, reniform, lobulated or, occasionally,

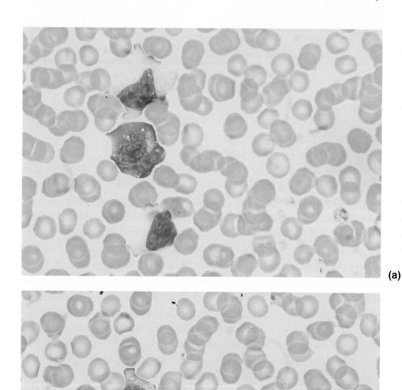

(a)

(b)

Fig. 9.4 Blood film in infectious mononucleosis showing atypical lymphocytes (atypical mononuclear cells): (a) pleomorphic cells, with plentiful cytoplasm – the largest cell has moderately basophilic vacuolated cytoplasm and a lobulated nucleus containing a nucleolus; and (b) a normal small lymphocyte and an atypical lymphocyte with voluminous cytoplasm and scalloped edges.

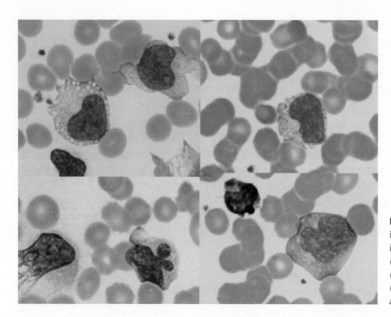

Fig. 9.5 Composite image of blood film in infectious mononucleosis showing two atypical lymphocytes, one of which is vacuolated (top left); atypical large granular lymphocyte (top right); smear cell and cloverleaf cell (bottom left); and apoptotic lymphocyte and atypical lymphocyte (bottom right).

clover-leafed. In one study 15% of patients had clover-leaf nuclei, an observation of low sensitivity but high specificity in patients with suspected infectious mononucleosis [9]. In the same study 30% of patients had smear cells, also a highly specific observation in this group of patients [9]. The chromatin pattern may be diffuse or partly condensed. The cytoplasm may be vacuolated, foamy or (occasionally) granulated, and moderately or strongly basophilic. Cytoplasmic basophilia may be generalised or confined to the cytoplasmic margins. When the atypical cells have contact with other cells the cytoplasmic margins sometimes appear scalloped. It should, however, be noted that both 'scalloping' and peripheral cytoplasmic basophilia can also be features of lymphoma cells. Some cells have a hand-mirror conformation. Binucleate cells and mitotic figures may be seen. Apoptotic cells may be present, infectious mononucleosis being the most common cause of apoptosis in circulating lymphocytes [10]. Large granular lymphocytes may be increased and there may be some plasmacytoid lymphocytes and plasma cells. In some patients sequential changes are observed with initially large granular lymphocytes (activated CD8-positive T cells that are not EBV-specific) and subsequently pleomorphic atypical lymphocytes (EBV-specific) [11]. The abnormal cells can have cytochemical abnormalities such as block-positivity on a periodic acid–Schiff (PAS) stain – usually a feature of ALL – and tartrate-resistant acid phosphatase (TRAP)

activity – usually a feature of hairy cell leukaemia. However, cytochemistry is not recommended in the diagnosis of infectious mononucleosis.

Changes in other cell lines are quite common, although they tend to be overshadowed by the abnormalities in the lymphocytes. In one series, 10% of patients had neutrophil counts of less than $1 \times 10^9/l$ [12]. Occasionally, neutropenia is very severe [13]. Neutrophilia can also occur. Neutrophils sometimes show toxic granulation, left shift and Döhle bodies; despite these changes, the neutrophil alkaline phosphatase (NAP) score is usually reduced. Reduction of the eosinophil count is usual; during recovery there is eosinophilia. Thrombocytopenia is not uncommon, the platelet count being less than $150 \times 10^9/l$ in about one third of patients. Severe thrombocytopenia that sometimes occurs is likely to be due to immune destruction of platelets. Haemolytic anaemia due to a cold antibody can occur and the blood film then shows red cell agglutination, some spherocytes and, later, the development of polychromasia. A larger number of patients show some red cell agglutination without overt haemolysis. Subjects with hereditary spherocytosis appear to be particularly prone to haemolysis during infectious mononucleosis. Some patients develop severe cytopenias consequent on virus-triggered haemophagocytosis. Aplastic anaemia is a rare complication, developing 1–6 weeks after presentation.

Not all patients with primary infection by EBV have the clinicopathological features of infectious mononucleosis. Young children have a greater degree of lymphocytosis and a lower percentage of atypical lymphocytes than older children, but the absolute count of atypical lymphocytes is similar in children under and over 4 years of age [14]. In older patients the degree of lymphocytosis and the percentage of atypical lymphocytes may be less than is usually observed in adolescents and young adults [15]. Rare patients with infectious mononucleosis have severe lymphopenia [16]. This is associated with severe disease and a worse prognosis.

Automated counters usually 'flag' the presence of suspected blast cells, atypical (or 'variant') lymphocytes or both. Depending on the instrument, there may be an increase in 'monocytes', 'mononuclear cells' or large unstained (i.e. peroxidase-negative) cells (LUC) or a factitious increase in 'basophils'. In one study of patients with a clinical suspicion of infectious mononucleosis who had, or did not have, a positive test for a heterophile antibody, a Coulter STKS instrument blast flag had a sensitivity of 41% for heterophile-positive disease, while an atypical lymphocyte flag had a sensitivity of 72%. For a Sysmex NE-8000, sensitivities were 43% and 16% respectively [9].

Differential diagnosis

The differential diagnosis of infectious mononucleosis includes other causes of atypical lymphocytes (Table 9.1) and, to a lesser extent, ALL and non-Hodgkin lymphoma.

Further tests

The finding of a blood film suggestive of infectious mononucleosis is an indication to test for a heterophile antibody that agglutinates sheep or horse red cells and differs from heterophile antibodies in other conditions in that it is adsorbed by ox red cells but not by guinea pig kidney. Rapid commercially available slide tests for heterophile antibodies are sensitive and very convenient, with a false-positive rate of 1–2%. At presentation, 60% of patients with infectious mononucleosis have a positive heterophile antibody test and up to 90% become positive if closely followed. In adolescents and adults, 'heterophile-negative infectious mononucleosis' most often represents either cytomegalovirus (CMV) or EBV infection. In one series of patients, 70% of cases represented CMV infection and 16% EBV infection [30]. In

Table 9.1 Some causes of atypical lymphocytes.

Viral infections
Infectious mononucleosis (Epstein-Barr virus infection), cytomegalovirus infection,* infectious hepatitis (hepatitis A infection),* measles (rubeola), German measles (rubella), echovirus infection, adenovirus infection,* chicken pox (varicella) and herpes zoster, herpes simplex infection, human herpesvirus 6 infection* [17], influenza, mumps, lymphocytic meningitis (lymphocytic choriomeningitis virus infection), human immunodeficiency virus (HIV) infection, human T-cell lymphotropic virus 1 (HTLV-1) infection, hantavirus pulmonary syndrome [18]

Bacterial infections
Brucellosis, tuberculosis, typhoid fever [19], syphilis, rickettsial infections* including tick typhus (*Rickettsia conorii*), scrub typhus (*Rickettsia tsutsugamushi*), murine typhus (*Rickettsia typhi*) [20,21], ehrlichia infections (including Sennetsu fever (Japan) and ehrlichiosis (USA)) [22], *Mycoplasma pneumoniae* infection

Protozoan infections
Toxoplasmosis,* malaria, babesiosis

Immunisations

Serum sickness (rarely)

Hypersensitivity to drugs*
Hypersensitivity to para-aminosalicylic acid, sulfasalazine, sodium phenytoin, mesantoin, dapsone, phenothiazines, streptokinase [23]

Angioimmunoblastic lymphadenopathy/angioimmunoblastic T-cell lymphoma [24]

Systemic lupus erythematosus [25]

Sarcoidosis [26]

Graft-versus-host disease

Graft rejection

Hodgkin lymphoma

Kawasaki syndrome [27]

Familial haemophagocytic lymphohistiocytosis [28]

Transient idiopathic proliferation of monoclonal atypical lymphocytes [29]

* Conditions that can be associated with sufficiently large numbers of atypical lymphocytes to be confused with infectious mononucleosis

another series, the percentages of patients with immunoglobulin (Ig) M antibodies to various viruses were 40% for EBV, 39% for CMV and 25% for human herpesvirus 6 [31], some patients having IgM antibodies to more than one virus; 3% of patients had toxoplasmosis. Well below one half of infants with primary EBV infection have heterophile antibodies [14], so that in this age group EBV infection is the commonest cause of heterophile-negative infectious mononucleosis. Specific serological tests for IgM antibodies to EBV and CMV can clarify the diagnosis in heterophile-antibody negative cases. Serological tests for toxoplasmosis are also indicated and, in high-risk groups, testing for human immunodeficiency virus (HIV) should be considered (see below).

HIV infection and AIDS

HIV infection causes an acute illness at the time of seroconversion followed by a phase of latent infection before the manifestations of chronic infection appear. Chronic infection is associated with development of the acquired immune deficiency syndrome (AIDS). A transient expansion of CD8-positive large granular lymphocytes may occur as chronic HIV infection becomes clinically evident. Less often there is a persistent increase in large granular lymphocytes associated with a syndrome that clinically resembles Sjögren syndrome, with lymphoid infiltration of salivary glands, lungs and kidneys [32].

Blood film and count

The acute illness can resemble infectious mononucleosis both clinically and haematologically, but in general the number of atypical lymphocytes (Fig. 9.6) is considerably less. Following recovery from the acute phase, the infected person is clinically and haematologically normal, often for many years. Isolated thrombocytopenia,

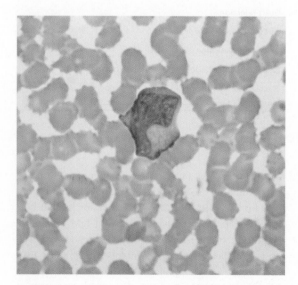

Fig. 9.6 Peripheral blood film showing an atypical lymphocyte during acute human immunodeficiency virus (HIV) infection.

resulting from immune destruction of platelets, can occur during this period of clinically latent infection.

Chronic infection is associated with a progressive decline in the number of CD4-positive lymphocytes and, usually, a decline in the total lymphocyte count. Reactive lymphocytosis consequent on an increase in CD8-positive lymphocytes (including CD8-positive CD57-positive large granular lymphocytes [32,33]) can initially mask the progressive decline in CD4-positive lymphocytes. The declining CD4-positive lymphocyte count is associated with a progressive decline in immune function, which eventually leads to opportunistic infection or neoplasia. The development of certain specified infective or neoplastic conditions defines the patient as suffering from AIDS. Haematological features then include both the effects of HIV infection and the effects of intercurrent infections. HIV infection itself causes a normocytic normochromic anaemia, thrombocytopenia and neutropenia with dysplastic neutrophils; one relatively specific neutrophil abnormality is the presence of detached nuclear fragments [34]. Dysplastic forms can include hypogranular and pseudo-Pelger neutrophils and neutrophils with large nuclei of abnormal shape (Fig. 9.7). Thrombotic thrombocytopenic purpura (TTP) may occur as a complication of HIV infection and the blood film then shows thrombocytopenia and red cell fragmentation. Recurrent infections contribute to the development of anaemia and are associated with increased rouleaux formation and increased background staining. Minor reactive changes in lymphocytes are common and may include cloverleaf forms. Bacterial infection can also be associated with toxic changes in neutrophils. Viral and mycobacterial infections can be associated with severe pancytopenia resulting from virus-associated haemophagocytosis. In the final stages of the disease there is a progressive pancytopenia.

Patients with HIV infection are also prone to iatrogenic haematological complications including macrocytosis and pancytopenia caused by zidovudine therapy, neutropenia caused by ganciclovir and oxidant-induced haemolytic anaemia caused by dapsone.

In patients with chronic HIV infection, the automated count with Siemens H.1 and Advia series counters can show increased peroxidase activity of neutrophils and a reduction of nuclear density seen as a reduced lobularity index. Both these features are indicative of dysplastic granulopoiesis. There can also be an increase in LUC.

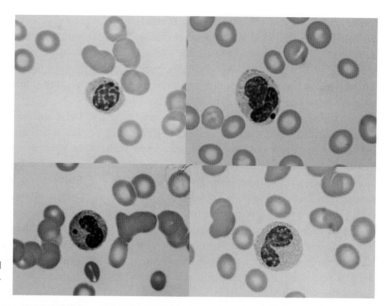

Fig. 9.7 Composite image of the peripheral blood film of an HIV-infected patient showing HIV-related neutrophil dysplasia.

Differential diagnosis

Depending on the stage of the disease and the specific haematological features, the differential diagnosis can include infectious mononucleosis and other viral infections, autoimmune ('idiopathic') thrombocytopenic purpura (ITP) and TTP. It is important to think of the possibility of HIV infection and consider performing specific serological tests in patients who present with these haematological features. An expansion of large granular lymphocytes can be confused with large granular lymphocyte leukaemia, particularly as up to a quarter of patients have evidence of a clonal expansion on T-cell receptor analysis [32]; the immunophenotype of the cells is CD8-positive, CD11a-positive, CD11c-positive and CD57-positive with strong expression of HLA-DR and negative reactions for CD16 and CD56. HIV infection is part of the differential diagnosis of chronic red cell aplasia, since immune deficiency can lead to failure to eliminate parvovirus B19 so that virus-induced red cell aplasia is chronic rather than transient. Late in the disease, confusion with myelodysplastic syndromes (MDS) and other causes of bone marrow failure can occur.

Further tests

Diagnosis is customarily by serological detection of antibodies to HIV. If there is chronic red cell aplasia in an HIV-positive patient, serological tests for parvovirus should be supplemented by tests for parvovirus deoxyribonucleic acid (DNA), since there may be a failure of specific antibody production.

Other viral infections

Viral infections may be acute or chronic. They cause a variety of effects on blood cells.

Blood film and count

Acute viral infections are associated with transient haematological abnormalities, most often lymphocytosis with reactive changes in lymphocytes. Large granular lymphocytes may be increased. With some viruses these changes can be sufficiently severe to simulate infectious mononucleosis (see Table 9.1). Other acute viral infections are associated with neutrophilia (see Table 6.4). The eosinophil count is reduced during acute infection and rises during recovery. Thrombocytopenia, as a result of platelet consumption, can occur during active viral infection. In the case of the viral haemorrhagic fevers, disseminated intravascular coagulation can cause severe thrombocytopenia. During recovery from some viral infections, e.g. rubella, there may be thrombocytopenia consequent on interaction of immune complexes with platelets. Acute haemolysis caused by the Donath–Landsteiner (anti-P) antibody can follow viral infections, e.g. measles, and acute haemolysis consequent on a cold agglutinin (anti-I or anti-i) can occur during other viral infections. Parvovirus infection in normal subjects causes acute, transient red cell aplasia associated with a slight fall in Hb and the disappearance of reticulocytes, and therefore a lack of polychromasia. In some patients there is associated neutropenia or thrombocytopenia. In patients with a shortened red cell lifespan, more severe but transient anaemia occurs. Some viruses, particularly herpesviruses, trigger a haemophagocytic syndrome, leading to pancytopenia. Infection by the Sin Nombre hantavirus has been observed to be associated with thrombocytopenia early in the illness, with severe cardiopulmonary malfunction being predicted by a constellation of five peripheral blood features – thrombocytopenia, the presence of myelocytes, lack of marked toxic granulation (even if there was marked neutrophilia), increased haematocrit (attributable to a capillary leak syndrome) and the presence of more than 10% immunoblast-like cells (of T lineage) or plasma cells [35].

The effects of chronic viral infection vary with the virus. There may be an increase of large granular lymphocytes. In chronic infection with human T-cell lymphotropic virus 1 (HTLV-1), there may be lymphocytosis with occasional atypical lymphocytes, including some with cloverleaf nuclei (Fig. 9.8). Immunologically incompetent subjects, not only those with HIV infection but also those with congenital or iatrogenic immunosuppression, can develop chronic parvovirus infection with resultant chronic red cell aplasia. An apparent viral hepatitis (non-A, non-B,

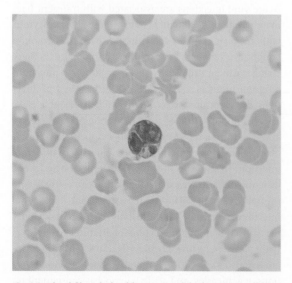

Fig. 9.8 Blood film of a healthy carrier of the human T-cell lymphotropic virus I (HTLV-1 virus) showing a lymphocyte with a flower-shaped nucleus.

non-C) [36] can be followed by aplastic anaemia. Patients with chronic infection by any of the hepatitis viruses can develop haematological abnormalities resulting from chronic liver disease and hypersplenism and those with hepatitis C infection can develop cryoglobulinaemia.

Differential diagnosis

The differential diagnosis of the haematological effects of viral infection is complex, since the abnormalities caused are very variable. The differential diagnoses include the various conditions that can cause lymphocytosis, atypical lymphocytes and thrombocytopenia.

Further tests

Tests for heterophile antibodies and serological tests for specific viruses should be performed when clinically appropriate.

Persistent polyclonal B-cell lymphocytosis

Persistent polyclonal B-cell lymphocytosis is a rare condition occurring mainly in women and mainly in cigarette smokers. There is an association with the HLA-DR7 tissue type. Familial cases have been reported, both in several sets of siblings and in a parent and a child. An association with EBV infection has also been suspected. A minority of patients have hepatomegaly, splenomegaly or lymphadenopathy, but most have only non-specific clinical features, such as fatigue. Occasional patients have massive splenomegaly [37]. There is an association with chromosomal instability and acquired chromosomal abnormalities, particularly i(3q), trisomy 3 and dup(3)(q26q29) [38,39], which, remarkably, are present in both kappa-expressing and lambda-expressing lymphocytes and therefore cannot be taken as indicative of clonality.

Blood film and count

The abnormal lymphocytes include both large lymphocytes with increased cytoplasmic basophilia, resembling those seen in viral infections, and bilobed and binucleated lymphocytes [40] (Fig. 9.9). The latter are strongly suggestive of this particular disorder. Some cells have nucleoli and among these there may also be some resembling prolymphocytes. Rarely the cells show ethylenediaminetetra-acetic acid (EDTA)-dependent agglutination [41]. The diagnosis can be made in patients without an absolute lymphocytosis if cytological and other features are typical. Such cases constituted 20% of patients in one series [42].

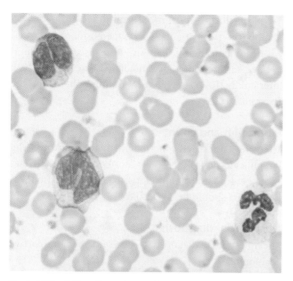

Fig. 9.9 Blood film of a patient with persistent polyclonal B-cell lymphocytosis showing lobulated lymphocytes.

Differential diagnosis

The differential diagnosis includes reactive lymphocytosis and non-Hodgkin lymphoma.

Further tests

Immunophenotyping is indicated to exclude a monoclonal proliferation of lymphocytes. The cells usually express IgM and IgD together with pan-B markers (such as CD19 and CD24), CD11c, CD21, CD25, CD27, CD95 and CD148 [43,44]. The proportion of B cells expressing CD5 and CD23 is lower than in normal controls, FMC7 is higher, and CD10 and CD38 are not usually expressed [43]. The abnormal cells appear to represent an expanded population of memory B cells [43], possibly analogous to marginal zone B cells [44]. Although the κ:λ ratio may be abnormal, the atypical population includes both κ-expressing and λ-expressing cells. The polymerase chain reaction (PCR) shows that single or multiple *BCL2- IGH* rearrangements are often present. There is often a polyclonal increase in IgM. In addition to i(3q) (leading to amplification of the *ATR* gene), del(6q), +8 and del(11q) have been observed [42]. There may be nodular or intrasinusoidal bone marrow infiltration [45].

Reactive eosinophilia

Reactive eosinophilia is common in a wide variety of allergic and parasitic conditions (see Chapter 6). Less often it represents a reaction to a neoplasm, e.g. carcinoma or sarcoma

Blood film and count

Eosinophilia varies from mild to marked. Eosinophils may be cytologically normal or show a greater or lesser degree of degranulation or vacuolation (Fig. 9.10). The blood film may also show lymphoma cells, blast cells or atypical lymphocytes. In reactive eosinophilia that occurs as a response to ALL, the leukaemic blasts may be very infrequent in the peripheral blood and the eosinophils very numerous.

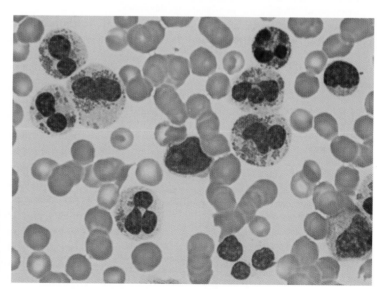

Fig. 9.10 Blood film of a patient with B-lineage acute lymphoblastic leukaemia and reactive eosinophilia. There is a leukaemic lymphoblast in the centre. Many of the eosinophils are hypogranular and some have trilobed nuclei.

When eosinophils are degranulated, automated instruments may fail to recognise them.

Differential diagnosis

The differential diagnosis includes eosinophilic leukaemia, T-cell mediated hypereosinophilia and the idiopathic hypereosinophilic syndrome. The latter diagnosis requires that no evidence of an underlying cause can be found (see below).

Further tests

The most important initial step in investigating unexplained hypereosinophilia is a full history including a travel and drug history followed by a physical examination. These procedures may provide clues indicating the direction of further investigation. If parasitic infection appears likely, a considerable range of investigations may be necessary, the precise choice of test depending on the travel history and on any relevant features in the medical history or found on physical examination. Investigations that may be useful in patients with eosinophilia are shown in Table 9.2.

Table 9.2 Investigations that may be useful in unexplained eosinophilia.

If parasitic infection is suspected [46]
Examination of stools for ova, cysts and parasites
Examination of urine for *Schistosoma haematobium*
Rectal biopsy for *Schistosoma mansoni*
Serology – antibody tests for strongyloidiasis, toxocariasis, schistosomiasis, filariasis and a variety of other parasites – or antigen tests for cysticercosis, filariasis or a variety of other parasites (depending on the travel history)
Examination of the blood for microfilariae
Duodenal aspiration
Assay of immunoglobulin E concentration
Chest radiology
Biopsy of skin or muscle

If neoplasia is suspected
Chest radiology
Computed tomography (CT) scan or other imaging of chest and abdomen
Bone marrow aspirate, trephine biopsy, cytogenetic analysis and molecular analysis (can be done on peripheral blood) for the *FIP1L1-PDGFRA* fusion gene
Biopsy of lymph node or other tissue
Immunophenotyping of peripheral blood lymphocytes or of any abnormal cell population in blood or bone marrow
T-cell receptor gene analysis to establish clonality of T lymphocytes

T-cell mediated hypereosinophilia

A proportion of patients with hypereosinophilia, often with cutaneous manifestations of the disease, are found to have eosinophilia that is mediated by cytokines (e.g. interleukin (IL) 5) secreted by immunophenotypically aberrant T cells.

Blood film and count

There are no specific peripheral blood features. The lymphocyte count is usually normal and, if it is elevated, eosinophilia secondary to T-cell non-Hodgkin lymphoma should be suspected.

Differential diagnosis

The differential diagnosis is the same as for reactive eosinophilia.

Further tests

Immunophenotyping shows a population of T cells with an aberrant phenotype, e.g. with failure to express CD3, with expression of CD3 but not CD4 or CD8, or with over- or under-expression of other T-cell associated antigens. Use of a panel of antibodies to variable domains of the T-cell receptor can provide evidence of clonality and clonal rearrangements of T-cell receptor genes can be demonstrated in about half of these patients. Cytogenetic abnormalities, e.g. 6q– or 10p–, can occur as secondary events. Serum immunoglobulin E concentration is usually increased and there may be polyclonal hyperimmunoglobulinaemia.

Idiopathic hypereosinophilic syndrome

The term idiopathic hypereosinophilic syndrome (HES) is used to describe a heterogeneous group of conditions characterised by persistent unexplained eosinophilia and tissue damage (e.g. involving the heart and nervous system) attributable to the release of eosinophil granule contents. The condition is much more common in males. Cases are arbitrarily classified as idiopathic HES when the eosinophil count is in excess of $1.5 \times 10^9/l$, when unexplained eosinophilia persists for at least 6 months and when there is associated tissue damage [47]. Some cases appear to be attributable to an abnormality of T lymphocytes, with eosinophilia provoked by lymphokines such as IL2, IL3, IL5 and IL15 [48–50] (see above). If the T lymphocytes can be shown to be clonal, the eosinophilia may be reactive to an overt or occult T-cell lymphoma, but if T cells are non-clonal, classification as 'idiopathic' remains appropriate. It is likely that certain other cases represent a myeloproliferative neoplasm with predominant eosinophilic differentiation, i.e. eosinophilic leukaemia, but if there is no proof of this, classification as 'idiopathic' is appropriate.

Blood film and count

The haematological features of idiopathic HES are currently ill-defined as previous series of patients included many who would now be recognised as having eosinophilic leukaemia. The description that follows should therefore be regarded as provisional.

There is a moderate or marked eosinophilia. Eosinophils often show marked degranulation and vacuolation, even including completely agranular eosinophils (Fig. 9.11). Granules are often smaller than normal. Eosinophil nuclei may be hyperlobated, hypolobated or ring-shaped. Other haematological features can include anaemia, anisocytosis, poikilocytosis (including teardrop poikilocytes), a leucoerythroblastic blood film, basophilia, thrombocytopenia, thrombocytosis, neutrophilia and the presence of neutrophils with heavy, rather basophilic granules (see Fig. 3.71). The latter abnormality may be so marked that the abnormal neutrophils are confused with basophils. A true increase in basophils can also occur [47]. The number of degranulated eosinophils is of prognostic significance. If they exceed

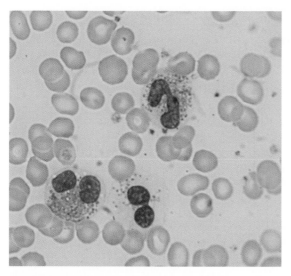

Fig. 9.11 Blood film of a patient with the idiopathic hypereosinophilic syndrome (HES); the three eosinophils show various degrees of degranulation.

$1 \times 10^9/1$ it is likely that cardiac damage is already present or will occur [51].

Differential diagnosis

Idiopathic HES is a diagnosis of exclusion. The diagnosis should not be made without excluding the presence of a *FIP1L1-PDGFRA* fusion gene, since many cases of what was previously classed as idiopathic HES are now know to represent eosinophilic leukaemia as a result of this fusion gene.

Many of the characteristic features are not specific. Tissue damage from the release of eosinophil granule contents can also occur both in reactive eosinophilia (see above) and in eosinophilic leukaemia. Degranulation and vacuolation of eosinophils can also be marked both in eosinophil leukaemia and in severe reactive eosinophilia. Peripheral blood features indistinguishable from idiopathic HES can occur in some patients who are subsequently found to have systemic mastocytosis [52], ALL or lymphoma. Making a distinction between idiopathic HES and chronic eosinophilic leukaemia (see below) at the onset of the disease can be difficult or even impossible.

Further tests

The patient should be appropriately investigated by history, physical examination and laboratory tests for known causes of eosinophilia. If no cause is identified, immunophenotypic analysis of peripheral blood lymphocytes should be performed to identify any population of lymphocytes expressing aberrant markers [49,50]. If an abnormal population is identified, T-cell receptor gene analysis should be performed to seek evidence that the abnormal population is clonal [49]. Bone marrow aspiration, a trephine biopsy and cytogenetic analysis are also indicated, since detection of increased blast cells or a clonal cytogenetic abnormality permits the diagnosis of eosinophilic leukaemia. Systemic mastocytosis or a lymphoma may also be diagnosed on the bone marrow aspirate or trephine biopsy sections.

Although cases without evidence of an abnormal T-cell clone or specific features that identify them as 'leukaemia' are best classified as idiopathic HES, some such patients subsequently show transformation of their disease to acute myeloid leukaemia (AML), providing evidence that the condition was neoplastic from the beginning. In others, an overt lymphoproliferative disorder subsequently becomes apparent. In some patients death occurs from the early or late effects of tissue damage without the true nature of the condition having become apparent.

Leukaemoid reactions

A leukaemoid reaction is a haematological abnormality that simulates leukaemia and thus may be confused with it, but that is, in fact, reactive to some other disease. In a leukaemoid reaction the abnormalities reverse when the underlying condition is corrected. In many of the early reports of leukaemoid reactions, the patient did not recover from the primary disease and correction of the haematological abnormality did not occur. In such cases, it is difficult to be sure that the patient did not have leukaemia coexisting with some other disease. This is so in many of the early reports of an apparent leukaemoid reaction with tuberculosis. Transient abnormal myelopoiesis in neonates with Down syndrome (see below) should not be described as a leukaemoid reaction. It is a neoplastic condition and is more correctly regarded as a spontaneously remitting leukaemia [53]. Leukaemoid reactions may be myeloid or lymphoid.

Myeloid leukaemoid reactions

Leukaemoid reactions rarely simulate chronic myelogenous leukaemia (CML), since the characteristic spectrum of changes (see below) is virtually never seen in reactive conditions. The differences are summarised in Table 9.3. The myeloid leukaemias that are most likely to be simulated by a leukaemoid reaction are AML, atypical Philadelphia-negative chronic myeloid leukaemia (aCML), chronic myelomonocytic leukaemia (CMML), juvenile myelomonocytic leukaemia (JMML), neutrophilic leukaemia and eosinophilic leukaemia. Causes of myeloid leukaemoid reactions (Fig. 9.12) include any strong stimulus to bone marrow activity such as severe bacterial infection (particularly if complicated by megaloblastic anaemia, alcohol-induced bone marrow damage or prior agranulocytosis), tuberculosis, certain viral infections, haemorrhage and carcinoma or other malignant disease (with or without bone marrow metastases). Leukaemoid reactions in carcinoma may precede other manifestations of the carcinoma, sometimes by a number of years [54]. Myeloid leukaemoid reactions have been recognised in ALL [55]. The diagnosis of

Table 9.3 Some features that may be useful in distinguishing chronic myelogenous leukaemia (CML) from reactive neutrophilia.

Feature	Reactive neutrophilia	CML
WBC	Rarely > 60 × 10⁹/l	Usually 20–500 × 10⁹/l or even higher
Left shift	May be moderate or marked; if slight in relation to neutrophilia supports reactive neutrophilia	Proportional to WBC; may be marked
White cell morphology	Toxic granulation, neutrophil vacuolation and Döhle bodies may be present	Toxic changes not present
Absolute eosinophil count	Usually reduced	Usually elevated; eosinophil myelocytes may be present
Absolute basophil count	Usually reduced	Almost invariably elevated: basophil myelocytes may be present
Absolute monocyte count	May be elevated	Usually moderately elevated, but not in proportion to the increase in the neutrophil count
Erythropoiesis	Anaemia may be present; usually normocytic and normochromic, but if hypochromic and microcytic supports a reactive neutrophilia; rouleaux may be present	Anaemia may be present; normocytic and normochromic
Platelet count	Thrombocytosis or thrombocytopenia can occur; if there is reactive thrombocytosis the platelets are usually small	The platelet count is usually normal or high; giant platelets may be present; platelets are large, even in the presence of thrombocytosis; circulating megakaryocytes may be present
NAP score	Usually elevated	Almost always reduced

NAP, neutrophil alkaline phosphatase; WBC, white blood cell count

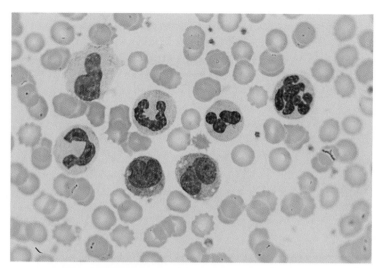

Fig. 9.12 Blood film of a patient with a leukaemoid reaction resulting from severe post-operative sepsis due to a Gram-negative organism. WBC was $92 \times 10^9/l$ with a neutrophil count of $74 \times 10^9/l$ and a monocyte count of $16 \times 10^9/l$; the film shows a band form, a macropolycyte and monocytes with increased cytoplasmic basophilia.

such reactions in AML is more problematical, often requiring cytogenetic and molecular genetic studies; the administration of growth factors or of high-dose chemotherapy can lead to pseudo-relapse, with circulating immature but non-leukaemic cells, but growth factors can also lead to the appearance of leukaemic cells in the blood. Leukaemoid reactions in neonates may result from congenital syphilis [56] and in infants may be consequent on the syndrome of thrombocytopenia with absent radii, particularly if complicated by haemorrhage [57]. Although it has been considered that there is an association between multiple myeloma, and other plasma cell neoplasms, and neutrophilic leukaemia, it appears more likely that the neutrophilia in these patients usually represents a leukaemoid reaction [58,59], mediated by G-CSF secreted by the myeloma cells [60]; however, in one such patient AML developed only one and a half years after presentation [61] (rather too short an interval for an alkylating agent-related leukaemia) and the exact nature of this condition is not always certain. Ectopic G-CSF secretion by other tumours can cause a neutrophilic leukaemoid reaction similar to that seen in multiple myeloma; this has been observed in sarcomas and in carcinomas of the lung, thyroid, stomach, gall bladder and urinary bladder [60,62,63]. A leukaemoid reaction can result from administration of growth factors such as G-CSF, granulocyte-macrophage colony-stimulating factor (GM-CSF) and IL3. If the clinical history is not known to the laboratory staff, CMML, aCML or eosinophilic leukaemia may be suspected. Cases may have up to 30% circulating myeloblasts so can also simulate AML [64]. Various infections in children can lead to a leukaemoid reaction that simulates JMML. These include histoplasmosis, toxoplasmosis, mycobacterial infection [65] and infection by *Mycoplasma pneumoniae* [66], EBV [67], CMV [68], human herpesvirus 6 [69] and parvovirus B19 [70]. The blood film in osteopetrosis may simulate JMML [71] (Fig. 9.13).

Useful features in making the distinction between leukaemia and a leukaemoid reaction include toxic changes, such as toxic granulation and vacuolation, a preponderance of more mature cells (in a leukaemoid reaction) and hypogranular neutrophils and the presence of a disproportionate number of myeloblasts (in many leukaemias). A low NAP score is strongly in favour of a diagnosis of leukaemia since it is almost invariably raised in leukaemoid reactions. If Auer rods are seen in blast cells, a confident diagnosis of leukaemia or MDS can be made.

If clinical and haematological features do not permit the distinction between leukaemia and a leukaemoid reaction, then bone marrow aspiration with cytogenetic analysis and microscopy and culture for *Mycobacterium tuberculosis* is indicated.

'Pseudo-relapse' resulting from growth factor administration can be distinguished from relapse of leukaemia by cytogenetic or molecular genetic analysis, which shows that a leukaemia-associated abnormality is no longer present.

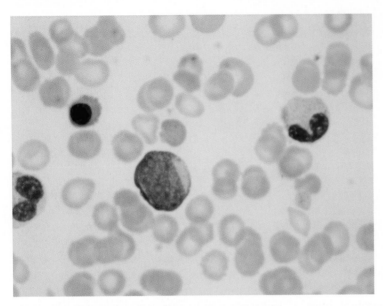

Fig. 9.13 Blood film of a child with a leukaemoid reaction as a result of early onset osteopetrosis, showing a blast cell a nucleated red blood cell and a neutrophil.

Lymphoid leukaemoid reactions

The blood film of whooping cough (Fig. 9.14) and of infectious lymphocytosis may simulate chronic lymphocytic leukaemia (CLL) but, since the clinical features and the age range of the two diseases are totally different, no problem occurs in practice. CLL has also been misdiagnosed in patients with post-splenectomy lymphocytosis. Knowledge of the high levels that the lymphocyte count can reach post-splenectomy and careful examination of the peripheral blood film for post-splenectomy features will avoid this

problem. Post-splenectomy lymphocytosis can also simulate large granular lymphocyte leukaemia, since the dominant cell can be a large granular lymphocyte (Fig. 9.15). Considerable numbers of large granular lymphocytes have also been reported in association with rituximab-induced autoimmune neutropenia [72]. Persistent polyclonal B-cell lymphocytosis can also be confused with CLL or non-Hodgkin lymphoma, occasionally even leading to inappropriate chemotherapy. Knowledge of this syndrome and detection of the characteristic cytological features (see above) allow a

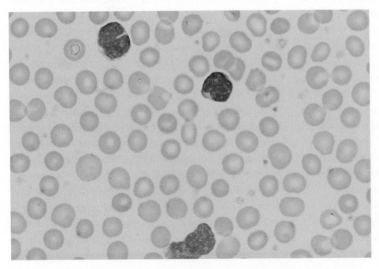

Fig. 9.14 Blood film of a child with whooping cough showing a cleft lymphocyte, a lymphocyte of normal morphology and a smear cell.

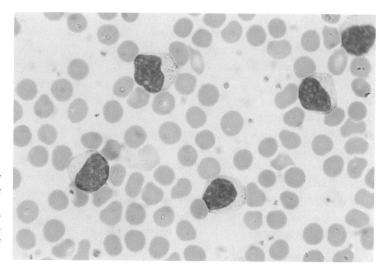

Fig. 9.15 Blood film following splenectomy for hereditary spherocytosis. The white blood cell count (WBC) was 29.3 × 10⁹/l and the lymphocyte count 24 × 10⁹/l. The lymphocytes were predominantly large granular lymphocytes. By courtesy of Dr J. Houghton, Salford.

distinction to be made. Hyper-reactive malarial sple-nomegaly can be associated with lymphocytosis with numerous villous lymphocytes and can thus simulate splenic lymphoma with villous lymphocytes (SLVL) [73]; however, immunophenotyping is essential to be certain that the patient does not in fact have SLVL, since this lymphoma occurs in the same geographical area and may represent a neoplasm arising, as a result of chronic antigenic stimulation, in a patient with prior hyper-reactive malarial splenomegaly. A peripheral blood picture resembling Sézary cell leukaemia has been observed as part of a drug reaction [74]. Circulating plasma cells sufficient to simulate plasma cell leukaemia have been reported in a patient with bone marrow aplasia preceding ALL [75].

ALL can be simulated by infectious mononcleosis and other viral infections that cause atypical lymphocytes to appear in the blood, by reactions to stress in children and by mycoplasma infection [66], tuberculosis and congenital syphilis. Lymphocytosis with immature lymphoid cells of T lineage has been described in acute HTLV-1 infection [76] and in ehrlichiosis [77]. When there is diagnostic uncertainty, immunophenotyping is required. However, it should be noted that phenotypically abnormal lymphoid cells can appear in the blood during lymphoid leukaemoid reactions, e.g. CD10-positive B-cell precursors or T cells co-expressing CD4 and CD8 [66].

Severe congenital neutropenia

Severe congenital neutropenia occurs either sporadically (most often) or as an autosomal dominant or, rarely, autosomal recessive or X-linked recessive inherited condition. In some patients it is the result of heterozygosity for a mutation in the *ELANE* gene at 19p13.3, encoding neutrophil elastase. Other causative mutations are shown in Table 6.22. Clinical presentation is with frequent severe bacterial infections in young infants, sometimes starting in the early neonatal period with infection of the umbilicus.

Blood film and count

Apart from changes related to infection, any neutrophils present are cytologically normal. There may be mild anaemia and thrombocytosis, both likely to be the result of infection. Monocytes and eosinophils are sometimes increased.

Differential diagnosis

The differential diagnosis includes other inherited and acquired causes of neutropenia in infants and children, particularly autoimmune neutropenia, cyclical neutropenia and Pearson syndrome (see Table 6.22).

Further tests

Bone marrow examination usually shows an apparent arrest of myelopoiesis at the promyelocyte stage. The diagnosis can be confirmed by DNA analysis.

Cyclical neutropenia

Cyclical neutropenia occurs as an autosomal dominant inherited condition or sporadically, usually in children under 1 year of age. This condition is the result of heterozygosity for a mutation in the *ELANE* gene. As a result of abnormal regulation of hae-mopoietic stem cells, the neutrophil count cycles with a periodicity of about 21 days, leading to recurrent infective episodes.

Blood film and count

Apart from changes related to infection, neutrophils are cytologically normal. The reticulocyte and platelet count may also cycle and sometimes also the eosino-phils and lymphocytes [78]. The monocyte count may cycle in opposite phase to the neutrophil count.

Differential diagnosis

The differential diagnosis includes other inherited and acquired causes of neutropenia in infants and children.

Further tests

Bone marrow examination shows cyclical changes, from an apparent arrest of myelopoiesis at the pro-myelocyte stage, preceding the neutropenia, to appar-ently normal maturation as the neutrophil count is rising. Diagnosis requires serial counts, three per week over a period of a month, and molecular genetic analysis.

Haematological neoplasms

Haematological neoplasms should be diagnosed and classified according to the World Health Organization (WHO) classification of tumours of haematopoietic and lymphoid tissues [79].

Acute myeloid leukaemia

AML is a disease resulting from proliferation of a clone of myeloid stem cells that show defective or absent maturation. Disease manifestations are those resulting from cell proliferation, such as hepatomegaly and sple-nomegaly, and those resulting from replacement of nor-mal bone marrow, such as anaemia and bleeding. The neoplastic clone is usually derived from a multipotent myeloid stem cell, but in some cases it may be derived either from a lineage-committed progenitor or a pluri-potent lymphoid–myeloid stem cell.

AML is further classified on the basis of peripheral blood and bone marrow features. For several decades the most generally accepted classification of AML was the French–American–British (FAB) classification

[80–84], but this has now been largely replaced by the WHO classification [79,85]. Because application of the WHO classification requires knowledge of cytogenetic and molecular genetic abnormalities, there is necess-arily some delay in making a definitive diagnosis. A preliminary morphological diagnosis based on the FAB classification therefore remains appropriate. The FAB classification also remains important in parts of the world where cytogenetic and molecular genetic analysis are not available. The most important dif-ference between these two classifications is that in the FAB classification the bone marrow blast cell percent-age must be at least 30% for a diagnosis of AML to be made, whereas in the WHO classification the defining criterion is a bone marrow or peripheral blood blast cell count (including promonocytes) of at least 20% (unless one of certain specified cytogenetic abnormali-ties is present). These classifications are summarised in Tables 9.4 and 9.5. Different FAB subtypes of acute leukaemia are illustrated in Figs 9.16–9.25 and various WHO categories in Figs 9.26–9.37. It should be noted that the WHO classification is hierarchical with cases first being assigned to the category of therapy-related AML, if appropriate, and then to other categories, in the order shown in Table 9.5.

Blood film and count

The majority of patients have leukaemic blast cells in the peripheral blood. These may be myeloblasts, monoblasts, megakaryoblasts, early erythroblasts or a mixed population. There may be some maturing cells. In some patients an abnormal promyelocyte is the dominant cell. Most patients are neutropenic, but in some types of AML there is maturation of the leukaemic clone with resultant neutrophilia or, less often, eosinophilia. Rarely, there is an increase in basophils. Most patients have a normocytic normo-chromic anaemia or, if there has been preceding MDS (see below), a macrocytic anaemia. Most patients are thrombocytopenic, but in a minority there is a nor-mal platelet count or even thrombocytosis. Peripheral blood cells may show dysplastic features similar to those of MDS. In a minority of patients, there is cyto-penia, usually pancytopenia, without any circulating immature cells.

Automated instruments flag suspected blast cells and may show that neutrophils have aberrant char-acteristics.

Table 9.4 The French–American–British (FAB) classification of AML [80–84]).

M1 (AML without maturation)
Blasts ≥ 90% of NEC; ≥ 3% of blasts positive for peroxidase or SBB; monocytic component ≤ 10% of NEC; granulocytic component ≤ 10% of NEC

M2 (AML with granulocytic maturation)
Blasts 30–89% of NEC; granulocytic component > 10% of NEC; monocytic component < 20% of NEC

M3 and M3 variant
Characteristic morphology

M4 (Acute myelomonocytic leukaemia)
Blasts ≥ 30% of NEC; granulocytic component (including myeloblasts) ≥ 20% of NEC

AND

EITHER	OR
BM monocytic component ≥ 20% of NEC and PB monocyte count ≥ 5 x 10^9/l	BM resembling M2 but PB monocyte count ≥ 5 x 10^9/l and lysozyme elevated*
OR	OR
BM monocytic component ≥ 20% of NEC and lysozyme elevated	BM resembling M2 but PB monocyte count ≥ 5 x 10^9/l and cytochemical demonstration of monocytic component in BM
OR	
BM monocytic component ≥ 20% of NEC and cytochemical confirmation of monocyte component in BM†	

M5 (acute monocytic/monoblastic leukaemia)

M5a (without maturation or acute monoblastic leukaemia)
Monocytic component ≥ 80% of NEC; monoblasts ≥ 80% of monocytic component

M5b (with maturation or acute monocytic leukaemia)
Monocytic component ≥ 80% of NEC; monoblasts < 80% of monocytic component

M6 (erythroleukaemia)
Erythroblasts ≥ 50%; blasts ≥ 30% of NEC

M7 (megakaryoblastic leukaemia)
Blasts demonstrated to be megakaryoblasts, for example by ultrastructural cytochemistry showing the presence of platelet peroxidase or by immunological cell marker studies showing the presence of platelet antigens

M0 (AML with minimal evidence of myeloid differentiation)
Peroxidase and SBB positive in < 3% of blasts but blasts demonstrated to be myeloid by immunophenotyping

BM, bone marrow; NEC, non-erythroid cells; PB, peripheral blood; SBB, Sudan black B.
* Lysozyme in serum or urine elevated threefold compared with normal.
† Positive for naphthol AS acetate esterase activity, with activity being inhibited by fluoride.

Table 9.5 The 2008 World Health Organization (WHO) classification of acute myeloid leukaemia (AML) [85].

AML and myelodysplastic syndromes, therapy-related
AML with recurrent cytogenetic/genetic abnormalities
    AML with t(8;21)(q22;q22); *RUNX1-RUNX1T1*
    AML with inv(16)(p13.1q22) or t(16;16)(p13.1;q22); *CBFB-MYH11*
    Acute promyelocytic leukaemia with t(15;17)(q22;q12); *PML-RARA*
    AML with t(9;11)(p22;q23); *MLLT3-MLL (MLLT3-KMT2A)*
    AML with t(6;9)(p23;q34); *DEK-NUP214*
AML with inv(3)(q21q26.2) or t(3;3)(q21;q26.2); *RPN1-EVI1 (RPN1-MECOM)*
AML (megakaryoblastic) with t(1;22)(p13;q13); *RBM15-MKL1*
AML with mutated *NPM1*
AML with mutated *CEBPA*
AML with myelodysplasia-related changes
    With prior myelodysplastic or myelodysplastic/myeloproliferative neoplasm
    With myelodysplastic syndrome-related cytogenetic abnormality
    With multilineage dysplasia*
AML not otherwise categorised
    AML with minimal differentiation
    AML without maturation
    AML with maturation
    Acute myelomonocytic leukaemia
    Acute monoblastic and monocytic leukaemia
    Acute erythroid leukaemia
    Acute megakaryocytic leukaemia
    Acute basophilic leukaemia
    Acute panmyelosis with myelofibrosis

* Defined as dysplastic features in more than 50% of cells in two or more cell lines

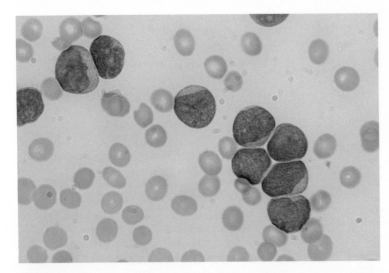

Fig. 9.16 Blood film in acute myeloid leukaemia (AML) without maturation (French–American–British (FAB) type M1). The blast cells have a fine chromatin pattern; they resemble lymphoblasts in having small nucleoli and a high nucleocytoplasmic ratio; in this patient only occasional blast cells had fine azurophilic granules but myeloperoxidase (MPO), Sudan black B (SBB) and chloroacetate esterase (CAE) were positive in a high percentage of cells.

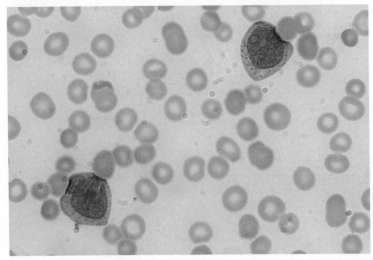

Fig. 9.17 Blood film in acute myeloid leukaemia with maturation (FAB type M2) showing leukaemic cells that are maturing beyond the blast stage. Both cells are promyelocytes, one with a nucleus of abnormal shape. Differentiation in M2 AML can be neutrophilic, eosinophilic, basophilic or any combination of these.

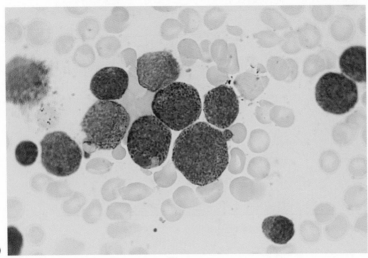

(a)

Fig. 9.18 Blood films of two patients with acute hypergranular promyelocytic leukaemia (FAB type M3) showing: (a) hypergranular promyelocytes, one of which has a giant granule. *Continued p.405*

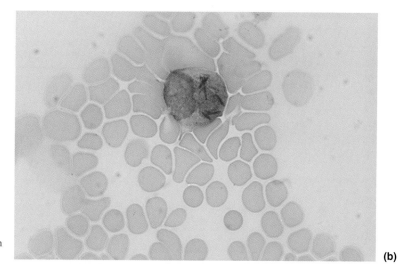

(b)

Fig. 9.18 *Continued* (b) a promyelocyte with few granules but stacks of Auer rods.

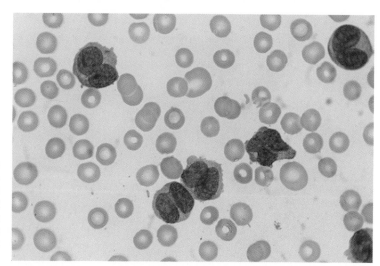

Fig. 9.19 Blood film in the hypogranular/ microgranular variant of acute promyelocytic leukaemia (FAB type M3 variant) showing cells with characteristic bilobed nuclei; only occasional cells have granules visible by light microscopy, but despite this there was strong cytoplasmic positivity with SBB, MPO and CAE.

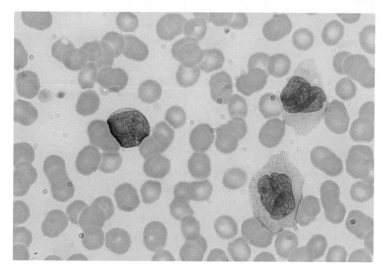

Fig. 9.20 Blood film of a patient with acute myelomonocytic leukaemia (FAB type M4) showing one myeloblast and two monoblasts; the monoblasts are large cells with lobulated nuclei, a fine lacy chromatin pattern, several nucleoli per nucleus and voluminous finely granulated cytoplasm, whereas the myeloblast is smaller with a higher nucleocytoplasmic ratio. In M4 AML the granulocytic differentiation may be neutrophilic, eosinophilic (see Fig. 9.21) or basophilic.

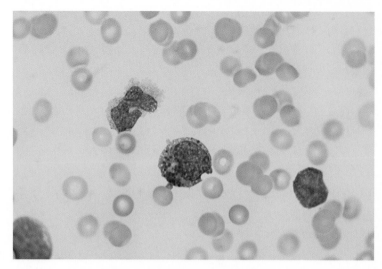

Fig. 9.21 Blood film in acute myelomonocytic leukaemia with eosinophilia (often designated 'M4 Eo', although this is not a FAB category) showing a myeloblast, a monocyte and an eosinophil myelocyte in which some granules have basophilic staining characteristics. By courtesy of the late Dr David Swirsky.

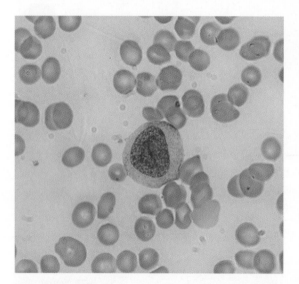

Fig. 9.22 Blood film in acute monoblastic leukaemia (FAB type M5a) showing a monoblast with a non-lobulated nucleus and a vesicular nucleolus. Monoblasts are usually strongly positive for non-specific esterase reactions, such as α-naphthyl acetate esterase (ANAE), and may have a few MPO and SBB-positive granules.

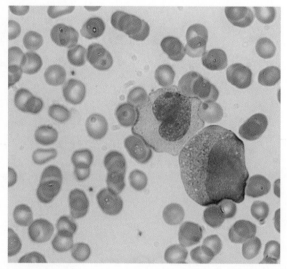

Fig. 9.23 Blood film in acute monocytic leukaemia (FAB type M5b) showing one promonocyte and one monocyte; the promonocyte has moderately basophilic cytoplasm, which is granulated and vacuolated; promonocytes are positive with SBB and for MPO and non-specific esterase.

Differential diagnosis

The differential diagnosis is mainly ALL, transformation of CML and other myeloproliferative neoplasms, MDS and other causes of bone marrow failure such as aplastic anaemia. Occasionally, it is necessary to distinguish between acute leukaemia and a leukaemoid reaction (see above).

Further tests

When AML is suspected, a bone marrow aspiration is indicated for cytological assessment and cytogenetic analysis. Immunophenotyping is indicated unless there is clear evidence of myeloid differentiation, in order to distinguish AML with minimal evidence of

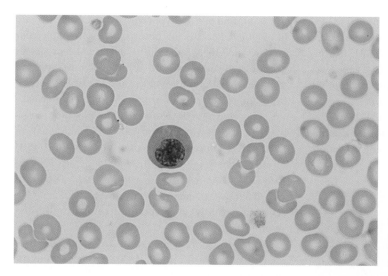

Fig. 9.24 Blood film in acute erythroleukaemia (FAB type M6) showing a circulating nucleated red blood cell (NRBC), which is megaloblastic.

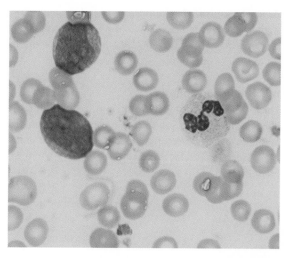

Fig. 9.25 Blood film in acute megakaryoblastic leukaemia (FAB type M7) showing a neutrophil and two blast cells; the blasts have no cytological features that permit their identification as megakaryoblasts, but they expressed platelet-associated antigens detectable on immunophenotyping; the giant hypogranular platelet adjacent to the neutrophil is the only clue that this leukaemia may be of megakaryocyte lineage.

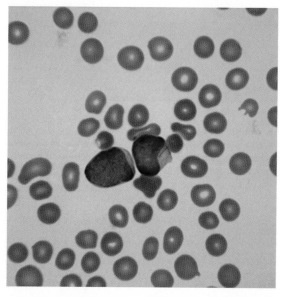

Fig. 9.26 Blood film from a patient with the World Health Organization (WHO) category, AML with t(8;21)(q22;q22); *RUNX1-RUNX1T1* showing two blast cells, one with a typical long Auer rod in the cavity of the nucleus.

differentiation and acute megakaryoblastic leukaemia from ALL. Immunophenotyping is also essential for the diagnosis of mixed phenotype acute leukaemia. Depending on local practice, immunophenotyping may be performed in all patients so that results can be applied in follow-up for minimal residual disease.

Cytochemical evaluation to confirm granulocytic or monocytic differentiation is used much less often since immunophenotyping became widely employed, but should not be neglected in circumstances when immunophenotyping is not readily available. The most useful reactions are myeloperoxidase (MPO) or

Sudan black B (SBB), to confirm granulocyte differentiation, and a 'non-specific' esterase reaction, such as α-naphthyl acetate esterase (ANAE), to confirm monocytic differentiation. A positive chloroacetate esterase (CAE) reaction confirms neutrophilic differentiation and can be combined with ANAE, as a combined esterase stain, for the easy identification of acute myelomonocytic (FAB M4) leukaemia. Trephine biopsy is of use in some patients in whom

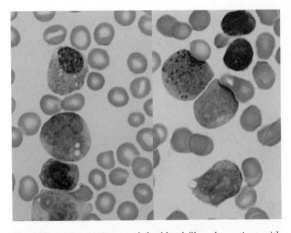

Fig. 9.27 Composite image of the blood film of a patient with the WHO category, AML with inv(16)(p13.1q22); *CBFB-MYH11*; note monocytic differentiation, a hypolobated eosinophil and an eosinophil precursor with purple proeosinophilic granules (see also Fig. 9.21).

the bone marrow is hypocellular or a poor aspirate is obtained because of fibrosis. Selective molecular genetic analysis is indicated to detect good prognosis genetic abnormalities (*CEBPA* bi-allelic mutation and mutated *NPM1* mutation in the absence of *FLT3* mutation) and to detect poor prognosis genetic abnormalities that need to be considered in planning treatment (e.g. *BCR-ABL1* fusion). If cytogenetic analysis fails, either fluorescence *in situ* hybridisation (FISH) or molecular analysis is needed to detect *RUNX1-RUNX1T1*, *PML-RARA* and *MYH11-CBFB*. The accurate diagnosis of acute promyelocytic leukaemia is required urgently since specific treatment (all-*trans*-retinoic acid) is needed. This is often possible on the basis of cytology but, if there is any doubt, FISH or analysis of the distribution of PML protein within the nucleus is needed [84].

Acute basophilic leukaemia

Acute basophilic leukaemia is a rare type of AML that is recognised as a specific *BCR-ABL1*-negative category in the WHO classification.

Blood film and count

There may be blast cells and mature basophils or blast cells alone. Some cases can be recognised cytologically because of characteristic basophil granules (see Fig. 9.34). Others need ultrastructural examination.

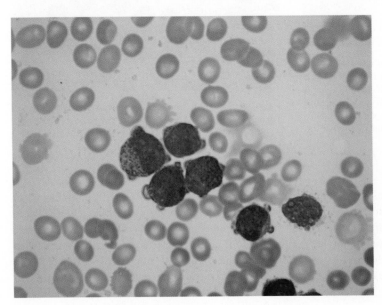

Fig. 9.28 Blood film in the WHO category, AML with t(15;17)(q22;q12); *PML-RARA*, which is equivalent to the FAB M3 category (see also Figs. 9.18 and 9.19). The case illustrated shows the hyperbasophilic variant of acute promyelocytic leukaemia. The intense cytoplasmic basophilia and the cytoplasmic blebs suggest possible acute megakaryoblastic leukaemia, but note that one of the leukaemic cells is hypergranular.

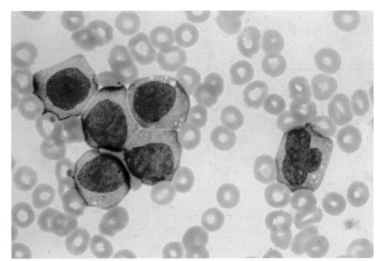

Fig. 9.29 Blood film in the WHO category, AML with t(9;11)(p22;q23); *MLLT3-MLL* (*MLLT3-KMT2A*) showing five monoblasts and one promonocyte. The FAB category was M5a.

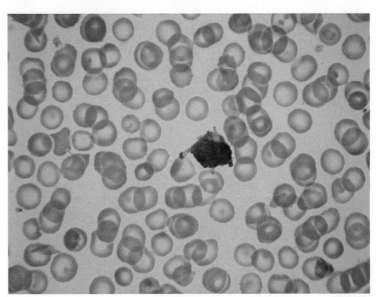

Fig. 9.30 Blood film in the WHO category, AML (megakaryoblastic) with t(1;22) (p13;q13); *RBM15-MKL1*, showing one megakaryoblast. The FAB category was M7. Cytoplasmic blebs, as shown in this cell, are often seen in acute megakaryoblastic leukaemia.

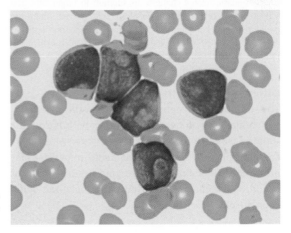

Fig. 9.31 Blood film in the WHO category, AML with mutated *NPM1* showing cup-shaped blast cells. By courtesy of Dr Mike Leach, Glasgow.

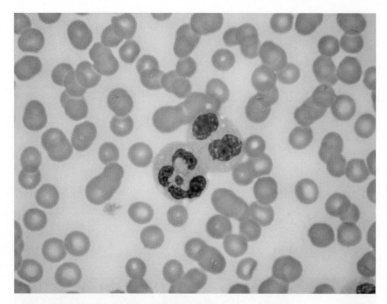

Fig. 9.32 Blood film in the WHO category, AML with myelodysplasia-related changes. There are two dysplastic neutrophils; both are macropolycytes, one having a single nucleus and the other having two Pelger nuclei. This case qualified for this category both because of a previous myelodysplastic syndrome (MDS) and because of myelodysplastic changes in more than 50% of cells of granulocyte lineage.

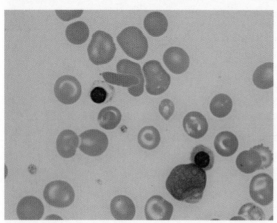

Fig. 9.33 Blood film from a patient with sickle cell anaemia who developed AML assigned to the WHO category, AML with myelodysplasia-related changes. In addition to target cells and a boat-shaped cell, reflecting the sickle cell anaemia, there are two erythroblasts and a myeloblast. One of the erythroblasts has defective haemoglobinisation and hypochromic microcytes were present. An iron stain confirmed the presence of ring sideroblasts.

Differential diagnosis

The differential diagnosis includes other AML in which blast cells have large granules with basophilic staining characteristics, particularly mast cell leukaemia and to a lesser extent acute hypergranular promyelocytic leukaemia. The granules in the latter condition are often reddish-purple rather than being deep purple.

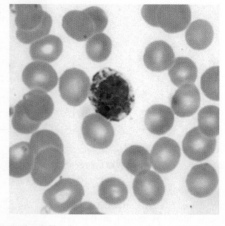

Fig. 9.34 Blood film from a patient with the WHO category of acute myeloid leukaemia, not otherwise specified, acute basophilic leukaemia. By courtesy of Robyn Wells, Brisbane.

Other tests

Most cases are MPO and SBB negative and Auer rods are absent [86]. CD13 and CD33 are positive and basophil markers, CD9 and CD25, may be positive [86].

Mast cell leukaemia

Mast cell leukaemia is a rare disease, which may occur *de novo* or as a complication of systemic mastocytosis. In the 2008 WHO classification, it is categorised with other neoplasms of mast cell lineage [79]. A mast cell leukaemia or mixed mast cell/basophil leukaemia can also occur as a terminal phase of CML [87].

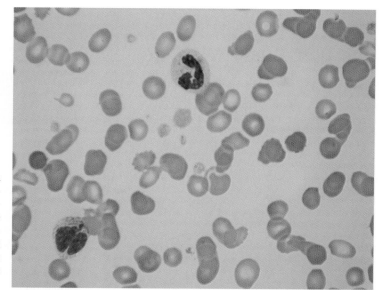

Fig. 9.35 Blood film from a patient with the WHO category of acute myeloid leukaemia, not otherwise specified, acute panmyelosis with myelofibrosis, showing large hypogranular platelets and a dysplastic granulocyte of uncertain lineage. The peripheral blood features of this category of AML are non-specific, the diagnosis resting on the bone marrow findings.

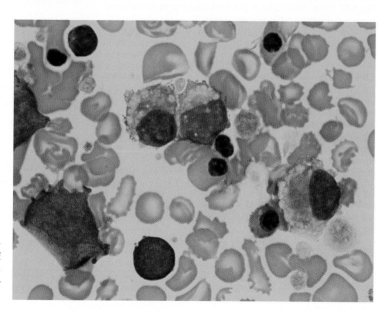

Fig. 9.36 Blood film showing the WHO category, transient abnormal myelopoiesis of Down syndrome. There are three micromegakaryocytes, a promyelocyte, a number of erythroblasts and several giant platelets.

Blood film and count

Normal mast cells have a small oval nucleus that is not obscured by the purple granules that pack the cytoplasm (see Fig. 3.154). In mast cell leukaemia (Fig. 9.38), some neoplastic cells may resemble normal mast cells, while others have larger nuclei or nuclei that are bilobed or multilobed. Granules vary in colour from red to dark purple and may or may not obscure the nucleus. They may fuse into homogeneous masses. Less mature cells may have scanty granules and a nucleus that is oval or kidney-shaped with nucleoli [88,89].

Differential diagnosis

The differential diagnosis includes other leukaemias with hypergranular neoplastic cells, specifically hypergranular promyelocytic leukaemia and basophilic leukaemia.

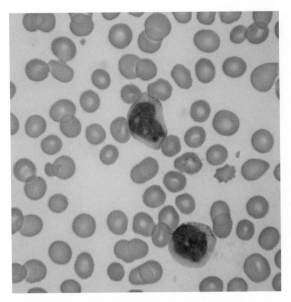

Fig. 9.37 Blood film in the WHO AML category of blastic plasmacytoid dendritic cell neoplasm showing two neoplastic cells, one with small cytoplasmic vacuoles. Bone marrow cells of this patient showed characteristic cytoplasmic tails.

The presence of multiple Auer rods suggests a diagnosis of acute hypergranular promyelocytic leukaemia.

Further tests

Bone marrow aspiration and cytochemistry (Table 9.6) are useful in confirming the diagnosis. Mast cells are negative for MPO and positive for CAE [86]. CD13, CD33, CD68 and CD117 are usually strongly positive and mast cell tryptase is expressed [86]. Mast cells can also be distinguished from basophils by electron

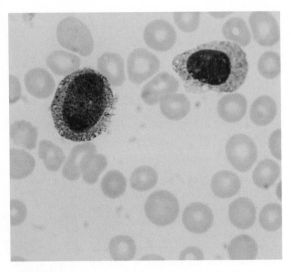

Fig. 9.38 Blood film of a patient with acute mast cell leukaemia showing two mast cells. By courtesy of Miss Desley Scott and Dr Ian Bunce, Brisbane.

microscopy, which shows basophils to have granules that are either of a uniform consistency or finely particulate, whereas mast cell granules are heterogeneous and contain whorled, scrolled, lamellate and crystalline structures. Serum tryptase is expected to be elevated, but it can also be elevated in other types of AML.

Transient abnormal myelopoiesis of Down syndrome

Transient abnormal myelopoiesis (TAM) of Down syndrome occurs during intrauterine life and in neonates.

Table 9.6 Some cytochemical tests and immunophenotypic markers that are useful in distinguishing between basophils, mast cells and hypergranular promyelocytes.

Cell type	Basophiloblast	Basophil	Mast cell	Hypergranular promyelocyte
Myeloperoxidase	–	– or +*	–	+++
Sudan black B	–	– or +	– or +	+++
Chloroacetate esterase	–	–†	+++	+++
Toluidine blue (metachromatic staining)	– or +	+++	+++	–
Usual immunophenotypic markers	CD123, CD203c, CD11b, usually CD9, CD25 variable, CD117–		CD25, CD68, CD117, mast cell tryptase	Myeloperoxidase, CD117 variable

* positive in basophil promyelocytes to metamyelocytes
† positive in basophil promyelocytes to metamyelocytes and may be positive in leukaemic basophils [90]
–, negative; +, weakly positive; +++, strongly positive

Cytogenetic and molecular evidence indicate that this disorder is actually spontaneously remitting AML, often with prominent megakaryocytic differentiation [91,92]. Remission occurs within a few weeks but, in a significant percentage of affected infants, AML develops, most often at 1–2 years of age. TAM is recognised as a specific entity in the WHO classification.

Blood film and count
The blood film resembles that of AML but often has distinctive features, particularly the presence of megakaryoblasts, megakaryocytes, micromegakaryocytes, giant or hypogranular platelets and immature erythroid precursors (see Fig. 9.36). The WBC may be moderately to greatly elevated with a high percentage of blast cells. There may be anaemia and thrombocytopenia.

Differential diagnosis
The differential diagnosis of TAM is congenital leukaemia of other types.

Further tests
Cytogenetic analysis is indicated in order both to confirm Down syndrome by demonstration of the constitutional trisomy 21 and to exclude specific cytogenetic abnormalities that may be associated with other cases of congenital leukaemias, e.g. t(4;11)(q21;q23). Molecular genetic analysis is indicated since a mutation in the *GATA1* gene is uniformly present [92]. Otherwise there are no laboratory investigations that will distinguish TAM from other forms of AML. In the absence of molecular analysis, this is achieved only by being aware of the typical morphological features of this disorder and by observing its clinical course.

Acute myeloid leukaemia of Down syndrome
The WHO classification recognises Down syndrome-associated AML as a further specific entity. It develops mainly in the first three years of life. The child may have suffered from TAM in the neonatal period and there can also be a myelodysplastic phase preceding acute leukaemia. The leukaemia often shows megakaryoblastic differentiation, but this is not necessarily so.

Blood film and count
The blood film has no distinctive features, other that cytological features of megakaryoblasts in some cases.

Differential diagnosis
The differential diagnosis is with other types of AML.

Further tests
Cytogenetic analysis may show only constitution trisomy 21, but sometimes there is an acquired trisomy 8 or another unbalanced abnormality. Molecular analysis shows a *GATA1* mutation; when paired samples are available this is found to be the same mutation as was present during preceding TAM.

The myelodysplastic syndromes
The MDS are a morphologically heterogeneous group of conditions that result from the proliferation of a clone of neoplastic haemopoietic cells showing abnormalities of proliferation and maturation that are less profound than those of AML. Haemopoiesis is functionally ineffective and morphologically dysplastic. MDS is potentially preleukaemic, although some patients die from complications of cytopenia without evolution to AML. MDS may arise *de novo* or follow exposure to mutagenic agents such as ionising radiation, benzene and anti-cancer agents, including alkylating agents. The FAB classification has now been supplanted by the WHO classification. This latter classification is hierarchical with cases first being assigned, if appropriate, to the group of therapy-related AML/MDS and then consecutively to the category of MDS with isolated del(5q), and then to other categories, as shown in Table 9.7. CMML, which in the FAB classifications was regarded as MDS, is assigned in the WHO classification to a category designated myelodysplastic/myeloproliferative neoplasms (see below).

Blood count and film
The peripheral blood film usually shows features suggesting the diagnosis (Figs 9.39–9.42). Most patients are anaemic with red cells being normochromic and either normocytic or macrocytic. Anisocytosis and poikilocytosis are usual. In patients with sideroblastic erythropoiesis, there is a minor population of hypochromic microcytes and Pappenheimer bodies are present; the dominant red cell population is usually macrocytic. Red cells may also show anisocytosis, poikilocytosis and basophilic stippling. There may be mild leucocytosis, leucopenia or a normal WBC. By definition, the WBC is less than 13×10^9/l

Table 9.7 The WHO classification of the myelodysplastic syndromes (MDS) [93].*

Disease	Peripheral blood findings	Bone marrow findings
MDS associated with isolated del(5q)	Anaemia, platelet count usually normal or elevated, < 1% blasts	Megakaryocytes in normal or increased numbers but with hypolobated nuclei, < 5% blasts, no Auer rods, 5q– as sole cytogenetic abnormality
Refractory cytopenia with unilineage dysplasia (RCUD) – mainly refractory anaemia, but also refractory thrombocytopenia and refractory neutropenia	Cytopenia affecting one or two lineages, blasts rarely seen and always less than 1%, monocytes $< 1 \times 10^9$/l	Dysplasia confined to one lineage, < 5% blasts, < 15% ring sideroblasts
Refractory anaemia with ringed sideroblasts (RARS)	Anaemia, no blasts, monocytes $< 1 \times 10^9$/l	Dysplasia confined to erythroid lineage, < 5% blasts, ≥ 15% ringed sideroblasts
Refractory cytopenia with multilineage dysplasia (RCMD)	Cytopenias (bicytopenia or pancytopenia), blasts < 1%, no Auer rods, monocytes $< 1 \times 10^9$/l	Dysplasia in ≥ 10% of the cells of two or more myeloid cell lineages, < 5% blasts, no Auer rods, ring sideroblasts may or may not be present
Refractory anaemia with excess blasts-1 (RAEB-1)	Cytopenias, < 5% blasts, no Auer rods, $< 1 \times 10^9$/l monocytes	Unilineage or multilineage dysplasia, 5–9% blasts, no Auer rods
Refractory anaemia with excess blasts-2 (RAEB-2)	Cytopenias, 5–19% blasts,[†] Auer rods sometimes present,[†] $< 1 \times 10^9$/l monocytes	Unilineage or multilineage dysplasia, 10–19% blasts,[†] Auer rods sometimes present
Myelodysplastic syndrome-unclassified (MDS-U)	May meet criteria for RCUD except for pancytopenia[‡]; may meet criteria for RCUD or RCMD except for 1% blasts in blood[‡]; blasts no greater than 1%, no Auer rods	Cytopenia with dysplasia being less than 10% in all lineages but there is a defined cytogenetic abnormality,[‡] < 5% blasts, no Auer rods

* Therapy-related cases are classified with therapy-related acute myeloid leukaemia as therapy-related myeloid neoplasms
† For a case to be categorised as RAEB-2 there must be **either** 5% or more peripheral blood blasts **or** 10% or more bone marrow blasts **or** Auer rods
‡ One of these three criteria must be met
WHO, World Health Organization

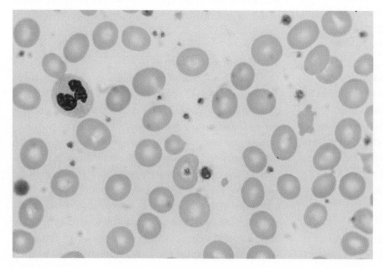

Fig. 9.39 Blood film of a patient with MDS – refractory anaemia (FAB classification)/refractory cytopenia with multilineage dysplasia (WHO classification), showing anisocytosis, macrocytosis and one poikilocyte; the neutrophil is hypogranular.

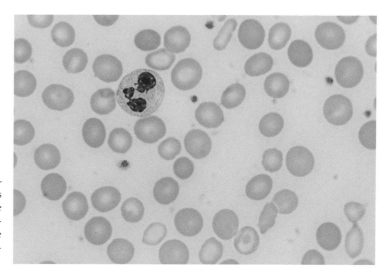

Fig. 9.40 Blood film of a patient with MDS – refractory anaemia with ring sideroblasts (FAB and WHO classifications), showing one target cell and several hypochromic microcytes; the remainder of the erythrocytes are normochromic cells, which are either normocytic or macrocytic; MCV was 103 fl.

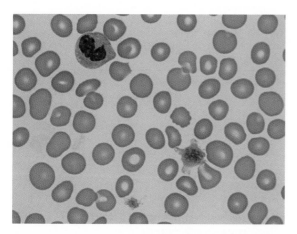

Fig. 9.41 Blood film of a patient with MDS – refractory anaemia (FAB classification)/refractory cytopenia with multilineage dysplasia (WHO classification), showing macrocytosis and evidence of dysplasia in the granulocytic and megakaryocyte lineages. There is a hypolobated neutrophil and of the four platelets present, one is giant and two are severely hypogranular.

or the case is categorised as myelodysplastic/myeloproliferative neoplasm (MDS/MPN). There may be monocytosis, but by definition the monocyte count is less than 1×10^9/l. Neutrophilia is uncommon. An increase of eosinophils or basophils is very uncommon. Blast cells may be present and they may contain Auer rods. There may be occasional promyelocytes, myelocytes or nucleated red blood cells (NRBC).

Neutrophils commonly show dysplastic features, particularly hypogranularity (see Fig. 9.42), the acquired Pelger–Huët anomaly (see Fig. 3.75) and excessive chromatin clumping. Detection of neutrophil hypogranularity requires that the blood film be correctly stained; a useful check is that at least some of the platelets have lilac granules. Neutrophil hypogranularity can be recognised in a manner that is reproducible between individuals if the criterion used is a reduction of granules by at least two-thirds [94]. The platelet count is often reduced but in a minority of patients it is increased; by definition the platelet count is less than 450×10^9/l or the case is categorised as MDS/MPN. Platelets may show dysplastic features such as large size and hypogranularity.

Automated instruments may flag blasts cells, show neutrophils with aberrant characteristics or show abnormal red cell populations. With Siemens Advia series instruments, increased normochromic macrocytes and increased hypochromic macrocytes unrelated to reticulocytosis can also provide evidence of dysplastic erythropoiesis. These instruments also demonstrate a particular pattern in a red cell cytogram that has been found to be predictive of the presence of ring sideroblasts (see Fig. 8.35).

Differential diagnosis

The differential diagnosis includes other causes of macrocytic anaemia and cytopenia, AML and non-neoplastic conditions causing dysplasia such as HIV infection, exposure to heavy metals and the direct rather than long-term effects of the administration of anti-cancer drugs.

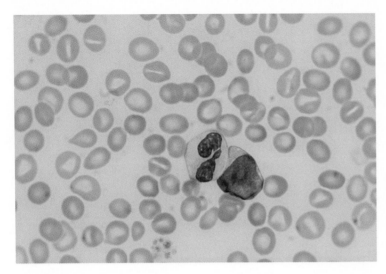

Fig. 9.42 Blood film of a patient with MDS – refractory anaemia with excess of blasts (FAB and WHO classifications), showing a myeloblast and a hypogranular neutrophil; the red cells show anisocytosis and poikilocytosis including teardrop cells and stomatocytes.

Further tests

Bone marrow aspiration is often necessary for diagnosis and is always necessary for further classification (see Table 9.7) and for determining prognosis. Either an MPO or an SBB stain is useful for the detection of Auer rods and a Perls' stain is essential for identification of ring sideroblasts. Trephine biopsy can be useful, particularly if the bone marrow is hypocellular or if a poor aspirate is obtained because of fibrosis. When cytological evidence is insufficient for a firm diagnosis, cytogenetic analysis or other investigations to establish clonality of haemopoietic cells may be essential for diagnosis. Cytogenetic analysis is also important for determining prognosis and is essential for applying the WHO classification. It is likewise essential for the recognition of cases associated with del(5q); recognition of such cases is clinically important because of their responsiveness to lenalidomide therapy.

Myeloproliferative and myelodysplastic/myeloproliferative neoplasms

The WHO classification recognises a group of myeloproliferative neoplasms (MPN) and another group of MDS/MPN (Table 9.8). Different types of chronic myeloid leukaemia are assigned to these two groups and, in addition, others are classified separately, according to the molecular genetic abnormality. The chronic myeloid leukaemias differ from AML in that there is effective maturation with production of granulocytes.

Table 9.8 The 2008 WHO classification of the myeloproliferative and myelodysplastic/myeloproliferative neoplasms [76]

Myeloproliferative neoplasms
Chronic myelogenous leukaemia, *BCR-ABL1* positive
Chronic neutrophilic leukaemia
Chronic eosinophilic leukaemia, not otherwise specified*
Primary myelofibrosis
Polycythaemia vera
Essential thrombocythaemia
Mastocytosis
Myeloproliferative neoplasm, unclassifiable
Myelodysplastic/myeloproliferative disorders
Chronic myelomonocytic leukaemia
Atypical chronic myeloid leukaemia
Juvenile myelomonocytic leukaemia
Myelodysplastic/myeloproliferative neoplasm, unclassifiable

* Cases with rearrangement of *PDGFRA*, *PDGFRB* or *FGFR1* are excluded
WHO, World Health Organization

Myeloproliferative neoplasms

Polycythaemia vera, primary myelofibrosis and essential thrombocythaemia have been dealt with in Chapter 8. Other MPN will be dealt with in this chapter.

Chronic myelogenous leukaemia

The specific entity, variously referred to as chronic granulocytic leukaemia, chronic myelogenous leukaemia and chronic myeloid leukaemia, is associated with a specific translocation, t(9;22)(q34;q11.2), giving rise to an abnormal chromosome 22, designated the Philadelphia (Ph) chromosome, and a specific fusion gene, *BCR-ABL1*. The designation 'chronic myeloid leukaemia' is widely used for this specific entity but the term is not ideal since it is also used as a generic term for a wider group of disorders. CML occurs at all ages, but incidence increases steadily with age. It is characterised clinically by anaemia, splenomegaly and hepatomegaly.

Blood film and count

The WBC is elevated, often markedly so. The differential count (Fig. 9.43) [95] and blood film (Fig. 9.44) are very characteristic, with myelocytes and neutrophils being the most frequent cells. In patients with a very high WBC, the blast cells may be as high as 15%, but nevertheless blasts remain less frequent than promyelocytes; similarly, promyelocytes are less frequent than myelocytes. There is an increase in the absolute basophil count in almost every case and an increase in the absolute eosinophil count in

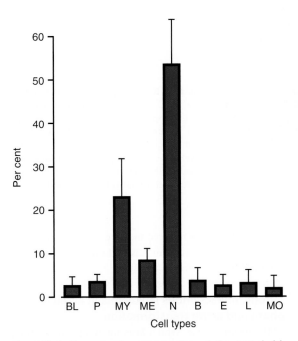

Fig. 9.43 A diagrammatic representation of the typical differential count in chronic myelogenous leukaemia (CML) based on 1500 cell differential counts in 50 patients with Philadelphia-positive CML [85]. BL, blasts; P, promyelocytes; MY, myelocytes; ME, metamyelocytes; N, neutrophils; B, basophils; E, eosinophils; L, lymphocytes; MO, monocytes.

more than 90% of cases. Some eosinophils may have a proportion of immature granules with basophilic staining characteristics. Monocytes are increased, but not in proportion to neutrophils. Some NRBC are present. Dysplastic features are minor. The platelet count is usually normal or increased, but in a minority of cases it is decreased. Platelet size is increased. Circulating megakaryocytes, mainly almost bare nuclei, are sometimes present.

A minority of patients present with isolated thrombocytosis.

Occasional patients with CML have striking cyclical changes in WBC with a periodicity of 50–70 days, and with the WBC varying from frankly leukaemic levels to almost normal. All myeloid cells participate in the cycles.

A minority of patients have bone marrow fibrosis at presentation and the typical peripheral blood features of myelofibrosis are then superimposed on the features of CML.

Many patients with CML present with symptoms and well-established disease. However, an increasingly large proportion of patients are diagnosed incidentally while still asymptomatic. Occasional patients who have developed the disease while being monitored haematologically have allowed the early stages of the disease to be defined. The first detectable peripheral blood features are an increase in the basophil count, thrombocytosis and a low NAP score. Following this, the neutrophil count and the WBC rise and small numbers of immature cells appear. With the progressive rise of WBC that follows, the percentage of immature cells steadily increases.

The natural history of CML is for the disease to terminate in acute transformation, also designated blast crisis (see below), often preceded by an accelerated phase. Secondary myelofibrosis can also occur. With the advent of effective tyrosine kinase inhibitor therapy, which leads to sustained remission in most patients, this type of disease evolution is less often seen.

Differential diagnosis

The differential diagnosis includes reactive neutrophilia, other types of chronic myeloid leukaemia and the early stages of polycythaemia vera and essential thrombocythaemia. Features useful in distinguishing CML from reactive neutrophilia are shown in Table 9.3 but, in practice, diagnostic difficulty only arises in early cases of CML.

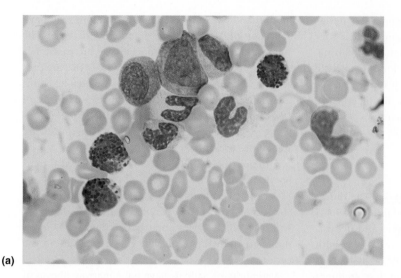

(a)

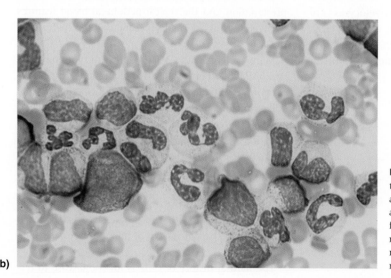

(b)

Fig. 9.44 Blood film in Philadelphia-positive CML showing: (a) a promyelocyte, an eosinophil myelocyte, three basophils and a number of neutrophils and band forms; and (b) a promyelocyte, several myelocytes, neutrophil band forms and neutrophils; the presence of a binucleate neutrophil is relatively uncommon.

Further tests

Cytogenetic and molecular analysis are indicated to confirm the diagnosis. The great majority of cases of CML are associated with t(9;22)(q34;q11.2). A minority of cases, clinically and haematologically indistinguishable, lack the classical microscopically detectable translocation, but nevertheless have a *BCR-ABL1* fusion gene. Molecular analysis is indicated since identification of the specific breakpoints leading to the fusion gene facilitates later monitoring of minimal residual disease. FISH analysis using *BCR* and *ABL1* probes is also a useful technique, particularly during follow-up.

The NAP score is reduced in more than 90% of cases of chronic phase CML, but it is no longer regarded as a useful test.

Chronic myelogenous leukaemia in accelerated phase and acute transformation

CML chronic phase, which lasts for weeks, months or years, can be followed by blast transformation. This is sometimes preceded by an accelerated phase. Clinical features of such disease evolution are pallor and bruising, increasing hepatomegaly and splenomegaly, lymphadenopathy or, less often, soft tissue tumours, bone pain and refractoriness to treatment.

Table 9.9 Some haematological abnormalities that may be detected during the accelerated phase of chronic myelogenous leukaemia.

Red cells and precursors
Anaemia (including that due to red cell aplasia in which reticulocytes are very infrequent or absent), macrocytosis, marked poikilocytosis (may be consequent on bone marrow fibrosis), vacuolated erythroblasts (PAS-positive), hypochromia and microcytosis
White cells and precursors
Refractory leucocytosis, increasing basophil count, disappearance of eosinophilia, increasing monocytosis, acquired Pelger–Huët anomaly of neutrophils or eosinophils, hypogranular neutrophils, vacuolated neutrophils, pseudo-Chédiak–Higashi anomaly (giant granules) of neutrophils and precursors, binuclearity and other dysplastic features of neutrophil precursors, increasing blast cell percentage with decreasing percentage of more mature cells, Auer rods in blast cells
Platelets and megakaryocytes
Thrombocytopenia, thrombocytosis, micromegakaryocytes, bare megakaryocyte nuclei
General
Pancytopenia (may be resultant on refractory splenomegaly or, rarely, bone marrow necrosis)

PAS, periodic acid–Schiff

Blood film and count

During the accelerated phase there may be anaemia, leucocytosis, thrombocytopenia, thrombocytosis, a rising basophil count, an increasing blast cell percentage and the appearance of dysplastic features (Table 9.9 and Fig. 9.45). Blast transformation can occur without any warning or be preceded by an accelerated phase. Blast transformation is lymphoblastic in about one quarter of cases and myeloid or mixed lymphoblastic and myeloid in the remainder (Table 9.10). Myeloid transformation is often megakaryoblastic or mixed myeloblastic/megakaryoblastic. A patient who remits from one blast crisis (e.g. lymphoblastic) may subsequently suffer a second blast crisis with cells of different lineage (e.g. megakaryoblastic).

Table 9.10 Types of transformation that can occur in chronic myelogenous leukaemia.

Myeloblastic transformation
Lymphoblastic transformation
Megakaryocytic transformation (with micromegakaryocytes and thrombocytosis)
Megakaryoblastic transformation
Erythroblastic transformation [96] and acquired sideroblastic erythropoiesis
Monoblastic transformation [97]
Basophil blast transformation [98]
Mast cell and mixed basophil/mast cell transformation [87]
Eosinophil blast transformation [99]
Hypergranular promyelocytic transformation [100]
Transformations with various mixtures of cell types
Acute myelofibrosis

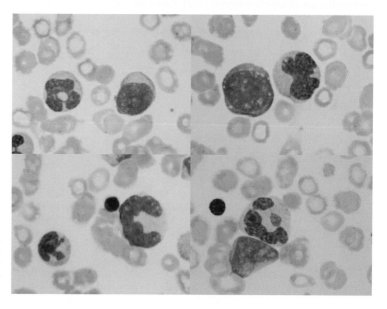

Fig. 9.45 Composite image of the blood film in CML in accelerated phase showing increased blast cells and a range of dysplastic features. There was associated cytogenetic evolution.

Differential diagnosis

Patients may present already in blast transformation, in which case the differential diagnosis is acute leukaemia. Patients presenting in accelerated phase can also simulate aCML or other myeloid neoplasms. In patients presenting in chronic phase, the likely diagnosis is usually readily evident from the clinical and haematological features.

Further tests

Bone marrow aspiration is indicated unless there are large numbers of blasts in the peripheral blood. Cytogenetic analysis is indicated since cytogenetic evolution often precedes or occurs simultaneously with the development of acceleration or acute transformation. Immunophenotyping of blast cells may be useful since there is more likelihood of a response to treatment in lymphoblastic transformation.

Chronic neutrophilic leukaemia

Chronic neutrophilic leukaemia is a rare condition characterised clinically by anaemia, splenomegaly and sometimes hepatomegaly.

Blood film

There is anaemia and a marked neutrophilia with very few circulating immature cells (Fig. 9.46). The WBC is usually of the order of 40–70 × 10^9/1. There is no basophilia, eosinophilia or monocytosis. Neutrophils may have both toxic granulation and Döhle bodies [101]. Ring neutrophils are relatively common [102]. Cases have also

been described with marked dysplastic features [103], but in the WHO classification these are excluded [104]. The disease may terminate in acute transformation.

Differential diagnosis

The differential diagnosis includes reactive neutrophilia (including neutrophilic leukaemoid reaction associated with multiple myeloma or monoclonal gammopathy of undetermined significance) and other chronic leukaemias and myeloproliferative neoplasms.

Further tests

Bone marrow aspiration and cytogenetic analysis are indicated. Serum protein electrophoresis should be performed to exclude reactive neutrophilia associated with a plasma cell neoplasm. The NAP score is usually high. When no clonal cytogenetic abnormality is present, a period of observation may be necessary to make the distinction from reactive neutrophilia.

Chronic eosinophilic leukaemia, not otherwise specified

Eosinophilia, which is sometimes very marked, can be a feature of AML. There are other cases of leukaemia in which the leukaemic cells are almost exclusively mature eosinophils or both mature and immature cells of eosinophil lineage, but with there being fewer than 20% bone marrow and peripheral blood blast cells. These cases are referred to as chronic eosinophilic leukaemia (CEL). The prognosis is variable and is related to the percentage of blast cells and to the extent of tissue damage consequent

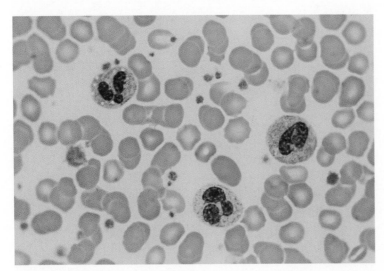

Fig. 9.46 Blood film in chronic neutrophilic leukaemia. The neutrophils show 'toxic' granulation and vacuolation. One giant platelet is present. Other neutrophils showed Döhle bodies and macropolycytes were present.

on the release of eosinophil granule contents. The WHO classification requires that the eosinophil count is greater than $1.5 \times 10^9/l$ and that **either** blast cells are greater than 2% in the blood or greater than 5% in the bone marrow **or** that there is cytogenetic or molecular genetic evidence of clonality [105]. Cases with a rearrangement of *PDGFRA*, *PDGFRB* or *FGFR1* are categorised separately [106,107], other cases being designated CEL, not otherwise specified [105].

Blood film and count

The blood film (Fig. 9.47) shows mature eosinophils and sometimes also blast cells, promyelocytes and eosinophil myelocytes. The mature eosinophils often show hypogranularity, vacuolation and hypolobation, but sometimes they are cytologically normal. Eosinophils and eosinophil myelocytes may contain some darkly staining proeosinophilic granules. In acute eosinophilic leukaemia, the blast cells and, occasionally, maturing cells may contain Auer rods, but these are not seen in CEL. Anaemia and thrombocytopenia are common. Neutrophils may be increased in number and often show heavy granulation. The monocyte count may be increased.

Differential diagnosis

The differential diagnosis includes reactive eosinophilia (see above), aCML or CMML with eosinophilia, and idiopathic HES. Idiopathic HES is only diagnosed if all other causes of eosinophilia are excluded after appropriate investigation. Reactive eosinophilia that can be confused with eosinophilic leukaemia includes that which occasionally occurs in ALL (Fig. 9.48) and non-Hodgkin lymphoma.

Further tests

Bone marrow aspiration, cytogenetic analysis and molecular genetic or FISH analysis for *FIP1L1-PDGFRA* are indicated. The bone marrow should be specifically examined for increased blast cells (either myeloblasts or lymphoblasts), lymphoma cells and abnormal mast cells. If there is doubt as to the diagnosis, a trephine biopsy should also be performed, since the features of lymphoma or systemic mastocytosis may be revealed. Cytogenetic analysis has shown a variety of clonal chromosomal abnormalities, including trisomy 8, del(20q), an isochromosome of 17q and rearrangements involving the long arm of chromosome 5. It can be useful to perform immunophenotyping of peripheral blood lymphocytes and T-cell receptor analysis, to establish T-cell clonality, in patients in whom there is neither evidence of an underlying cause of reactive eosinophilia nor conclusive morphological or cytogenetic evidence that the eosinophilia represents eosinophilic leukaemia. The diagnosis of eosinophilic leukaemia is readily established in those cases in which there is a significant increase in blast cells and other immature cells, dysplasia of other lineages, a clonal cytogenetic abnormality or other evidence of clonality of myeloid cells. The presence of soft tissue tumours composed of immature myeloid cells also confirms the diagnosis. In cases with

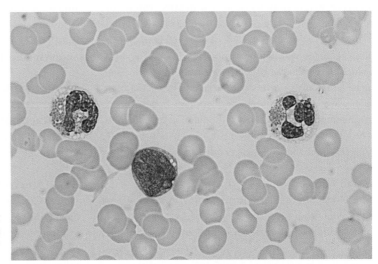

Fig. 9.47 Blood film in chronic eosinophilic leukaemia, not otherwise specified, showing a blast cell and two vacuolated and partly degranulated eosinophils.

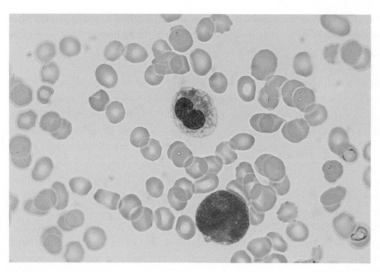

Fig. 9.48 Peripheral blood film of a patient with acute lymphoblastic leukaemia (ALL) with reactive eosinophilia showing a lymphoblast and a partially degranulated hypolobulated eosinophil. It is important in such cases to establish the lineage of the blast cells by immunophenotyping.

predominantly mature eosinophils, the diagnosis can be difficult to establish. The presence of marked morphological abnormalities confined to eosinophils is *not* useful in diagnosis since such abnormalities can be seen also in reactive eosinophilia and in systemic mastocytosis. In some cases, which cannot initially be clearly identified as eosinophilic leukaemia, subsequent evolution of the disease confirms the true nature.

Cases that are found to be *BCR-ABL1*-positive, a rare occurrence, are classified as variants of CML and treated accordingly.

Mastocytosis

Since the mast cell is derived from a multipotent myeloid stem cell, mastocytosis is classified as an MPN. This is usually an indolent disorder, characterised by systemic symptoms resulting from the release of mast cell granule contents. Patients with lymphadenopathy and eosinophilia, associated myelodysplastic features or other associated myeloid neoplasm involving other lineages have a more aggressive course. A minority of patients have urticaria pigmentosa, resulting from skin infiltration by mast cells. The disease may terminate in transformation to AML, which is more often of lineages other than mast cell.

Blood film and count

The blood film and count may show proliferative or dysplastic features such as eosinophilia, monocytosis and thrombocytosis or anaemia and thrombocytopenia. There may be small numbers of circulating mast cells, which may be cytologically abnormal (Fig. 9.49).

Differential diagnosis

The differential diagnosis is broad, including other MPN, myeloid neoplasms associated with rearrangement of *PDGFRA*, *PDGFRB* or *FGFR1* and MDS. CEL or aCML with eosinophilia associated with a *FIP1L1-PDGFRA* fusion gene is important in the differential diagnosis, since this condition is often associated with increased bone marrow mast cells and increased serum tryptase.

Further tests

A bone marrow aspirate for cytogenetic and molecular genetic analysis and a trephine biopsy are required for diagnosis. Cytogenetic analysis may show a clonal abnormality and molecular genetic analysis shows a *KIT* mutation in the majority of patients. Trephine biopsy histology shows infiltration by cytologically abnormal mast cells with aberrant expression of CD2 and CD25. Serum mast cell tryptase is increased.

Myelodysplastic/myeloproliferative neoplasms

Atypical chronic myeloid leukaemia

Atypical CML (aCML) is a disease of adults. The clinical features are similar to those of CML.

Blood film and count

Patients are anaemic and have a moderate to marked elevation in the WBC. On average, patients with aCML present with a lower Hb and a lower WBC than patients with CML. Peripheral blood features (Fig. 9.50) differ from those of CML in that monocytosis and

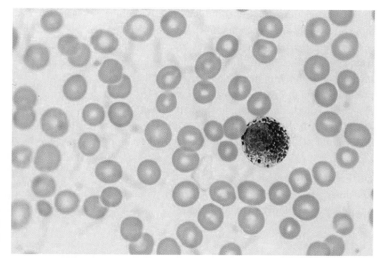

Fig. 9.49 Blood film in mastocytosis show-ing a circulating mast cell, which has a larger nucleus and is less granular than a normal mast cell.

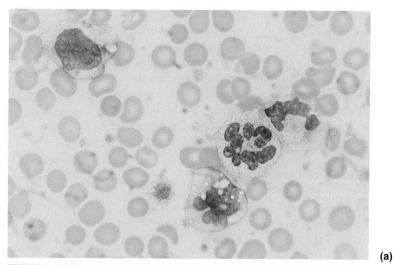

(a)

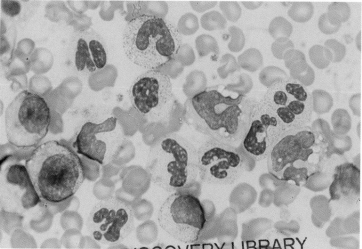

Fig. 9.50 Blood film in atypical *BCR-ABL1*-negative chronic myeloid leukaemia (aCML) showing: (a) a normal neutrophil, a macropo-lycyte, a monocyte and a somewhat imma-ture monocyte – there is one large platelet; (b) numerous neutrophils, band forms, monocytes and hypogranular myelocytes.

(b)

thrombocytopenia are more common while basophilia and eosinophilia are less common. Granulocyte precursors are present. Dysplastic features are common. In comparison with CMML, there are more granulocyte precursors in the peripheral blood, monocytes are less prominent and dysplasia is more prominent. The WHO diagnostic criteria are shown, in comparison with those of CMML, in Table 9.11.

Atypical CML may terminate in blast transformation.

Differential diagnosis

The differential diagnosis includes leukaemoid reactions and other types of myeloid leukaemia.

Further tests

Bone marrow aspiration and cytogenetic analysis may be useful in diagnosis, e.g. for assessing erythropoiesis and megakaryopoiesis and to exclude a diagnosis of AML. However, generally the peripheral blood features are more important than the bone marrow in categorising the MDS/MPN. The Philadelphia chromosome is not detected but other clonal cytogenetic abnormalities may be present. The *BCR-ABL1* fusion gene is absent. The NAP score is low in the majority of patients but elevated in a minority and is not a useful test.

Chronic myelomonocytic leukaemia

CMML is mainly a disease of the elderly, characterised by anaemia, hepatosplenomegaly and, occasionally, significant tissue infiltration by leukaemic monocytes.

Table 9.11 The 2008 WHO criteria for diagnosing aCML and CMML and for distinguishing between them [108,109].

	ACML*	CMML*
Peripheral blood monocytes	Less than 10% of leucocytes	Greater than 1 × 10⁹/l, almost always greater than 10% of leucocytes
Peripheral blood immature granulocytes (promyelocytes, myelocytes and metamyelocytes)	At least 10% of leucocytes	Usually less than 10% of leucocytes
Dysplasia	Granulocytic dysplasia	Dysplasia in at least one myeloid lineage or alternative supporting criteria must be met†

* In both conditions t(9;22) and *BCR-ABL1* are absent and peripheral blood blast cells plus promonocytes are less than 20%
† If there is not dysplasia in at least one lineage either a clonal cytogenetic abnormality must be present **or** the monocytosis must persist for at least 3 months **and** all other causes of monocytosis must be excluded
aCML, atypical chronic myeloid leukaemia; CMML, chronic myelomonocytic leukaemia; WHO, World Health Organization

Blood film and count

The blood film (Fig. 9.51) shows monocytosis and most patients also have anaemia and neutrophilia. By definition, the monocyte count is greater than $1 \times 10^9/1$ (see Table 9.11). The monocytes may be somewhat

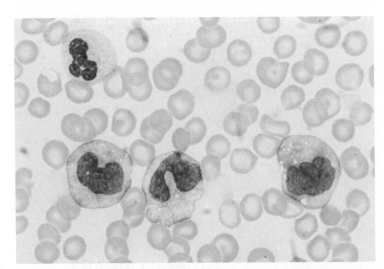

Fig. 9.51 Blood film in chronic myelomonocytic leukaemia (CMML) showing a hypogranular neutrophil and three abnormal monocytes.

immature, with cytoplasmic basophilia or nucleoli. Granulocyte precursors may be present but they are usually less than 5% of white cells, whereas in aCML there are significant numbers of immature granulocytes, often over 15% and almost always over 5%. Basophilia and eosinophilia are quite uncommon. Bone marrow blast cells plus promonocytes are less than 20%. Dysplastic features in other lineages are often but not invariably present.

CMML may terminate by evolving into AML.

Differential diagnosis

The differential diagnosis includes reactive conditions, other chronic myeloid leukaemias, MDS and MPN. The response to administration of G-CSF can simulate CMML. A careful distinction between promonocytes and immature or atypical monocytes is necessary to avoid misclassification as acute monocytic leukaemia.

Further tests

Bone marrow aspiration, trephine biopsy and cytogenetic analysis are useful in diagnosis. The Philadelphia chromosome and the *BCR-ABL1* fusion gene are not detected, but other clonal cytogenetic abnormalities may be present.

Juvenile myelomonocytic leukaemia

Children can develop typical Philadelphia-positive CML, although it is rare before adolescence. Children below the age of 5 years can also develop a distinctive, Philadelphia-negative condition previously known as juvenile CML and now designated juvenile myelomonocytic leukaemia. JMML encompasses also the childhood monosomy 7 syndrome. Usual clinical features are anaemia, splenomegaly, sometimes hepatomegaly, lymphadenopathy and a rash. JMML is more prevalent among children with neurofibromatosis or Noonan syndrome.

Blood film and count

The blood count shows anaemia, neutrophilia and monocytosis. In comparison with CML, the WBC is usually lower and myelocytes are less frequent, while monocytosis, thrombocytopenia and circulating NRBC are common features. Monocytosis is particularly important in diagnosis since it is almost always present. Dysplastic features are present (Fig. 9.52). Diagnostic criteria proposed by the WHO are shown in Table 9.12. A high blast count, large numbers of NRBC and a low platelet count are indicative of a worse prognosis [111].

The disease may terminate in acute transformation, but slow progression and death without transformation are more usual.

Differential diagnosis

The differential diagnosis includes reactive conditions that can cause monocytosis and dysplasia in infants and young children, particularly viral and bacterial infections. It should be noted that children with Noonan syndrome, as well as having an increased incidence

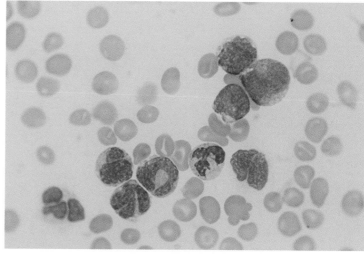

Fig. 9.52 Blood film in juvenile myelomonocytic leukaemia (JMML) showing several neutrophils, a blast, a promyelocyte and several very dysplastic cells, which may be of monocyte lineage. By courtesy of Dr O. Oakhill and Dr G.R. Standen, Bristol. The patient was a child of 6 months with hepatosplenomegaly, WBC 94 × 10⁹/l, Hb 102 g/l, platelet count 28 × 10⁹/l, NAP score 10 and haemoglobin F concentration 11%.

Table 9.12 The 2008 WHO criteria for diagnosing juvenile myelomonocytic leukaemia (JMML) [110].

1. Monocyte count greater than 1×10^9/l
2. Blasts plus promonocytes less than 20% in peripheral blood and bone marrow
3. No Ph chromosome or *BCR-ABL1* fusion gene
4. Two or more of the following
   Haemoglobin F percentage increased for age
   Immature granulocytes in the peripheral blood
   White cell count greater than 10×10^9/l
   Clonal chromosomal abnormality present
   Myeloid progenitors hypersensitive to GM-CSF in vitro

GM-CSF, granulocyte-monocyte colony-stimulating factor; Ph, Philadelphia chromosome; WHO, World Health Organization

of JMML, can develop a spontaneously remitting condition that resembles JMML.

Further tests

Bone marrow aspiration, cytogenetic analysis and quantification of haemoglobin F are indicated. Cytogenetic analysis is often normal at presentation but monosomy 7, trisomy 8 or other clonal cytogenetic abnormality may be present or may appear during disease evolution. Molecular analysis is indicated since there is often mutation of *NRAS*, *KRAS*, *PTPN11*, *ASXL1* or *CBL* or bi-allelic inactivation of *NF1*. In addition to an increased haemoglobin F percentage, there may be other features associated with fetal haemopoiesis, specifically low haemoglobin A_2, low red cell carbonic anhydrase, reduced expression of the red cell I antigen and increased expression of the red cell i antigen. Serum immunoglobulin concentration may be increased. The NAP score may be high, normal or low, so is not useful.

Myelodysplastic/myeloproliferative neoplasm, unclassifiable

This condition has overlapping features between MDS and MPN, but does not meet the criteria of the conditions already described above [112]. Included in this category is refractory anaemia with ring sideroblasts and thrombocytosis.

Blood film and count

The blood film and count may show proliferative features such as a WBC of 13×10^9/l or more and a platelet count of 450×10^9/l or more. There may be blast cells but they are less than 20% of leucocytes. In addition there are dysplastic features affecting one or more lineages. In patients with refractory anaemia with ring sideroblasts and thrombocytosis there may be hypochromic cells and Pappenheimer bodies (Fig. 9.53).

Differential diagnosis

The differential diagnosis includes MDS, MPN and other MDS/MPN.

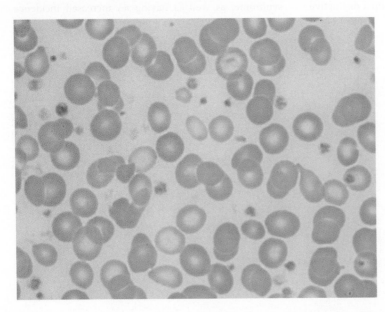

Fig. 9.53 Blood film is refractory anaemia with ring sideroblasts and thrombocytosis showing dimorphic red cells and thrombocytosis with large platelets or variable granularity.

Further tests

Tests indicated include a bone marrow aspirate, trephine biopsy, cytogenetic analysis and molecular analysis for a *JAK2*, *MPL* or *CALR* mutation.

Lymphoid and myeloid neoplasms with abnormalities of *PDGFRA*, *PDGFRB* or *FGFR1*

This group of neoplasms is defined by their specific molecular abnormalities [107]. Haematological features differ. The most common abnormality leading to *PDGFRA* rearrangement is a cryptic interstitial deletion leading to a *FIP1L1-PDGFRA* fusion gene. This condition most often manifests as CEL but can also present with a secondary AML or with T-lymphoblastic lymphoma. Cases with rearrangement of *PDGFRB*, including those with t(5;12)(q31~33;p12) and *ETV6-PDGFRB*, usually present with a myeloid neoplasm resembling aCML or CMML, often with eosinophilia. Cases with *FGFR1* rearrangement, among which the most common is t(8;13)(p11;q12) with *ZNF198-FGFR1*, can present with CEL, AML, T-lymphoblastic lymphoma or B-lymphoblastic lymphoma.

Blood film and count

Eosinophilia is common but not invariable (Fig. 9.54). Other haematological features vary according to the specific genes that are involved.

Differential diagnosis

It is important that these conditions are distinguished from other MPN and MDS/MPN with similar haematological features, since cases associated with rearrangement of *PDGFRA* and *PDGFRB* are responsive to tyrosine kinase inhibitors.

Further tests

Rearrangements of *PDGFRB* and *FGFR1* are detected by cytogenetic analysis. However, *FIP1L1-PDGFRA* fusion is cytogenetically silent, being due to an interstitial deletion, and detection requires FISH or molecular analysis, specifically a nested polymerase chain reaction.

Acute lymphoblastic leukaemia

ALL is most common in children under 10 years of age but continues throughout childhood, adolescence and adult life, with a second rise in incidence in later adult life. Clinical features are those due to leukaemic cell proliferation, such as bone pain, hepatosplenomegaly and lymphadenopathy, and those that are an indirect consequence of bone marrow infiltration, such as pallor and bruising. ALL may be of T or B lineage. The FAB classification of ALL was based on cytology [80], whereas the WHO classification is based on immunophenotyping and, to some extent, on molecular genetic analysis and is designated B or T lymphoblastic

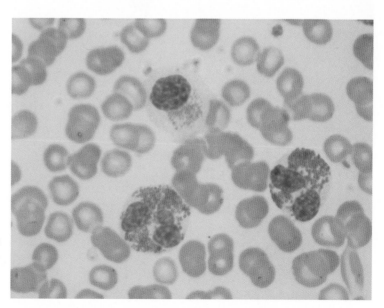

Fig. 9.54 Blood film in a patient with chronic eosinophilic leukaemia associated with a *FIP1L1-PDGFRA* fusion gene showing eosinophils with varying degrees of degranulation, one of which is non-lobulated.

leukaemia/lymphoma [79]. The FAB group categorised ALL morphologically as L1, L2 and L3. In L1 ALL (Fig. 9.55) the blast cells are small to medium in size and are fairly uniform in appearance. Larger cells have diffuse chromatin and sometimes small nucleoli, whereas the smaller blasts have no visible nucleolus and show some chromatin condensation. Cytoplasm is scanty and weakly to moderately basophilic. There may be a few cytoplasmic vacuoles. In L2 ALL (Fig. 9.56) the blasts are larger and more pleomorphic with more irregular nuclei, more prominent nucleoli and more abundant cytoplasm. Cytoplasm is weakly to strongly basophilic

and may contain some vacuoles. L3 ALL (Fig. 9.57) is characterised by moderately intense cytoplasmic basophilia and variable but usually heavy cytoplasmic vacuolation. The FAB classification of ALL is now of little consequence except that it is a reminder of the significance of cytology. Cases with L1 cytology have a very high probability of being ALL, whereas cases with L2 cytology are sometimes AML without evidence of differentiation. Noting L3 morphology alerts the observer to the fact that often, but not always, the case represents the leukaemic phase of Burkitt lymphoma rather than ALL. The WHO classification is shown in Table 9.13.

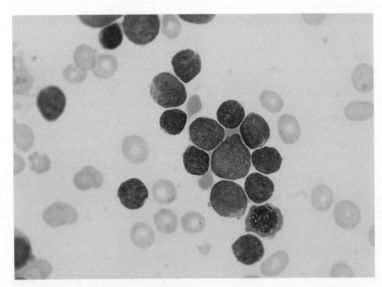

Fig. 9.55 Blood film in FAB L1 ALL showing lymphoblasts and one NRBC. The lymphoblasts vary in size but are relatively uniform in morphology. The smaller blast cells show some chromatin condensation, which can be a feature of lymphoblasts but not of myeloblasts. This case was shown on immunophenotyping to be of B lineage.

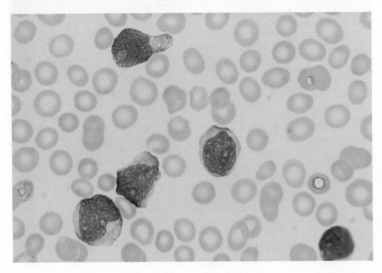

Fig. 9.56 Blood film in FAB L2 ALL. The blast cells are larger and more pleomorphic than in L1 ALL and in this case have a more diffuse chromatin pattern; one of the blasts has a hand-mirror conformation. This case was shown on immunophenotyping to be of T lineage.

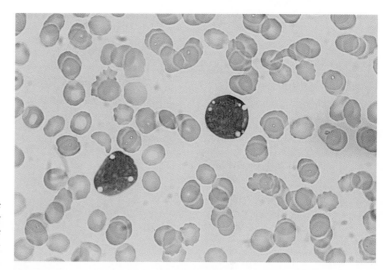

Fig. 9.57 Blood film in FAB L3 ALL. The blast cells are medium sized with strongly basophilic vacuolated cytoplasm. This case was shown to have a mature B-cell immunophenotype.

Table 9.13 The 2008 WHO classification of precursor lymphoid neoplasms (acute lymphoblastic leukaemia/lymphoma) [79].

B lymphoblastic leukaemia/lymphoma, not otherwise specified
B lymphoblastic lymphoma with recurrent genetic abnormalities
B lymphoblastic leukaemia/lymphoma with t(9;22)(q34;q11.2); *BCR-ABL1*
B lymphoblastic leukaemia/lymphoma with t(v;11q23); *MLL (KMT2A)* rearranged
B lymphoblastic leukaemia/lymphoma with t(12;21)(p13;q22); *ETV6-RUNX1*
B lymphoblastic leukaemia/lymphoma with hyperdiploidy
B lymphoblastic leukaemia/lymphoma with hypodiploidy
B lymphoblastic leukaemia/lymphoma with t(5;14)(q31;q32); *IL3-IGH*
B lymphoblastic leukaemia/lymphoma with t(1;19)(q23;p13.3); *TCF3-PBX1*
T lymphoblastic leukaemia/lymphoma

WHO, World Health Organization

Blood film and count

Some cases present with anaemia and thrombocytopenia without any circulating leukaemic cells. Others have variable numbers of lymphoblasts in the peripheral blood, with the WBC sometimes being greatly elevated. There is usually anaemia, neutropenia and thrombocytopenia, but occasionally there are normal numbers of neutrophils, platelets or both. Occasional patients have an increased platelet count [113]. Reactive eosinophilia is present in a minority of patients. The WHO categories of ALL do not have any distinctive features, with the exception of B-lineage ALL with t(5;14)(q31;q32), when there

is striking reactive eosinophilia as a result of dysregulation of the *IL3* gene by proximity to the *IGH* locus (Fig. 9.58).

Differential diagnosis

The differential diagnosis is mainly AML and reactive lymphocytosis.

Some cases of ALL have a few azurophilic granules and some cases of AML lack any granules or other light microscopy signs of myeloid differentiation, so that reliable differentiation of the two conditions requires further tests. Typical childhood cases of ALL (FAB L1) can usually be distinguished from AML on cytological features. There are usually some quite small blast cells, barely any bigger than a normal lymphocyte, and these cells show some chromatin condensation, whereas the blasts of AML are rarely this small and usually have a diffuse chromatin pattern. Cases of small cell tumours of childhood with circulating neoplastic cells are sometimes confused with ALL. Immunophenotyping may be necessary to make the distinction.

In cases of ALL with only small numbers of circulating blasts, it is sometimes necessary to do further tests, e.g. a bone marrow aspiration, to distinguish ALL from lymphocytosis with atypical lymphocytes resulting from infection.

In cases with no circulating leukaemic cells the differential diagnosis includes aplastic anaemia and other causes of bone marrow failure. Concern is often expressed as to whether children with severe thrombocytopenia, consistent with autoimmune thrombocytopenic purpura, are

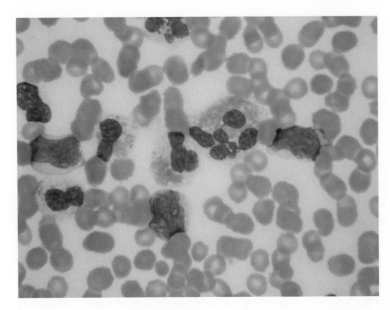

Fig. 9.58 Blood film in ALL associated with t(5;14)(q31;q32) showing leukaemic lymphoblasts and reactive eosinophilia. The eosinophils are cytologically abnormal, one having a hyperlobated nucleus and granule numbers being reduced.

actually suffering from ALL. When there are no atypical lymphoid cells and no anaemia this is possible, but is quite uncommon and unless there are atypical features or corticosteroid therapy is to be given, bone marrow aspiration is not usually considered necessary.

Further tests

Bone marrow aspiration and immunophenotyping of either peripheral blood or bone marrow blast cells are essential to confirm the diagnosis of ALL (Table 9.14). Cytogenetic analysis to identify prognostically relevant subgroups is important for patient management. Molecular analysis is becoming increasingly important, both to identify good prognosis cases, in which stem cell transplantation in first remission is inappropriate, and to identify poor prognosis cases, in which intensive and innovative forms of therapy are justified. Cytogenetic or molecular analysis is essential to identify Ph-positive, *BCR-ABL1*-positive cases (25–30% of adult patients), who require therapy with tyrosine kinase inhibitors.

Chronic lymphoid leukaemias and lymphomas

Both chronic lymphoid leukaemias and lymphomas are lymphoid neoplasms. By definition, in chronic lymphoid leukaemias there are circulating leukaemic cells, whereas lymphomas primarily involve lymph nodes and other tissues. Lymphomas may, however,

Table 9.14 Typical immunophenotypic findings in acute lymphoblastic leukaemia (expression is on the surface membrane unless otherwise specified).

B-lineage	T-lineage
Expression of CD19, CD22, CD24, CD79a* and HLA-DR; TdT† and CD45 usually expressed; variable expression of CD34, CD10, CD20, CD79b and cytoplasmic μ chain; FMC7 not expressed; surface membrane immunoglobulin is generally not expressed and cases showing expression are better classified as non-Hodgkin lymphoma rather than acute lymphoblastic leukaemia	Expression of CD7, CD45, cytoplasmic CD3 and nuclear TdT†; variable expression of CD1a, CD2, membrane CD3, CD5, CD4, CD8, CD10 (weaker than in B-lineage ALL) and T-cell receptor αβ or γδ; HLA-DR more often not expressed

* Monoclonal antibodies in use detect a cytoplasmic epitope
† Terminal deoxynucleotidyl transferase, nuclear expression

have a leukaemic phase, either at presentation or with disease progression. The term 'lymphoproliferative disorder' includes both leukaemias and lymphomas. Cytology is very useful in the differential diagnosis of these disorders [104], but it is not always possible to arrive at a definitive diagnosis on the basis of cytological features alone. Diagnosis should be based on clinical features, blood count, cytology and immunophenotype, supplemented when necessary by

Table 9.15 Typical immunophenotypic findings in chronic lymphoid leukaemias and non-Hodgkin lymphoma of B-lineage.*

Condition		Immunophenotype	
Chronic lymphocytic leukaemia		Weak expression of SmIg; expression of CD5 and CD23; lack of expression or weak expression of CD20, CD22 and CD79b; CD35 and FMC7 not expressed; CD200 strong	
Prolymphocytic leukaemia, hairy cell leukaemia and non-Hodgkin lymphoma	Prolymphocytic leukaemia	Moderate or strong expression of SmIg; lack of expression of CD23; expression of FMC7, CD20, CD22, CD35 and CD79b; variable expression of CD5 and CD10	
	Hairy cell leukaemia		SmIg strong, expression of CD11c, CD25, CD103 and CD123; CD22 and CD200 strongly expressed
	Follicular lymphoma		CD10 most often expressed in this subtype
	Mantle cell lymphoma		Expression of CD5 and nuclear cyclin D1, CD200 weak
	Splenic lymphoma with villous lymphocytes		CD11c and CD103 sometimes expressed
	Large cell lymphoma		Variable expression of CD5 and CD10
Plasma cell leukaemia		Expression of monotypic (κ or λ) cytoplasmic immunoglobulin (but not SmIg); expression of CD38 and CD138	

* All this group of disorders are likely to express surface membrane immunoglobulin (SmIg), CD19 and CD79a (cytoplasmic epitope detected); they express CD37 strongly whereas it is expressed weakly by T cells; they express CD40, which is expressed by some myeloid cells but not by T cells; terminal deoxynucleotidyl transferase is not expressed.
SmIg, surface membrane immunoglobulin

cytogenetic and molecular genetic analysis. In some patients, histological examination of the bone marrow or lymph nodes is also necessary. Only peripheral blood features will be discussed in any detail here. For further information on immunophenotype and histology the reader is referred to Tables 9.15 and 9.16 and references 84 and 114–116.

B-lineage lymphoproliferative disorders
Chronic lymphocytic leukaemia
CLL is a chronic condition characterised by accumulation of mature small B cells with consequent development of lymphadenopathy, hepatomegaly and splenomegaly. In early cases there may be no abnormal physical findings and the diagnosis is made incidentally

Table 9.16 Typical immunophenotypic findings in chronic T-lineage and natural killer (NK)-lineage lymphoproliferative disorders.

Condition	Immunophenotype	
T prolymphocytic leukaemia	Variable expression of CD2, CD3, CD5 and CD7; CD1 and TdT not expressed; expression of T-cell receptor αβ or γδ	CD4 and CD7 usually expressed
Sézary syndrome/mycosis fungoides		CD4 usually expressed
Adult T-cell leukaemia/lymphoma		CD4 and CD25 usually expressed; HLA-DR expressed in half and CD38 in two-thirds of patients
Large cell lymphoma		
Large granular lymphocyte leukaemia –T-cell		Most often expression of CD2, CD3, CD8, CD57 and T-cell receptor αβ; CD4 and CD16 usually not expressed
Large granular lymphocyte leukaemia –natural killer cell	CD3 and T-cell receptors not expressed; CD1a and TdT not expressed	Variable expression of CD2 and CD8; CD4 usually not expressed; expression of CD11b, CD16, CD56 and sometimes CD57; expression of CD158a, CD158b or CD158e or failure to express any CD158 epitope

TdT, terminal deoxynucleotidyl transferase

on a routine blood count. The peripheral blood and bone marrow are always involved.

Blood film and count

The WBC and lymphocyte count range from just above normal to greatly elevated. The Hb and platelet count may be normal or reduced. In the untreated patient, the neutrophil count is rarely reduced. The lymphocytes are similar in size to normal lymphocytes but are more uniform in appearance (Fig. 9.59). The chromatin is usually clumped and nucleoli are small and inconspicuous. Cytoplasm is scanty and weakly basophilic. In some cases there are cytoplasmic crystals (Fig. 9.60), globular inclusions [117] or azurophilic granules [118]. Vermiform inclusions representing immunoglobulin in dilated cisternae of the endoplasmic reticulum have also been described [119]. Because CLL cells have increased mechanical fragility, there are increased numbers of smear cells. There may be a small number of larger cells with prominent nucleoli resembling the cells of prolymphocytic leukaemia (PLL). If there are more than 10% of prolymphocytes or the degree of pleomorphism is greater than usual, the diagnosis of CLL of mixed cell type (CLL/PL) is preferred [115]. Anaemia is usually normocytic and normochromic. If there is complicating autoimmune haemolytic anaemia there are spherocytes and polychromasia.

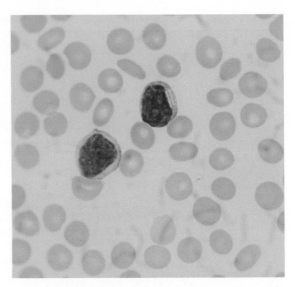

Fig. 9.60 Blood film in CLL showing two lymphocytes, one of which contains two crystals. By courtesy of Professor Daniel Catovsky, London.

Automated instruments show increased lymphocytes with there sometimes also being a flag for atypical lymphocytes or an increase in large unstained (i.e. peroxidase-negative) cells. There may be pseudobasophilia. When there is an associated autoimmune haemolytic anaemia, red cell cytograms show the presence of hyperchromic erythrocytes (Fig. 9.61).

Differential diagnosis

The differential diagnosis includes other chronic lymphoproliferative disorders, particularly follicular lymphoma, SLVL/splenic marginal zone lymphoma, mantle cell lymphoma and the small cell variant of T-lineage PLL. Benign conditions that can be confused with CLL include post-splenectomy lymphocytosis and lymphocytosis induced by acute stress. If the blood film is examined in isolation without reference to the age and clinical features, then whooping cough and infectious lymphocytosis can also be confused with CLL.

Further tests

The diagnosis should be confirmed by immunophenotyping (Table 9.15), which may be supplemented by cytogenetic analysis (particularly FISH) and trephine biopsy of the bone marrow.

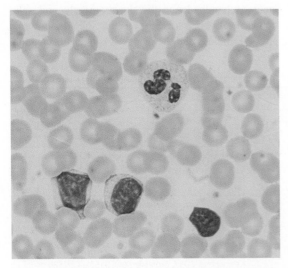

Fig. 9.59 Blood film in chronic lymphocytic leukaemia (CLL) showing a neutrophil, two mature lymphocytes and a smear cell.

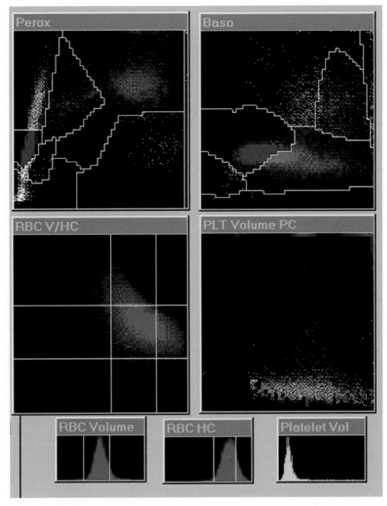

Fig. 9.61 Histograms and red cell cytogram from a patient with CLL complicated by autoimmune haemolytic anaemia. The lymphocyte count was 59.26 × 10⁹/l, with a large unstained cells (LUC) count of 3.14 × 10⁹/l. There was a mild pseudobasophilia ('basophil' count 0.55 × 10⁹/l). 15% of red cells were identified as hyperchromic and there was also an increase of macrocytes, attributable to reticulocytosis. By courtesy of Professor Gina Zini, Rome.

Monoclonal B-cell lymphocytosis

Monoclonal B-cell lymphocytosis or monoclonal lymphocytosis of undetermined significance is an asymptomatic condition that is sometimes detected in apparently healthy people. The clonal B-cells may have the immunophenotype of CLL or of non-Hodgkin lymphoma, either CD5-positive or CD5-negative, including cases with the immunophenotype of splenic marginal zone lymphoma. The probability of this condition evolving into an overt lymphoproliferative disorder is not yet known, although it is known that in the short term the condition may regress, be stable or progress.

Blood film and count

The blood count may be normal or there may be a mild increase in the total lymphocyte count. A few smear cells may be seen.

Differential diagnosis

The differential diagnosis is with overt lymphoproliferative disorders. Criteria have been proposed to help make this distinction [120].

Further tests

The diagnosis will only be made if immunophenotyping is carried out either in individuals with a mild lymphocytosis or, as part of a research project, in individuals who are apparently haematologically normal. The condition has been detected as the result of observation of crystalline inclusions in lymphocytes, leading to immunophenotyping [121]. A paraprotein is sometimes present at a low concentration. No further tests are indicated.

B-lineage prolymphocytic leukaemia

B-lineage prolymphocytic leukaemia (B-PLL or PLL) is characterised clinically by marked splenomegaly with trivial lymphadenopathy. The peripheral blood and bone marrow are always involved. There may be anaemia and other cytopenias. The disease is more rapidly progressive than CLL.

Blood film and count

The WBC is usually greatly elevated. The neoplastic cells are larger than those of CLL and often show more variation in size. They are predominantly round with round nuclei and weakly basophilic cytoplasm, which is more abundant than in CLL (Fig. 9.62). Many cells, particularly the larger ones, have large and prominent nucleoli. There is moderate chromatin condensation, which is enhanced around the large nucleolus, giving it a 'vesicular' appearance. If blood films are dried too slowly, cell shrinkage can lead to artefactual hairy projections and a less conspicuous nucleolus [122].

Differential diagnosis

The differential diagnosis includes other chronic lymphoproliferative disorders, particularly CLL/PL, mantle cell lymphoma and T-lineage PLL. The best morphological criterion to separate PLL from CLL/PL is that in PLL prolymphocytes are at least 55% of circulating lymphoid cells [123]. The possibility of a diagnosis of mantle cell lymphoma should be excluded by immunophenotyping, including investigation of cyclin D1 expression, and by FISH or molecular studies. In T-lineage PLL, the cells are more irregular in shape, more pleomorphic and often smaller than in B-lineage PLL. Occasionally, the leukaemic phase of large cell lymphoma resembles PLL, but generally the degree of pleomorphism is much greater in large cell lymphoma. Plasma cell leukaemia can also occasionally be difficult to distinguish, but usually there are some cells with more evident plasma cell features such as an eccentric nucleus and cytoplasmic basophilia with a paranuclear Golgi zone.

Further tests

Immunophenotyping (see Table 9.15) supports a provisional diagnosis of PLL and permits a distinction from plasma cell leukaemia. Cytogenetic analysis may show clonal cytogenetic abnormalities including trisomy 3 and rearrangements with a 14q32 breakpoint. t(11;14)(q13;q32) has been described, but such cases are better considered as mantle cell lymphoma.

Hairy cell leukaemia

Hairy cell leukaemia is a chronic disorder characterised by splenomegaly without lymphadenopathy. Early cases may have no abnormal physical findings and diagnosis may then be made incidentally because of cytopenia.

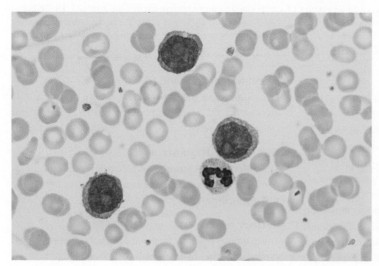

Fig. 9.62 Blood film in B-lineage prolymphocytic leukaemia (PLL) showing a neutrophil and three prolymphocytes with characteristic vesicular nucleoli.

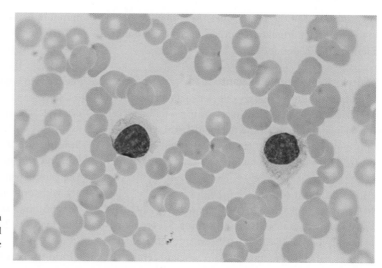

Fig. 9.63 Blood film in hairy cell leukaemia showing two hairy cells; both have plentiful cytoplasm with irregular margins and in one cell fine hair-like projections are present.

Blood film and count

The WBC is usually not elevated and hairy cells (Fig. 9.63) are infrequent in the peripheral blood. When they are very infrequent, making a buffy coat preparation can be useful.

There is usually normocytic anaemia and marked monocytopenia. In more advanced disease there is also neutropenia and thrombocytopenia. Hairy cells are larger than normal lymphocytes. They have abundant weakly basophilic cytoplasm with irregular 'hairy' margins. Occasionally there are cytoplasmic inclusions, which represent the ribosomal-lamellar complex that has been identified on electron microscopy; on light microscopy these inclusions appear as two indistinct parallel lines (Fig. 9.64). The nucleus may be round, oval, dumbbell-shaped or bilobed. It has a bland appearance with little chromatin condensation and sometimes an indistinct nucleolus.

Differential diagnosis

The differential diagnosis includes other lymphoproliferative disorders, particularly the variant form of hairy cell leukaemia, and SLVL. Hairy cells do not have the prominent nucleolus of the neoplastic cells in the variant form of hairy cell leukaemia and have more plentiful cytoplasm than the cells of SLVL. Since there may be pancytopenia with very infrequent leukaemic cells, hairy leukaemia can also be confused with aplastic anaemia. The disproportionate reduction of the monocyte count is a useful indicator of the correct diagnosis. A condition similar to hairy cell leukaemia but with a higher WBC and a different immunophenotype has been reported from Japan [124]. In addition, rare cases of polyclonal hairy B lymphocyte proliferation have been reported in Japanese people [124].

Further tests

The diagnosis is confirmed by immunophenotyping [114] (see Table 9.15), TRAP activity and a highly characteristic trephine biopsy in which neoplastic cells are spaced apart. Molecular genetic analysis shows

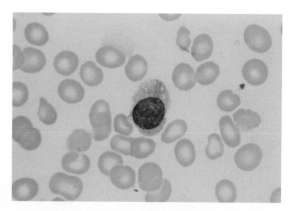

Fig. 9.64 Blood film in hairy cell leukaemia showing a hairy cell containing a ribosomal–lamellar complex. These structures are more readily observed by ultrastructural examination, but can occasionally be identified by light microscopy as two parallel basophilic lines. By courtesy of Dr Laura Sainati, Padua, and Professor Daniel Catovsky.

rearrangement of the *BRAF* gene. There may be clonal cytogenetic abnormalities, but no specific rearrangement has been identified.

Hairy cell leukaemia variant

A variant form of hairy cell leukaemia has been described. It has similar clinical features to hairy cell leukaemia, but some of the haematological, cytological and immunophenotypic features differ and it is better regarded as a distinct condition.

Blood film and count

In hairy cell leukaemia variant, the WBC is often elevated and neoplastic cells are numerous. Severe monocytopenia is not a feature. Otherwise haematological features are similar to those of hairy cell leukaemia. The neoplastic cells have similar cytoplasmic characteristics to hairy cells, but have a prominent vesicular nucleolus, resembling that of the prolymphocyte (Fig. 9.65).

Differential diagnosis

The differential diagnosis is hairy cell leukaemia and SLVL. In SLVL the neoplastic cells have less abundant cytoplasm and the nucleolus, if visible, is less prominent than in hairy cell leukaemia variant.

Further tests

Immunophenotyping, cytochemistry and a trephine biopsy are useful in confirming the diagnosis. The immunophenotype of hairy cell variant differs from that of hairy cell leukaemia and TRAP activity is generally negative. The trephine biopsy usually does not show the spaced cells that are almost invariable in hairy cell leukaemia. SLVL has a similar immunophenotype to hairy cell leukaemia variant, so that distinction is mainly on cytological features.

Splenic lymphoma with villous lymphocytes (splenic marginal zone lymphoma)

The clinical features of SLVL are prominent splenomegaly with only minor lymphadenopathy. In the WHO classification, SLVL is regarded as a variant of splenic marginal zone lymphoma.

Blood film and count

The WBC varies from normal to moderately elevated. The blood film (Fig. 9.66) shows variable numbers of mature small lymphocytes, which are not as uniform in appearance as those of CLL. The nucleus is round with chromatin clumping and sometimes an inconspicuous nucleolus. Cytoplasm is scanty to moderate in amount and weakly to moderately basophilic. In cases categorised as SLVL, some of the neoplastic cells have irregular or 'villous' margins, sometimes at one pole of the cell. Other cases of splenic marginal zone lymphoma do not have any distinguishing features. Some neoplastic cells show plasmacytoid differentiation. Some cases show increased rouleaux formation, indicating the presence of a paraprotein.

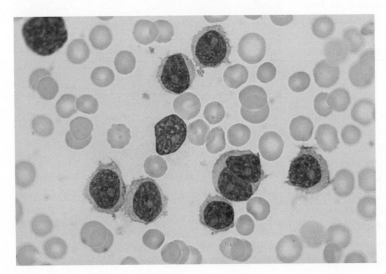

Fig. 9.65 Blood film in the variant form of hairy cell leukaemia showing cells with the cytoplasmic characteristics of hairy cells but with a prominent nucleolus. There is one binucleate cell. By courtesy of Professor Daniel Catovsky.

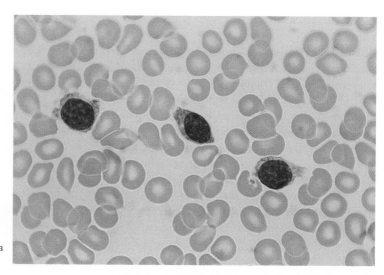

Fig. 9.66 Blood film in splenic lymphoma with villous lymphocytes (SLVL).

Differential diagnosis

The differential diagnosis is CLL and the variant form of hairy cell leukaemia.

Further tests

The immunophenotype is useful in making the distinction from CLL (see Table 9.15). Analysis of serum immunoglobulins may demonstrate a paraprotein.

Lymphoplasmacytic lymphoma

Lymphoplasmacytic lymphoma, as defined by the WHO group, is a lymphoma in which some cells show differentiation to plasma cells. This condition has previously often been referred to as lymphoplasmacytoid lymphoma. Lymphoplasmacytic lymphoma is usually a disease of lymph nodes and sometimes of the spleen and other lymphoid organs. A proportion of cases have involvement of the peripheral blood and bone marrow. There is often secretion of a paraprotein, most often but not always IgM. Sometimes the paraprotein is a cryoglobulin or shows cold agglutinin activity. The term 'Waldenström macroglobulinaemia' is sometimes used interchangeably with lymphoplasmacytic lymphoma, but in fact what Waldenström described was lymphoplasmacytic lymphoma with a marked increase in plasma IgM concentration leading to hyperviscosity.

Blood film and count

When the bone marrow is infiltrated, a normocytic normochromic anaemia is common and other cytopenias can also occur. The blood film may show only rouleaux and increased background staining, reflecting the presence of a paraprotein, or there may be circulating lymphoma cells (Fig. 9.67). In a minority of cases, there is red cell agglutination or cryoglobulin deposition. Circulating lymphoma cells resemble small lymphocytes, but show some plasmacytoid features such as cytoplasmic basophilia or an eccentric nucleus. Mature plasma cells must also be present (in peripheral blood or other tissues) to meet the WHO criteria for this diagnosis. Sometimes cells have cytoplasmic crystals or globular inclusions.

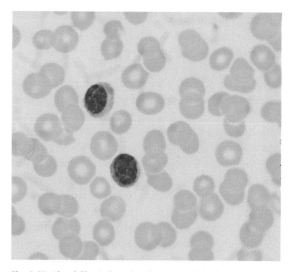

Fig. 9.67 Blood film in lymphoplasmacytic lymphoma.

Differential diagnosis

The differential diagnosis includes CLL and SLVL. Waldenström macroglobulinaemia (as described by Waldenström) and chronic cold haemagglutinin disease represent subsets of lymphoplasmacytic lymphoma in which the dominant clinical and haematological features are caused by hyperviscosity and cold-induced red cell agglutination respectively. In chronic cold haemagglutinin disease the lymphoma itself is often very low grade and sometimes clinically inapparent. Type I and type II cryoglobulinaemia also are lymphoid neoplasms in which a paraprotein is either a cryoglobulin (type I) or has rheumatoid factor activity, complexing with polyclonal immunoglobulin to form a cryoglobulin (type II). Many patients with type II cryoglobulinaemia have chronic hepatitis C infection. The neoplastic clone may be occult in cryoglobulinaemia, sometimes becoming clinically apparent during the course of the illness. Diagnosis of these three conditions rests on assessment of all disease features rather than just the peripheral blood abnormalities.

Further tests

Bone marrow aspiration and trephine biopsy, immunophenotyping and investigations for a serum paraprotein and for urinary Bence–Jones protein (free monoclonal immunoglobulin light chains) are indicated. The immunophenotype is similar to that of other non-Hodgkin lymphomas, but there may be, in addition, cytoplasmic immunoglobulin and expression of CD38.

Follicular lymphoma

Follicular or centroblastic/centrocytic lymphoma is mainly a disease of the lymph nodes, although in advanced disease the liver and spleen are also involved. Circulating neoplastic cells may be present at diagnosis or a leukaemic phase may develop with disease progression.

Blood film and count

The WBC varies from normal to greatly elevated. The Hb and platelet count may be normal but, in advanced disease, anaemia and thrombocytopenia can develop. Circulating lymphoma cells may be rare or present in large numbers. Lymphoma cells (Fig. 9.68) are often very small with scanty, almost inapparent, weakly basophilic cytoplasm. Some nuclei show notches or deep narrow clefts. These cytological features are particularly typical of cases with a high WBC. Other cases have larger,

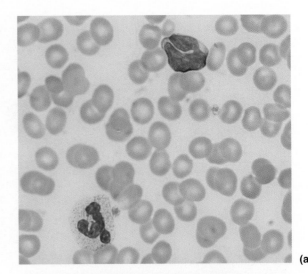

(a)

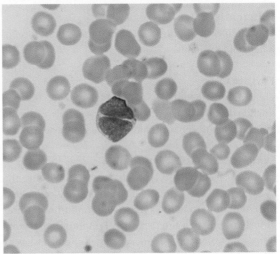

(b)

Fig. 9.68 Blood film in follicular lymphoma showing: (a) a neutrophil and a cleft lymphocyte; and (b) a cleft lymphocyte.

more pleomorphic cells, some of which have small but distinct nucleoli. Again there are notches or clefts in a proportion of cells. Smear cells are not a feature. Rarely the cells contain crystals [125].

Differential diagnosis

The differential diagnosis includes CLL and other non-Hodgkin lymphomas, particularly mantle cell lymphoma.

Further tests

Immunophenotyping is very useful in making the distinction between follicular lymphoma and CLL. The immunophenotypes of follicular lymphoma and mantle cell lymphoma are more similar, but mantle cell lymphoma is characteristically CD5-positive whereas follicular lymphoma is CD5-negative and is much more likely to be CD10-positive (see Table 9.15). When cytological features are insufficient to make a diagnosis, lymph node biopsy or cytogenetic/molecular genetic analysis may be needed.

Mantle cell lymphoma

Mantle cell lymphoma, previously known as diffuse centrocytic lymphoma and lymphoma of intermediate differentiation, is mainly a lymph node disease but the peripheral blood is involved in one fifth to one quarter of cases.

Blood film and count

Lymphoma cells vary from small to medium in size (Fig. 9.69). Some cases have been confused with CLL but, in general, the cells are more pleomorphic. Cells are variable in shape and nucleocytoplasmic ratio. Some have cleft or irregular nuclei. Chromatin condensation is less than in CLL and some cells appear blastic. Some cells are nucleolated. In the blastoid variant, most cells resemble blast cells.

Differential diagnosis

The differential diagnosis includes other non-Hodgkin lymphomas, CLL and CLL/PL. In the blastoid variant a differential diagnosis of ALL may also have to be considered

Further tests

The immunophenotype is quite distinct from that of CLL and shows subtle differences from that of other non-Hodgkin lymphomas (see Table 9.15). In general, cytological and immunophenotypic features are not sufficiently distinctive for a definite diagnosis and either lymph node histology or cytogenetic/molecular genetic analysis is needed for confirmation. This lymphoma is characterised by t(11;14)(q13;q32) (detectable by FISH analysis), rearrangement of *BCL1* and expression of cyclin D1 (detectable immunohistochemically and by flow cytometry).

Other B-lineage lymphomas

Burkitt lymphoma may involve the peripheral blood. In endemic Burkitt lymphoma, leukaemia usually occurs only in advanced disease. In non-endemic and AIDS-associated Burkitt lymphoma, peripheral blood involvement is much more common. When a leukaemic phase occurs, the cells have the cytological features described by the FAB group as 'L3 ALL'.

A leukaemic phase is much less common in B-lineage large cell lymphomas than in the low grade lymphoproliferative disorders described above. When it occurs, the cells have a diameter about three times that of a red cell (Fig 9.70). They are usually pleomorphic with abundant moderately basophilic cytoplasm [126]. Nuclei are often lobulated and there may be prominent nucleoli. In some cases the cells resemble monoblasts. A case of intravascular large B-cell lymphoma has been reported

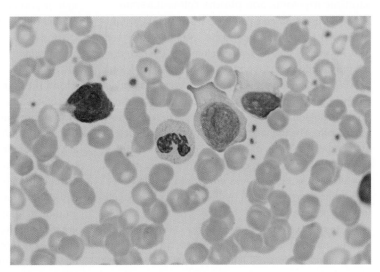

Fig. 9.69 Blood film of a patient with mantle cell lymphoma showing a neutrophil and three highly pleomorphic lymphocytes. By courtesy of Dr Estella Matutes, Barcelona.

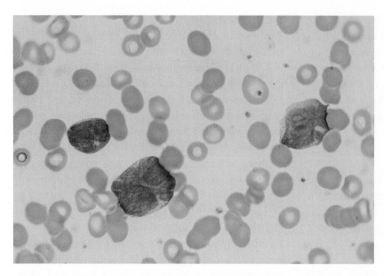

Fig. 9.70 Blood film of a patient with large cell lymphoma (centroblastic) showing large pleomorphic lymphoma cells with cleft nuclei.

in which diagnosis followed observation of clumps of lymphoma cells in a blood film [127].

Certain low-grade lymphomas, e.g. mucosa-associated lymphoid tissue (MALT) type lymphoma and monocytoid B-cell lymphoma, rarely have a leukaemic phase although occasional cases have shown peripheral blood dissemination. In monocytoid B cell lymphoma, the circulating neoplastic cells may have voluminous cytoplasm and somewhat irregular nuclei [18].

The haematological features of μ heavy chain disease are similar to those of CLL, including the presence of smear cells [128].

Multiple myeloma and plasma cell leukaemia

Multiple myeloma and plasma cell leukaemia are disseminated plasma cell neoplasms. Multiple myeloma, also known as plasma cell myeloma, is characterised by proliferation of abnormal plasma cells (myeloma cells) in the bone marrow and, in the great majority of patients, secretion of a monoclonal immunoglobulin or immunoglobulin light chain, which is referred to as a paraprotein. The monoclonal immunoglobulin is detectable in the serum. The monoclonal light chain, being of low molecular weight, is excreted in the urine, where it is referred to as Bence–Jones protein. In multiple myeloma there may be some 'spillover' of neoplastic cells into the peripheral blood.

The term 'plasma cell leukaemia' indicates that significant numbers of neoplastic plasma cells are circulating in the blood. Plasma cell leukaemia may occur *de novo*

or as the terminal phase of multiple myeloma. The FAB group [115] suggested that this term be restricted to a *de novo* presentation in leukaemic phase, but others, including the WHO expert group, have used it more generally [129,130]. Plasma cell leukaemia has been arbitrarily defined as an absolute plasma cell count of more than $2 \times 10^9/1$, with the plasma cells also being more than 20% of peripheral blood cells [129]. In the 2008 WHO classification, either of these criteria is considered sufficient for the diagnosis [130]. Plasma cell leukaemia is particularly common in IgD myeloma.

The picture of plasma cell leukaemia can also occur transiently when infection occurs in a patient with multiple myeloma, probably as a result of stimulation of plasma cells by IL6 [131].

The most typical clinical features of multiple myeloma are anaemia, bone pain, hypercalcaemia and renal failure.

Blood film and count

The blood film in multiple myeloma usually shows normocytic normochromic anaemia, but sometimes there is macrocytosis. In the majority of cases in which there is a serum paraprotein there is also increased background staining and increased rouleaux formation (Fig. 9.71). Cases with Bence–Jones protein but no serum paraprotein do not have increased rouleaux or increased background staining, so the absence of these features does not exclude the diagnosis. The WBC and platelet count are usually not elevated and may be reduced. There may be occasional NRBC and immature granulocytes.

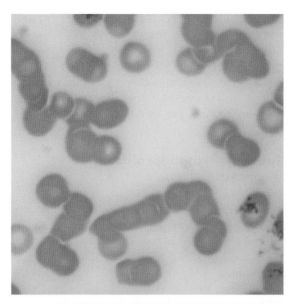

Fig. 9.71 Blood film in multiple myeloma showing rouleaux formation.

Circulating myeloma cells may be absent, infrequent or numerous. Circulating myeloma cells may be cytologically normal, but often they show abnormalities such as nuclear immaturity (a diffuse chromatin pattern and a nucleolus), high nucleocytoplasmic ratio, reduction of cytoplasmic basophilia and poorly developed Golgi zone, mitotic figures, binuclearity and dissociation of maturation of the nucleus and the cytoplasm. The number of circulating myeloma cells has been found to

be of prognostic significance, with 4% or more plasma cells being indicative of a worse prognosis [132].

In plasma cell leukaemia (Fig. 9.72), the neoplastic cells may resemble mature plasma cells or, particularly in cases with a *de novo* presentation, may be highly abnormal with an immature chromatin pattern, nucleoli and minimal features of plasma cell differentiation.

In some patients with multiple myeloma, the paraprotein is a cryoglobulin or has cold agglutinin activity. In such cases, precipitated cryoglobulin or red cell agglutinates may be noted in blood films.

When paraproteins are cold agglutinins or cryoglobulins they may cause factitious results with automated blood cell counters (see Chapter 4).

Differential diagnosis

In patients with circulating myeloma cells the differential diagnosis is reactive plasmacytosis. Both conditions may have increased rouleaux formation and background staining. These abnormalities are usually, but not always, much more striking in multiple myeloma. Neutrophilia, monocytosis, thrombocytosis and reactive changes in neutrophils are often present in patients with reactive plasmacytosis, but they are quite uncommon in multiple myeloma. However, rarely, there is a neutrophilic leukaemoid reaction in myeloma. Marked cytological abnormalities in plasma cells are indicative of a neoplastic condition.

The differential diagnosis in cases without circulating plasma cells includes other causes of normocytic nor-

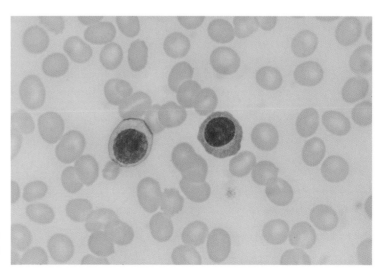

Fig. 9.72 Blood film of a patient with plasma cell leukaemia showing two neoplastic plasma cells.

mochromic anaemia, particularly conditions, such as AIDS, chronic inflammation and cirrhosis of the liver, in which an increased concentration of plasma proteins leads to increased rouleaux formation.

When the neoplastic cells are cytologically very atypical, the differential diagnosis includes prolymphocytic leukaemia and non-Hodgkin lymphoma.

Further tests

The ESR is often markedly elevated in multiple myeloma and is often used as a screening test for this condition. However, it should be noted that, if there is marked hyperviscosity, the ESR may be normal and in cases without a serum paraprotein the ESR may not show much elevation. When multiple myeloma is suspected, tests indicated to confirm the diagnosis are bone marrow aspiration, a radiological survey or magnetic resonance imaging of the skeleton, serum calcium, creatinine and uric acid estimation and investigation for serum and urinary paraproteins. Suitable tests include serum protein electrophoresis and immunofixation, immunofixation of a concentrated urine sample and nephelometry for assessment of the ratio of free kappa chain to free lambda chains in the serum. The latter technique will detect an abnormality in patients with Bence–Jones myeloma and in the majority of patients with non-secretory myeloma [133]. Immunophenotyping is not needed unless there is any reason to doubt that the plasma cells are neoplastic, in which case use of anti-κ and anti-λ reagents will give evidence of clonality. Peripheral blood immunophenotyping can also be used to identify small

number of circulating clonal plasma cells, an indicator of worse prognosis [134]. Immunophenotyping is also useful when there is doubt as to whether highly abnormal circulating cells are neoplastic or when their lineage is not apparent. The immunophenotype of the terminally differentiated plasma cell differs from that of non-Hodgkin lymphoma cells (see Table 9.15).

T-lineage lymphoproliferative disorders

T-lineage lymphoproliferative disorders are less common than B-lineage disorders. Precise diagnosis requires immunophenotyping and, sometimes, cytogenetic analysis or histological examination of lymph nodes, skin or other tissues.

T-lineage prolymphocytic leukaemia

T-lineage prolymphocytic leukaemia (T-PLL) is most often a disease of elderly people. Splenomegaly is the commonest clinical feature. A rash, indicative of skin infiltration, is sometimes present.

Blood count and film

The WBC is moderately to greatly elevated. T-lineage prolymphocytes (Fig. 9.73) are smaller and more pleomorphic than B-lineage prolymphocytes. Nuclei are irregular or lobulated. Cytoplasm is often scanty and may be moderately basophilic. Some cases cells have protruding cytoplasmic 'blebs'. Nucleoli may be

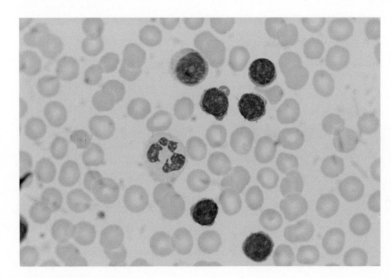

Fig. 9.73 Blood film of a patient with T-lineage prolymphocytic leukaemia (T-PLL) showing lymphocytes with irregular hyperchromatic nuclei, inconspicuous nucleoli and scanty moderately basophilic cytoplasm, which in one cell is forming blebs. Only one of the cells resembles those of B-lineage PLL, being larger with a moderate amount of cytoplasm and a more prominent nucleolus.

inapparent or prominent, but are rarely as large or as prominent as in B-lineage PLL.

Differential diagnosis

The differential diagnosis is mainly CLL and B-lineage PLL.

Further tests

Immunophenotyping is essential to confirm a diagnosis. Cells characteristically express CD7, which is usually negative in other T-lineage lymphoproliferative disorders (see Table 9.16).

Cutaneous T-cell lymphomas

Mycosis fungoides and Sézary syndrome are T-cell lymphomas that characteristically infiltrate the skin. The presence of circulating lymphoma cells is essential for the diagnosis of Sézary syndrome, in which there is widespread disease dissemination at diagnosis, whereas in mycosis fungoides circulating lymphoma cells are seen only in patients with advanced-stage disease. The cytological features do not differ between Sézary syndrome and mycosis fungoides, although they differ greatly between cases.

Blood count and film

The blood count may be normal, apart from sometimes showing lymphocytosis. Sometimes there is also eosinophilia. Lymphoma cells, known as Sézary cells, may be predominantly either small (Fig. 9.74) or large (Fig. 9.75) or a case may show a mixture of large and small cells. The most characteristic feature of the Sézary cell is a convoluted or cerebriform nucleus with tightly intertwined nuclear lobes. The cytoplasm is weakly basophilic and may contain a ring of vacuoles, which has been likened to rosary beads. In the small Sézary cell, there is scanty cytoplasm and a compact nucleus, the surface of which appears grooved. In large Sézary cells, there is more plentiful cytoplasm and a larger nucleus with more obvious nuclear lobes. The percentage and, particularly, the absolute number of circulating Sézary cells are of prognostic significance.

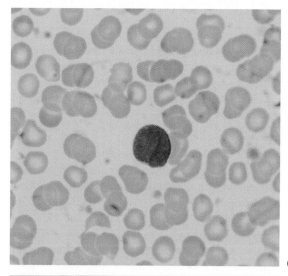

(a)

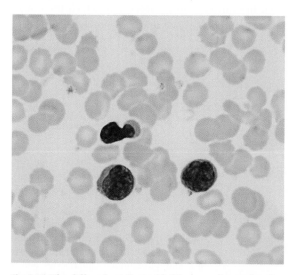

Fig. 9.74 Blood film of a patient with Sézary syndrome showing small Sézary cells with hyperchromatic convoluted or cerebriform nuclei.

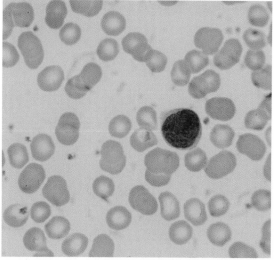

Fig. 9.75 Blood film of a patient with Sézary syndrome showing large Sézary cells.

(b)

Differential diagnosis

The differential diagnosis includes other lymphomas and benign dermatological conditions, in which cells resembling Sézary cells are sometimes seen [135]. 'Sézary cell leukaemia', in which skin infiltration is absent, is now thought to be a variant of T-PLL.

Further tests

Skin biopsy and immunophenotyping (see Table 9.16) are useful in diagnosis. Intra-epidermal lymphocyte accumulations (Pautrier micro-abscesses) are characteristic. It is sometimes difficult to recognise small Sézary cells by light microscopy. Ultrastructural examination can be useful in such cases since the complex nuclear form is then readily apparent (see Fig. 7.18). Because cells resembling small Sézary cells can be seen in benign inflammatory skin conditions, morphology alone is sometimes insufficient for diagnosis. In some cases demonstration of a clonal T-cell population is necessary for confirmation.

Adult T-cell leukaemia/lymphoma

Adult T-cell leukaemia/lymphoma (ATLL) is a disease that develops in a minority of adults who are long-term carriers of the HTLV-1 retrovirus. Such carriers mainly live in, or originate from, Japan and the Caribbean, but the disease is also found in Taiwan, the Middle East, Central and West Africa, South America, the south-eastern USA and in Native Americans in North America. In the majority of cases the disease manifests itself as leukaemia and in a minority as a lymphoma. In those who present with leukaemia there is usually lymphadenopathy and sometimes hepatomegaly and splenomegaly. Skin infiltration and hypercalcaemia are common. Patients with ATLL are also prone to opportunistic infections.

Blood count and film

The WBC is often greatly elevated. Leukaemic cells are generally medium sized to large and very pleomorphic. Nuclei are often polylobated, their shape resembling a flower or a cloverleaf (Fig. 9.76). Some nuclei have condensed chromatin while others have a diffuse chromatin pattern. Some cells are nucleolated. There is a variable amount of cytoplasm, which may be basophilic. A minority of cells can resemble those of Sézary syndrome. Some patients have associated eosinophilia. Anaemia and thrombocytopenia may be minimal at diagnosis.

Differential diagnosis

The differential diagnosis is cutaneous T-cell lymphoma and other lymphomas of mature T cells. The degree of pleomorphism and the presence of at least a minority of cells with flower-shaped nuclei are useful in the differential diagnosis. The typical acute form of ATLL should also be distinguished from smouldering or chronic ATLL, which generally lacks organomegaly, cytopenia and biochemical abnormalities. It also needs to be distinguished from the carrier state for HTLV-1 in which there may be small numbers of polyclonal atypical lymphocytes in

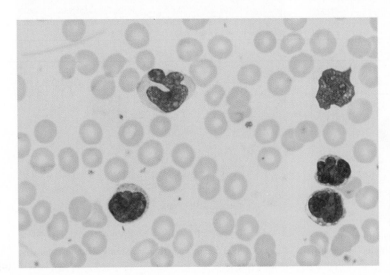

Fig. 9.76 Blood film of a patient with adult T-cell leukaemia/lymphoma (ATLL) showing four pleomorphic lymphocytes and a smear cell; one of the lymphoma cells has a flower-shaped nucleus and two others have convoluted nuclei.

the peripheral blood, including some lymphocytes with polylobated nuclei.

Other tests

Serological tests for HTLV-1 are indicated (not forgetting that a patient who is seropositive for HTLV-1 may develop another type of lymphoma or lymphoid leukaemia). Immunophenotyping is also useful in the differential diagnosis, since CD25 is commonly positive whereas it is usually negative in other leukaemias and lymphomas of phenotypically mature T cells (see Table 9.16).

Large granular lymphocyte leukaemia

Large granular lymphocyte leukaemia is a heterogeneous group of disorders in which the neoplastic cells have the cytological features of large granular lymphocytes and the immunophenotypic features of either cytotoxic T cells or natural killer cells. The clinical course is variable. Some patients have little organomegaly and a slowly progressive disease, but the course may be complicated by the effects of cytopenia, most often neutropenia. Other patients, particularly those whose cells have the phenotype of natural killer cells, have more typical features of lymphoma and a more rapid clinical course.

Blood count and film

In most cases the leukaemic cells are cytologically very similar to normal large granular lymphocytes (Fig. 9.77) with a small nucleus with condensed chromatin,

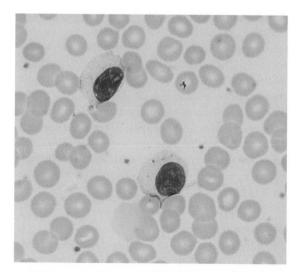

Fig. 9.77 Blood film of a patient with large granular lymphocyte leukaemia showing two large granular lymphocytes.

plentiful weakly basophilic cytoplasm and prominent azurophilic granules in at least some of the cells. Sometimes cells are larger with some nuclear irregularity and cytoplasmic basophilia. Sometimes there is neutropenia or, less often, anaemia or thrombocytopenia. Cytopenias may be profound, being the result of abnormal immune responses rather than bone marrow infiltration.

Differential diagnosis

The differential diagnosis is a reactive increase of large granular lymphocytes, e.g. that caused by a chronic viral infection, occurring post-splenectomy or associated with rituximab-induced autoimmune neutropenia.

Other tests

When the diagnosis is in doubt, immunophenotyping and tests to demonstrate clonality can be of use. Cells usually express CD2 and CD8 and do not express CD4 (see Table 9.16). In T-lineage cases, they express CD3, T-cell receptor antigens and usually CD57. Natural killer (NK)-lineage cases do not express CD3 or T-cell receptor antigens; they may express CD11b, CD16 and CD56 and, less often, CD57. A very uniform immunophenotype is suggestive of clonality and therefore of neoplasia. Clonality can be demonstrated in CD3-positive cases by molecular genetic analysis to demonstrate rearrangement of T-cell receptor genes. In NK, CD3-negative cases, cytogenetic analysis demonstrates an abnormal clone in some cases. In a larger group, analysis of CD158a, CD158b and CD158e (Killer Inhibitory Receptor) expression provides indirect evidence of clonality [136]. Polyclonal NK cells express all three antigens (on different cells), whereas monoclonal NK cells uniformly express one or none.

Other T-cell lymphomas

T-cell lymphomas are less common than B-cell lymphomas and less often have a leukaemic phase.

Blood count and film

Circulating lymphoma cells are often medium sized or large and quite pleomorphic (Figs 9.78 and 9.79).

Differential diagnosis

T-cell lymphomas cannot be reliably distinguished from certain B-cell lymphomas, particularly mantle cell lymphoma and B-lineage large cell lymphomas. Occasionally, they can also be confused with AML, particularly acute monoblastic leukaemia.

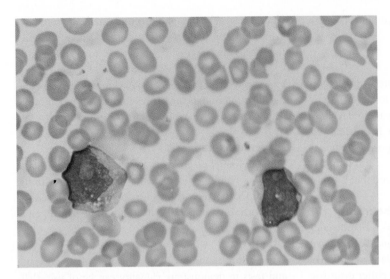

Fig. 9.78 Peripheral blood film of a patient with large cell lymphoma of T lineage showing two large lymphoma cells.

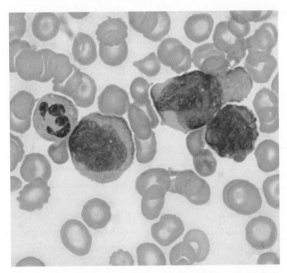

Fig. 9.79 Peripheral blood film of a patient with large cell anaplastic lymphoma of T lineage showing very large pleomorphic lymphoma cells. By courtesy of Dr David Clark, Grantham.

Other tests

Immunophenotyping is indicated and confirms the diagnosis. Cells express T-cell markers but the immunophenotype is often aberrant. Molecular analysis shows rearrangement of T-cell receptor genes.

Hodgkin lymphoma

Hodgkin lymphoma (Hodgkin's disease) is of B-lymphocyte origin. The disease is now divided into two major categories, nodular lymphocyte-predominant Hodgkin lymphoma and classical Hodgkin lymphoma. The former is clearly of B-cell origin, whereas in the latter the neoplastic cells (Reed–Sternberg cells and mononuclear Hodgkin cells) are defective B-cells that fail to express many B-lineage associated surface antigens. Classical Hodgkin lymphoma is further divided into nodular sclerosing Hodgkin lymphoma, mixed cellularity Hodgkin lymphoma, lymphocyte-depleted Hodgkin lymphoma and lymphocyte-rich classical Hodgkin lymphoma. The usual clinical presentation is with lymphadenopathy, with or without systemic symptoms.

Blood count and film

Hodgkin lymphoma can cause anaemia, leucocytosis, neutrophilia, eosinophilia, lymphopenia and thrombocytosis. The anaemia may be normocytic and normochromic or microcytic and hypochromic, with the characteristics of anaemia of chronic disease. There may also be increased background staining and increase rouleaux formation. When there is bone marrow infiltration there may be anaemia, leucopenia or pancytopenia. On multivariate analysis, an elevated WBC and a reduced lymphocyte count correlate with worse prognosis [137].

Differential diagnosis

The differential diagnosis includes non-Hodgkin lymphoma and a variety of infective and inflammatory conditions. There are no specific peripheral blood features to point to a diagnosis of Hodgkin lymphoma.

Other tests

The ESR is increased, serum iron and transferrin concentration are reduced and serum ferritin is normal or elevated. Diagnosis usually requires a lymph node biopsy, although occasionally a bone marrow aspirate and trephine biopsy give the diagnosis, particularly in patients with immunodeficiency as a result of HIV infection.

TEST YOUR KNOWLEDGE

Visit the companion website for MCQs and EMQs on this topic:
www.wiley.com/go/bain/bloodcells

References

1 Leibovici L, Drucker M, Samra Z, Konisberger H and Pitlik SD (1995) Prognostic significance of the neutrophil count in immunocompetent patients with bacteraemia. *Q J Med*, **88**, 181–189.

2 Gombos MM, Bienkowski RS, Gochman RF and Billett HH (1998) The absolute neutrophil count: is it the best indicator of bacteremia in infants? *Am J Clin Pathol*, **109**, 221–225.

3 Lascari AD (1984) *Hematologic Manifestations of Childhood Diseases*. Theme-Stratton, New York.

4 Manroe BL, Weinberg AG, Rosenfeld CR and Browne R (1979) The neonatal blood count in health and disease. I. Reference values for neutrophilic cells. *J Pediatr*, **95**, 89–98.

5 Christensen RD and Rothstein G (1978) Pitfalls in the interpretation of leukocyte counts in newborn infants. *Am J Clin Pathol*, **72**, 609–611.

6 Morris CDW, Bird AR and Nell H (1989) The haematological and biochemical changes in severe pulmonary tuberculosis. *Q J Med*, **73**, 1151–1159.

7 Glasser RM, Walker RI and Herion JC (1990) The significance of hematologic abnormalities in patients with tuberculosis. *Arch Intern Med*, **125**, 691–695.

8 Hoagland RJ (1960) The clinical manifestations of infectious mononucleosis: a report of two hundred cases. *Am J Med*, **240**, 21–29.

9 Brigden ML, Au S, Thompson S, Brigden S, Doyle P and Tsaparas Y (1999) Infectious mononucleosis in an outpatient population: diagnostic utility of 2 automated hematology analyzers and the sensitivity and specificity of Hoagland's criteria in heterophile-positive patients. *Arch Path Lab Med*, **123**, 875–881.

10 Lach-Szyrma V and Brito-Babapulle F (1999) The clinical significance of apoptotic cells in peripheral blood smears. *Clin Lab Haematol*, **21**, 277–280.

11 Kahl C and Freund M (2010) Peripheral blood alterations in a patient with infectious mononucleosis. *Br J Haematol*, **150**, 2.

12 Cantow EF and Kostinas JE (1966) Studies on infectious mononucleosis. IV. Changes in the granulocytic series. *Am J Clin Pathol*, **46**, 43–47.

13 Habib MA, Babka JC and Burningham RA (1973) Profound granulocytopenia associated with infectious mononucleosis. *Am J Med Sci*, **265**, 339–346.

14 Sumaya CV and Ench Y (1985) Epstein–Barr virus infectious mononucleosis in children. I. Clinical and general laboratory findings. *Pediatrics*, **75**, 1003–1010.

15 Carter JW, Edson RS and Kennedy CC (1978) Infectious mononucleosis in the older patient. *Mayo Clin Proc*, **53**, 146–150.

16 Bar RS, Adlard J and Thomas FB (1975) Lymphopenic infectious mononucleosis. *Arch Intern Med*, **135**, 334–337.

17 Akashi K, Eizuru Y, Sumiyoshi Y, Minematsu T, Hara S, Harada M *et al.* (1993) Severe infectious mononucleosis-like syndrome and primary human herpesvirus 6 infection in an adult. *N Engl J Med*, **329**, 168–171.

18 Foucar K (2001) *Bone Marrow Pathology*, 2nd edn, ASCP Press, Chicago.

19 Piankijagum A, Visudhiphan S, Aswapokee P, Suwanagool S, Kruatrachue M and Na-Nakorn S (1977) Hematological changes in typhoid fever. *J Med Assoc Thai*, **60**, 828–838.

20 McDonald JC, MacLean JD and McDade JE (1988) Imported rickettsial disease: clinical and epidemiologic features. *Am J Med*, **85**, 799–805.

21 Wilson ME, Brush AD and Meany MC (1989) Murine typhus acquired during short-term urban travel. *Am J Med*, **57**, 233–234.

22 McDade JE (1990) Ehrlichiosis—a disease of animals and humans. *J Infect Dis*, **161**, 609–617.

23 Chesterman CN (1992) Late adverse effects of streptokinase. *Aust NZJ Med*, **22**, 106–108.

24 Cullen MH, Stansfeld AG, Oliver RTD, Lister TA and Malpas JS (1979) Angio-immunoblastic lymphadenopathy: report of ten cases and review of the literature. *Q J Med*, **48**, 151–177.

25 Delbarre F, Le Go A and Kahan A (1975) Hyperbasophilic immunoblasts in the circulating blood in chronic inflammatory rheumatic and collagen diseases. *Ann Rheum Dis*, **34**, 422–430.

26 Daniele R and Rowlands DT (1976) Lymphocyte subpopulations in sarcoidosis: correlation with disease activity and duration. *Ann Intern Med*, **85**, 593–600.

27 Craig J and Isaacs D (1993) Kawasaki syndrome in a Sydney hospital. *Aust NZ J Med*, **23**, 440.

28 Karandikar NJ, Kroft SH, Yegappan S, Rogers BB, Aquino VM, Lee KM *et al.* (2004) Unusual immunophenotype of CD8+ T cells in familial hemophagocytic lymphohistiocytosis. *Blood*, **104**, 2007–2009.

29 Nakahara K, Utsunomiya A, Hanada S, Takeshita T, Uozumi K, Yamamoto K *et al.* (1998) Transient appearance of

CD3+CD8+ T lymphocytes with monoclonal gene rearrangement of T-cell receptor beta locus. *Br J Haematol*, **100**, 411–414.

30 Horwitz CA, Henle W, Henle G, Polesky H, Balfour HH, Siem RA *et al.* (1977) Heterophile-negative infectious mononucleosis and mononucleosis-like illnesses. *Am J Med*, **63**, 947–957.

31 Tsaparas YF, Brigden M, Mathias R, Thomas E, Raboud J and Doyle PW (2000) Proportion positive for Epstein–Barr virus, cytomegalovirus, human herpesvirus 6, *Toxoplasma*, and human immunodeficiency virus types 1 and 2 in heterophile-negative patients with an absolute lymphocytosis and an instrument-generated atypical lymphocyte flag. *Arch Pathol Lab Med*, **124**, 1324–1330.

32 Smith PR, Cavenagh JD, Milne T, Howe D, Wilkes SJ, Sinnott P *et al.* (2000) Benign monoclonal expansion of CD8+ lymphocytes in HIV infection. *J Clin Pathol*, **53**, 177–181.

33 Milne TM, Cavenagh JD, Macey MG, Dale C, Howes D, Wilkes S and Newland AC (1998) Large granular lymphocyte (LGL) expansion in 20 HIV infected patients; analysis of immunophenotype and clonality. *Br J Haematol*, **101**, Suppl. 1, 107.

34 Bain BJ (2008) Dysplastic neutrophils in an HIV-positive woman. *Am J Hematol*, **83**, 738.

35 Koster F, Foucar K, Hjelle B, Scott A, Chong Y-Y, Larson R and McCabe M (2001) Rapid presumptive diagnosis of hantavirus cardiopulmonary syndrome by peripheral blood smear review. *Am J Clin Pathol*, **116**, 665–672.

36 Pol S, Thiers V, Driss F, Devergie A, Berthelot P and Bréchot C (1993) Lack of evidence for a role of HCV in hepatitis-associated aplastic anaemia. *Br J Haematol*, **85**, 808–810.

37 Bosch Benitez JM, Piris M, Peri V, Martin L, Marrero M, Mollejo M *et al.* (2011) Persistent B cell polyclonal lymphocytosis (PPBL) with massive splenomegaly mimicking marginal zone lymphoma. *Haematologica*, **96**, Suppl. 2. 569.

38 Mossafa H, Malaure H, Maynadie M, Valensi F, Schillinger F, Garand G *et al.* (1999) Persistent polyclonal B lymphocytosis with binucleated lymphocytes: a study of 25 cases. Groupe Français d'Hématologie Cellulaire. *Br J Haematol*, **104**, 486–493.

39 Callet-Bauchu E, Gazzo S, Poncet C, Pages J, Morel D, Alliot C *et al.* (2000) Distinct chromosome 3 abnormalities in persistent polyclonal B-cell lymphocytosis. *Genes Chromosomes Cancer*, **26**, 221–228.

40 Deplano S, Nadel-Melsió E and Bain BJ (2014) Persistent polyclonal B lymphocytosis. *Am J Hematol*, **89**, 224.

41 Lesesve J-F, Cornet E, Mossafa H and Troussard X (2011) EDTA-dependent lymphoagglutination in persistent polyclonal B-cell lymphocytosis. *Br J Haematol*, **154**, 668.

42 Mossafa H, Tapia S, Flandrin G, Troussard X and the Groupe Français d'Hématologie Cellulaire (GFHC) (2004) Chromosomal instability and the ATR amplification gene in patients with persistent and polyclonal B-cell lymphocytosis (PPBL). *Leuk Lymphoma*, **45**, 1401–1406.

43 Himmelmann A, Gautsschi O, Nawrath M, Bolliger U, Fehr J and Stahel RA (2001) Persistent polyclonal B-cell lymphocytosis is an expansion of functional IGD+CD27+ memory B cells. *Br J Haematol*, **114**, 400–405.

44 Salcedo I, Campos-Caro A, Sampalo A, Reales E and Brieva JA (2002) Persistent polyclonal B lymphocytosis: an expansion of cells showing IgVH gene mutations and phenotypic features of normal lymphocytes with the CD27+ marginal zone B-cell compartment. *Br J Haematol*, **116**, 662–666.

45 Del Giudice I, Pileri SA, Rossi M, Sabattini E, Campidelli C, Starza ID *et al.* (2009) Histopathological and molecular features of persistent polyclonal B-cell lymphocytosis (PPBL) with progressive splenomegaly. *Br J Haematol*, **144**, 726–731.

46 Leder K and Weller PF (2000) Eosinophilia and helminth infections. *Baillière's Clin Haematol*, **13**, 301–317.

47 Chusid ML, Dale DC, West BC and Wolff SM (1975) The hypereosinophilic syndrome. *Medicine*, **54**, 1–27.

48 Cogan E, Schandené L, Crusiaux A, Cochaux P, Velu T and Goldman M (1994) Clonal proliferation of type 2 helper T cells in a man with the hypereosinophilic syndrome. *N Engl J Med*, **330**, 535–538.

49 Simon H-U, Plotz SG, Dummer R and Blaser K (1999) Abnormal clones of T cells producing interleukin-5 in idiopathic eosinophilia. *N Engl J Med*, **341**, 1112–1120.

50 Means-Markwell M, Burgess T. de Keratry D, O'Neil K, Mascola J, Fleisher T and Lucey D (2000) Eosinophilia with aberrant T cells and elevated serum levels of interleukin-2 and interleukin-15. *N Engl J Med*, **342**, 1568–1571.

51 Spry C (1980) Discussion: Management of the idiopathic hypereosinophilic syndrome. In: Mahmoud AAF, Austere KP and Simon AS (eds). *The Eosinophil in Health and Disease*, Grune & Stratton, New York.

52 Parker RI (1991) Hematologic aspects of mastocytosis. II. Management of hematologic disorders in association with systemic mast cell disease. *J Invest Dermatol*, **96**, 52S–53S.

53 Bain B (1991) Down's syndrome—transient abnormal myelopoiesis and acute leukaemia. *Leuk Lymphoma*, **3**, 309–317.

54 Ferrer A, Cervantes F, Hernåndez-Boluda JC, Alvarez A and Montserrat E (1999) Leukemoid reaction preceding the diagnosis of colorectal carcinoma by four years. *Haematologica*, **84**, 671–672.

55 Olipitz E, Strunk D, Beham-Schmid C and Sill H (2004) Neutrophilic leukaemoid reactions as the presenting feature of de novo and therapy-related acute leukemias. *Acta Haematologica*, **111**, 233–234.

56 Stevens MCG, Darbyshire PJ and Brown SM (1987) Early congenital syphilis and severe haematological disturbance. *Arch Dis Child*, **62**, 1073–1075.

57 Willoughby MLN (1977) *Paediatric Haematology*. Churchill Livingstone, Edinburgh.

58 Standen GA, Steers FJ and Jones L (1998) Clonality of chronic neutrophilic leukaemia associated with myeloma: analysis using the X-linked probe M27β. *J Clin Pathol*, **46**, 297–298.

59 Nagai M, Oda S, Iwamoto M, Marumoto K, Fujita M and Takahara J (1996) Granulocyte-colony stimulating factor concentrations in a patient with plasma cell dyscrasia and clinical features of chronic neutrophilic leukaemia. *J Clin Pathol*, **49**, 858–860.

60 Kohmura K, Miyakawa Y, Kameyama K, Kizaki M and Ikeda Y (2004) Granulocyte colony stimulating factor-producing multiple myeloma associated with neutrophilia. *Leuk Lymphoma*, **45**, 1475–1479.

61 Dinçol G, Nalçaci M, Dogan O, Aktan M, Küçükkaya R, Agan M and Dinçol K (2002) Coexistence of chronic neutrophilic leukemia with multiple myeloma. *Leuk Lymphoma*, **43**, 649–651.

62 Marui T, Yamamoto T, Akisue T, Hitora T, Yoshiya S and Kurosaka M (2003) Granulocyte colony-stimulating factor–producing undifferentiated sarcoma occurring in previously fractured femur. *Arch Pathol Lab Med*, **127**, e186–e189.

63 Sonobe H, Ohtsuki Y, Ido E, Furihata M, Iwata J, Enzan H *et al.* (1997) Epithelioid sarcoma producing granulocyte colony-stimulating factor. *Hum Pathol*, **28**, 1433–1435.

64 Reykdal S, Sham R, Phatak P and Kouides P (1995) Pseudoleukemia following the use of G-CSF. *Am J Hematol*, **49**, 258–259.

65 Pinkel D (1998) Differentiating juvenile myelomonocytic leukemia from infectious disease. *Blood*, **91**, 365–367.

66 Beigelman A, Moser AM, Shubinsky G, Ben-Harosh M, Alon H, Benjamin G and Kapelushnik J (2003) The leukaemoid reaction – clinical and molecular characterization in the pediatric population. *Blood*, **102**, 53b.

67 Herrod HG, Dow LW and Sullivan JL (1983) Persistent Epstein–Barr virus infection mimicking juvenile chronic myelogenous leukemia: immunologic and hematologic studies. *Blood*, **61**, 1098–1104.

68 Kirby MA, Weitzman S and Freedman MH (1990) Juvenile chronic myelogenous leukemia: differentiation from infantile cytomegalovirus infection. *Am J Pediatr Hematol Oncol*, **12**, 292–296.

69 Lorenzana A, Lyons H, Sawal H, Higgins M, Carrigan D and Emanuel P (1997) Human herpes virus-6 (HHV-6) infection in an infant mimicking juvenile chronic myelogenous leukemia (JCML). *J Pediatr Hematol Oncol*, **19**, 370.

70 Yetgin S, Çetin M, Yenicesu I, Özaltin F and Uçkan D (2000) Acute parvovirus B19 infection mimicking juvenile myelomonocytic leukemia. *Eur J Haematol*, **65**, 276–278.

71 Toren A, Neumann Y, Meyer JJ, Mandel M, Schiby G, Kende G *et al.* (1993) Malignant osteopetrosis manifested as juvenile chronic myeloid leukemia. *Pediatr Hematol Oncol*, **10**, 187–189.

72 Papadaki T, Stamatopoulos K, Stavroyianni N, Paterakis G, Phisphis M and Stefanoudaki-Sofianatou K (2002) Evidence for T-large granular lymphocyte-mediated neutropenia in Rituximab-treated lymphoma patients: report of two cases. *Leuk Res*, **26**, 597–600.

73 Bates I, Bedu-Addo G, Rutherford TR and Bevan DH (1997) Circulating villous lymphocytes—a link between hyperreactive malarial splenomegaly and splenic lymphoma. *Trans R Soc Trop Med Hyg*, **91**, 171–174.

74 Jabbar A and Siddique T (1998) A case of pseudolymphoma leukaemia syndrome following cefixime. *Br J Haematol*, **101**, 209.

75 Kikuchi M, Ohsaka A, Chiba Y, Sato M, Muraosa Y and Hoshino H (1999) Bone marrow aplasia with prominent atypical plasmacytic proliferation preceding acute lymphoblastic leukemia. *Leuk Lymphoma*, **35**, 213–217.

76 Ehrlich GD, Han T, Bettigole R, Merl SA, Lehr B, Tomar RH and Poiesz BJ (1988) Human T lymphotropic virus type I-associated benign transient immature T-cell lymphocytosis. *Am J Hematol*, **27**, 49–55.

77 Caldwell CW, Poje E and Cooperstock M (1991) Expansion of immature thymic precursor cells in peripheral blood after acute bone marrow suppression. *Am J Clin Pathol*, **95**, 824–827.

78 Zeidler C (2005) Congenital neutropenia. *Hematology*, **10**, Suppl. 1, 306–311.

79 Swerdlow SH, Campo E, Harris NL, Jaffe ES, Pileri SA, Stein H, Thiele J and Vardiman JW (eds) (2008) *WHO Classification of Tumours of Haematopoietic and Lymphoid Tissues*. IARC, Lyon.

80 Bennett JM, Catovsky D, Daniel M-T, Flandrin G, Galton DAG, Gralnick H and Sultan C (1976) Proposals for the classification of the acute leukaemias (FAB cooperative group). *Br J Haematol*, **33**, 451–459.

81 Bennett JM, Catovsky D, Daniel MT, Flandrin G, Galton DAG, Gralnick H and Sultan C (1985) Proposed revised criteria for the classification of acute myeloid leukemia. *Ann Intern Med*, **103**, 620–625.

82 Bennett JM, Catovsky D, Daniel M-T, Flandrin G, Galton DAG, Gralnick H and Sultan C (1985) Criteria for the diagnosis of acute leukemia of megakaryocyte lineage (M7): a report of the French–American–British Cooperative Group. *Ann Intern Med*, **103**, 460–462.

83 Bennett JM, Catovsky D, Daniel M-T, Flandrin G, Galton DAG, Gralnick H and Sultan C (1991) Proposal for the recognition of minimally differentiated acute myeloid leukaemia (AML M0). *Br J Haematol*, **78**, 325–329.

84 Bain BJ (2010) *Leukaemia Diagnosis*, 4th edn, Wiley-Blackwell, Oxford.

85 Vardiman J, Brunning RD, Arber DA, Le Beau MM, Porwit A, Tefferi A *et al.* (2008) Introduction and overview of the classification of the myeloid neoplasms. In: SwerdlowSH, CampoE, HarrisNL, JaffeES, PileriSA, SteinH *et al.* (eds) *WHO Classification of Tumours of Haematopoietic and Lymphoid Tissues*. IARC, Lyon.

86 Lichtman MA and Segel BG (2005) Uncommon phenotypes of acute myelogenous leukemia: basophilic, mast cell, eosinophilic, and myeloid dendritic cell subtypes: a review. *Blood Cells Mol Dis*, **35**, 370–383.

87 Soler J, O'Brien M, Tavaras de CJ, San Miguel JF, Kearney L, Goldman JM and Catovsky D (1985) Blast crisis of chronic granulocytic leukemia with mast cell and basophil precursors. *Am J Clin Pathol*, **83**, 254–259.

88 Coser P, Quaglino D, de Pasquale A, Colombetti V and Prinoth O (1980) Cytobiological and clinical aspects of tissue mast cell leukaemia. *Br J Haematol*, **45**, 5–12.

89 Efrati P, Klajman A and Spitz H (1957) Mast cell leukemia? Malignant mastocytosis with leukemia-like manifestations. *Blood*, **12**, 869–882.

90 Parwaresch MR (1976) *The Human Blood Basophil. Morphology, Origin, Kinetics, Function and Pathology*. Springer-Verlag, Berlin.

91 Bain BJ (1994) Transient leukaemia in newborn infants with Down's syndrome. *Leuk Res*, **18**, 723–724.

92 Hitzler JK, Cheung J, Yue LI, Scherer SW and Zipursky A (2003) GATA1 mutations in transient leukemia and acute megakaryoblastic leukemia of Down syndrome. *Blood*, **101**, 4301–4304.

93 Brunning RD, Orazi A, Germing U, Le Beau MM, Porwit A, Baumann I et al. (2008) Myelodysplastic syndromes/neoplasms, overview. In: Swerdlow SH, Campo E, Harris NL, Jaffe ES, Pileri SA, Stein H *et al.* (eds) *WHO Classification of Tumours of Haematopoietic and Lymphoid Tissues*. IARC, Lyon.

94 Goasguen JE, Bennett JM, Bain BJ, Brunning R, Vallespi MT, Tomonaga M *et al.*; International Working Group on Morphology of MDS (IWGM-MDS) (2014) Proposal for refining the definition of dysgranulopoiesis in acute myeloid leukemia and myelodysplastic syndromes, *Leuk Res*, **38**, 447–453.

95 Spiers ASD, Bain BJ and Turner JE (1977) The peripheral blood in chronic granulocytic leukaemia. Study of 50 untreated Philadelphia chromosome-positive cases. *Scand J Haematol*, **18**, 25–38.

96 Srodes CH, Hyde EH and Boggs DR (1973) Autonomous erythropoiesis during erythroblastic crisis of chronic myelocytic leukaemia. *J Clin Invest*, **52**, 512–515.

97 Ondreyco SM, Kjeldsberg CR, Fineman RM, Vaninetti S and Kushner JP (1981) Monoblastic transformation in chronic myelogenous leukemia. *Cancer*, **48**, 957–963.

98 Rosenthal S, Schwartz JKH and Canellos GP (1977) Basophilic chronic granulocytic leukaemia with hyperhistaminaemia. *Br J Haematol*, **36**, 367–372.

99 Marinone G, Rossi G and Verzura P (1983) Eosinophilic blast crisis in a case of chronic myeloid leukaemia. *Br J Haematol*, **55**, 251–256.

100 Hogge DE, Misawa S, Schiffer CA and Testa JR (1984) Promyelocytic blast crisis in chronic granulocytic leukaemia with 15;17 translocation. *Leuk Res*, **8**, 1019–1023.

101 You W and Weisbrot IM (1984) Chronic neutrophilic leukemia, report of two cases and review of the literature. *Am J Clin Pathol*, **72**, 233–242.

102 Kanoh T, Saigo K and Yamagishi M (1986) Neutrophils with ring-shaped nuclei in chronic neutrophilic leukemia. *Am J Clin Pathol*, **86**, 748–751.

103 Zoumbos NC, Symeonidis A and Kourakli-Symeonidis A (1989) Chronic neutrophilic leukemia with dysplastic features: a new variant of myelodysplastic syndromes? *Acta Haematol*, **82**, 156–160.

104 Bain B, Vardiman JW, Brunning RD and Thiele J (2008) Chronic neutrophilic leukaemia. In: SwerdlowSH, CampoE, HarrisNL, JaffeES, PileriSA, SteinH *et al.* (eds) *WHO Classification of Tumours of Haematopoietic and Lymphoid Tissues*. IARC, Lyon.

105 Bain BJ, Gilliland DG, Vardiman JW, Brunning RD and Horny H-P (2008) Chronic eosinophilic leukaemia, not otherwise specified. In: Swerdlow SH, Campo E, Harris NL, Jaffe ES, Pileri SA, Stein H *et al.* (eds) *WHO Classification of Tumours of Haematopoietic and Lymphoid Tissues*. IARC, Lyon, 2008.

106 Cools J, DeAngelo DJ, Gotlib J, Stover EH, Legare RD, Cortes J *et al.* (2003) A tyrosine kinase created by the fusion of the PDGFRA and FIP1L1 genes as a therapeutic target of imatinib in idiopathic hypereosinophilic syndrome. *N Engl J Med*, **348**, 1201–1214.

107 Bain BJ, Gilliland DG, Horny H-P and Vardiman JW (2008) Myeloid and lymphoid neoplasms with eosinophilia and abnormalities of *PDGFA*, *PDGFRB* or *FGFR1*. In: Swerdlow SH, Campo E, Harris NL, Jaffe ES, Pileri SA, Stein H *et al.* (eds) *WHO Classification of Tumours of Haematopoietic and Lymphoid Tissues*. IARC, Lyon.

108 Orazi A, Bennett JM, Germing U, Brunning RD, Bain BJ and Thiele J (2008) Chronic myelomonocytic leukaemia. In: Swerdlow SH, Campo E, Harris NL, Jaffe ES, Pileri SA, Stein H *et al.* (eds) *WHO Classification of Tumours of Haematopoietic and Lymphoid Tissues*. IARC, Lyon.

109 Vardiman JW, Bennett JM, Bain BJ, Brunning RD and Thiele J (2008) Atypical chronic myeloid leukaemia, *BCR-ABL1* negative. In: Swerdlow SH, Campo E, Harris NL, Jaffe ES, Pileri SA, Stein H *et al.* (eds) *WHO Classification of Tumours of Haematopoietic and Lymphoid Tissues*. IARC, Lyon.

110 Baumann I, Bennett JM, Niemeyer CM, Thiele J and Shannon K (2008) Juvenile myelomonocytic leukaemia. In: Swerdlow SH, Campo E, Harris NL, Jaffe ES, Pileri SA, Stein H *et al.* (eds) *WHO Classification of Tumours of Haematopoietic and Lymphoid Tissues*. IARC, Lyon.

111 Castro-Malaspina H, Schaison G, Passe S, Pasquier A, Bergen R, Bayle-Weisgerber C *et al.* (1984) Subacute and chronic myelomonocytic leukemia in children (juvenile CML). *Cancer*, **54**, 675–686.

112 Vardiman JW, Bennett JM, Bain BJ, Baumann I, Thiele J and Orazi A (2008) Myelodysplastic/myeloproliferative neoplasm, unclassifiable. In: Swerdlow SH, Campo E, Harris NL, Jaffe ES, Pileri SA, Stein H *et al.* (eds) *WHO Classification of Tumours of Haematopoietic and Lymphoid Tissues*. IARC, Lyon.

113 Blatt J, Penchansky L and Horn M (1989) Thrombocytosis as a presenting feature in acute lymphoblastic leukaemia of childhood. *Am J Hematol*, **31**, 46–49.

114 Bain BJ and Catovsky D (1994) The leukaemic phase of non-Hodgkin's lymphoma. *J Clin Pathol*, **48**, 189–193.

115 Bennett JM, Catovsky D, Daniel M-T, Flandrin G, Galton DAG and Gralnick H and Sultan C (1989) Proposals for the classification of chronic (mature) B and T lymphoid Leukaemias. *J Clin Pathol*, **42**, 567–584.

116 Bain BJ, Clark D and Wilkins BS (2010) *Bone Marrow Pathology*, 4th edn. Wiley–Blackwell, Oxford.

117 Metzgeroth G, Schneider S, Hofmann W-K and Hastka J (2013) Globular intracytoplasmic inclusions in a patient with chronic lymphocytic leukaemia. *Br J Haematol*, **161**, 302.

118 Merino A, Rozman M and Esteve J (2006) Chronic (B cell) lymphocytic leukaemia with unusual granulation. *Br J Haematol*, **133**, 354.

119 Dorion RP and Shaw JH (2003) Intracytoplasmic filamentous inclusions in the peripheral blood of a patient with chronic lymphocytic leukemia: a bright-field, electron microscopic, immunofluorescent, and flow cytometric study. *Arch Pathol Lab Med*, **127**, 618–620.

120 Girodon F, Poillot N, Martin I, Carli PM and Maynadie M (2004) Crystalline inclusions in B monoclonal lymphocytes. *Haematologica*, **89**, ECR40.

121 Marti GE, Rawstron AC, Ghia P, Hillmen P, Houlston RS, Kay N *et al.* on behalf of The International Familial CLL Consortium (2005) Diagnostic criteria for monoclonal B-cell lymphocytosis. *Br J Haematol*, **130**, 325–332.

122 Nguyen D and Diamond L (2000) *Diagnostic Hematology: a Pattern Approach*. Butterworth-Heinemann, Oxford.

123 Melo JV, Catovsky D and Galton DAG (1986) The relationship between chronic lymphocytic leukaemia and prolymphocytic leukaemia. I. Clinical and laboratory features of 300 patients and characterisation of an intermediate group. *Br J Haematol*, **63**, 377–387.

124 Machii T, Yamaguchi M, Inoue R, Tokumine Y, Kuratsune H, Nagai H *et al.* (1997) Polyclonal B-cell lymphocytosis with features resembling hairy cell leukemia-Japanese variant. *Blood*, **15**, 2008–2014.

125 Groom DA, Wong D, Brynes RK and Macaulay LK (1991) Auer rod-like inclusions in circulating lymphoma cells. *Am J Clin Pathol*, **96**, 111–115.

126 Bain BJ, Matutes E, Robinson D, Lampert IA, BritoBabapulle V, Morilla R and Catovsky D (1991) Leukaemia as a manifestation of large cell lymphoma. *Br J Haematol*, **77**, 301–310.

127 Cobcroft R (1999) Images in haematology: diagnosis of angiotropic large B-cell lymphoma from a peripheral blood film. *Br J Haematol*, **104**, 429.

128 Liapis K and Apostolidis J (2012) Empty, but heavy, plasma cells. *Blood*, **120**, 4282.

129 Kyle RA, Maldonado JE and Bayrd ED (1974) Plasma cell leukaemia. Report on 17 cases. *Arch Intern Med*, **133**, 813–818.

130 McKenna RW, Kyle RA, Kuehl WM, Grogan TM, Harris NL and Coupland RW (2008) Plasma cell neoplasms. In: Swerdlow SH, Campo E, Harris NL, Jaffe ES, Pileri SA, Stein H *et al.* (eds) *WHO Classification of Tumours of Haematopoietic and Lymphoid Tissues*. IARC, Lyon.

131 Murayama K, Sawamura M and Tamura K (1993) Transient plasmacytosis with acute infection in myeloma. *Br J Haematol*, **82**, 475.

132 Witzig TE, Gertz MA, Lust JA, Kyle RA, O'Fallon WM and Greipp PR (1996) Peripheral blood monoclonal plasma cells as a predictor of survival in patients with multiple myeloma. *Blood*, **88**, 1780–1787.

133 Drayson M, Tang LX, Drew R, Mead GP, Carr-Smith H and Bradwell AR (2001) Serum free light-chains measurements for identifying and monitoring patients with nonsecretory multiple myeloma. *Blood*, **97**, 2900–2903.

134 Nowakowski GS, Witzig TE, Dingli D, Tracz MJ, Gertz MA, Lacy MQ *et al.* (2005) Circulating plasma cells detected by flow cytometry as a predictor of survival in 302 patients with newly diagnosed multiple myeloma. *Blood*, **106**, 2276–2279.

135 Duncan SC and Winkelman RK (1978) Circulating Sézary cells in hospitalized dermatology patients. *Br J Dermatol*, **99**, 171–178.

136 Morice WG, Kurtin PJ, Leibson PJ, Tefferi A and Hanson CA (2003) Demonstration of aberrant T-cell and natural killer-cell antigen expression in all cases of granular lymphocytic leukaemia. *Br J Haematol*, **120**, 1026–1036.

137 Portlock CS, Donnelly GB, Qin J, Straus D, Yahalom J, Zelenetz A *et al.* (2004) Adverse prognostic significance of CD20 positive Reed-Sternberg cells in classical Hodgkin's disease. *Br J Haematol*, **125**, 701–708.

Index

Page numbers in *italics* denote Figures; those in **bold** denote Tables.

Blood Cells A Practical Guide, Fifth Edition. By Barbara J. Bain © 2015 John Wiley & Sons, Ltd. Published 2015 by John Wiley & Sons, Ltd.
Companion Website: www.wiley.com/go/bain/bloodcells